KT-140-665

Occupational Therapy in Psychiatry and Mental Health

Fourth Edition

WM 640

Occupational Therapy in Psychiatry and Mental Health

Fourth Edition

Edited by

Rosemary Crouch PhD Occupational Therapy
Medical University of Southern Africa (MEDUNSA),
MSc Occupational Therapy, University of the Witwatersrand

and

Vivyan Alers MSc Occupational Therapy
University of the Witwatersrand, BA Social Work
University of Stellenbosch

MEDICAL LIBRARY
WATFORD POSTGRADUATE
MEDICAL CENTRE
WATFORD GENERAL HOSPITAL
VICARAGE ROAD
WATFORD WD1 8HB

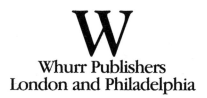

Whurr Publishers
London and Philadelphia

© 2005 Whurr Publishers Ltd
First published 2005
by Whurr Publishers Ltd
19b Compton Terrace
London N1 2UN
England

Reprinted 2005 and 2006

All rights reserved. No part of this publication may be
reproduced, stored in a retrieval system, or transmitted
in any form or by any means, electronic, mechanical,
photocopying, recording or otherwise, without the
prior permission of Whurr Publishers Limited.

This publication is sold subject to the conditions that it
shall not, by way of trade or otherwise, be lent, resold,
hired out, or otherwise circulated without the publisher's prior consent in any form of binding or cover other
than that in which it is published and without a similar
condition including this condition being imposed
upon any subsequent purchaser.

British Library Cataloguing in Publication Data

A catalogue record for this book is available from the
British Library.

ISBN-10 1 86156 420 1 p/b
ISBN-13 978 186156 420 7 p/b

Typeset by Adrian McLaughlin, a@microguides.net
Printed and bound in the UK
by Athenæum Press Ltd, Gateshead, Tyne & Wear.

Contents

Contributors

Vivyan Alers BA Social Work (Stellenbosch University), Nat. Dip. Occupational Therapy (Vona du Toit College, Pretoria), MSc Occupational Therapy (University of Witwatersrand). Qualifications in paediatric and psychiatric Sensory Integrative Therapy (SAISI). Private practitioner in psychiatry, paediatrics and trauma with children, adolescents and adults. Director Acting Thru Ukubuyiselwa (NPO) and occupational therapist treating trauma survivors in the community in Gauteng, South Africa. Co-editor of *Occupational Therapy in Psychiatry and Mental Health*, 3rd and 4th editions.

Romy Ancer BA Psychology (University of Pretoria), B. Occupational Therapy (University of Pretoria), Diploma Group Activities and Counselling (University of Pretoria). Occupational therapist and counsellor with the South African Department of Education and the Department of Social Services, Gauteng, South Africa.

Sylvia Birkhead BSc Occupational Therapy (University of Witwatersrand), MOT Occupational Therapy (University of Pretoria). Private practitioner in occupational therapy with children with ADHD and learning problems in Johannesburg, South Africa, part-time lecturer in the Department of Occupational Therapy at the University of Witwatersrand, and Consultant to Headway (head-injured clients), Stroke Aid, ARDA, MND Society and MS Society.

Candace Lee Bylsma BSc Occupational Therapy (University of Cape Town). Qualifications in paediatric Sensory Integrative Therapy (SAISI). Private practitioner in paediatric occupational therapy, in Johannesburg, South Africa.

Rosemary Crouch MSc Occupational Therapy (University of Witwatersrand) with distinction, PhD Occupational Therapy (Medical University of Southern Africa, MEDUNSA). Private practitioner in adult psychiatry and addictions in Johannesburg, South Africa, part-time senior lecturer in the Department of Occupational Therapy at the Medical University of Southern Africa (MEDUNSA) and the University of Pretoria. Editor of the first two editions of *Occupational Therapy in Psychiatry and Mental Health* and co-editor with Vivyan Alers of the 3rd and 4th editions.

Patricia de Witt MSc Occupational Therapy (University of Witwatersrand). Senior lecturer in the Department of Occupational Therapy at the University of Witwatersrand, Johannesburg, South Africa, and Head of Department.

Madeleine Duncan MSc Occupational Therapy (University of Cape Town), BA Hons Psychology (University of Durban-Westville). Senior lecturer in occupational therapy in the Department of Occupational Therapy at the University of Cape Town, South Africa.

Louise Fouché M. Occupational Therapy (University of Pretoria). Postgraduate diploma in groups and interpersonal communication – cum laude (University of Pretoria). Lecturer in psychiatry and group work in the Department of Occupational Therapy at the University of Pretoria, South Africa.

Stephanie Homer BSc Occupational Therapy (University of Witwatersrand). Has worked for ten years with the Community Rehabilitation Research and Education (CORRE) Programme of the University of Witwatersrand. At present working on a pilot programme to increase access to disability grants offered by the South African Department of Social Security and Population Development in Mpumalanga, South Africa.

Robin Joubert Nat. Dip. Occupational Therapy (Vona du Toit College, Pretoria), BA (UNISA), M. Occupational Therapy (University of Durban-Westville). Senior lecturer in the Department of Occupational Therapy at the University of KwaZulu-Natal, South Africa.

Rae Labuschagne Nat. Dip. Occupational Therapy (Vona du Toit College, Pretoria). Dip. Ed. Ther. Voc. (Pretoria), MSc Gerontology (Leonard Davis School of Gerontology, University of Southern California). Consulting gerontologist in private practice in South Africa.

Michelle Moore B. Occupational Therapy (University of the Free State). Manager of the occupational therapy department of the Free State Psychiatric Complex, including the Forensic Department, in Bloemfontein, South Africa.

Deidre Niehaus B. Occupational Therapy (University of Pretoria). Qualifications in paediatric Sensory Integrative Therapy (SAISI). Private practitioner in the field of paediatric occupational therapy with children with socio-emotional problems and developmental delays, in Richards Bay, South Africa.

Ann Nott B. Occupational Therapy (Hons) (MEDUNSA). Head occupational therapist at Headway in Johannesburg (a brain injury support group). Private practitioner in the field of psychiatry and neurology in Gauteng, South Africa.

Marita Rademeyer MA Clinical Psychology (Rand Afrikaans University – RAU). Private practitioner in Gauteng, South Africa, in the field of learning and developmental delays, as well as trauma, in children. Director of Kinder Trauma Kliniek in Pretoria, South Africa.

Lee Randall BSc Occupational Therapy, with distinction (University of Witwatersrand), MA (Tufts, USA), Postgraduate Dip. in Vocational Rehabilitation (University of Pretoria). Private practitioner in Johannesburg, South Africa, in the field of disability, vocational rehabilitation and medicolegal work.

Lyndsey Swart BSc Occupational Therapy (University of Witwatersrand), M. Occupational Therapy (University of the Free State), Postgraduate Diploma in Vocational Rehabilitation (University of Pretoria), Certificate in Advanced Labour Law (UNISA). Private practitioner in disability equity, disability management and vocational rehabilitation, in Gauteng, South Africa.

Annamarie van Jaarsveld M. Occupational Therapy (University of the Free State), qualifications in paediatric and psychiatric Sensory Integrative Therapy (SAISI). Lecturer in the Department of Occupational Therapy at the University of the Free State.

Dain van der Reyden Nat. Dip. Occupational Therapy (Vona du Toit College), Dip. Ed. Voc. Ther. (University of Pretoria), BA (UNISA). Senior lecturer in the Department of Occupational Therapy, University of KwaZulu-Natal, South Africa.

Lana van Niekerk M. Occupational Therapy (University of the Free State). Associate Professor and Head of the Division of Occupational Therapy, University of Cape Town, South Africa.

Erla Venter Nat. Dip. Occupational Therapy (Vona du Toit College), B. Arb. Hons (University of Pretoria). Head of the Occupational Therapy Department at Sterkfontein State Psychiatric Hospital in Krugersdorp, South Africa for 19 years.

Lisa Wegner BSc Occupational Therapy (University of Witwatersrand), MSc Occupational Therapy (University of Cape Town). Senior lecturer in the Department of Occupational Therapy at the University of the Western Cape, South Africa.

Kobie Zietsman B. Occupational Therapy (University of Stellenbosch). Chief Occupational Therapist at the Randfontein Care Centre (Life Care Hospital) for the mentally ill, Randfontein, South Africa.

Preface

Advances in the thinking, practice and professionalism of occupational therapists in the psychosocial field have heralded the fourth edition of this book. Added to this is the extreme good fortune of finding our international publisher, Colin Whurr, who was generously introduced to us by our friend and colleague, Jennifer Creek. This edition of the book is intended to complement Jennifer's work rather than echo it.

New and old authors have been encouraged to include a much more international bias in their chapters, whilst still maintaining the unique work of South African occupational therapists. We extend our grateful thanks to all the authors who willingly met the deadlines, and would like to acknowledge the exceptional contribution of our colleague Madeleine Duncan and her expertise based on the International Classification of Functioning, Disability and Health (ICF) (WHO, 2001a).

The context shapes practice, and the South African context is motivated by a concern with primary healthcare and community practice (developing countries context) and the private health sector (developed countries context). Acknowledgement of the models of occupation and occupational therapy, and the need for a paradigm shift from the medical model to the occupational model, have been encouraged. The inclusion of clinical reasoning, post-traumatic brain injury, vocational rehabilitation, trauma, occupational science, HIV/AIDS and sexual rehabilitation, in the mental health field, have greatly enhanced the breadth of information in this edition.

Whilst acknowledging the theoretical premise of the profession we have also striven to retain an aspect of the book that has been very successful in the past, namely the educational, or more specifically, prescriptive, aspect. In the past occupational therapy students, as well as occupational therapists moving into the psychiatric field after a break or for the first time, have used this book extensively as a good guide to actual practice. We hope that this state of affairs continues.

We anticipate that this edition of an educational tool that has hitherto been so successful in South Africa will now reach a much wider international professional population.

Our intention is to enhance and further the profession of occupational therapy in taking its rightful place as a vital service in the field of psychiatry and mental health. Encouraging expertise and good practice of occupational therapy in the mental health field will ensure that the profession receives the acknowledgement that it so justly deserves worldwide.

Rosemary Crouch and Vivyan Alers

Foreword

It is indeed an honour to write the foreword to the fourth edition of *Occupational Therapy in Psychiatry and Mental Health*.

Rosemary Crouch and Vivyan Alers must be congratulated for their dedication and perseverance in bringing about the publication of this revised edition.

This book is still, after 14 years, the only publication of its kind in the psychosocial field of occupational therapy in South Africa – a truly remarkable achievement.

The book makes it possible for expert occupational therapists to share their ideas and knowledge. At the same time guidance is provided to occupational therapy staff for their service delivery to patients and clients in the various psychosocial areas.

The 'right mix' of information in the various chapters of the book will contribute to determining the quality of services delivered in this field. Improving and updating knowledge is the cornerstone for the empowerment of all practitioners and for the continuous development of the profession.

The relevance and the variety of topics covered in the book makes it a valuable source for use by undergraduate and postgraduate students in occupational therapy.

The publication of this revised edition has given stature to work done by occupational therapists in the psychosocial field. The what, why and how of occupational therapy are verified in the various chapters.

After a decade and a half it still gives one a heartwarming feeling to see *Occupational Therapy in Psychiatry and Mental Health* on the shelves of libraries and bookshops.

Susan Beukes

Head of Training, Department of Occupational
Therapy, University of Stellenbosch
August 2004

PART ONE
THE SCIENCE OF OCCUPATIONAL THERAPY

Chapter 1
Creative ability: a model for psychosocial occupational therapy

PATRICIA DE WITT

The theory of creative ability was elaborated upon during the 1970s by Vona du Toit, a key figure in the development of occupational therapy in South Africa. The theory provides a framework to evaluate a client's occupational performance according to the skills he has attained in the personal, social, work and recreational occupational performance areas. (Throughout this chapter both the client and occupational therapist will be referred to as 'he'. The term 'individual' is used when referring to people in general and 'client' is used when referring to a person in a therapy setting.)

Creative ability also provides guidelines for treatment by:

- identifying treatment priorities
- proposing principles that guide treatment so it is appropriate to the client's level
- determining expectations for performance, as well as how and when to up- or downgrade the treatment.

This theory is particularly useful for occupational therapists who work with large groups of heterogeneous clients in mental health settings, where the client group is very diverse in terms of age, cultural group, language and diagnosis. Creative ability is helpful in coping with this extent of diversity as it enables the occupational therapist to categorize clients efficiently in terms of their occupational performance needs and this enables the correct treatment to be administered at the right time and in the most cost-effective manner.

As an occupational therapist, Vona du Toit ascribed to the belief, central to professional philosophy, that occupational therapy actively engages a client in meaningful occupation in order to improve or maintain occupational performance and quality of life (du Toit, 1991). Creative ability theory does not dictate specific activities/occupations – only the characteristics they should have to be appropriate to the client's level of performance. This model presupposes that occupational therapists will select activities that are appropriate to the client's individual profile and are considered meaningful, purposeful and goal-directed in the context of the client's life.

Creative ability does not represent the whole of occupational therapy for a client. It has an assessment aspect which determines the level on which the client functions and then provides a stratified guide to increase the client's level of performance. This acts as the baseline from which all of the client's individually identified problems (both occupational performance and psychopathological) can be addressed. So it brings the specific treatment to his level of individual functioning.

History

The inception of creative ability theory was based on Vona du Toit's belief that a client's ability to behave creatively has a pronounced effect on his engagement in treatment, the resolution of his problems and/or adjustment to disability. She was influenced by the work of Buber, Rogers and Piaget and by her own belief that the quality of human participation in purposeful activities influences the meaning of life (du Toit, 1991). Du Toit's initial work on creative ability was first recorded in 1962 in a dissertation entitled 'Initiative in Occupational Therapy' (du Toit, 1991, p. i). Her idea of consequential stages of creativity seems to have been influenced by work carried out in Israel with psychiatric patients who were divided into four levels of occupational development (Weinstein and Schossberger, 1964). Although she read many papers at national and international conferences, her first recorded publication was in 1972 (du Toit, 1991). The initiative to develop this model further was lost by du Toit's untimely death in 1974.

In spite of the fact that this model is widely used clinically in South Africa, no substantial research has evaluated its reliability and validity. There have been approximately 12 publications on the subject (van der Reyden, 1994), and a National Conference on its application in occupational therapy, but only two research projects have been undertaken on aspects of the theory (Casteleijn, 2001; de Witt, 2003).

Fundamental concepts in the theory of creative ability

Creative ability as defined by du Toit (1991) is **'the ability to present oneself, freely, without anxiety, limitations or inhibitions'. It is also being prepared to function at one's maximal level of competence and being free from self-consciousness.**

Although du Toit did not limit creative ability to occupational performance, her guidelines are couched in occupational terms.

According to du Toit, creative ability develops within the context of one's 'creative capacity'. Creative capacity is defined as the maximal creative potential an individual has, and which could possibly develop under optimal circumstances.

Creative capacity varies from one individual to another and is influenced by factors such as intelligence, personality structure, mental health, environmental opportunities and security. As with all other concepts that denote human potential, individuals seldom reach their full potential, and there is always some capacity in reserve for growth.

To grow in a creative ability sense the individual has to exert maximal effort. *Maximal effort* refers to the exertion of creative effort at the boundary of an individual's creative ability to achieve growth. Exertion of maximal creative effort therefore extends that individual's creative ability, but in order for this to occur three other aspects also need to be evident:

1) *Creative response*
This reflects the positive attitude or response, which an individual displays towards any opportunity offered to him. It precedes creative participation. It also reflects the individual's preparedness to use all his resources to participate, for anticipated pleasure, gain or acknowledgement, in spite of some anxiety about capabilities and outcomes.

2) *Creative participation*
Creative participation is the process of being actively involved in all activities concerned with everyday living. This concept refers to taking an active rather than a passive role in the activities of life, and engaging in such a way that it challenges his abilities and resources.

3) *Creative act*
This is the final result of an individual's creative response and creative participation, in terms of producing a final end product, be it tangible or intangible.

Therefore to behave creatively and extend the level of creative ability an individual has to:

- have a positive attitude towards an opportunity offered to him by an activity, despite some anxiety (creative response);
- be actively engaged in 'doing' the activity (creative participation); and
- work towards producing an end product, be it tangible or intangible (creative act).

While much has been written in occupational therapy literature about occupational performance and how to achieve it, no author has so succinctly defined how to achieve growth in a client's occupational ability.

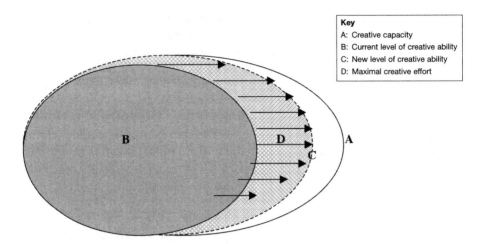

Figure 1.1 The relationship between creative capacity and creative ability, and the influence of maximal effort on creative ability.

While occupational growth would be the best outcome of occupational therapy, it does not occur independently. Occupational therapists need to manipulate the therapy situation to the best advantage of the client, select the most appropriate activity, apply therapeutic methods and techniques and recognize that it takes hard work on the part of both the client and the occupational therapist to achieve positive outcomes.

Du Toit proposed *volition* as being a central concept within creative ability theory.

She described volition as having two components: *motivation and action*. These two components are intrinsically linked. The motivational component represents the energy source for occupational behaviour and the action component the conversion of energy into action or occupational behaviour. Thus motivation governs action since it is only possible to express the motivation that exists within the individual.

Motivation

This may be defined as **the inner condition of the organism that initiates or directs behaviour towards a goal** (Coleman, 1969). While this was the working definition used by du Toit, the definition of 'intrinsic motivation' given by Kielhofner (2002) and Wilcock (1993) is more precise. **Intrinsic motivation is the biological or innate urge to explore and master the environment through occupation. This intrinsic motivation is the underlying source of energy for occupational behaviour.**

Du Toit believed that motivation was not static but had different focuses at different stages of occupational development. This led to the describing of six different and sequential levels of motivation, each with its own qualities and directed at developing specific life tasks.

The levels of motivation are:

- tone
- self-differentiation
- self-presentation
- participation
- contribution
- competitive contribution.

These levels indicate what motivates an individual. They also indicate the strength of motivation as it develops intrinsically throughout life.

Action

Action is defined as **the exertion of motivation into mental and physical effort, which results in occupational behaviour and the creation of a tangible or intangible end product that is the outcome of doing** (du Toit, 1991). Like motivation, action can be classed into levels.

These levels describe the sequential differences in the quality of the individual's ability to form relational contact with others, events, materials and objects in the environment as well as the characteristics of engagement in occupations. The levels describe the individual's development of occupational behaviour and performance, which influences his ability to live, work and play in the community.

Levels of action are:

- predestructive
- destructive
- incidental constructive action
- explorative
- experimental
- imitative
- original
- product centred
- situation centred
- society centred.

Creative ability phases

During the course of both the levels of motivation and action, the individual accomplishes a very wide range of skills and occupational behaviours. It is important therefore to be able to distinguish where he is within a particular level – at the beginning of the level, in the middle or at the end, or moving towards the next level.

The following phrases are used to describe this and can be applied at each level of both motivation and action.

Therapist-directed phase

This indicates that the individual is demonstrating skills and occupational behaviour characteristic of both the previous and current level. However, without support, structure and encouragement, he may not be able to maintain the functioning characteristic of this level and occupational behaviour could easily regress to that of an earlier level.

Patient-directed phase

This indicates that the individual's occupational behaviour is generally characteristic of the requirements of that level. He can maintain this occupational behaviour relatively independently.

Transitional phase

This indicates that the individual is demonstrating some behavioural and occupational characteristics of the next level, but only under optimal conditions; his overall occupational behaviour remains characteristic of the current level.

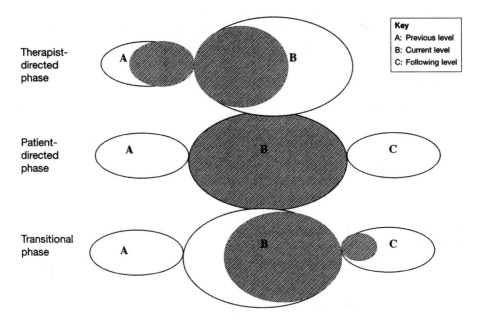

Figure 1.2 Diagrammatic representations of the three phases of creative ability.

Development of creative ability

The development of creative ability describes how occupational performance develops along a continuum from existence and egocentrism to contribution to the community and society at the highest level.

While the continuum represents the optimal level of occupational performance, few individuals reach this ultimate goal due to the limitations on their creative potential, internal capacities and environmental opportunities. In addition individuals seldom use all their potential. Current creative ability reflects that aspect of their creative capacity that is available to them to use in their everyday occupational performance.

Development starts at birth and continues throughout life. Although development is usually progressive, it need not always be so. Development is not always consistent, with growth taking place in spurts followed by periods of consolidation while the individual remains in a comfort zone.

A dynamic relationship exists between the external world and the development of creative ability. While the external environment provides the challenges and opportunities for creative growth, new opportunities and circumstances may create stress that leads to regression. Development of creative ability is therefore dependent on the fit between readiness of the individual to grow creatively (i.e. creative, response, creative participation and creative act) and the 'just right' challenge that the environment provides (de Witt, 2002).

The normal developmental process may be limited or disrupted, either temporarily or permanently, by illness, disability, trauma or barriers which may lead to a delay in development or regression of varying levels of severity.

Illness, disability or trauma may limit or disrupt the development of creative ability because of difficulties within the human system which fail to support appropriate occupational behaviour. On the other hand, there may be barriers in the external environment such as *occupational deprivation*, which is a situational barrier, like lack of funds or sufficient objects, opportunity or time, or *occupation injustice* where there are institutional barriers which limit individuals from opportunity (Wilcox, 1998).

There are also internal barriers that impact on development, such as attitudes, perceptions and past experiences (Bruce and Borg, 1993).

Like all other developmental models, creative ability is subject to the following theoretical assumptions:

- Human development occurs in an orderly fashion throughout life.
- Steps within the developmental process are sequential and cannot be omitted.
- An individual has an innate drive to encounter his world and master its challenges.
- As an individual goes through life, changing events and changes in the internal and external environment will demand adjustment and reorganization. Confrontation with change creates tension, disequilibrium and stress, which represent a necessary developmental task.
- An individual's response to the demands for change can result in adaptation and mastery, attempts at maintaining the status quo, or regression and dysfunction.

- An individual's ability to master developmental tasks is influenced by his physical and psychological capacity, learned skills, life experiences and the availability of resources and opportunity.
- Successful adaptation usually leads to self-satisfaction and societal approval.
- Successful adaptation promotes future success in meeting challenges.
- Purposeful use of activity enables the individual to learn or relearn the skills and behaviours necessary for coping with developmental demands.

Activities are purposeful when they meet the individual's needs, interests, abilities and purpose within his life and when they provide sufficient opportunity for growth and change (Bruce and Borg, 1993).

While these assumptions are important in understanding the characteristics of creative ability, they also form the underlying principles of the intervention to re-establish creative ability, should it be delayed or disrupted.

Characteristics of creative ability

Creative ability has three main characteristics.

Sequential development

The growth and recovery of creative ability follows a constant and sequential pattern. This means that growth and recovery of both the motivation and action components follow a stable and sequential pattern in which no level or phase may be omitted.

Levels of motivation develop in the following sequence: tone, self-differentiation, self-presentation, participation (passive, imitative, active, competitive) contribution and competitive contribution.

Levels of action develop in the following sequence: predestructive, destructive, incidentally constructive action, explorative, experimental, imitative, original, product centred, situation centred and society centred.

Motivation governs action

The motivation and action components are inseparable, but the motivation component governs the action. Action is therefore a direct manifestation of the motivational component of an individual's creative ability.

The levels of motivation and action relate to one another in a stable and sequential manner, as indicated in Table 1.1.

The exception is when an individual's motor capacity is severely interfered with. For example, if he cannot speak, it may not be possible for him

Table 1.1 The relationship between levels of motivation and action

Level of motivation	Level of action
Tone	Predestructive
Self-differentiation	Destructive
	Incidental constructive action
Self-presentation	Explorative
Participation: Passive	Experimental
Imitative	Imitative
Active	Original
Competitive	Product centred
Contribution	Situation centred
Competitive contribution	Society centred

to express his abstract thoughts, no matter how creative they are. If a quadriplegic client desires to brush his teeth he may not have the physical capacity to do this. Under these circumstances there may be a marked discrepancy between the motivation and action components.

Creative ability is dynamic

Creative ability is not static but varies with the individual's circumstances, confidence, anxiety level and the demands that the situation makes on his creative ability. Thus there is a forward and backward flow between the levels of creative ability, which is related to security in the lower level and stress in higher level. This tends to be a gentle forward and backward flow between two levels, rather than a violent movement across the continuum of all levels.

Creative ability and the mentally ill patient

While creative ability theory is applicable to all fields of practice the psychiatric occupational therapist's interest in this theory stems from its developmental possibilities, and its emphasis on occupation. Psychiatric illness impacts markedly on overall occupational performance and creative ability theory gives a precise way of describing functioning eluded to in the Global Assessment of Function (GAF) described in the DSM-IV-TR™ (American Psychiatric Association, 2000). Clients can be grouped easily according to creative ability and the use of creative ability theory helps in improving or maintaining the client's occupational performance, mental health and quality of life.

Assessment of level of creative ability

The assessment of a client's level of creative ability involves three sequential steps:

1. evaluation of the client's current skills and abilities in each occupation performance area;
2. establishing the client's level of action;
3. drawing a conclusion about the client's level of motivation from the level of action.

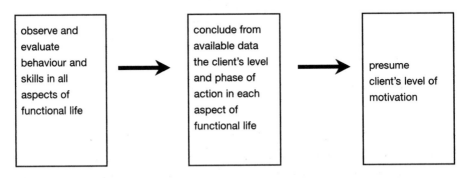

Figure 1.3 The steps involved in the assessment of a client's creative ability.

Step 1: Evaluation of skills and behaviour

This step should be included in the client's initial assessment prior to commencement of treatment. It should be part of the ongoing monitoring of their condition, so that the developmental momentum of creative ability can be maintained in all facets of intervention.

Initial assessment of the client's level of creative ability should be based on observation and evaluation of his skills and behaviour in as wide a variety of situations as possible. This assessment should not be based on what the client reports he can do, but on a practical evaluation of his current behaviour and skill in all four occupational performance areas (personal management, social ability, work ability and constructive use of free time). While the client's occupational history is pertinent in trying to establish treatment goals, it is what the client is currently able to do that is relevant in this assessment.

What to assess

The following aspects need to be explored:

Personal management

This is the client's ability to:

- care for both himself and his personal business, according to the norms and culture of his society;

- acquire skills such as toileting, washing, dressing, caring for personal belongings, grooming and refined forms of self-care, and managing himself independently within society.

Social ability

This is the client's ability to:

- communicate and interact socially with others who are familiar and unfamiliar (social skills)
- form acquaintances, make friends and develop some lasting, stable, intimate and mature relationships
- read and comply with overt and covert norms governing social behaviour in all situations and all life roles.

Work ability

This is the client's ability to be productive, and includes the ability to:

- initiate projects or tasks at the right time and see them through to conclusion, developing new ideas and methods when appropriate in both a work and home setting
- manage himself, his workload and resources effectively in the work/home situation, be it in an open, sheltered, protective or educational setting
- work effectively according to the norms set, and
- be critical of his performance through realistic judgement.

Constructive use of free time

This is the ability to use free time in a balanced, constructive, recreational and socially acceptable manner to attain pleasure and to de-stress.

How to carry out the assessment

In order to treat the client effectively a comprehensive assessment is required. The following describes the process to enable the occupational therapist to execute this assessment efficiently and reasonably quickly.

In addition to collecting background information during the initial interview, discuss the client's skills and behaviours, and the problems encountered in each occupational performance area, before he became ill and now that he is ill. Understanding premorbid functioning and abilities is useful when planning treatment and expected outcomes. Information on current function is used as a screen to approximate current skills so as to direct the detailed practical assessment at the right level. The interview should not replace practical evaluation, as often the psychiatric client's judgement of his abilities is poor due to limited insight. If a client is unable to give an accurate account of himself, or cannot communicate effectively, the interview may not be a very helpful tool for collecting data, but may be used to obtain clinical observations.

Following the interview, involve the client in an activity to determine his current occupational performance and the psychopathological symptoms that are compromising his performance. The nature of his engagement and the quality of performance will determine his level of action. Select an activity in consultation with the client, taking into account interests and aptitudes. The activity should preferably be unfamiliar yet within his frame of reference, be challenging, be completed within 45 minutes, have a concrete end product and encourage active participation. The activity should be carefully analysed to ensure it is appropriate to the occupational performance area or symptom being assessed.

Observe the client executing the activity and note the nature of his task concept, engagement and prevocational skills. Facilitate discussion about what he is doing, steps needed to complete the activity, what the end product will be, what he will do with it and his opinion of his performance. Structure the situation in such a way to enable independence, but intervene if the client appears to need support. Present the activity so that the client has to think about what has to be done and how to do it, offering assistance only if the client becomes anxious. Evaluate the social occupational performance area by including the client in a structured evaluative group. Including an activity from either occupational performance area could cover personal management and leisure. Also observing the client in the ward, during meals and unstructured periods gives the occupational therapist important data about functional performance.

When evaluating a client's creative ability, consider the following:

- attitude to and ability to make relational contact with materials, objects, people and events in the environment
- ability to plan, initiate and sustain effort until the activity is complete, or to continue at the same level of performance if the activity or task is repetitive
- quality of performance and his ability to evaluate what he has done and the standard he sets for himself
- ability to do activities with or without supervision, the amount of environmental structure required for adequate participation and ability to set and meet norms
- ability to control anxiety when faced with routine tasks and new challenges
- ability to act with originality to solve problems and act on decisions made
- response to engagement and emotional response to performance and the end product – particularly his personal causation (Kielhofner 1985, 2002).

This assessment must take cognisance of the client's stage of development and life tasks as well as his cultural background and environment, in terms of opportunities and barriers. This systematic assessment will give the occupational therapist a sound understanding of the client's skills and the occupational behaviour of which he is capable. It will also indicate skills that need to be encouraged to promote growth and recovery, or what should be maintained to support quality of life and wellness.

Step 2: Establishing the level of action

Because each level of action defines the skills and behaviour characteristics of that level of action, it is possible to categorize the client's behaviour and skill in the occupational performance areas. This is usually done on a grid system, such as the one in Table 1.2.

Table 1.2 An example of a grid system that can be used to establish the level of action

	Personal management	Social ability	Work ability	Use of free time
Predestructive				
Destructive				
Incidental				
Explorative				
Experimental				
Imitative				
Original				
Product centred				
Situation centred				
Society centred				

Using the information gathered about the client's skills and occupational behaviour, analyse his level of action in each occupational performance area. Make a cross in the grid in the appropriate column, positioning it to indicate whether the action is in the therapist-directed, patient-directed or transitional phase. For example, make a cross at the top of the square to indicate therapist-directed and at the bottom to indicate transitional phase.

Note that although there is often variation in the level of action between the four occupational performance areas, this is not usually marked. The variation is usually between two subsequent levels of action, or three at the most. If there are marked fluctuations, review the assessment data to ensure that it represents the client's overall pattern of functioning, rather than his splinter skills.

Step 3: Establishing the level of motivation

As motivation is difficult to observe and measure directly, one must presume the client's level of motivation from the quality and nature of his observable behaviour or actions. We know that there is a stable correlation between the levels of motivation and the levels of action (Table 1.1). Using the data recorded on the level of action grid completed in Step 2, make a presumption about the client's level of motivation.

Where the level of action in all four occupational areas is clustered, the presumption is straightforward, as in the example in Table 1.3. Data in Table 1.3 shows that the client's skills and behaviours are explorative in all four occupational performance areas, but are in the patient-directed phase in three occupational performance areas (social and work ability and use of free time). In one occupational area (personal management) the phase is transitional. This indicates that although behaviour and skills are largely reflective of the explorative level, there are some skills and behaviours that are associated with the experimental level of action under optimal circumstances. Thus, using the principle of majority rule, the client's level of motivation is 'self-presentation-patient-directed phase'.

Table 1.3 An example of a clustered level of action

	Personal management	Social ability	Work ability	Use of free time
Predestructive				
Destructive				
Incidental				
Explorative	X	X	X	X
Experimental				
Incidental				
Imitative				
Original				
Product centred				
Situation centred				
Society centred				

The data in Table 1.4 indicate that although all occupational performance areas are within the experimental level, personal management and social ability fall within the patient-directed phase, while work and leisure fall within the therapist-directed phase. The majority usually determines the phase. However, when there are two occupational performance areas marked in one phase and two in another, the following principles can be applied: social ability has the most impact on occupational performance, followed by work ability. Since the social occupational performance area has a governing influence, the overall phase would be patient-directed.

Table 1.4 An example of a grid system that can be used to establish the level of action

	Personal management	Social ability	Work ability	Use of free time
Predestructive				
Destructive				
Incidental				
Explorative				
Experimental	X	X	X	X
Incidental				
Imitative				
Original				
Product centred				
Situation centred				
Society centred				

However, where there is variation in the client's level of action in the four occupational performance areas, the presumption of the level of motivation is more complicated. See the example in Table 1.5. The data in this table indicate a variation in the level of skills and behaviours in four occupational performance areas. In the social area this client's skill is mostly explorative and he is in the patient-directed phase; in both the work and free time areas, skills are characteristically experimental, except in the work area where there are a few indications of skill and behaviours in the imitative level (transitional phase).

In the personal management area, although skill and behaviour are predominantly imitative in nature, some experimental behaviours may be evident (therapist-directed).

Thus the client's overall level of motivation is passive participation – fluctuating between the therapist-directed and transitional phases. Clustering usually occurs within the level or across two levels, so the data shown in Table 1.5 would be unusual.

Fluctuations in the level of action between the different occupational performance areas are not lost when classifying the client's level of motivation. When treating the client, these variations are accounted for in planning the programme as the levels of action are used when planning treatment, rather than the levels of motivation. The occupational therapist therefore mixes and matches the principles of treatment so that they fit the client's needs and reflect the variation in the action grid.

Table 1.5 An example showing a variable level of action

	Personal management	Social ability	Work ability	Use of free time
Predestructive				
Destructive				
Incidental				
Explorative		X		
Experimental			X	X
Imitative	X			
Original				
Product centred				
Situation centred				
Society centred				

Application of creative ability to psychosocial occupational therapy

Mental illness has a negative influence on the client's ability to live efficiently and to behave in a creative manner. Some psychiatric disorders have a more disorganizing effect on occupational performance than others. In some the disorganization may be temporary, while in others it may be permanent. The same psychiatric disorder may influence the occupational performance of two individuals differently, or there may be some differences in the same individual from one episode of illness to another. Psychosocial occupational therapy aims to improve or maintain the occupational performance of mentally ill clients. This is done by improving or maintaining skills and abilities within the occupational performance areas to improve functioning and reduce the chances of regression. It is also done to control or improve the psychiatric symptoms that are having a disorganizing effect by involving the client in meaningful activities that control and manage the psychopathology.

A client's level of creative ability forms the platform from which the occupational therapist manages both the specific occupational performance and the psychopathological problems. For example, if two clients both have low self-esteem, but the first client functions on a self-presentation level patient-directed phase and the other is on a passive-participation level transitional phase, the methods and techniques used to improve self-esteem will be similar, but the level of occupational performance will be qualitatively different. Therefore the treatment will need to be different. The same is true if two clients have destructive use of leisure time but are on different levels and phases of creative ability.

Creative ability theory can be applied to all categories of psychiatric disorder, on both Axes I and II of the DMS IV classification, and can be aligned to the International Classification of Function (ICF). It can be applied to both acute and chronic conditions. It can also be used equally effectively in most treatment settings.

The levels of creative ability

As described previously, creative ability represents a continuum of occupational behaviour from total dependence and egocentricity to contribution to the community with little expectation of personal rewards. This broad continuum can be divided into six levels of motivation, each with their corresponding levels of action. Because of similarities in the overall purpose of levels they can be divided into three quite distinct groups (see Table 1.6).

Table 1.6 The groups into which creative ability can be divided

Stages of motivation	Stages of action
Group 1: Preparation for constructive action	
Tone Self-differentiation	Predestructive Destructive Incidental constructive action
Group 2: Behaviour and skill development for norm compliance	
Self-presentation Participation: Passive Imitative	Explorative Experimental Imitative
Group 3: Behaviour and skill development for self-actualization	
Participation: Active Competitive Contribution Competitive contribution	Original Product centred Situation centred Society centred

Group 1: preparation for constructive action

This group includes the predestructive, destructive and incidental levels of action where the main purpose is the development of functional body use. This includes grasp and more refined hand function, muscle control, coordination, visual fixation and tracking, sensory identification and adequate motor response patterns. On a psychological level the individual develops knowledge of who he is and what he can do with his body, his relationship to the environment and an awareness of others and events. His occupational performance is quite limited and he is not able to engage in productive occupation performance.

Group 2: behaviour and skill development of norm compliance

This includes the explorative, experimental and imitative levels of action. These levels all concentrate on developing the necessary psychological, physical, social and work skills, as well as occupational behaviours, necessary to live and be productive in the community and comply with the prescribed norms of the society and group within which the client lives.

Group 3: behaviour and skill development for self-actualization

This includes the original, product centred, situation centred and society centred levels of action. These levels concentrate on developing leadership skills and behaviours that are novel, in any aspect of life. It may involve developing new products, methods of doing things, technology, problem-solving processes, or solutions to a tricky or complex situation. Motivation for this type of action is directed towards the benefit of self in the early levels and later towards others in a specified group of people and then towards society at large. These levels demand personal dedication, self-motivation and continuous critical self-evaluation.

The rewards for one's effort may not be tangible and one may have to wait for many months, years or even a lifetime to see results.

The characteristics of each level of creative ability will be discussed using these groups.

Group 1

In this group the first level of motivation is tone and the level of action associated with this is predestructive.

Tone

Motivation on this level is directed at 1) establishing and maintaining the will to live – du Toit (1980) called this positive tone; and 2) establishing and maintaining biological tone, which is the starting point from which all human systems needed in occupational performance develop.

Predestructive action

Clients on this level are defenceless, dependent, incapable and like new-born babies they have to be protected, cared for and nurtured. Their activity is mainly automatic and appears purposeless and not goal-directed, but their actions contribute to the development of the internal human (biological) systems.

They lack an awareness of themselves as being separate from the world around them. Occupational performance skills are extremely limited.

Personal management

These clients are unable to provide, defend or care for themselves in any way. They have very little or no control over their bodies and bodily functions. They need to be washed, dressed, toileted, fed, cared for and protected.

Social ability

The clients have little awareness of others. They attempt to communicate their basic needs of discomfort, hunger or thirst, but this is non-specific; for example they may grunt or shout, but this does not identify the problem or the extent of the distress. Language is frequently absent or if present, is unintelligible. They usually respond positively to nurturing and are usually able to recognize their caregivers. They appear to be unable to identify different situations, other than a momentary awareness of strangeness or familiarity.

Work ability and use of free time

These clients are totally non-productive in an occupational sense and have no concept of productivity. There is little evidence of intention or effort. They can focus their attention momentarily on stimuli and physical movements are uncoordinated, often reflexive and haphazard. These movements, while seeming purposeless, are directed at establishing and maintaining biological tone. They are unable to produce an end product of any sort under any circumstances. They have no concept of free time.

Clients with psychiatric illness who regress to this level are usually severely disordered. They are disorientated and severely impaired in all the psychosocial internal sub-systems, which totally incapacitates them.

Treatment

The treatment outcomes on the predestructive level are to encourage positive tone and biological tone by stimulating the client maximally via all his sensory modalities, in a consistent and continuous manner.

To achieve this outcome it is important for all members of the multi-disciplinary team to adopt a uniform treatment approach, which should be used by all the caregivers that come into contact with the client. Clients on this level are so occupationally incapacitated that a specific programme of activities is not practical. However all interactions with the client should focus on stimulating awareness of his own body, making him aware of things and others in the environment and stimulation of the sensory and motor system to promote biological tone.

Handling principles

The occupational therapist's interaction with the client should be warm and caring and the client should be treated with dignity. He must be accepted unconditionally. The occupational therapist or occupational therapy auxiliary must give everything in the relationship and expect nothing in return, not even recognition of himself as an individual. He should also be patient and persistent, making regular contact with the client to try to bring him into contact with the world, even if only momentarily. This is done by talking continuously to him, in a slightly raised voice to attract his attention, making physical contact (but with discretion), calling him by name and by describing the environment, objects and events in it. All processes involved in caring for the client should be verbalized.

Structuring of treatment

These clients are usually treated in their room or a familiar room in ward.

The treatment area should be stimulating but should not distract or overwhelm him. The external stimuli should be changed from time to time to prevent habituation. If practical, the client should not sit in the same place all day; he should be seated in places with different environmental stimuli. If at all possible he should be taken out of doors from time to time. Clients should be actively encouraged to move around, if that is possible. However if they are very mobile and tend to get lost, they should be contained within the ward area.

Clients should not be exposed to continuous therapeutic intervention. Therapy should be divided into a few short sessions (two to five minutes), spread throughout the day, but also included in caring interventions like feeding, dressing, bathing and other activities carried out by the nursing staff.

Presentation principles

Clients should also be exposed to objects and materials from the environment. These should be presented singly, in a consistent manner, with much repetition. The object or material should be placed in his hands and the occupational therapist or occupational therapy auxiliary should verbalize its basic concepts and properties to him, encouraging him to focus attention on it all the time he is in contact with it.

Activity requirements

Objects and materials should be from the client's own environment. They should stimulate the senses and allow for physical interaction within his capabilities. The materials and objects should be non-toxic in case he puts them into his mouth. They should also be non-breakable in case the client handles them in an uncoordinated manner. Do not expect him to interact purposefully with the object or materials during this stage. The only purpose is for him to focus on it momentarily; once his concentration span is exceeded the object/material will probably be discarded.

Grading

If the client shows signs of becoming more receptive to stimulation, it should be gradually and carefully upgraded. It can be upgraded by:

* increasing the frequency of the stimulatory sessions
* increasing their duration
* increasing the number of objects and materials to which the client is exposed, both in a session and over a period of time and
* encouraging the client to focus his attention on the object or material more frequently and for longer.

If the client shows signs of becoming less receptive to stimulation, the programme can be downgraded by reversing the principles listed above.

There are three criteria that should be used to evaluate whether the client is ready to move to the next level. These criteria are:

1. receptiveness to environmental stimuli;
2. ability to focus attention fleetingly; and
3. indications that interaction with materials and objects is becoming destructive.

Self-differentiation

The second level of motivation in Group 1 is self-differentiation. There are two levels of action associated with this, namely destructive and incidentally constructive.

On the level of self-differentiation, motivation is directed at three areas:

1. establishing and maintaining self-awareness as a separate entity from the environment and the objects and people in it;
2. achieving control over the body and learning the basic skills involved in using the body to interact with the world and integrating these into coordinated behaviours;
3. learning basic social behaviours such as greetings, making requests and complying with commands.

Destructive action

Destructive action is the first level of action to appear in self-differentiation. It is the most primitive interaction that the client has with the world. Destructive action aims to assist him to define his body boundaries and to practise the basic skills necessary for material and objects handling. Clients are not destructive by intention, but handle materials and objects destructively due to lack of abilities. Destructive actions help develop basic human system skills needed for occupational performance on later levels.

These skills are, for example, focusing of attention, basic concept formation, thinking, body concept, perception, coordination and hand function. This in turn stimulates primary intention and construction that occur coincidentally on the next level of action.

Destructive action has the following characteristics:

* Individuals are receptive to external stimulation and are prepared to make contact with the environment using their bodies.
* Action is of short duration (a minute or two) and the individual shows an inability to sustain effort.
* Action is non-constructive, in that no end product is produced other than fragments or a change in the form or volume of the material, owing to the client's destructive interaction with it. This interaction is unplanned, non-specific and does not take the properties of the materials or objects into account. It is, however, the first step in the exploration of materials and objects, and ability to interact with them. In all occupational performance areas, the client on a destructive level of action remains incapable, dependent and defenceless.

Personal management

He is still not able to do any personal tasks for himself, or even assist with them. However, because the client is more receptive to environmental stimuli, the interaction between the environment and the body in activities of personal management makes him aware of his body and its functions. Verbal reinforcement facilitates this. For example, when the client is bathed, the contact with the water, the facecloth, soaps and the towel makes him aware of his body and its boundaries. He can use his hands to splash the water or hold the soap and he can use his mouth to suck the facecloth and eat or lick the soap, even if it does not taste good.

Social ability

In the social environment, clients are more open to social contact. They are able to recognize the caregivers as familiar or unfamiliar. They respond positively to nurturing.

Communication remains erratic. They are unable to communicate their needs effectively, even though language may be present. They sometimes use simple words and gestures to communicate. Clients have no concept of social norms. They are still unable to recognize situations as being markedly different, and consequently behaviour is not differentiated from one situation to another.

There may be evidence of bizarre behaviour resulting from psychotic phenomena.

They learn to respond to simple commands such as 'sit here' and 'take that out of your mouth'.

Emotions are feebly displayed and, although there is a differentiation between the expression of positive and negative emotions, there is little variation in intensity. Anxiety is apparent if the client is distressed or frightened, but if he is distracted this, like all other emotions, dissipates quickly.

Work ability and use of free time

These clients tend to be more active and mobile than those on the previous level but they seldom venture out of their immediate environment. Their action remains non-constructive but there is evidence of conscious direct physical interaction with materials and objects in the environment. This results in a change of volume, shape or fragmentation of materials and a change of the position of objects. Destructive interaction with materials and objects may be sustained for short periods. Material and object handling still does not appear to reflect any active thinking or demonstrate intelligence, although such clients are attracted by colour and shape, indicating a developing awareness of basic concepts. The destructive interaction with materials and objects is the first step in the development of the part–whole concept. As the client's basic concepts are further developed so he is able to recognize and match shapes, colours, size, textures of objects and materials. He usually cannot name them until the next level, however.

Clients still have no concept of the use of free time.

Treatment

The treatment outcomes for clients on the destructive level are to:

* stimulate body awareness especially body boundaries
* stimulate the physical awareness of people and objects in the environment and the sense of familiarity/non-familiarity
* stimulate the focusing of attention for short periods, as well as physical and psychological abilities needed for basic interaction with the world.

As with clients on the predestructive level, for treatment to be successful, all caregivers should be involved in the treatment programme regardless of their discipline. All caregivers should be actively involved in the planning of the treatment so that principles are consistently applied in all care-giving activities even though they might take more time. Stimulation needs to be applied according to a specific plan to avoid habituation and over-stimulation.

Handling principles

* These clients should be handled in a caring, nurturing and dignified way. On this level accept the client unconditionally, as well as his unacceptable behaviour.
* Greet him regularly and talk to him.
* Verbalize all activities to the client, stimulating basic orientation to person and place and all basic concepts. Call all objects and people by their correct name. Ensure that you have the client's attention and encourage him to look at you, which will help to bring him into contact with reality.
* Encourage cooperation in all caregiving activities and facilitate body action to help the client participate in these activities, e.g. lift arms when dressing, open mouth when feeding.

Structuring of treatment

* Clients should be contained within the ward area but should be moved to different areas within the ward for different activities. The ward should be stimulating but not overwhelming or distracting. Make the clients aware of changes in the environment, e.g. a new flower arrangement.
* Encourage them to extend their world by looking out of the window and making them aware of the objects/people outside.
* Clients should be grouped with clients on the same level for short stimulation groups – usually only a single session a day.

Presentation principles

Treatment materials should be presented one at a time, and the client should be made familiar with the basic concepts of the material and objects. Verbalize the texture, form, shape and size of the material or object, while encouraging the client to make relational contact with it via his senses. He should look at, hold, feel, taste, listen to and smell the item in question, verbalizing the involved body part.

Activity requirements

* Actively encourage destructive action and don't expect constructive action.
* Objects and materials used should, where possible, come from the basic material group. They should demand no prior knowledge for the client to interact with them and should be edible, non-toxic and safe if mishandled. They should fall within his frame of reference and be part of his environment.
* Objects and material should not require fine coordination or skilled action or present much physical resistance.

Grading

During the course of this level, treatment needs to be adjusted as the client's physical and psychological abilities improve.
Grade physical activities by:

- increasing the range of movement from small to larger
- increasing the coordination expected during interaction with objects and materials, although coordination will still be poor and
- increasing the rate of movement from very slow to a little faster and increasing the control of his actions.

Grade psychological activities by:

- extending the period for which the client can keep his attention focused
- awareness of objects and people in the environment
- upgrading the amount and quality of cooperation in caregiving activities.

Should the client show signs of deterioration the above grading principles can be reversed to accommodate the deterioration.

The following criteria need to be met before the client is ready to move on to the next level:

- the client is able to interact destructively with all materials and objects and shows some indication of intention
- basic concepts are evident
- the client is more aware of his immediate environment and is orientated to person.

Incidentally constructive action

This is the second level of action to develop on the self-differentiation level. It is characterized by unplanned, unintentional, constructive action that results, by chance, in an immediate, recognizable end product. This one-task activity stimulates the development of the part–whole concept. There is a tendency for incidental action to be repeated in both the same and other situations, which stimulates generalization. Du Toit (1980) saw this as the essential precursor to constructive activity participation.

Personal management

Although clients on this level still remain dependent on others for care, safety and security, they establish the basic skills necessary to care for themselves, although they are not yet able to do this without supervision.

As the client's body concept becomes consolidated, so he is able to learn the basic skills and behaviours involved in care and control of his body, hygiene, dressing and feeding.

During this stage the client achieves competence in the practical skills involved in these activities but continues to have difficulty with the following:

- Timing of toileting – he must go to the toilet the minute he has the urge.
- Putting shoes on the correct feet and coping with fastenings.
- Carrying out the above tasks independently and at an acceptable level of performance.

Clients learn to do these hygiene activities within a specific routine set by caregivers. This stimulates the start of the concept of temporal organization of activities. Clients often become distressed when the routine is disturbed as it provides a sense of security and predictability in their lives.

Sociability

In the social situation, the awareness of familiar people is extended to those other than caregivers, which helps to extend their orientation to person. They can be very demanding.

Communication becomes more coherent and they are able to communicate their needs more efficiently, although the communications are egocentric and simple.

Clients continue to have little awareness of social norms, although they do start to differentiate between right and wrong from the response of the caregiver. For example, they may be praised for eating their food but reprimanded for spitting on the floor. Behaviour continues to be undifferentiated from one situation to another and bizarre behaviour again may be evident in response to psychotic phenomena.

Tantrums may occur if the client's needs are not met as soon as he would like or if he is restricted or refused what he desires.

Work ability and use of free time

He is able to focus his attention on his activity for longer. Initially five minutes and extending to ten minutes towards the end of the level.

He can interact with materials and objects, usually more than one or two at a time, unintentionally producing an immediate, clearly recognizable end product, which is a direct result of his interaction with the world. Although he demonstrates no desire to do anything with the end product he has produced, he might practise this incidental response a number of times, not always immediately, but within a few hours or days.

Basic concepts are usually consolidated on the therapist-directed phase with clients able to name objects. Elementary concepts also develop and by the transition phase clients can state the function and use of most common objects within their environment.

These clients are often quite mobile and are reluctant to sit for long periods of time.

They appear to want to be of help and can do simple tasks/chores if directed by the caregiver.

They are more aware of the environment. They can recognize different people and can identify the different rooms where activities take place. They can identify their own bed area and become very possessive about their possessions. Their orientation to person and place is improved but they are quite sensitive to changes in the environment, although they often can not identify the nature of the change.

Clients on this level continue to have no concept of free time.

Mentally ill clients who deteriorate to the self-differentiation level show evidence of severe, incapacitating psychopathology. Frequently the expression of this psychopathology is more evident because the client is more active and more verbal than on the level of tone. Disorganization of thinking, language impairments, aggressive and bizarre uncontrolled behaviour are common. Clients on this level are usually found in chronic institutions, which provide habilitation and rehabilitation.

Treatment

The treatment outcomes with clients on the level of incidentally constructive level are:

- The consolidation of body concept; making the client aware of his body parts; awareness of shape, size and functions by using sensory stimulation during hygiene and other tasks involving movement and interaction with materials and objects.
- The improvement of his awareness of the physical presence of others in the environment by exposing him to people other than caregivers, for example other clients and staff, and focusing his attention on them during the treatment process.
- The development or improvement of the physical and cognitive skills necessary for constructive action by encouraging incidentally constructive interaction, with possibilities for practice and repetition.
- Basic orientation to person, place and time.
- The achievement of basic skills of personal care.

Occupational therapy programmes for these clients can be planned by an occupational therapist and executed by a trained occupational therapy auxiliary. As on the previous levels, for treatment to be really successful all caregivers should be involved in the programme so that the client has specific, consistent stimulation in all situations in which he finds himself. The caregivers should be actively involved in the planning of the programme and should be encouraged to use the principles of treatment effectively, even if this is more time-consuming. A specific programme of activities should be introduced into a ward programme, and therapy sessions can be introduced as well so that treatment is now extended beyond caregiving activities.

Handling principles

- Clients should be handled in a caring and dignified way but one should reward good behaviour and reprimand unacceptable behaviour, such as defecating on the floor, in a kind and non-punitive manner.
- It is important to talk to the client clearly, in a slightly raised voice to attract his attention, but you should not shout.
- Continuously orientate the client in terms of person and place. Make him aware of others, call him by name and verbalize his actions. Make him aware of the environment and the different activities that occur there.
- Stimulate orientation to time by orientating him to the day, date, year, time of day and seasons and the events that take place in each.
- Verbalize the client's activity to him and also tell him what others are doing, to encourage the development of basic and elementary concepts and body concept.
- Ensure that you have the client's attention when stimulating him. Call him by name and encourage him to look at you at the same time. This will help bring him into contact with reality.

Structuring principles

The treatment situation should be stimulating, but there should be no external stimuli that unduly overwhelm or distract the client. External stimuli can be increased as the client's ability to focus attention improves.

Although some of the treatment should be carried out in the ward environment, the client can also be taken to an occupational therapy department or out into the garden, as long as these areas are in fairly close proximity as mobility may be a problem.

Treatment time should be broken up into a number of short sessions of between ten and 20 minutes. These should be repeated a number of times during the day. Treatment may also be part of some of the caregiving processes such as bathing, washing and eating. Treatment will only be effective if it occurs on a daily basis.

Clients should be treated in small groups with other clients on the same level of action. The group should consist of no more than six members and the group leader needs to be consistent. Group treatment assists in developing awareness of others and the environment. The therapist should encourage introductions and an awareness of the activity of each member of the group.

Treatment situations must be well organized before the clients arrive so that the session starts immediately. Materials and equipment must be at hand and the workplace should be carefully structured, taking safety and ergonomic factors into account. Where possible no tools should be used and clients must be encouraged to make direct contact with the materials and objects.

When treatment does not incorporate caregiving processes and is outside the ward, remember to include time for basic hygiene such as hand washing and regular toileting.

Both the ward and occupational therapy areas should be planned or structured to promote orientation. This is particularly important during the later phases of the incidental level. Calendars and clocks should be correct and clearly displayed. All doors should be clearly marked, especially the toilet door.

Presentation principles

The client must be given clear, simple, direct, step-by-step instructions. Instructions should be repeated frequently in exactly the same way every time, so that the client does not have to deal with new elements that were not present earlier.

When teaching the client a new skill or stimulating him to use an old one demonstrate by physically moving his body through the desired movements, until he has the idea. Then repeat the action until he is able to do it alone. Remember that the quality of what he does will be poor and he will still need help.

Activity requirements

Incidental constructive activities should be planned, prepared and structured for the client. All that should be required of him is to interact with the materials and objects in the activity to produce an end product that he did not expect. Activities must give immediate gratification. An edible end product often has more impact. Activities should clearly show the impact of his effort and the difference between the parts and the whole. All that can be expected is that he should interact with materials and objects.

The activities should be concrete and simple, and should facilitate the client's knowledge and control of his body as well as pre-functional physical and psychological skills.

The activities also need to help develop basic self-care skills.

Grading

- Therapy is centred on all caregiving activities to specific therapy sessions.
- Treatment is only within the ward setting to therapy in occupational therapy department and outside.
- Cooperation in basic self-care activities to development of skills but still requires supervision.
- Upgrade the physical demands of activities: increase rate, control and range of movement.

- Upgrade the psychological demands of activities on:

  - Body concept: Grade from body awareness to identification of body parts and their function to more functional use of the body and control of body processes.
  - Concentration: As the client's active and passive attention span improves, so treatment time can be extended from five to ten minutes. As the level of distractibility decreases so more external stimuli can be introduced.
  - Awareness: Grade from minimal awareness of self and familiar others, to more consistent awareness of both self and others and their temporal and spatial relationship to the client. For example before and after tea, and spatial concepts, such as sitting next to, in front of or on the left or right of the occupational therapist/occupational therapy auxiliary.
  - Orientation: Grade from orientation to person, place and basics of time.

Should the client show an indication of deterioration the above principles can be reversed to accommodate this.

- The following criteria have to be met before the client is ready to move on to the next level:

  - Body concept must be consolidated.
  - He must be able to go to the toilet independently.
  - The client must have the necessary skill to carry out hygiene tasks, although the quality of performance may be poor.
  - There should be awareness of self and others and the temporal and spatial relationship between them.
  - The client should be able to interact with materials and objects incidentally and should show interest in more explorative action.
  - The client should be orientated to person and place and has some understanding of orientation to time.

Group 2

This group consists of the following levels of motivation: self-presentation, passive and imitative participation.

Self-presentation

On this level, motivation is directed towards:

- Development of individuality but at the same time a sense of belonging to a group.

- Developing the basic components of self-concept.
- Presentation of self to others and developing the most basic and fundamental skills involved in social interaction and interpersonal relationships (social awareness, judgement, basic social skills, relating, and socially acceptable behaviour).
- Exploring the ability to influence the environment and be constructive and to discriminate interests.
- Basic elements of productivity and occupational performance in all occupational performance areas (achieving task concept, an awareness of pre-vocational skills and a concept of leisure).

Throughout this stage clients demonstrate a readiness to present the newly differentiated self to others, to explore the world and define its reality. This exploration of the world is a prerequisite for constructiveness and productivity that develop in this and the subsequent levels.

Explorative action

This level of action coincides with self-presentation. It can be defined as the intentional investigation of materials, objects and others in the environment.

This exploration is directed towards establishing the particular properties of materials and objects and the way in which they can be influenced. It is also the reaction of the materials, objects and others in the environment to the client and marks the first step towards productivity. The more he interacts with others and objects in the environment, the more he learns about his effectiveness as an occupational being. It is the start of the development of personal causation (Kielhofner, 2002).

During this stage the limitations placed on occupational performance by a client's psychological and environmental resources are evident in how he interacts with the environment. During the course of this level the client learns many of the skills needed for independent living, but his need for structure, encouragement, support and outside organization precludes him from using these skills independently.

Clients with mental illness often regress to this level of action during acute exacerbations and plateau on this level in the chronic phase of illness. Symptoms in all of the psychosocial subsystems of man can impact on a client's ability and limit occupational performance to the explorative level. Although symptoms are less gross than on the earlier levels, psychopathology remains of moderate intensity. Clients on this level can be found in acute units, mental hospitals and care centres. When their psychiatric condition is controlled they can also live in halfway houses, or a protective environment or within a protective family unit, provided they have the resources to cope with them. They can seldom work in the open labour market unless the job is low level, undemanding and highly supervised, but they can work in industrial therapy, sheltered or protective workshops.

Personal management

In the therapist-directed phase of this level clients consolidate their basic hygiene, which had to be supervised on the previous level. The quality and efficiency of performance become more socially acceptable. While they cannot organize these skills into a routine and need reminders to carry them out, they can execute them independently.

In the therapist-directed phase, clients can dress themselves efficiently. They can select clothes but they are not really concerned about the appropriateness of the clothes, regular changes of clothing or the state of the clothes and often wear the same soiled clothes for several days. The less choice there is available to the client, the more appropriate his clothes tend to be.

In the patient-directed phase clients learn the need and skills to care for their clothes, personal belongings and their immediate surroundings. They develop an awareness of the need to be presentable and then the skills to wash, iron, sew on a button, keep personal belongings safe and orderly, etc. In spite of this, they still wear clothes for several days, but they recognize the fact that they should change. They like to have their own belongings and develop preferences for clothes, which reflect their individuality. Choice may still not be socially appropriate. All these tasks need supervision by the occupational therapist or nursing staff and washing and repairs are usually done by caregivers on a regular basis.

In the transitional phase clients develop an interest in and explore refined forms of self-care and grooming. They start to become concerned about how they look and the need to be dressed appropriately for the situation, weather and activity. They also develop some basic skills for independent living, e.g. making the bed, making tea and sandwiches, sweeping, and washing dishes. Clients usually change their clothes regularly. If facilities are available, clients can do their own washing, although relatives frequently do this if a client is hospitalized. Care of clothing and belongings is more regular, but the quality is not always socially appropriate.

Throughout this stage clients master some of the skills associated with independent living. However, they often manage themselves poorly when not supervised. They have difficulty organizing their activities into a routine, using their time effectively and organizing their resources, for example finances, and therefore cannot live independently. However, if relatives or caregivers organize a routine, clients are able to execute these personal domestic activities, although the quality is generally poor, as is their persistence and discipline.

Social ability

Clients come into the explorative level with an awareness of the physical presence of others. This is further refined in the therapist-directed phase; they recognize other clients from their ward, and can sometimes name them. They can differentiate between staff and other clients. In the patient-directed phase they become aware of the fact that others in the environment have needs and feelings. During the transition phase, their recognition of the needs and feelings of others becomes more accurate as their judgement improves, but they have difficulty in responding to these cues appropriately.

Throughout this stage the client develops basic social skills. The quality and appropriateness of verbal and non-verbal skills improve towards the transitional phase. Conversation remains superficial and egocentric throughout the level. Conversation also tends to reflect the client's psychopathology and they have difficulty in dealing with interpersonal anxiety.

In the patient-directed and transitional phase, clients tend to form egocentric, superficial, childlike, transient relationships with people within their immediate environment and they develop dependency relationships with caregivers. Relationships with others tend to be short-lived and they tend not to tolerate absences and differences of opinion.

Social behaviour within the relationship is often inconsistent and they often disregard the feelings of others.

Relationships with family members may be strained especially if there is a history of aggression, conflict about delusions and other behaviours associated with illness.

Clients often have a disturbed sense of belonging to groups. Either they feel quite detached from family and secondary group or are over-dependent on one or other group.

Work ability

The most important development in this level is the emergence of the 'task concept', which is essential for doing activities independently and for being productive (de Witt, 2003).

Initially task concept was described as having five distinct parameters which together contributed towards a client's occupational performance, moving from being incidental and purposeless to being goal-directed, purposeful and product-centred in his engagement in activities.

The five parameters were understanding the task as a whole, identifying with the task, task execution, task completion and task satisfaction. The emergence of the five concepts was plotted within the explorative level and helped the therapist to understand how the client functioned within the range of the explorative level. The occurrence of one of these parameters was consistent with the beginning of the level (i.e. therapist-directed phase). Having two or three parameters was consistent with the middle of the level (i.e. the patient-directed phase) and when all five parameters were evident the client was at the end of the explorative level, i.e. the transitional phase, and ready to move on to the experimental level which followed. From clinical experience it was assumed that understanding of the task as a whole develops first and satisfaction last, but this has never been tested scientifically.

Recent research suggests that there are two separate but complementary components that are pertinent to the development of a client's ability to engage efficiently in activities; these components are slightly different from the previous ideas about task concept and task engagement (de Witt, 2003). The first is the *task concept*, which appears to have two interacting subsections:

1. Understanding the process of the activity, which is aligned to understanding the activity as a whole.
2. Understanding the influence of his effort, having a sense of engagement in the activity and that the activity is the product of his effort. This appears to be the same concept as identifying with the task.

These two subsections are influenced by a client's interest in and recognition of the task at hand. This implies that the development of an understanding of the task is more likely to be facilitated when the activity is within both his range of interests and frame of reference. This links well with Reed's belief that in order for activities to be of value to a client they need to:

- be meaningful in terms of his or her personal needs and environment demands;
- be purposeful, which implies the activities are valued, sanctioned by the socio-cultural group;
- be goal directed in the sense that the occupation should have purpose which is both valued and meaningful; and
- provide the 'just right' challenge to stimulate interest and fully engage energy levels and resources (Reed 1994).

The second component relevant to how well a client engages in activities is the nature of a client's engagement in the activity. The following five interacting aspects describe the process of a client's engagement that is essential for productive action:

1. *Task selection* relates to the activities in which the client chooses to engage in. Task selection implies that the decision 'to do' needs to be made, as well as deciding between the options that the environment offers. Task selection is the most difficult in the therapist-directed phase. However, throughout the explorative level occupational therapists should offer clients the opportunity and resources to engage in activities that are meaningful, purposeful, goal-directed and within their abilities. However, a client must make the decision to engage even though he may need structure, support and some coercion to do this.
2. *Task execution* relates to how a client goes about the process of the task. This includes how a client interacts with the activity resources and uses his internal capacities to work through the steps in the activity, as

well as the level of motivation required to keep to the task at hand and sustain effort until the task is complete. This is poor at the beginning of the explorative level and improves considerably towards the end.

3. *Task completion* indicates that a client is aware that the end of the activity has been reached and no more work is needed or desired. In the therapist-directed phase clients want an end product, but cannot conceptualize the end, often believing the activity is complete after only one step. In the patient-directed phase they seem more concerned with the process than the end, while in the transitional phase the client knows what is needed for completion, although he does not necessarily act on this, but acknowledges that more could be done.

4. *Task evaluation* indicates a client's capacity to evaluate the quality of what has been done, as well as the effort that is needed. This evaluation is not robust, nor is it accurate; rather there is the capacity to look at what has been done in an evaluative manner. Thus a client exercises his interpretative and evaluative skills in relation to his own performance in order to develop his sense of personal causation. This, in turn, impacts on his concept of self and influences the nature of future engagement in all similar activities. While task satisfaction is important in normal activity participation there are many clients who seldom achieve task satisfaction due to their inadequate self-concept, resultant low self-esteem and unrealistically high need for perfection. The challenge for the occupational therapist is to assist the client to develop belief in his capacity to do activities effectively and so strengthen his occupational sense of self (de Witt, 2003).

5. *Task satisfaction* usually implies a client has the ability to gain a positive emotional response from engagement that should reinforce his participation. However, emotions in relation to engagement seem to be quite conflicting, e.g. frustration and disappointment when the end product is not exactly what was expected, but pleasure at the fact that something was achieved. An emotional response with regard to engagement is very important in helping a client determine his strengths and weaknesses as an occupational being. This develops not only from the quality of the end product but also from the nature of the effort as well as the feedback received from others.

Throughout this level the client's participation is goal-directed. Although an end product is usually produced, the emphasis is on the process of exploring the materials, objects and people encountered during the process, rather than on the end product itself. However, the production of a reasonable end product is important to support personal causation and fragile self-esteem.

The exploration, although gaining information about the properties of materials and objects, is also directed at the way in which he can influence or affect other situations and things in the world to find out about himself and his abilities.

Throughout this level, activity participation is influenced by psychopathology, a poorly developed self-concept and a poor ability to make considered decisions. Clients have difficulty with concrete decisions where there are more than two or three options and where the options are very similar (positive to positive) or equally poor (negative to negative). Clients also have difficulty with all decisions of an abstract nature. Clients have difficulty in working at an acceptable rate – they work either too quickly and impulsively or too slowly. Due to inadequate prevocational skills the quality of their work is usually poor and they cannot judge performance effectively. In addition they have difficulty in delaying gratification for long periods of time and their ability to confront and cope with obstacles in the activity process is poor.

Use of free time

During this level clients start to develop leisure interests. This is facilitated by their discrimination of activities, based on their past experience. At the same time they begin to develop the understanding that some activities are for the purpose of work or survival while others are only for pleasure and recreation. In the patient-directed phase the concept of leisure is firmly established and in the transitional phase they develop or regain a few isolated interests, but are not able to pursue their interests and leisure activities independently. They often intend to participate but they need structure and support to do so.

Throughout the explorative level characteristics of the client's personality and his background are more evident and need to be considered more specifically in the activities selected in the treatment programme.

Clients may also be aware of their occupational incapacity, but seldom realize the reason for it or what needs to be done to improve it. This limited insight often prevents clients from fully understanding the implications of the occupational therapy programme. This influences their ability to cooperate fully, and they need continual encouragement to do so.

Treatment

There are three main outcomes for treatment for clients on this level:

1. To give the client the opportunity to present himself to others in different situations in order to facilitate his awareness of others. To practise both verbal and non-verbal social skills, and to gain an impression of his ability to interact with and react to others, and to form relationships with others and caregivers.
2. To give the client the opportunity to explore his ability to influence the materials and objects in his environment so as to gain an impression of his abilities. This will help develop his concept of himself and his feelings of competence as an occupational being (personal causation).
3. To consolidate the task concept and facilitate engagement.

Handling principles

The occupational therapist needs to be encouraging and supportive of the client as a person. Because of his poor self-concept, he frequently feels insecure and doubts his ability. Patience is needed as this insecurity is usually reflected in all behaviours.

The client's individuality should be facilitated and emphasized in all interactions. This can be done by:

- asking the client for his opinions and ideas, and acting on these if practical
- sharing the client's contribution or pointing out his achievements to others. This helps to develop the external feedback system needed in the development of self-esteem and effective occupational performance
- executing the client's wishes if they are realistic and fall within therapeutic goals, and discussing those that do not
- giving the client the opportunity to make decisions concerning his activities and actions, and encouraging him to take responsibility for them if this is realistic.

Expectations for behaviour and occupational performance should be made clear to the client. As the client's social judgement is poor, covert norms need to be made overt but the expectation for compliance remains low. These norms should be used to help the client's judgement of performance and situations. However, actions that may be harmful or destructive to others must be firmly handled.

Clients are frequently reticent about being involved in occupational therapy. They should be firmly encouraged but not forced. The occupational therapist can facilitate involvement by using a roundabout method of inclusion and by sharing the responsibility for the activity with the client. A clear, simple explanation about the role of occupational therapy within his total treatment and the setting of objectives that measure improvement may also help.

The occupational therapist should actively encourage the client to present himself to others. He should be given many opportunities to do this and the occupational therapist should facilitate communication between the client and others.

The occupational therapist should also actively encourage exploration of his ability by giving him the opportunity to make relational contact with materials, objects and others. He must direct his interaction and focus his attention on the effect of his actions.

The occupational therapist should help the client to direct his energy towards active engagement in a wide variety of activities and interaction should facilitate the development of the task concept. Throughout this level prevocational skills should be stimulated to develop awareness, rather than to actively improve these skills.

Structuring principles

Treatment should be carried out in an area in which the client feels safe and secure. Special care must be taken to orientate the client to a new treatment environment, and the expectations for behaviour should be made clear to him.

Treatment situations should be varied and appropriate to the activity at hand.

The occupational therapist should always be on hand to give assistance, encouragement and support, and to dissipate anxiety that the situation or activity may provoke.

Other clients should be included in the treatment environment, but they should be involved in their own activities. This is important to promote interaction, to give feedback and to help the client to learn to share the time and attention of the occupational therapist with others.

He should also be included in groups, both structured and spontaneous, where the activity is concrete.

The treatment session should last approximately 45 minutes, but this will depend on the client's ability to explore. The treatment situation should be stimulating, but external stimuli should be adjusted to the client's level of distractibility.

The occupational therapist should prepare the selected activity and should structure the workplace to promote good prevocational skills, safety and ergonomic working. In the transitional phase the client should be encouraged to assist with this. The occupational therapist should clear up and pack away, but she can direct the patient to do some aspects of the clearing up to promote awareness. These clients should be encouraged to label and store their own activities in a safe place.

The treatment situation should be well organized with set locations for tools and materials. It is important to give the client security and to help organize his actions in relation to the environment.

The client should be given a copy of his treatment programme. Initially he will need reminders to attend but towards the transitional phase he should be encouraged to be more independent and be expected to report to the occupational therapist if he is unable to attend.

Presentation of activity

On this level, all activities should be presented in a way that evokes a feeling of anticipation and competence.

Presentation and teaching should facilitate the development of the task concept and engagement. Instructions should make the client aware of the processes or steps to be followed to complete the task, and their order. The client should be encouraged to contribute his ideas to the activity in order to facilitate identification and individuality.

He should be encouraged to evaluate his performance on a concrete level and to recognize the point at which the activity, or his participation in it, is complete.

Demonstration should be used with discretion so as not to form a model for interaction with materials, others and objects, and thus reduce exploration.

Throughout the treatment session, emphasis should be placed on the client's effort and involvement with the materials and processes, and not on the end product. Although the emphasis is not on the end product, it is important that the results of the client's interaction are positive. Thus it is important to direct the client's participation at the activity's key points of controls in order to ensure success.

In the therapist-directed phase, no norms should be set for quality or rate of performance. In the patient-directed and transitional phases, clients should be made aware of the norms relating to quality of performance. Compliance to these should be facilitated but not expected.

The programme should be graded from a number of short single-treatment sessions repeated throughout the day, to one where he is occupied for half of the day, while still allowing for adequate rest. It is desirable to have a number of individual sessions, where the treatment is directed towards his most important problem, as well as one group session per day.

Activity requirements

All activities should enable the client to behave exploratively.

As the client's task concept is not consolidated, it is acceptable for him to do only some aspects of an activity, with the occupational therapist doing most of the planning and preparatory steps. The client should do the execution and completion steps. Each step can consist of between four and seven tasks.

Activities must be carefully selected so that they assist in the development of task concept and facilitate engagement. Activities should be within the interests and frame of reference of the client, be purposeful and meaningful to him. Although the client may only do some aspects of the total activity, he should be encouraged to make some decisions about the end product, e.g. colour, what will be done with it, etc.

The activities should encourage tool and material handling and should be infallible or easily controlled with a good end product, although this should not be emphasized.

Try to use unfamiliar activities so that the client cannot compare current ability with previous skill. Also try to choose a unique activity that nobody else is doing to ensure that modelling does not reduce exploration, and also to encourage positive feedback.

The activity used should not include elements of competition or actively compare the client's skills or performance with that of others. The activity should also be concrete and simple so as not to raise the client's anxiety unduly, but should challenge him not to be childish.

Grading

Grading should take place in the following areas:

- *Interpersonal contact.* Social situations should be concrete and structured but the people to whom the client is exposed and with whom interaction is facilitated should vary from known selected people, to known unselected people, to unknown and unselected people.
- *Attendance.* In the therapist-directed phase the client needs to be fetched for treatment. In the patient-directed phase the client should be encouraged to attend treatment with other clients, even if he needs reminding. In the transitional phase the client can usually attend treatment independently, but needs to have the time and venue clearly stated. Frequent reminders are needed. Inconsistencies in punctuality must be tolerated.
- *Engagement.* This needs to be actively facilitated throughout the level. However, in the therapist-directed phase exploration should be actively facilitated, whilst in the patient-directed phase the client should be given the opportunity to direct his own exploration. In the transitional phase some opportunities for experimental action should be introduced into activities that remain predominantly explorative.
- *Behavioural expectations.* Initially all behavioural disturbances should be tolerated, but the therapist should make it clear to the client in a tactful and supportive way that his behaviour is not socially appropriate or acceptable. He should be given some alternative suggestions for more acceptable behaviour. In the two later phases the client should be given the opportunity to try out and explore the alternative behaviours suggested. The effectiveness of these should be discussed with the client on a concrete basis, either individually or in a small group – whichever is more acceptable to the client. Handle this with kindness and understanding and never in a punitive manner.

Should the client fail to progress and show signs of deterioration the grading principles mentioned above can be reversed.

The criteria which mark the movement to the passive participation level are:

- the consolidation of the task concept and an interest in being involved in all aspects of the activity, particularly the end product or ultimate purpose of his engagement
- an interest in the rules or norms which govern behaviour and activity participation in all spheres of life
- an ability to work through an activity without constant supervision and individual attention
- the consolidation of basic social skills and an increase in awareness of people and social situations and a keen interest in the norms governing social behaviour.

Passive participation

This is the first of the four levels of participation. Motivation on this level is directed at establishing the rules and norms acceptable to the group and the society in which the client lives, and according to which behaviour in all occupational performance areas is judged. Motivation is more extensive and becomes more goal-directed as the client shows interest in the totality and purpose of activities but is not yet able to initiate these independently. However, he does demonstrate the ability to sustain interest and effort in activities that are structured and initiated by others. Effort, ability and behaviour are characteristically erratic. The client is easily influenced by others who he believes demonstrate socially acceptable behaviour.

During this level ideals and morals are more evident. Clients functioning on this level become aware of the interpersonal, social, political and economic factors influencing their immediate environment and also the macro-environment. This awareness leads to the identification of potentially threatening environmental stress factors. Their poor anxiety control and limited behavioural resources negatively influence spontaneous participation, particularly in unfamiliar situations.

During this level the client's emotional repertoire is also much improved. More refined emotions such as regret, pride, sympathy and loyalty are evident. The client is more in control of his emotional response although when provoked, threatened or stimulated strongly, emotional control is tenuous.

Experimental level

The level of action that coincides with the passive participation level is experimental. Behaviour tends to be both passive and erratic. Clients on this level tend to be the followers, doing what others do and say; they do not want to singled out from the crowd.

However, on a psychological level they are very active – they watch and listen to everything going on around them. They do this to establish those behaviours that are both acceptable and unacceptable to their group and to society, and to determine the effects of both compliance and non-compliance. They actively experiment with their own behaviour, by following what others do to establish how society will react and how acceptable their behaviour will be.

On the occupational performance level the client has, and is developing, the following skills:

Personal management

The client has a well-ordered hygiene routine that is carried out independently and efficiently. The skills acquired on the previous level for the care of his clothing and belongings are consolidated on this level. However, the quality of performance is negatively influenced by his poor prevocational skills. Organization of these skills into a practical routine is poor.

Clients have a tendency to need structure in order to become organized, or they leave the activity until they are pressurized into doing it because of a definite need; for example, doing washing and ironing only when they have no more clothes to wear.

They show an interest in refined forms of self-care, grooming and fashion. In the therapist-directed phase, their interest needs to focus on these issues, while in the patient-directed phase they actively experiment with them when encouraged. In the transitional phase, patients tend to experiment more independently. Throughout the phase, however, behaviour with regard to self-care is erratic – sometimes it is insufficient and inappropriate and at other times appropriate and sufficient.

Ability to budget time and funds for everyday living is erratic and there is a tendency to buy impulsively. Organization of personal business, for example accounts and income tax, tends not to be very efficient.

Throughout the level clients express the desire for independence, but they need outside supervision and structure to achieve this competently.

Social ability

Interpersonal activity is directed towards being accepted and belonging. Communication is usually rational and logical and they can discuss a wide range of subjects, although clients demonstrate a reluctance to give their opinion if they are unsure of the opinion of the group. Conversation can be maintained effectively if other parties take most of the responsibility for it. Clients are able to form interpersonal relationships with others but do so for egocentric purposes such as feeling more accepted, adequate or important. They tend to relate to stronger personalities or more functional people who direct their behaviour. Clients on this level find group situations quite anxiety-provoking. They like to be involved with the group but not to be singled out to give an individual opinion or make a suggestion. They tend to take on a spectator role in groups but are nevertheless actively involved in the group process although they offer little, unless specifically invited to do so. Because of their desire to be 'one of the crowd' they have difficulty in being assertive. Assertive skills tend to start developing during this level. They have difficulty in dealing with difference of opinion and therefore find resolving conflict difficult.

Work ability

Occupational behaviour becomes progressively more product centred. The consolidated task concept facilitates the client's interest in all aspects of the activity and his desire to work through an activity from beginning to end. Although clients are eager to participate they have difficulty in initiating activities. They are also reluctant to participate in any activity where success is not ensured.

During the course of activity they need less rigorous supervision than previously but they still need to have the steps and sequence confirmed. Throughout this level they are concerned with what prevocational work skills are required to make their activity acceptable.

Judgement of their performance is poor throughout the level, although it improves towards the transitional phase. They tend to judge their performance in terms of good or bad, but do not look at the reasons for the quality of their performance.

If the end product is unsuccessful, some clients tend to blame the materials, tools or environmental factors rather than how they contributed to the problem (external locus of control), while others have an unrealistic desire for perfection and excellence which they are not able to meet.

Clients are able to sustain effort over a period of time. They are able to deal with some obstacles which may occur during the course of the activity, but are unable to demonstrate initiative. Quality of performance tends to improve towards the transitional phase, but may be erratic on a day-to-day basis throughout the level.

Domestic or survival skills are the focus of attention on this level. In the early phase the client can be given responsibility for caring for his bed area or room and personal possessions. He is able to take care of his room, clean up and pack things away, but the quality of these actions varies and the organization of these activities is poor. He is frequently interested in cooking and with encouragement and structure, is able to make nutritious meals. However, motivation to do this on a regular basis is poor.

Clients who have achieved this level may be able to work on the open labour market, but the work environment will have to be very structured and organized and the individual will require a great deal of supervision. The job should be such that variations in quality and rate of performance should not be too important to job security.

Use of free time

A greater range of interests in recreation develops throughout this level. Clients' discrimination of interests is largely dependent on those of their friends or caregivers. They will actively participate with others if organized and encouraged. If others are not available to encourage them, they tend to use their time unproductively or are involved in passive recreational activities such as watching television.

There is a percentage of the adult population who never develop beyond the experimental level. They live successfully in the community if they have familial support and structure and if not too much is expected of them in their everyday performance. If familial support is not available, they need to live in a situation where most of their basic needs are met by the efforts of others.

High-functioning individuals can regress to a level of experimental action as a result of psychiatric illness. The illness is usually of mild to moderate proportions and the psychopathology has an individualized presentation. These clients may be hospitalized in acute medium-term units and are often in a predischarge phase. Well mentally ill clients on this level may also be found in the community, participating in daycare or other rehabilitation facilities.

Treatment

The main outcomes for treatment are:

- To make clients aware of, learn or experiment with those behaviours and skills which will make them acceptable to the society in which they live and prepare them for the imitative level which follows, where compliance to norms will be expected. For example, they should be shown how to work neatly and accurately and should be shown what behaviours or methods will help achieve this.
- To be able to care for themselves within a protected and structured environment.
- To work and live productively within a sheltered setting and to develop sufficient coping skills to deal with the environmental demands.
- To use leisure time constructively.

Handling principles

- Clients should be handled with patience and understanding and one should be tolerant of their inconsistent effort and inability to produce behaviour and work of consistent standard.
- Clients should continuously be made aware of norms, both overt and covert, as well as the acceptability of their own and the group's behaviour and performance.
- Clients should be encouraged to participate actively in their treatment, but the occupational therapist should remember that the quality of the participation will be passive. Clients will need extra support to initiate activities, and encouragement will be needed from time to time until the task or activity is complete.
- Clients need encouragement with reading cues for socially appropriate behaviour and understanding why behaviour is inappropriate. They need help with assertiveness, conflict resolution, problem solving and value clarification, as well as understanding of the consequences of inappropriate or socially unacceptable behaviour.
- Clients need to be given opportunities and assisted in developing acquaintance relationships into a more meaningful relationship. They need to learn and practise the skills related to this.
- During this level prevocational skills should be actively trained or retrained, although compliance should not always be expected.

Prevocational skills can be divided into three categories:

1. *Personal presentation.* This refers to the individual's ability to attend punctually at the predetermined time; work for the time allocated; dress and behave in a manner appropriate to the situation.
2. *Social presentation.* This refers to the individual's ability to relate to the occupational therapist or supervisor in an appropriate way; relate to other clients in the work area in an appropriate manner; and behave in a manner appropriate to the norms laid down for the treatment situation.
3. *Work competence.* This refers to the client's ability to carry out the activity at hand, safely and accurately. This includes accurate, safe use and care of tools; accurate and economical use and storage of materials; error recognition and correction; judgement of effort and performance; and neat, accurate and effective working.

Structuring principles

Clients should be included in a full-day programme. It should be balanced and allow clients adequate opportunity to develop their skills in all occupational areas. The programme should be extended beyond the time for occupational therapy and should help clients to structure their free time.

The programme should include both individual and group activities, both task-centred and socio-emotional.

Any appropriate treatment area can be used. For group work, the atmosphere needs to be accepting and permissive, while for individual activities a work-related atmosphere should be created, allowing for experimentation. Others should be included and be involved with work-orientated or work-related activities.

The treatment area should be structured in keeping with the client's concentration. Preparation of the activity and workplace should be done together with the occupational therapist.

The client should be given the responsibility for cleaning up, packing away and storage of the tools, materials and activities. The occupational therapist should, however, direct and check this.

Presentation of activities

The client should be given comprehensive instructions that clearly define the sequence of steps and the contents of each step. The occupational therapist should ensure that he grasps what needs to be done and how it should be done before starting. He should be given some resource material to check his progress, for example a book with instructions, whilst working. Allow clients to decide when the activity or step is complete.

The client should be given practice at following all types of instructions: written, verbal and diagrammatic.

The occupational therapist must help the client to evaluate his effort, and the quality and progress of his work, as well as the reasons for success or failure. Assist clients with their judgement by giving them concrete suggestions for improvement. In the therapist-directed phase, the client finds this difficult and it is necessary to focus the evaluation on the properties of the activity such as the size, colour or texture, and he may be given an example to evaluate his work against. In the patient-directed phase, the evaluation should be done at the end of the activity because of the client's inability to tolerate negative feedback and his fear of failure. In the transitional phase, evaluation of quality can be introduced during the course of the steps of the activity.

Activity requirements

The activities used in treatment should be concrete, experimental, should stimulate the client's interest and should take note of diversity markers. He should be involved in all steps. The activities must be successful and gain approval from others.

They should also give the client the opportunity to improve his pre-vocational skills initially and later his vocational skills, but should not expect any initiative.

Activities should help the client to identify the norms and the cues to understand socially acceptable behaviour.

Activities should enable the client to learn and practise the higher-order social skills such as assertiveness, conflict resolution, etc.

Activities should give the client the opportunity to form relationships with people who were previously acquaintances.

Grading

On this level the treatment is graded through the following:

- As the client moves towards the transitional level he is expected to display more consistent behaviour and also to initiate some familiar activities independently.
- The complexity of the activities is increased, as well as the expectation for consistent prevocational skills and effort. Abstract elements can also be introduced into activities on the patient-directed phase.
- Vocational skills can be introduced in the patient-directed phase.
- The client should meet the following criteria before moving to the imitative level:

  - He should start to initiate familiar activities consistently.
  - He should demonstrate the desire to comply with the norms of all situations or activities.
  - He should become less dependent on environmental structure to direct his actions and activities.
  - Prevocational skills should be consolidated.

Imitative participation

The imitative level is the final level in the behaviour and skills development for norm compliance group (Group 2).

During this level motivation is predominantly directed at complying with the norms set by society for socially acceptable behaviour. The client actively seeks to be part of the group to which he belongs and does not wish to be identified as being different from others in terms of independence, life tasks and life roles, although individuality is evident. Motivation is product centred and directed towards productiveness but there is little evidence of initiative and there is a reluctance to compete actively and compare skills with those of others. Judgement of situations and of others is more refined, resulting in his being able to select the behaviour or skills that he needs to imitate in order to be accepted. Clients on this level are very stressed by the unknown and unfamiliar and any situation where the norms are unclear.

The major development that takes place during this particular level is separation from the caregiver and establishing an independent, self-supporting and self-sustaining lifestyle, which is defined by the group in which the client lives.

Imitative level of action

The level of action that coincides with this level of motivation is also called imitative. Imitative action indicates that people do what is asked of them – no more and no less. There is some variation in the skills and the activities that have to be achieved, depending on the age, gender and life tasks of an individual within his particular group. Bear these factors in mind when evaluating the client's capacity for imitative behaviour.

Although there are individual and cultural variations, there are some general trends in functional ability that are significant.

Personal management

In the personal management occupational performance area, behaviour concerning hygiene and care of clothes and belongings is usually consistent and efficient. Refined forms of self-care and grooming are usually fair, with the client developing a high level of awareness of fashion and suitability of dress for a wide variety of situations and occasions. There may, however, be a tendency to follow fashion, whether it suits the client or not, but it does create a sense of belonging or being part of the group.

Management of personal business usually improves in the sense that financial obligations are attended to in time. However, there may be impulsive spending to buy things that will improve their social acceptability, e.g., clothing, a car, the latest fad.

Social ability

All social behaviour is directed towards belonging. More mature, intimate relationships tend to develop during this level, but egocentric needs are still evident. Relationships tend to be dramatic with on/off elements. Communication is usually efficient and basic social skills are good. However, assertiveness skills are not yet consolidated especially in situations where the individual feels unsure or insecure.

Clients tend to function well socially in familiar situations but poorly in unfamiliar situations and in situations where the norms are not very clear. High anxiety is evident in these situations. They tend to be followers rather than leaders and acceptance by others is important. They are very susceptible to group pressures and sensitive to acceptance or rejection by other group members.

During the patient-directed phase, clients become aware of the shortcomings of others, and in the transitional phase they are often able to tolerate and compensate for these inadequacies. However, they still have difficulty in dealing with interpersonal and group conflict.

Independent living and productivity are the main focus of attention on this level and the client practises the independent living skills learnt during the passive level. This includes setting up and maintaining a home, either alone or with somebody else. It also involves organizing and managing household chores and activities in an orderly, hygienic and effective manner within the required financial restraints. In the therapist-directed phase, the client quite often experiences a certain amount of difficulty in coping with the stress of being responsible for himself and in managing the chores in an orderly and effective manner, but this tends to improve towards the transitional phase.

In the work situation, the client's performance is goal-directed and norm-compliant. He is able to do what is asked of him efficiently, provided that the activities are straightforward, do not have any unexpected hitches, and do not demand any initiative or problem solving on his part. Prevocational skills are good and vocational skills develop due either to formal or informal vocational training. While work tolerance and endurance are more robust than on the previous level, clients often feel overwhelmed by their workload, even if it is not extensive, and battle to manage their time appropriately.

Use of free time

In the recreational sphere clients generally have, or are developing, a wider variety of interests and skills. They have a tendency to be involved in those activities which are in vogue, and which are currently being done by other members of the group. This does not imply that the activity is a group task; it could just as well be an individual activity such as knitting in which other group members also indulge.

Much of the population functions on this level of action, and they live occupationally independent lives, doing what has to be done but contributing little beyond this.

There is a group of higher-functioning individuals who may regress to this level as a result of psychiatric illness.

Due to this independence few clients on this level are inpatients. They may receive treatment as outpatients on a regular or infrequent basis. These clients may, however, be seen in some specialized units for substance abuse or eating disorders.

As with the previous level, psychopathology, although characteristic of the condition, usually has an individualized presentation. Psychopathology may be of mild to moderate intensity as social, occupational and recreational performance may be interfered with, but the client is not occupationally incapacitated.

Although all routine assessments should be carried out, a more detailed individualized personal living skills and vocational assessment needs to be done.

Treatment

The outcomes of treatment are:

- To help clients comply with norms in all occupational performance areas appropriate to the group and society in which they live.
- To look after themselves independently.
- To be productive and be able to work effectively and efficiently.
- To use their leisure time constructively.

Handling principles

The therapeutic relationship should have more qualities of maturity than previously, being based on mutual trust and respect, with elements of both give and take. The occupational therapist should handle the client firmly in terms of norm compliance, while being sensitive to the anxiety this may cause.

Expectations should be negotiated and clearly stated so that he understands what is expected of him, and these expectations should be generalized to as many treatment situations as possible.

It is important to give the client recognition for imitative responses. If he is unable to comply, handle him supportively, helping him to explore the reasons for his failure, and propose some alternative behaviours for him to try that may increase the possibility of success.

Structuring of treatment programme

Plan the programme with the client in order to gain his cooperation and at the same time to establish the goals and norms, so that he knows what he has to work towards.

Where practical, the client should have a full-day programme where he is given the responsibility for his attendance or lack thereof.

The treatment programme should be balanced and should include:

- Work-related or work-simulated activities for approximately half the treatment time.
- Sport and recreational activities for approximately one-sixth of the treatment time.
- Group activities for the rest of the time. These should include task-centred, discussion and socio-emotional group work where the emphasis is on:
  - personal independence;
  - mature relationships where loyalty, cohesion and conformity to group norms is reinforced, but at the same time supporting individuality and assertiveness;
  - consolidation of prevocational skills and development of vocational skills;
  - stress management, problem solving, conflict resolution and value clarification.

If the client only attends sessions most time will be spent on a group programme as above. It is, however, important to help the client to balance his occupational performance so that it meets the criteria for Activities Health (Cynkin and Robinson, 1990).

Presentation of activities

All activities used in the treatment programme should be presented as a whole. The client should use written, diagrammatic and verbal instructions, although technical skills may need to be demonstrated.

Instructions should be logically presented and should emphasize the purpose of the activity. Instructions should outline the technique and method to be used, and give tips for success.

Instructions should clearly indicate the norms against which performance will be judged as acceptable.

When possible a completed, high-quality end product should be on hand so that he has something against which to rate his performance.

Activity requirements

All activities must have imitative characteristics and should facilitate norm compliance.

Grading

As the client moves from the therapist-directed phase, so the demands of the activities should be increased. Increasing the number of steps, the elements of fallibility and the complexity of the method can do this.

Elements of problem solving can also be introduced once the patient-directed level has been achieved.

- Gradually upgrade the demands for norm compliance in all occupational performance areas.
- Decrease structure, support and increase demands for independent personal management and lifestyle.
- Increase the demands for productive and vocational ability.
- Increase demands for constructive use of leisure time.
- Increase demands for effective use of coping skills in the face of environmental demands.

The following are the indications that the client is ready to move to the next level:

- He should be able to structure and execute familiar activities, consistently meeting the norms set efficiently.
- He should be prepared to meet the challenge of unfamiliar situations in spite of some anxiety.
- He should start to become aware of shortcomings within the current method of an activity or behaviour, and have an interest in exploring possibilities for improvement or change.

Group 3

The levels that fall into this group are least well described. This is probably because we see so few clients who fall into this group needing assistance, whether in hospital or in the community. This does not mean that they are immune to psychiatric disorders, but that any treatment needed is carried out intermittently by psychiatrists or psychologists and clients are seldom hospitalized.

Although there may be some reduction in their occupational performance from their premorbid state, these individuals are seldom dysfunctional in any area. For this reason, the levels falling in the group will be described but no treatment regime will be included.

Active participation

This is the first motivational level in this group. On this level motivation is directed towards improving or changing aspects of activities or behaviour that the individual has identified as a problem. However, this improvement is usually based on his personal egocentric needs, although others may derive indirect benefit from it. The main purpose is to save personal time, gain attention from others, earn a promotion or earn more money.

This improvement occurs as a result of initiative, original thought and a developing ability to think broadly considering more macro-issues rather than focusing specifically on just the activity at hand.

Original action

The level of motivation that coincides with the level of action is called original, due to the fact that originality is the level's main characteristic.

Personal management

In the personal sphere these individuals are able to cope independently. They are aware of norms, but some individuality may develop in dress and grooming that is peculiar to them. For example, some may develop a sophisticated manner of dressing that reflects the fashion. Others dress and behave in an eccentric way but are aware of their differing behaviour and style. They cope well with living independently and have developed a quite distinctive lifestyle.

Social ability

They are able to form interpersonal relationships that are consistent and lasting. They have a circle of acquaintances and are usually able to inter-act quite efficiently. They still tend to prefer subordinate positions, but will take responsibility for and manage group projects, and may bring some creative ideas to the group if asked. They may become involved in projects in the community, but they need to be asked to do things rather than initiating them.

Although the element of loyalty and intimacy is more prevalent than on the previous level there is still an element of egocentricity. They continue to have difficulty in expressing negative feelings within relationships, being their own person and solving interpersonal conflicts. Self-assertion may still be a problem and they may have difficulty expressing beliefs/opinions that are different from the prevailing view.

Work ability

In the work situation, if given authority they may lack sensitivity to the needs of their subordinates and this may cause conflict.

In their activity execution they are norm-compliant but are able to analyse activities so as to identify the shortcomings and work out possible original solutions. Although they are able to plan in a concrete sense, they have difficulty in synthesizing a lot of abstract information into an inte-grated whole. They can persist with tasks until they are complete, but they do need to see some concrete result from and be rewarded for their effort. They do not always know when they need help and may not go for advice when they need it. Specific vocational skills may still be develop-ing, and much energy is expended in grasping and practising these.

Their anxiety control is better than on the previous level if they have warn-ing of impending crises or stress, but they cope poorly in unpredictable and unexpected situations. Their range of emotional responses to situations/stimuli is greater and they are able to express subtle emotions more readily.

Use of free time

Individuals on this level have a fairly wide range of interests. Many participate in one or more activities for recreation. Frequently, family responsibility and other commitments may limit time spent on recreation tasks. Personal gratification and social acceptance still remain important factors in these activities.

The indication for transition to the next level is a willingness to compete actively with others and openly compare skills with those of other people.

Competitive participation

The next level of motivation is competitive participation and the level of action that coincides with this is product-centred action. On this level, individuals have self-confidence and they have a realistic cognitive and ideal self. The individual's motivation reflects the desire either to do better than others (compete actively against others). Self-esteem is high enough to tolerate failure and they deal with it in a realistic and socially acceptable fashion. Improved judgement enables them to evaluate reasons for success and failure correctly. The competitive edge which encourages effort varies according to the individual's mental and physical abilities, personality and environmental resources, and occurs in some or all occupational performance areas.

Product-centred action

Action is competitive in nature. Behaviour demonstrates self-discipline and is governed by the standards that the individual aims to surpass. However, the individual still requires concrete evidence on the quality of performance through feedback.

Effort can be sustained over extended periods of time – months or even years – in working towards a specific goal. Frequently the individual works steadfastly towards the goal despite considerable personal sacrifice.

Personal management

Individuals have competent hygiene and adequate life skills. Clients often have individual styles of refined forms and grooming. Many have a highly personalized style that is individualistic and can recognize that it is different from the norm but feel comfortable with this. They may compete with others for money, possessions or attention. They use materials creatively, demonstrate ability and success. They may have difficulty in managing finances in their attempt to be competitive or show they are successful.

Social ability

Relationships are mostly consistent and often predictable. There may, however, be an element of selfishness and self-advancement which may negatively influence a relationship when the individual has his sights set on a specific goal which may demand maximum effort and sacrifice. In spite of this, these individuals do demonstrate a greater capacity to compensate for the inadequacies of others and show a wide range of adaptive behaviour. In the patient-directed phase individuals usually become acutely aware of the needs of others and on the transitional phase they are able to modify their behaviour for their benefit.

Work ability

Activity execution is good but still essentially product-centred. Individuals are able to take responsibility and work independently on defined long-term projects. They can draw on the experience of others but with the purpose of doing something better. Synthesis of information into an integrated whole is better than previously, but the focus of attention is narrow and based on egocentric needs. In the work occupational performance area individuals compete actively with their peers for promotion or for acknowledgement from superiors or others. Although they are disappointed by failure, they are not devastated by it and can evaluate the reason for failure and propose alternative behaviours and approaches.

Use of leisure time

Clients have a wide range of leisure activities and they recognize the value of leisure in the context of their life. Work and other demands may limit the time spent on leisure activities. Sometimes leisure activities are used to network and for personal advancement rather than solely for relaxation and stress reduction. On the other hand there are individuals who pursue leisure activities very actively to compensate for limiting factors in productive activities. Leisure may be a strong focus of their life and be quite time and energy consuming. Such activities often have a community focus.

The major indication for movement to the next level is:

* Being able to put others' needs above their own.
* Competitiveness not so much for personal gain but for that of other people.
* Objectivity and the ability to see the 'big picture'.

Contribution and competitive contribution

Contribution and competitive contribution are the two final levels of motivation.

These two levels are very similar, in that one of the major features is the individual's ability to sublimate his own needs for those of others. In the case of the former level, he concentrates on the needs of individuals in his immediate situation or group. As a result the level of action that corresponds with this is called situation centred. In the case of the latter, he concentrates on the more global needs of society at large. The level of action that corresponds with this is called society centred.

The rare individuals who achieve these levels constitute true leaders. They may demonstrate leadership and exceptional skills in the work, social or recreational realms or maybe even in all three. These individuals are far-sighted with broad vision. They are able to set long-range goals and plans from which they may derive no benefit or which may not come to fruition for many years.

Personal management

These individuals are perfectly capably of looking after themselves. However, because of the many demands on their skills and time, these skills are often delegated to others. They have a high level of awareness of their self-presentation and often develop unique styles of dress and behaviour that set trends for others.

Social ability

They develop excellent relationships, which are characterized by diplomacy, sharing, loyalty and maturity. They are usually tolerant and are able to guide, lead and fulfil the needs of others. They have the ability to delegate responsibility.

Situation and society centred action is time-consuming, emotionally and cognitively demanding. It demands a high degree of consultation, data collection, synthesis, integration, problem solving and conflict resolution.

Work ability

These individuals are usually considered experts in their chosen field of work. They are highly productive and leaders in their field. They have a vision and are able to develop strategies to develop their chosen field further, not for personal gain but for the benefit of the people.

Use of free time

Organization of time for adequate relaxation and leisure is often a problem although they do recognize the need for stress reduction, for pleasure and for time to rebuild their energy reserves.

Table 1.7 Summary of the levels of creative ability (Reproduced with permission from D. van der Reyden)

	Tone	Self-differentiation	Self-presentation	Passive participation	Imitative participation	Active participation	Competitive participation
Action	Undirected, unplanned	Incidentally constructive or destructive (1–2 step task)	Explorative (3–4 step task)	Product centred (5–7 step task)	Product centred (7–10 step task)	With originality – transcends norm expectations	Product centred
Volition	Egocentric to maintain existence	Egocentric to differentiate self from others	To present self – unsure	Robust. Directed to attainment of skill	Directed to product, a good product, acceptable behaviour	Directed to improvement of product, procedures, etc.	Directed to participation with others to compare and evaluate self in relation to others
Handle tools and materials	Not evident	Only simple everyday tools (e.g. spoon)	Basic tools for activity participation – poor handing	Appropriate skill	Good	With initiative	Very good
Relate to people	No awareness	Fleeting awareness	Identification selection, makes contact tries to communicate, superficial	Communicate	Communicate/interact	Close interpersonal relationships, intimacy, can assist others, adapt, allowances, consideration	Adapt, allowance, consideration, close interpersonal relationships, intimacy, can assist others
Handle situations	No awareness of different situations	No awareness or ability	Stereotypical handling makes effort but unsure or timid	Follower, variety of situations, participates in a passive way	Manages a variety of situations, appropriate behaviour	Can evaluate adopt, adjust according to need, can deal with problems	Can evaluate, adjust according to need, can deal with problems

Table 1.7 contd.

	Tone	Self-differentiation	Self-presentation	Passive participation	Imitative participation	Active participation	Competitive participation
Task concept	No task concept, basic concepts	No task concept, basic and elementary concepts	Partial task concept, compound concepts	Total task concept, extended compound (abstract element concepts)	Comprehensive task concept, integrated abstract concepts	Abstract reasoning	Abstract reasoning
Product	None	None	Simple – familiar activities, poor quality product	Product of fair quality (aware of expectations)	Product good quality (according to expectations)	Quality – can adapt, modify exceed, have expectations, evaluate, upgrade	Quality – can adapt, modify exceed, have expectations, evaluate, upgrade
Assistance or supervision needed	Total assistance and supervision (24-hour)	Physical assistance and constant supervision	Constant supervision needed for task completion	Regular supervision	Guidance, supervision, regular for new activities, occasional for known activities	Guidance, formal training – (own responsibility), help to supervise others	Guidance, formal training (own responsibility), help to supervise others
Behaviour	Bizarre, disorientation	Bizarre, little reaction, disorientation	At times strange behaviour, hesitant, unsure willing to try out	Follower, but will participate passively – occasionally strange	Socially acceptable behaviour, generally controlled	Acceptable, shows originality	Socially acceptable or correct, variety of situations, adaptable, plan action behaviour
Norm awareness	None noted	None noted	Starts to be aware of norms	Norm awareness (aware of expectations}	Norm compliance (do as expected, required standard)	Norm transcendence (to do better or more than the norm) and to adapt effectively. This graded from activities or situations to a variety of situations	Norm transcendence (to do better or more than the norm) and to adapt effectively. This graded from activities or situations to a variety of situations

Table 1.7 contd.

	Tone	Self-differentiation	Self-presentation	Passive participation	Imitative participation	Active participation	Competitive participation
Anxiety and emotional responses	Limited responses	Limited uncontrolled basic emotions. Comfort and discomfort are easily evident.	Varied, usually low self-esteem and anxiety, poor control	Full range of emotions, mostly controlled, makes effort	Subtle differences compassion and self awareness, anxiety used	New situations – anxiety, normal emotional responses (anxiety motivator)	
Initiative effort	None noted	Fleeting, minimal	Effort inconsistent, not sustained not maintained, decreased frustration tolerance	Varies	As expected, required sustained	Consistent and original	Consistent and original

Questions

1. Define the following in your own words and the relationship between them:

   a) creative capacity
   b) creative response
   c) creative participation
   d) creative act.

2. Define in your own words the concept of 'creative ability'.
3. Define in your own words the term 'maximal creative effort' and state its relationship to creative ability.
4. Define the terms:

   a) therapist-directed phase
   b) patient-directed phase
   c) transitional phase.

   Discuss their function in terms of levels of motivation and action.
5. Make a table indicating the relationship between the levels of motivation and action.
6. Describe how to execute all the steps in the assessment of creative ability.
7. Make a table indicating the similarities and differences in occupational performance between each of the following levels of action:

   a) Predestructive
   b) Imitative
   c) Destructive
   d) Original
   e) Incidental
   f) Product centred
   g) Explorative
   h) Situation centred
   i) Experimental
   j) Society centred

8. Make a table indicating the similarities and differences in the principles of treatment that would be used in the first seven levels of action. Take specific note of the principles required for handling, structuring the treatment situation, presentation and teaching of the activity, activity requirements and principles of grading.

Chapter 2
Occupational science and its relevance to occupational therapy in the field of mental health

LANA VAN NIEKERK

In this chapter, the potential impact of occupational science on the practice of occupational therapy will be explored. Occupational science as a discipline holds particular benefits for the profession, including the provision of language, a focus on occupation, an interface of varied theoretical perspectives, research directions for the profession and a broad perspective for the development of services across levels of care and sectors. Zemke and Clark introduced occupational science as 'an academic discipline, the purpose of which is to generate knowledge about the form, the function, and the meaning of human occupation' (Zemke and Clark, 1996, p. vii).

Occupational therapists' concern with occupational behaviour – concretized as participation in work, leisure, play and personal life skills – together with the role it plays in achievement of wellness has been well debated and documented (Meyer, 1922; Pratt et al., 1997; Steward, 1997; Strong, 1998). This chapter will not focus on occupation as such, but rather on the potential influence of occupational science on the practice of occupational therapy and its relevance in the field of mental health.

The thinking shared in this chapter, as well as some of the examples, are based on a qualitative research study that the author undertook to explore *the influences that impact on the work-lives of people with psychiatric disability*. Quotes presented also originate from this study.

The character of occupational science

Occupational science is a basic science devoted to the study of the human as an occupational being. As a basic science it is free to pursue the widest and deepest questions concerning human beings as actors who adapt to the challenges of their environments via the use of skill and capacities organized or categorized as occupation (Yerxa, 1993, p. 5).

Yerxa introduced 'occupational science' by putting forward the working definition cited above. In doing so, she emphasized that it was a basic science and she made the point that occupational science could not be 'constrained in its development by preconceptions of how its knowledge will be applied in occupational therapy clinical practice' (Yerxa, 1993, p. 5). Yerxa identified the following assumptions:

- Skill is an essential capacity of human beings and is a vital component of occupation.
- People's experience of engagement in occupations influences both their satisfaction with performance and intrinsic motivation.
- Occupation is engaged in by whole human beings who should not be reduced to cells or organ systems (holism).
- The occupational human is a complex living system that interacts with multiple environments.
- Occupational science represents an important focus of study and, as such, a legitimate scholarly resource.

Hocking (2000), who explored the contribution made by occupational science, contended that it had a broad focus. She summarized the diverse domain of occupational science into perspectives, namely the elements of occupation, occupational processes and the relationship of occupation to other phenomena such as health. The potential of occupational science to influence occupational therapy practice, particularly to better address the needs of people with mental health concerns, will be the focus of this chapter.

Occupational therapists and occupational scientists alike concern themselves 'with the relationship between occupation and other phenomena such as health, quality of life, identity, social structures and policies, and more recently, the relationship between doing and being' (Hocking, 2000, p. 60).

The impact of occupational science on occupational therapy will be best felt in the opportunities it affords to give language to practice, to broaden and delineate the scope of our practice, the interface between theories that are relevant to practice, the emphasis placed on the environment and the fact that development across system boundaries is fostered. One of the most immediate consequences of occupational science is a renewed concern with the use of natural occupations. The understanding and use of *natural* occupations within naturalistic contexts, as differentiated from *constructed* occupations that are used within institutional contexts, is increasingly the focus of occupational therapists. An argument could be made that natural occupations are most often used to address occupation as an *end*, used here as defined by Trombly (1995). Natural occupation, by necessity, would involve a strong partnership between the occupational therapists and the individual, group or population. Conversely, constructed occupations have traditionally been used to meet particular therapeutic outcomes within occupational therapy practice settings, including hospitals. Occupational science presses for a focus on, and the use of, natural occupations.

Interventions designed to make adaptations to the natural occupations of people with mental illness hold obvious advantages. Provisional results from the above-mentioned study confirmed this view. Experiences associated with having a psychiatric disability, together with subsequent service interventions, made participants aware of the need to approach aspects of their lives differently. Participants highlighted their need to change particular behaviour patterns and/or coping strategies that they identified as less than ideal. Participants drew close associations between stress that resulted from occupational behaviour demands, and their illness experience. They often attributed the origin of their psychiatric illness, as well as subsequent relapse, to stress that they perceived to result from expectations to meet demands at work or at home. Participants used terms such as 'over-tired', 'burn-out', 'too busy' or 'did too much' when they were explaining what was for them an obvious link between their doing and their illness. Participants had an ongoing awareness, for some even a preoccupation, with the demands that participation in particular occupations would place on them. The need to balance occupational expectations and their own ability to tolerate the stress that resulted from such participation, emerged as a strong concern. For many participants, finding such a balance was motivated by a need to prevent the horror of having to live through another relapse.

Those participants in the study who had had the benefit of working closely with an occupational therapist remarked on the benefit of advice that helped them make decisions about balancing the demands of participation in occupation with their own abilities at each stage of their recovery:

> we did a lot of work at occupational therapy ... charts that fill up your hours of the day, and you know suddenly when you actually put it in black and white ... like that ... you suddenly realize that (snap), I spent my time working 16 hours a day, was this madness, of course I'm going to be exhausted, of ... you ... um ... I can't keep up that pace. So um ... you know like taking time out for leisure, and um, and if I'm not available, I pull the plug out of the telephone and um ... the answering machine still takes the... the ... messages ... so it's also just having time and I've got and ... um ... I'm also learning to say no, you know I can't do this, or I can't do that, or I can't come to this function, or I can't do that, because I need rest.

Similarly, a positive outcome was identified by a participant whose occupational therapist focused on providing assistance within naturalistic settings in order to optimize participation in chosen occupation.

> [Occupational therapist] put me in sheltered employment for two weeks, cutting out picnic squares for a blanket, and then they took me to the

[name of library] and by some miracle I fitted in immediately, I did six months voluntary, and now I've been working a second six months period, at a salary of £X a month. Now the problem is, I told them I had no stamina because I'm on so many psychiatric drugs, I have no stamina ... so I work 4 mornings a week, and 4 mornings a week I can manage easily. Work starts at 9 and ends at 12. So I have time to get up in the mornings, have breakfast, have medication, take the bus to work, and on Thursday afternoon when I finish for the week, I am tired.

I was never able to work until I found a job in a disabled capacity. And fortunately I knew exactly what to do ... I've done proof reading, they put me on a 10-day computer course, which I managed to pass, um ... every day there is something new to do, and I ... just all my talents have come back.

Giving language to practice

The question 'what do occupational therapists do?' is often asked by confused members of the general public or consumers of occupational therapy services. There is an expectation that a ready-made answer to this question exists. Occupational therapists themselves have described their dilemma when trying to capture the essence of occupational therapy or when attempting to delineate the occupational therapist's role (Sachs and Labovitz, 1994; Van Niekerk, 1998). This elusiveness may be attributed to difficulties in delineating the boundaries of professional role and defining occupational therapy in diverse practice settings. According to Yerxa, confusion could be attributed to 'the uniqueness of occupational therapists' ways of perceiving people and their needs and a different way of thinking from that of many other health professionals' (Yerxa, 1993, p.4).

The development of language that clarifies concepts considered in the study of occupation brings opportunities for collaborative research and easier sharing of research findings. It furthermore provides a focus that could ultimately shape occupational therapy practice. Spin-off effects could include:

- Definitions for occupation and concepts related to occupation that are broadly understood and as such facilitate sharing and understanding.
- Foregrounding humans as occupational beings.
- Linking occupational therapists' concern directly to the occupational engagement of the people we work with (instead of this being a secondary focus that follows a concern with disability or impairment).
- Shaping of occupational therapy identity as a profession that is concerned with optimizing human health and potential through the use of occupation.
- Marketing occupational therapy by foregrounding its link with occupation, thereby liberating the profession from the medical model that limits its scope and reduces its contribution.

Broadening and delineating scope of research and practice

> As occupational science expands, new insights concerning the nature of occupation and the manner in which it enriches people's lives are expected to emerge; such insights will spur the development of improved therapeutic techniques and thereby generate important yields both to the profession and to the clients whom it serves (Clark et al., 1993, p. 184).

This quote shows clearly how developments in occupational science ultimately would impact on occupational therapy practice. The scope of occupational science is not limited by a focus on illness and health – instead it encompasses a study of occupation in its broadest sense. Contributors to the field of study include researchers who are not occupational therapists.

Yerxa (1993) was discussing the dilemmas of occupational therapy practice when she identified 'a major question confronting societies' (p. 3), namely 'What is the relationship between human engagement in a daily round of activity (such as work, play, rest and sleep) and the quality of life people experience including their healthfulness?' (p. 3). This question would suggest occupational therapists' concern with the goal of restoring the occupational engagement of people who have lost their *ability to do*, due to the experience of impairment or disability. It also implies a concern for people who have reduced opportunity to participate in occupation due to macro-contextual influences such as high unemployment, limited access to education, discrimination (including gender restrictions) or inequality and deprivation (including issues associated with living in poverty). Yerxa considered this to be a dilemma; she stated that 'the profession may not be fully achieving its rich potential in making a difference in people's lives' (Yerxa, 1993, p. 4). She states the reason for this dilemma being that many occupational therapists still 'practice in hospitals and clinics in which the traditional medical view of illness and disability predominates' (Yerxa, 1993). With the medical model's priority concern being alleviation of symptoms, it often brings a limitation in focus that does not include the occupational engagement of people within their natural contexts. Certainly, those people whose healthfulness or quality of life is reduced by influences other than chronic impairment or disability would not be the concern of occupational therapists practising in traditional settings. Occupational science could provide a vehicle to broaden the scope of occupational therapy practice through its concern to understand better occupation in domains outside traditional practice settings, such as community projects for the mentally ill, e.g. farming projects, home industries, etc.

This issue is particularly relevant when the client population have mental health problems. The focus of the health team tends to be on the alleviation of symptoms associated with psychiatric impairment. Often society would accept, without question, that people with psychiatric disability are not able to participate in chosen occupations, for example work. Negative stereotypes held by society, and by some health professionals, often go undetected or unchallenged. Without conscious awareness of the stereotypes that influence decisions and actions, the focus of service providers tends to be dominated by a short-term focus on illness and associated symptoms. Emphasis on an occupational perspective, as opposed to a medical model perspective, insists on a broader focus.

One example was a Participatory Action Research (PAR) project that was initiated in order to inform and monitor the effective development of the Community-based Disability Entrepreneurship Project in Khayelitsha and Nyanga, Cape Town, South Africa. People with mental health concerns formed the Noluntu group which, together with two other groups, worked to develop entrepreneurial skills. Activities of the Noluntu group included leatherwork, knitting, electrical repairs, shoe repairs and sewing. Partners in the project were the entrepreneurship groups, an NGO called the South African Christian Leadership Assembly Rehabilitation Project, Disabled People South Africa and occupational therapists from the Division of Occupational Therapy from the University of Cape Town. The focus was on developing opportunities for people with mental illness to participate actively within their respective communities. The occupational therapists' role was to assist participants in the project with the challenges they faced during the development of their businesses.

Research by occupational scientists has shown variety in the forms of inquiry used. Research designs, other than those with a positivist focus, are being utilized to understand the complexities and subtleties that shape occupational behaviour. An example of such research is the work done to understand the meaning and purpose of leisure for adolescents living in an area of low socio-economic development. High levels of boredom, substance abuse and an environment characterized by poverty, crime and violence provided the context for the study. The findings of the study painted a picture of the leisure environment and opportunities available to the adolescents who participated in the study (Wegner and Magner, 2002). Research such as this provides contextual detail and information about occupational opportunities to guide decisions about interventions such as health promotion initiatives.

Interfacing relevant theories to inform practice

The way I see it, occupational scientists study people's occupational natures across a broad spectrum of concern, that is, they explore any other perspective, philosophy or idea from the point of view of the human need for occupation. So, for example, they reconsider, research and advise on politics, spirituality, education, social structures, science and technology, the media, work, growth, development and creativity, and health from an occupational perspective. If they are thorough, that will encompass reductionist as well as holistic perspectives and exploratory methods (Wilcock, 2001, p. 416).

Zemke and Clark (1996) defended concerns that occupational science overlaps with other sciences by sharing occupational scientists' view that it is the unique subject matter with an emphasis on occupation that sets it apart. Wilcock agreed, suggesting that 'We need to establish ourselves as advisors at all levels of society to increase awareness and understanding' (Wilcock, 2001, p. 416). She goes on to say that 'for the discipline to grow and develop most effectively and quickly, it would be best for it to be studied internationally across many disciplines' (Wilcock, 2001, p. 416). It is the focus on occupation that makes occupational science distinctive, rather than the use of particular research methodologies or the delineation of particular domains of concern. The flexibility of approaches used to generate knowledge situates it to allow an easy interface between different theories and disciplines. This is different from other social sciences that historically 'establish their distinctiveness not by their formal description but by their emphases and traditions' (Zemke, 1996, p. ix). What this means is that occupational scientists can draw on several different theories and disciplines to inform their efforts to understand better the occupational behaviour of people within the mental health field.

> Occupational science is distinct because it demands a fresh synthesis of interdisciplinary perspectives to provide a coherent corpus of knowledge about occupation. Although it is true that in the traditional disciplines, a researcher occasionally addresses issues of relevance to occupation, such efforts are interpreted in ways that do not ultimately place the focus on occupation (Zemke and Clark, 1996, p. ix).

The relationship between occupational therapy and occupational science should be comfortable and flexible so that it is to the benefit of the occupational therapy profession. The freedom afforded by occupational science to scholars who wish to study occupation for the sake of better understanding such occupation, will be available to inform the practice of occupational therapists.

An example is a study that explored the occupations of women living in poverty (Fourie, 2002) that could greatly increase occupational therapists' understanding of the range of occupations that women who live in poverty engage in, to ensure survival for themselves and their families. Knowledge generated not only provides direction in terms of the contextual realities that are faced by women who live in poverty, but also point to a range of needs that occupational therapists are well equipped to meet, and that fall outside the traditional domain of health provision. Similarly a study that explored the live-in domestic worker's experience of occupational engagement (Galvaan, 2000) could inform the practice of occupational therapists in mental health contexts, who work alongside domestic workers diagnosed with psychiatric impairment. At the same time it called for occupational therapist involvement in the alleviation of occupational injustice experienced by live-in domestic workers resulting from work contexts that fostered occupational deprivation and alienation. While the research examples mentioned here were conducted by occupational therapists, rich information that could inform occupational therapists' understanding of occupation emerged in fields such as psychology, sociology and anthropology. Occupational science provides a lens through which scientists from varied backgrounds can look at occupation.

Foreground environment

> Occupations do not occur in a vacuum, rather interdependent participation occurs. Because occupations are more than an abstraction of the mind, occupations occur in real-life contexts grounded in real time and real places, using real equipment, materials, and supplies with real people. Furthermore, occupations occur in a context of invisible occupational determinants and forms that determine possibilities and limits for occupational participation (Townsend and Wilcock, 2004, p. 256).

Occupational scientists concern themselves with studying the impact of the environment, and the contexts within which occupation takes place, on the occupational behaviour of people and populations. This focus could press for the creation of knowledge on the impact of broader-based issues, e.g. the effect of poverty on the occupational behaviour of people, thereby impacting on health and wellness in particular ways. Occupational risk factors, such as occupational deprivation, occupational imbalance and occupational alienation (Wilcock, 1998a), are a result of negative environmental impacts of on occupational opportunities (Townsend and Wilcock, 2004). Environmental factors, such as high unemployment, would therefore increase the vulnerability of those who are already at risk, such as people living with psychiatric impairments.

The occupational therapy profession has done well to understand and develop mechanisms to assist occupational behaviour within particular environments, i.e. assistive technology, but has not done sufficient research to understand better the impact of the environment on occupation, particularly in the mental health field.

Cross-system boundaries

> We need to establish ourselves as advisers at all levels of society to increase awareness and understanding (Wilcock, 2001, p. 416).

Several authors highlight the centrality of a systems approach as being a core characteristic of occupational science. Henderson identifies 'the physical, biological, information processing, socio-cultural, symbolic evaluative, and transcendental systems' as being included in the human system (Henderson in Zemke and Clark, 1996, p. 420).

Occupational research focuses increasingly on the exploration of occupation as an end, as opposed to occupation as a means. A concurrent shift from intervention focused on the improvement of performance component deficits, usually to treat symptoms associated with conditions and disorders, towards intervention designed to optimize the occupational performance domains of individuals, groups and populations, has been initiated. This further implies a shift away from the human as an individual system towards systems that impact on the wellness of groups, communities and populations.

The development of new language to capture developments in occupation-based practice and research stimulates research and service initiatives to address occupational risk factors, such as occupational deprivation, imbalance and alienation. At the same time potential strategies to address occupational risk factors, for example occupational empowerment, are being developed. Occupational empowerment as a strategy to address risk factors that impact on occupational performance areas has particular relevance. Townsend describes occupational justice as: economic, political and social forces that create equitable opportunity and the means to choose, organise and perform occupations that people find useful or meaningful in their environment (Townsend, 1999, p. 154). Occupational justice as a domain of concern for occupational therapists to become involved in is of particular relevance to the developing world.

Integration and participation of people with disabilities in society

Psychiatrically disabled people, and those with chronic impairments, confront many barriers when they attempt to participate in a world that is constructed by and for people without disabilities. In such a world, those with disabilities are often assumed to be 'second-class' citizens, i.e. less worthy and less competent without there necessarily being any evidence for such assumptions. This is particularly true for people with psychiatric disability, because of the fear and stigma that is often associated with psychiatric impairments. Barriers confronted by people with psychiatric impairment are therefore not limited to the restrictions imposed by a particular impairment, but are multiplied as a result of society's inability to ensure integration and accommodation of those with special needs. While some attention is being given to the removal of obvious environmental barriers, usually those that limit the participation of people with physical disabilities, not enough is done to confront attitudinal barriers that prevent the participation of people with psychiatric disability.

An important realization that emerged from the research project introduced earlier was to understand that participants in the study were all attempting to achieve their ultimate goal: *to live a 'normal' life*, with a regular job in an environment in which they belonged. The achievement of this goal, taken for granted by many people, dominated much of the participants' reflection and decision-making. To help people with psychiatric disabilities to achieve integration and participation, occupational therapy practice will have to situate itself better across those sectors that could influence occupational opportunities.

Occupational therapy practice was developed in the traditional health sector in which service delivery was focused on medical model practice. Traditional mental health practice focuses on vocational assessment and rehabilitation in settings outside real job environments and rehabilitation programmes that rely on technique-based skills training interventions. Developments should focus on sectors such as education, labour, social welfare and community development, as well as housing and sport and recreation. Such developments would help support the attempts of people who are at risk to become fully integrated in the work and leisure opportunities within their respective communities. It is in these developments that the discipline of occupational science would ideally inform occupational therapy practice.

Considering the centrality of a systems approach in occupational science, research and service could be guided to better understand and remove the barriers that hinder occupational behaviour at different system levels within society. Too much focus on alleviating problems of the human system at the individual level restricts occupational therapy from challenging attitudes, practices, policies or misinformation that hinder integration and participation of disabled people. Society, with the systems that operate within it, should be scrutinized to ensure the removal of barriers and to find strategies that will assist the participation of psychiatrically disabled people within natural occupational contexts, in accordance with their own needs.

Occupation and health for all

Because of the dominance of this medical science view of health, it is seldom that adequate recognition is given to the health-promoting effects of occupational wellbeing or to the susceptibility to ill-health that results from occupational injustice, deprivation, alienation or imbalance (Wilcock, 2001, p. 416).

Occupational therapists have traditionally concerned themselves with people who have health problems and are in need of occupational therapy intervention. Increasingly, the need for health prevention and health promotion strategies is being realized. The consumers of occupational therapy services are therefore shifting from people experiencing ill-health to those that are considered to be 'at risk'. With the introduction of occupational science, occupational therapists' concern should be broadened to include the impact of negative environmental influences on the occupational opportunities and behaviour of all populations that are considered to be occupationally at risk.

One example is the occupational enrichment programmes that are offered to learners who live in Lavender Hill, a socially disorganized community on the outskirts of Cape Town. Occupational opportunities available to children in this area are skewed towards occupations that are high-risk, such as gangsterism and substance abuse (Luger et al., 2003; Wonnacott, 2003; Mapham et al., 2004). When children's occupational opportunities are limited to occupations of which the dimensions are mostly unhealthy, e.g. those that emphasize violence, normalize abuse or demand immediate gratification, they are at risk. Occupational enrichment programmes as a health promotion strategy are therefore appropriately offered to all learners, including those who do not have immediate health concerns.

Conclusion

Departing from the premise that humans are occupational beings and that environments impact on occupational behaviour in ways that affect health and wellness, the macro-influences shaping occupational opportunities then become an important concern of occupational therapists. Occupational risk factors and issues of occupational justice have not been at the forefront of occupational therapy practice. This challenge would best be addressed by a repositioning of occupational therapy across all sectors in such a way that it could shape the provision of occupational opportunities. Health prevention and promotion strategies should continue to address the concerns of those populations at risk of ill-health, but should also include those populations that are occupationally at risk. More should be done to facilitate equity with regard to opportunities for people with disabilities to participate at all levels in society, including work. This is a particularly relevant issue for people with psychiatric disability.

The generation of knowledge that explores and explains 'what people do', 'how they do it' and the 'impact of such doing on the human system and the environment' is fostered within the discipline of occupational science. Knowledge obtained could then be applied in prevention and promotion programmes. The important contribution of occupational science is that it can bring together researchers and practitioners across professional boundaries and across theoretical perspectives to explore together the occupational opportunities and occupational behaviour of individuals, groups and populations. Occupational therapists will be in a position to use such knowledge to inform their practice.

Questions

1. Explain the character of occupational science as a discipline.
2. How is the discipline of occupational science shaping the scope of occupational therapy practice?
3. How could occupational science promote collaboration?
4. What should be the focus of health promotion programmes offered by occupational therapists?
5. Are people with psychiatric disability more likely to experience occupational risk factors than other disabled people?
6. Why are people with psychiatric disability best served by occupational therapists with an occupational focus (as opposed to a medical model focus)?

Chapter 3
Clinical reasoning in psychiatric occupational therapy

VIVYAN ALERS

Critical thinking

Vision without action is only a dream,

Action without vision is just passing time,

Action with vision can change the world.

Imagine you are walking along a beach on the high sand-dunes. You can feel the sea breeze and see the seashore below you. The long beach below is deserted except for one person seemingly doing exercises. You stand watching for a long time. (This relates to 'vision without action') You then walk down onto the beach and over thousands of starfish that have been washed up onto the sand. You approach the man and see that he is throwing the starfish back into the sea. You do not understand how and why this could possibly help the situation. (This relates to the action without vision) Approaching him, you ask him why he is throwing the starfish back into the sea. He answers you 'It helps with this one, and this one too, they will live to see another tide. For every one returned to the sea will live a longer productive life.' (This relates to the 'action with vision') http://www. CuttyhunkRose/inspirations (Starfish, 2004).

In psychiatric practice it is often the small pervasive signs of progress in a client that make the most impression in clinical practice, and these may sometimes be few and far between. These individual gems of improvement need to be remembered and the 'reflection on action with vision' needs to be considered. This is how occupational therapists can develop their clinical reasoning powers to progress from being a novice to an expert.

Clinical reasoning is a complex procedure incorporating personal knowledge, theoretical background and an application of cognitive abilities, together with tacit knowledge to integrate information for treatment intervention. This process is greatly enhanced by clinical and life experience. Clinical reasoning is the 'what?', 'how?' and 'why?' for 'best practice' in occupational therapy. These questions are all interchangeable for the 'best practice' model to emerge from the clinical reasoning. Clinical reasoning also involves the processing of constantly changing data and circumstances (Sinclair, 2003). Critical thinking is a foundation for this process to happen.

The elements of critical thinking are the generic starting point for clinical reasoning. Paul (1996) outlined an eight-step critical thinking process that leads the person to factual evidence, to be able to proceed to the clinical reasoning process:

1. Purpose – this is the goal, which needs to be realistic and achievable. The range of the purpose can be significant to trivial and it needs to be consistent and not be contradictory.
2. Question at issue – this is the problem to be solved. The importance of the problem needs to be considered, as well as the requirements for solving the problem.
3. Assumptions – these are the things that are taken for granted. When looking at assumptions they need to be recognized and articulated clearly; it should be considered whether they are justifiable or not, crucial or extraneous, consistent or contradictory.
4. Implications – further implications and consequences will always arise, no matter where the reasoning is ended. It is necessary to identify whether the implications are significant and realistic.
5. Inferences – these are the steps of reasoning. This refers to the logical progression of 'since this happens, that will also occur'.
6. Point of view – this is a frame of reference. The point of view should be broad, flexible, fair and adhered to consistently.
7. Concepts – this is the conceptual dimension of reasoning, including theories, principles, axioms and rules implicit in the reasoning.

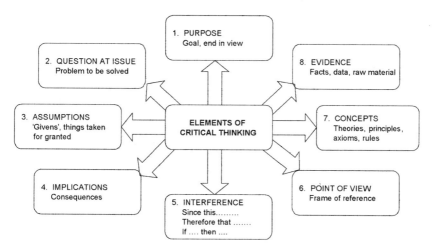

Figure 3.1 The eight sequential stages of critical thinking (www.criticalthinking.org).

8. Evidence – this is the empirical dimension of reasoning, namely the experiences, data or raw material. This needs to be reported clearly, fairly and accurately.

The eight-step process is easily illustrated with a riddle:

You cradle me, when you pick me up I purr for you, sometimes I cry, I enjoy being talkative, most times I am quiet, I can be very useful. What am I?

The *Purpose* is to solve the riddle by integrating all the information. The *Question at issue* is 'what is the answer?' These two steps are very similar. The *Assumptions* are that a cat purrs, and a baby is cradled and cries. The *Implications* are that the answer cannot be both a cat and a baby. The *Inferences* are that since cats cannot talk it must be a baby. The *Point of view* relates to the frame of reference that the answer to the riddle is functional. The *Concepts* relate to it not being an occupational therapy theory, but that metaphors are being used. The integration of these concepts needs to combine the metaphors and use lateral thinking to solve the riddle. Finally the *Evidence* is the culmination of the information of the metaphors. (Cradle = cradle a baby and a phone has a cradle on which to hang the handpiece, a mobile phone is cradled in the hand. Purr = a cat purrs and a phone purrs with a dialling tone. Cry = baby cries and a phone cries when it rings.) The evidence is integrated through prior knowledge and experience. Cats do not cry or talk. Babies are not useful, and usefulness suggests that it is an object. This then changes the mindset to think laterally and solve the riddle to answer it as 'a telephone' or a 'mobile phone'. These critical thinking processes are not often consciously thought about when solving the riddle.

When assessing critical thinking it is important to note:

- How clearly and completely the problem is stated.
- How logically and consistently a position is defended.
- How flexibly and fairly other points of view are articulated
- How significant and realistic the purpose is.
- How precisely and deeply the question at issue is articulated (Paul, 1996).

Clinical reasoning

The evidence of a clinical case using the biopsychosocial model is the factual information of the person, their illness, their mental and emotional state, their social and cultural context and their functional development into the future. This is what is used for the clinical reasoning process. Mattingly and Flemming (1994) describe the therapist's three-track mind model with its procedural, interactive and conditional tracks.

The *procedural track* is the thinking about the illness/condition/disability and its effect on the occupational performance, together with what actions are needed to perform effective treatment. The *interactive track* is thinking about the client as an individual and trying to see the illness/disability/situation from his point of view, also incorporating the client's illness experience. This relates to the interaction between the therapist and the client, and the therapist's empathy. This also includes the client's values and beliefs. The *conditional track* is thinking about the client and his condition within the broader social and temporal contexts. This includes the meaning attribution of the illness to the client as well as to the family, social and physical contexts. The temporal context implies how the illness could change/develop over time, and the future potential of the client (Mattingly and Flemming, 1994; Neistadt, 1998). Case Smith (2001) describes clinical reasoning as having four parts: procedural, interactive, intuitive and conditional reasoning. *Intuitive reasoning* is the occupational therapist's understanding of the client's mood, interests and intentions. This intuitive reasoning is the intrinsic motivational factor that the occupational therapist recognizes in the client, and may differ as the activity progresses. Neistadt (1998) includes also narrative reasoning and pragmatic reasoning. *Narrative reasoning* includes the occupational story of the client and the shared story of the client and occupational therapist (how the client's preferences are incorporated into the therapy to build a meaningful future). *Pragmatic reasoning* considers all the practical issues that will have an influence on the occupational therapy intervention. This includes 'the treatment environment, the therapist's values, knowledge, abilities and experiences; the client's social and financial resources; and the client's potential discharge environment' (Neistadt, 1998, p. 228). Pragmatic reasoning is very important in the developing countries as resources and finances are often severely lacking in rural areas or informal settlements in urban areas. The sophisticated, westernized hospital setting and the undeveloped rural setting that the client returns to is also a consideration with pragmatic reasoning. Chapter 19 of this book (Madeleine Duncan's contribution on anxiety and somatoform disorders) also discusses ethical reasoning. *Ethical reasoning* considers the human rights, ethical (beneficence, non-maleficence, veracity, justice and autonomy) and moral responsibilities, accountability and professionalism involved.

Tacit knowledge uses all the clinical reasoning constructs to view the occupational therapy intervention in a holistic manner. This informs 'best practice' in occupational therapy. Neistadt (1998) suggests that acquiring a thinking frame of clinical reasoning needs explicit explanation of that frame, and varied practical application of the clinical reasoning in occupational therapy fieldwork. Thus it is imperative for universities to engender a culture of clinical reasoning early in the curriculum. Occupational therapists need to use meta-cognition (thinking about their own thinking) and carry out self-evaluation of their clinical reasoning in their reflection about the client. A rating scale is also effective, using a seven-pronged diagram. A useful scale to use for this rating scale is the headings from the Sinclair Matrix (Sinclair, 2003), see Figure 3.2.

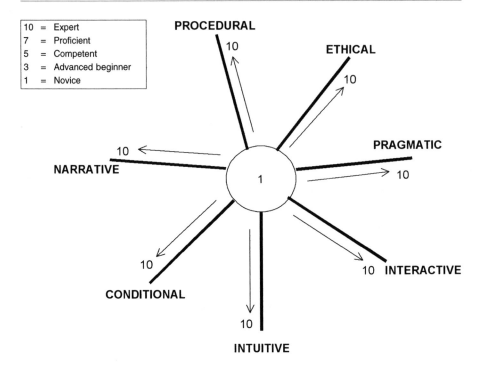

Figure 3.2 Self-rating of clinical reasoning skills (1–10 legend taken from Sinclair, 2003).

Reflective journals

The value of reflection is that it guides and informs the clinical reasoning process. Reflection helps increase the practitioner's awareness to enable questioning of the validity of actions within practice. Reflection contributes to professional development by enabling practitioners to learn and develop through experience. A reflective journal may be used as a measure over time to record and evaluate self-development, and due to the meta-cognition about the experiences, it enhances the learning curve for the practitioner. For the occupational therapy student a reflective learning journal can assist the development of clinical reasoning. This may take the form of an 'inter-active journal' between a student and a tutor/mentor, where the student can respond to the tutor/mentor comments (Tryssenaar, 1995). When considering the academic merit of a reflective journal it is important to consider that the experiences and feelings may be negative, and that the student–tutor/mentor relationship creates constraints. Students feel guarded about disclosing personal details to fellow students and to the tutor/mentor. Formal marking of reflective journals makes students anxious about how their performance might affect their marks at the end of the year. Thus reflective journals for students should be rated and not marked, so that a deep learning approach is encouraged (Alers and Smuts, 2002). The rating scales could include comments such as 'vague, incomplete, coherent, thorough' or 'superficial, adequate, sophisticated' (Randall, 1999). Students' reflective journals need to be incorporated into the clinical practice or fieldwork as a compulsory task even though a formal mark is not allocated. A reflective diary can be a useful tool to ensure that reflection becomes part of the work ethic in the workplace. Reflection relates to interpreting experiences rather than analysing them (Creek, 2002). Reflective practice certainly encourages analytical thinking, learning and subsequent clinical credibility. Tryssenaar (1995) found that interactive journals in academic courses promote reflection and increase the students' awareness and openness, revealing positive changes in attitude associated with new knowledge and experiences.

According to Sinclair (2003), to enable the student to become a reflective, expert practitioner, questions and challenges need to be set to promote ethical and creative ways of improving intervention quality: 'Student learning should take place in the context of a supportive teaching and learning environment and in a curriculum which allows for development of clinical reasoning. Interactive teaching and learning must provide support to the development of cognitive skills, knowledge and experience' (Sinclair, 2003, chapter 14, p. 26).

A current trend in medical education around the world is to move away from the didactic type of curriculum to a problem-based learning (PBL) curriculum. The key concepts underpinning the PBL approach are 'life-long learning' and that the student takes a greater responsibility for their own learning. This 'life-long learning' concept has been further incorporated in many countries where practitioners need to comply with rules relating to continued professional development (CPD). Professional skills, personal values and ethical practice contribute to practitioners who are confident, competent and creative in their occupational therapy practice.

A useful format for a reflective journal for students is:

1. Description of the critical incident.
2. Reasoning process of the critical incident – the central problem and the central tasks.
3. Assumptions and presuppositions.
4. Tapping into existing knowledge.
   a) Prior experiences including knowledge, skills, feelings and attitudes.
   b) Procedural track, Interactive track, Conditional track, Ethical track, Pragmatic track, Narrative track.
5. Key learning that occurred.
   a) What hindered learning.
   b) What assisted learning.
6. Reflection in action. (Intuitive track) (The use of tacit knowledge and practitioner's adaptive responses/reactions.) (Andrews, 2000)
7. Reflection on action. (The use of theoretical knowledge, and to evaluate professional skills used.) (Andrews, 2000)
8. Use of the self-rating clinical reasoning skills diagram.

Table 3.1 Qualities of a reflective practitioner in a nutshell (Randall, 1999)

Key concepts	A reflective practitioner
(R) esearch	... hypothesizes, acts with curiosity, looks for answers
(E) valuation	... judges her own professional knowledge and can identify where this is lacking
(F) lexibility	... adapts her knowledge to new challenges and circumstances
(L) ooking	... looks for the bigger picture
(E) limination	... reduces 'messiness' and untangles confusion, cutting out irrelevant information and extracting what is important
(C) onnection	... connects the scientific basis of his/her professional knowledge to the demands of real-world practice
(T) acit knowledge	... uses unconscious 'knowing -in-action' as well as conscious knowledge
(I) dentification	... identifies what is 'best practice' in a particular situation
(V) alues	... is conscious of the value system and frame of reference that he/she is using, and that other value systems may also be valid
(E) xceptions	... is awake to the fact that there are exceptions to every rule and is willing to tailor his/her approach to each unique situation

Example of a Reflective Journal

An example of an assignment by a final-year occupational therapy student. Acknowledgement to Anupa Singh, BSc Occupational Therapy (University of Witwatersrand, South Africa).

Description of the critical incident

During a fieldwork placement in a rural area of South Africa I never quite understood how happy people could be in the context of poverty and nothingness. I wanted to experience working in the real community setting and was not keen on remaining confined to treatment of the district hospital patients. One of the hospital patients allocated to me was a middle aged female, Sophie, diagnosed with Guillain Barré Syndrome (Pedretti and Early, 2001). The onset of the syndrome was in January, leading up to admission in June. She was transferred to the district hospital due to sepsis as a result of pressure sores. She spoke Shangaan, so my communication with her was an artistic sign language. This hampered our inter-personal relationship quite considerably. I would see her daily, mainly to check on the progress of the activities given to her under the guidance of the occupational therapy auxiliary, and to complete some basic personal management activities. I found that I was demotivated by the lack of resources at the hospital.

At the midweek ward round the sister approached me saying that due to lack of bed space, Sophie was to be discharged by the doctor and if I consented on behalf of the rehabilitation unit, she could go home. It was then that reality struck me. I was no longer a learning student with a supervisor to lean on. I had to deal with my obvious neglect of a patient whom I had not even considered in a predischarge phase. I had to consent to a discharge of a patient who had limited bed mobility, could not transfer, had no wheelchair to transfer onto, could not dress herself or get to the toilet herself. These were her immediate physical needs, and I had not considered any psychological needs. She would be returning to live with her aged parents, to sleep on a 12 cm sponge mattress on a cement floor (bed sores and all) and had to somehow get to an outside 'long drop' toilet if she needed the toilet.

This came to me as a flooding torrent of panic, knowing that I had seen her for ten days but had done nothing about this, yet I had the power to consent to her discharge at this stage. To me it was not acceptable for her to be discharged home and my need to experience a 'rural culture' was not an excuse for me not channelling my energy in a case where my professional expertise could bear such an impact, such that it could make someone else's life more liveable.

Over the next few days I explained to the patient and the medical staff that she needed a few more days of rehabilitation. I then managed my time to fulfil the community commitments that I had initiated yet come back to the hospital to see her. During the next four days I worked to build her assistive devices to aid her dressing, I had her transferring at every opportunity that was practical, I organized a wheelchair against all odds, and built an adapted commode low enough to transfer off from a 12 cm mattress. During this time I also somehow communicated with her about the necessity for her to be as independent as possible, and that her role in her family was still very worthwhile despite her disability. She managed to explain that her children would help her at home, that she could delegate duties to be done, that she felt more empowered to try to do things for herself where possible and that she felt less depressed about her situation. I liaised with the family, provided education and information about her illness and her rehabilitation process, and began the process of organizing a temporary disability grant. Four days later both Sophie and I felt more confident about her discharge from hospital.

As I wished her goodbye, I realized that my communication had evolved into something phenomenal – even though my Shangaan had not improved. A magic had happened for me. I had realized my capabilities as a competent occupational therapist and realized that this honour must not be taken for granted.

I left for home a few hours before Sophie went home. As I wished her well, she sat beaming, upright in her bed with an odd-looking packet slung over her wrist by her mother. As I said goodbye she raised her wrist with all the power inside of her, and offered me this packet in gratification of my duty and also the maternal relationship that had evolved. Inside the packet was a home grown paw-paw. The best gift I had ever received!

Reasoning process of the critical incident

New information presented during the critical incident. The most interesting new information that I was presented with was the question of my own competence, my own abilities and my own priorities.

There was also the realization that occupational therapy could not be confined to a perspective of physical dysfunction. Why had I not tapped into her anxiety, her depressive state, her motivation? Why had I not viewed her holistically?

The central problem and task. The problem facing me was to reach the goals of independence that I had set for my patient without reaching burnout myself. In a culture of poverty and disempowerment, people in the rural setting are not as motivated to reach independence in the light of obvious limitations and constraints. Fortunately, although Sophie originally intended to rely on her parents and her children, she understood my intentions of providing ways in which she could maintain her independence and self-worth so she soon became a participant in the treatment process.

A wheelchair needed to be hired and a commode needed to be built. I found an old adapted paper technology (APT) (Packer, 1995) toilet trainer and adapted and strengthened it. My final case presentation involved her sponge painting her commode using an adapted applicator made from polystyrene and sponge. Sophie felt empowered as she dignified the commode for her own use.

There was also the task of dealing with her psychosocial problems without having a medium of communication. International literature states that an efficient occupational therapist must understand the language, objects and culture of an individual in order to perceive the individual holistically. I could not even start to understand this for Sophie. I could not even ask her what her traditional Shangaan name was. Fortunately dealing with the primary physical problems had dissipated many psychosocial problems. A basic humanness and warmth from another health professional soon put her on a path to deal with residual psychosocial problems.

Assumptions and presuppositions I assumed that the rural setting was more laissez faire than the urban one, and was not prepared for the severity of the cases to be treated. I did not understand that there was the same internal performance component needs, physically and emotionally, within quite a different external environment. Like many students, I treated a physical case in a physical setting and neglected the psychosocial aspects that are pertinent to the case.

Tapping into existing knowledge

Procedural track
Although Sophie was in the restorative phase she needed to be prepared for discharge. My priority list changed together with becoming more client centred. To her, going to the toilet was going to be very undignified and unpleasant, thus this became a primary aim. Dignity falls within integrity and self worth, which feeds into quality of life experiences. Many psychosocial problems were linked to her lack of capacity, deprivation of dignity and increased independence on others.

Interactive track
Sophie had a fighting spirit and a cultured and dignified upbringing. Her hospitalization had dis-empowered her and made her dependent on care staff. She tried her best to maintain her dignity, but months of hospitalization had led her to adopt a sick role. She needed to rid herself of this role and my enthusiasm gave her the incentive she needed.

Conditional track
The prognosis for Guillain Barré Syndrome is promising. However, if Sophie was to return home with poor mobility and depression there would be a greater possibility of further bed sores. Her depression would also negatively effect her reintegration into the family. Practical follow-up sessions with the consultant occupational therapist were arranged.

Key learning that occurred

I learnt that I am an eligible candidate for burnout if I allow myself to lose sight of my priorities. I learnt that I have the capacity to make such an impact on a patient's/client's life, be it negative or positive. I also learnt that belief in my own ability and competence is imperative.

What hindered learning
My panic experienced when I found out that she was to be discharged. My inability to identify and treat psychosocial problems linked to a physical case.

What assisted learning
My self-introspection is becoming an acquired skill which I intend to develop. This helped me to think through what I was doing and evaluate my attempts. A greater understanding that occupational therapy is

not found within the confines of a medical institution. The understanding that human spirit is enough to make significant changes.

Reflection in action
I panicked and experienced an awareness of the necessary work competence.

Reflection on action
The reflective journal has been self-affirming and has given me a heightened awareness of a commitment to a positive work ethic for the benefit for all my patients and the realization that I am able to treat a patient holistically.

The reflective journal shown here demonstrates obvious self-growth, with the accompanying affirmation of value systems and professional beliefs. It is only through a concrete example of writing down the reflective journal that these realizations can be achieved. Many occupational therapists just think about their achievements or learning curve with their clients' improvements, but these thoughts are lost in the mists of memory and cannot be used concretely to show development towards becoming an expert as described in the Sinclair Matrix (Sinclair, 2003). Reflective journals are not only geared to describe positive outcomes of treatment; they can be used just as effectively when a negative outcome (client relapse) occurs. In the latter case it is affirming to make a detailed note of what interventions and their effects were carried out. The insight that the occupational therapist may gain is that expectations for improvement/maintenance/realignment of function need to be made more realistic. So often occupational therapists have overly high expectations for the improvement of their clients (relating to their own value systems instead of having a client-centred approach and the accompanying client's value system). Thus they do not realistically evaluate their intervention outcomes.

The Sinclair Matrix

Sinclair used the Benner's Skill Acquisition Model together with King and Kitchner's Model of Reflective Judgement to develop the facets of clinical reasoning for the Sinclair Matrix (Sinclair, 2003). Sinclair states that reflective judgement is an integral part of clinical reasoning: 'Reflective judgement indicates the personal ability to weigh arguments and make "best" decisions. Epistemological beliefs lay the foundation for judgement in all situations, including clinical encounters. Understanding one's own beliefs and biases is fundamental in developing into an expert reflective practitioner' (Sinclair, 2003, chapter 14, p. 3).

The Sinclair Matrix explains the qualities and abilities of the practitioner's development of clinical reasoning from a novice to an expert as a five-part progression (novice, advanced beginner, competent, proficient, expert). These stages indicate increasingly sophisticated assumptions about knowledge to make sense of experiences, and prior learning informs the level of understanding. The various aspects of reasoning correlating to this development are portrayed as a five-part skill acquisition that is used for meta-cognition (evidence discovery, theory application, decision making, judgement and ethics).

According to Sinclair, 'Expert practitioners incorporate technical and procedural efficiency and effectiveness with values and ethics. Professional thinking and clinical reasoning involve judgement which incorporates an understanding of a person's experience with, and response to an illness or disabling situation while at the same time understanding family concerns' (Sinclair, 2003, chapter 14, p. 3).

The Sinclair Matrix (Sinclair, 2003) describes *evidence discovery in occupational therapy* as the data-gathering and evidence-seeking stage. This is recognizing clinical cues and their relationship to other cues, and testing/verifying them through further examination and management (Dutton in Sinclair, 2003). Sinclair states that the identification of a client's problems is not a linear process. Objective, subjective, historical and current data are gathered about the client, verified and interpreted. The *theory application in occupational therapy* incorporates the theoretical concepts to contextualize the information for better understanding. *Decision making in occupational therapy* involves personal values and beliefs and the application of theoretical concepts. 'Clinical reasoning involves processing constantly changing data and circumstances' (Sinclair, 2003, chapter 14, p. 11). Client-centred practice is the participation in decision making by both the client and the occupational therapist. *Judgement in occupational therapy* is drawing inferences and conclusions justified by evidence. Clinical reasoning uses professional judgement, which includes reflective judgement that contextualizes and evaluates all the aspects presented. *Ethics in occupational therapy* refers to safety, reliability, responsibility, justice and beneficence. Ethical reasoning is essential for the protection of vulnerable clients, especially in the mental health field. The capability of the occupational therapist is then described against the above headings, showing the development of their clinical reasoning *from novice to advanced beginner, to competent, proficient and eventually expert.*

The data for the Sinclair Matrix was not confined to a specific field of occupational therapy, nor is it culture-specific. Its relevance is to the occupational therapy process and thus it can be contextualized to all countries.

Clinical reasoning demands three basic attributes, science, ethics and artistry (Rogers in Turner et al., 1999). The science relates to the knowledge base that is theoretical or experiential, the ethics relates to the therapist's philosophy about human dignity, and the artistry relates to the therapist's ability to use personal skills and the ability to guide decisions impartially. Clinical reasoning includes the therapeutic relationship and

Table 3.2 Sinclair Matrix of clinical reasoning (Sinclair 2003)

Clinical reasoning skills	Novice	Advanced beginner	Competent	Proficient	Expert
Evidence Discovery Problem sensing, formulation and definition	May be distracted by irrelevant information Not able to sort evidence, not looking for evidence	Seeking evidence, facts or knowledge by identifying relevant sources	Gathers objective, subjective, historical and current data in organized manner Distinguishes essential from non-essential data	Obtains data from all sources. Verifies relevant information. Identifies logical inconsistencies or fallacies. Interprets data back to client	Diligent and focused in inquiry – takes new evidence and applies it to current situations. Clear understanding of issues. Recognizes multiple perspectives. Identifies missing data. Questions the accepted
Theory Application Knowledge and concept development	Dependent on theory to guide thinking Objective attributes recognized without situational experience such as objective measurable parameters Limited and inflexible context-free application of rules	Incorporates contextual information into rule-based thinking. Recognizes differences between theoretical expectations and presenting problems (but unable to respond to situation quickly)	Relating theoretical concept (condition, nature, form or function) to context. Interprets data using relevant theoretical constructs	Combines different diagnostic and procedural approaches with flexibility and creativity. Putting it all together. No longer relies on guidelines to direct appropriate action for situation. Recognizes assumptions	Cognitive reasoning is quick and intuitive with solutions to ill-structured problems. Can predict multiple outcomes. Engages global view and applies theory in a global way. Recognizes meaningful patterns and determines generalizations

Table 3.2 contd.

Clinical reasoning skills	Novice	Advanced beginner	Competent	Proficient	Expert
Decision making Evaluating, planning, prioritizing, predicting Treatment approach	Uses rule-based procedural reasoning to guide 'actions' but doesn't recognize cues and therefore is not skilful in adapting rules to fit situation. Responds to every need and request with almost equal intensity and speed (not able to prioritize)	Still procedural, but can recognize some patterns of behaviour or symptoms, so doesn't prioritize data well or identify what is most important	Procedural aspects more automatic and organized, so able to prioritize problems and plan deliberately, efficiently, and in response to urgency and contextual issues (including background, relationships and environment) relevant to situation. Can see actions in terms of long-range goals. Selects tactics pragmatically.	Perceives situations as wholes, can anticipate situation and avoid irrelevant information. Prioritize issues Predicts multiple outcomes. Evaluates action, recognizes relationship of action and inaction. Supervisory responsibilities. Liaises with outside organizations for benefit of others.	Shows confidence in own reasoning abilities; schema-based, abilities; automated processing. Rapid, methodical and critical evaluations of solutions. Takes nothing for granted. Meets multiple patient requests and care needs or crisis management without losing important information or missing significant needs. Prioritizes quickly and efficiently. Mentors others in decision making skills
Judgement including reflective judgements	Unable to use discriminatory judgement Unreflective – informed by routine. Unable to deal with unfamiliar situations	Unable to determine priorities, makes judgement based on established criteria/rules if at all	Drawing inferences or conclusions that are supported or justified by evidence Professional autonomy in decision making. Conscious deliberation	Receptive to divergent views and sensitive to own biases. Recognizes ramifications of actions	Shows confidence in own reasoning abilities. Applies judgement prudently in relevant context. Integrates feedback from others to improve practice. Insight into societal conditions generating a patient's illness

Table 3.2 contd.

Clinical reasoning skills	Novice	Advanced beginner	Competent	Proficient	Expert
Ethics including client orientation and documentation	Recognizes overt ethical issues. Defends views based on preconceptions	Begins to to recognize more subtle ethical issues, judging according to established personal, professional or social rules or criteria	Recognizes ethical dilemmas. Recognizes individual differences. Sensitive to client's views. Contextual considerations. Equality of practice -- same rules for all	More sophisticated in recognizing situational nature of ethical reasoning. Provides options, explains outcomes, outlines time sequences for client	Demonstrates clear understanding of ethical issues and practises ethically, uses practical wisdom. Honest in facing personal bias. Evaluates soundness of conclusions and worth of action to clients and others

the therapeutic use of self, together with all the facets of the situation presented. Clinical or fieldwork experience is integral in the development of clinical reasoning. An example of this (showing the integration of the occupational therapy knowledge of the physical and psychiatric conditions of clients and the group work process, together with the therapeutic relationship) is the adaptation of a situation to fulfil the physical, psychological and group process needs of the group by encouraging discussion in an innovative, creative manner. A paraplegic group showed resistance to talking about their present emotive issues relating to their traumatic incident causing the paraplegia. This resistance was not expected due to the high cohesion of the group, so the occupational therapist used a teddy bear as a prop to which each person could relate their story. This was reflection in action, to encourage the locomotion of the group (forward movement of the group process) and increase the meaning attribution of the activity. Through quick and intuitive reasoning the therapist was able to counteract the resistance.

According to Rogers, clinical reasoning has a four-stage process (Rogers in Turner et al., 1999). Andrews (2000) uses this process through preparatory reflection, reflection in action and reflection on action.

1. Deduction – ideas formulated about the problem possibilities from pre-assessment information.
2. Induction – adjustment to these ideas due to the specific information gained from the assessment.
3. Dialectic reasoning – logical interpretation of the evidence supporting or refuting each alternative solution based on knowledge. This knowledge uses observation, experience and reflection.
4. Ethical reasoning – considering with the client the priorities of the solutions (Rogers in Turner et al, 1999).

The **STEP-SI** Model of intervention for sensory modulation dysfunction is an application of clinical reasoning in occupational therapy (Bundy et al., 2002). This is clinical reasoning based on sensory integration theory, specifically for use in treating children with sensory modulation dysfunction and other individuals with sensory integration dysfunction. Thus the clinical reasoning has been structured for a specific occupational therapy field of practice. The STEP-SI dimensions are:

(S) Sensation (Sensory modalities – tactile, vestibular, proprioception, audition, vision, taste, olfaction, oral input and respiration. Quality of sensation – duration, intensity, frequency, complexity and rhythmicity)
(T) Task (Structure, complexity, demand for skill and sustained attention, level of engagement, fun, motivation and purposefulness)
(E) Environment (Organization, complexity, perceived comfort and safety, possibilities for engagement exploration, self-challenge)
(P) Predictability (Novelty, expectation, structure, routine, transitions and congruency, level of control)

(S) Self-monitoring (Moving from dependency on external supports and cues to self directed and internally organized ability to modify own behaviour and manage challenges)

(I) Interactions (Interpersonal interaction style, including responses to supportive, nurturing styles versus more challenging, authoritative styles, locus of control, and demands or expectations for engagement) (Bundy et al., 2002, p. 438)

This example of structure to assist the clinical reasoning process can give further depth to the interpretation of the information gathered. It also gives an example of the type of structure that can be used by practitioners to be comprehensive in the clinical reasoning process. This type of structure could assist reflection in and on action.

A structure to assist the clinical reasoning process in psychiatric occupational therapy could be the use of the Model of Human Occupation (MOHO) (Kielhofner, 1995) as a construct. The aspects of habituation, values and beliefs, internal performance components (physical and psychological), occupational performance components and the feedback mechanisms could form a basis for information for clinical reasoning.

Conclusion

Clinical reasoning is a complex and skilled process that develops with experience and meta-cognition of reflection in and on the action. There is a number of constructs inherent in the clinical reasoning process. This process has been described together with the evaluative ability of the practitioner. Reflective journaling is an integral part of clinical reasoning, and a format for this reflective journaling is suggested. The case study suggests that all aspects of a client need to be considered in the reflective journal (namely the physical, psychological/psychiatric aspects, mobility, family concerns, the home context, a client-centred approach considering the beliefs and values of the client, and ethical considerations) together with the clinical reasoning process. Reflective practitioners are able to evaluate their practice and learn from experiences to develop 'best practice' and practical wisdom. Thus the abilities of the occupational therapy practitioner can develop from novice to expert.

Reflective practice demands time and dedication to self-growth. With the increasing case loads and time and resource constraints in occupational therapy, together with the complexities of community-based work, practitioners may find that time spent on clinical reasoning may not be a priority. The trend for countries to have health professionals undertake continued professional development impresses the importance of self-development and the personal responsibility of maintaining and developing professional competence. Clinical reasoning is an integral part of this development and needs to be given the attention it deserves.

Questions

1. Explain the process of critical thinking and why it is a foundation for clinical reasoning.
2. Describe the different facets of clinical reasoning.
3. What is the difference between reflection-in-action and reflection-on-action? Use a case to illustrate this.
4. Use a case from your own experience and write a reflective journal, together with a self-rating of your own clinical reasoning skills.
5. Use the Sinclair Matrix (2003) to consider your self-growth regarding clinical reasoning.

PART TWO
SPECIFIC ISSUES IN OCCUPATIONAL THERAPY

Chapter 4
HIV/AIDS in psychiatry: the moral and ethical dilemmas and issues facing occupational therapists treating persons with HIV/AIDS

DAIN VAN DER REYDEN AND ROBIN JOUBERT

It is important to put on record the authors' decision to avoid the use of the term 'client' when referring to the individual with HIV/AIDS. We believe that the term 'client' is both out of place and lacks the inference of unbiased caring so essential in the treatment of such a patient. The term 'individual' is used in the context of a community setting.

Because Africa is the epicentre of the HIV/AIDS pandemic with by far the largest numbers of cases in the world, much of the information in this chapter is related to the African context where the need is greatest. However the information is relevant and applicable to any situation in the world where occupational therapists treat individuals with HIV/AIDS-related conditions.

This chapter is of particular significance due to considerable concern within the profession about the increasing number of HIV/AIDS infected persons being referred to occupational therapy departments and the dearth of literature on occupational therapy and HIV/AIDS.

The chapter's foundations are based upon a literature search and a survey of occupational therapy clinicians working in rural and urban government hospitals in KwaZulu-Natal, South Africa (Joubert and van der Reyden, 2003). This survey revealed that an estimated 70 per cent of patients currently being treated in occupational therapy departments in state hospitals were HIV/AIDS infected. The majority of respondents in the survey also admitted that the knowledge that a patient had HIV/AIDS impacted upon their approach and handling. Most, as supported by our literature review, also agreed that occupational therapists working with these clients require advice on how to deal with ethical and moral dilemmas that arise in the process and felt they would like counselling and debriefing on a regular basis.

In the year 2000, HIV surpassed all other pathogens to become the leading infectious cause of death in the world (Farmer et al., 2001). It is debatable whether there has ever been another disease comparable to HIV/AIDS which has had such an incrementally devastating impact upon not only the sufferers but also their partners, relatives, friends, society in general and those caring for them. In the HIV-positive phase the disease's pathophysiology proceeds in a very unobtrusive and asymptomatic manner, which is misleading not only its victims but also those treating them.

The virus is classified among the lentiviruses, a family of viruses characterized by their tendency to cause chronic neurological disease (which may present with both physical and psychiatric symptoms) in their hosts. Neurological complications in HIV-infected patients are common and not confined to opportunistic infections. It is estimated that about 60 per cent of patients in the advanced stages of the disease will have clinically evident neurological dysfunction (McGuire, 2003). This in turn leads to occupational dysfunction and it is thus common practice for them to be referred for occupational therapy. It is also not uncommon for patients who are HIV-infected and asymptomatic to be referred to occupational therapy departments for other reasons, such as spinal cord injury, resulting in occupational dysfunction.

In addition a possible combination of factors such as an increased HIV-1 proliferation, a heavy 'viral burden' in the brain and a macrophage-initiated cascade of events can lead to brain dysfunction and clinical dementia. The activated macrophages are capable of secreting potent neurotoxins which can destroy brain cells. Thus, apart from the neuropathies and opportunistic infections and diseases that are brought about by HIV infection, with their debilitating effect on function, the victim also frequently suffers from psychiatric disorders associated with HIV/AIDS (McGuire, 2003).

As if the often devastating physical and psychiatric symptoms caused by the virus and compromised immune system were not enough, stigmatization of those with the disease may result in social isolation and ostracization by the communities in which they live. This often leads to a sense of despair and desperation with its concomitant problems of loneliness, poor sense of self-worth, fear and anxiety. Crawford (in Crossley 1997) refers to some of the negative symbolism surrounding AIDS and our implicit images of those with HIV/AIDS such as: *contagious, sexually deviant, addicted and irresponsible*. Pandya (1997, pp. 49–55) notes that:

> for many patients, the ward of a public hospital is the last stopping place of a dismal journey of stigmatization. Patients with AIDS are driven from their communities by fearful neighbours, pushed from one hospital to another by doctors and staff members reluctant to treat them and, finally, approaching death in the AIDS ward.

The individual with HIV/AIDS

Pathophysiological neurological and neuro-psychiatric manifestations of HIV and AIDS that impact upon occupational performance

General pathophysiological manifestations

It is now well known that human-immunodeficiency (HIV) infection, which ultimately leads to acquired immunodeficiency syndrome (AIDS), is caused by a retrovirus which specifically targets and ultimately destroys cells in the body that have CD4 receptors on their surface membranes, T4 helper lymphocytes (CD4+) and cells of the gastrointestinal tract, central nervous system and uterine cervix (American Journal of Psychiatry, 2000).

The HIV virus infects the CD4+ helper T lymphocytes which are responsible for the initiation of nearly all immunological responses to pathogens. Gradual attrition of the CD4 cell population (normal > 1000/mm³ of blood) occurs as the condition worsens, resulting in increasing failure of most immune functions and in particular cell-mediated immunity (Haslett et al., 1999). Peripheral neuropathy occurs at a CD4 count of 50–100 and dementia occurs at a very low CD4 count of 0–50, (American Journal of Psychiatry, 2000).

The four stages of HIV infection are identified in Table 4.1.

Table 4.1 The four stages of HIV infection (Pizzi and Burkhardt, 2003, p. 822)

Stage	Description	Signs and symptoms
1.	Acute infection	Short-lived and manifests in influenza-like symptoms
2.	Asymptomatic disease	HIV continues to replicate in the body but not sufficiently to cause signs and symptoms
3.	Symptomatic	Signs and symptoms now become evident
4	Advanced disease or AIDS	The immune system is now severely compromised

As a result of the disease progression shown in the table, the HIV-infected patient becomes prone to a multitude of opportunistic viral, fungal and bacterial infections each with their own series of mildly to severely unpleasant symptoms such as malaise, fatigue, diarrhoea and oral candida, amongst some of the most common. Cytomegalovirus (CMV) infection is responsible for inflammation and infection in parts of the eye, which results in perivascular haemorrhages and exudates and usually leads to rapid blindness. CMV encephalitis usually presents with personality change, poor concentration, headaches and insomnia (Haslett et al., 1999).

Pain caused by a variety of etiologies complicates HIV disease and McGuire (2003, p. 6) maintains that 'patients with AIDS have pain comparable in prevalence and intensity to pain in patients with cancer'. Fatigue is also a common, chronic symptom in HIV disease and may be associated with physical disability and depressed mood.

Common neurological manifestations

Clinical neurological disease in HIV-infected individuals presents most commonly with cerebral symptoms (McGuire, 2003). Altered mental status and generalized seizures may occur in global cerebral disease whereas the focal disease manifestations often result in hemiparesis, hemisensory loss, visual field cuts or disturbances in language use.

According to McGuire (2003) there is a variety of neuromuscular disorders resulting in peripheral neuropathy. In summary, these are:

- *Distal symmetric polyneuropathy*, which can disable otherwise healthy HIV patients with various paresthesias and mild weakness of limb muscles.
- *Mononeuropathy multiplex* presents as multifocal or asymmetric sensory and motor deficits as well as cranial neuropathies.
- *Inflammatory demyelinating polyneuropathy* presents with progressive, usually symmetrical, weakness in the upper and lower extremities.
- *Progressive lumbosacral polyradiculopathy* as a result of the CMV infection, which appears to have a predilection for the lumbosacral roots resulting in weakness and flaccid paraplegia as well as sensory and sphincter disturbances (McGuire, 2003).

There are other less common pathological manifestations resulting in physical disturbances.

Psychological responses, neuro-psychiatric disorders and syndromes

Psychological responses

The diagnosis of HIV infection and the development of the disease process undoubtedly has a devastating and far-reaching effect on the individual's life. Grimes and Grimes in Pedretti and Early, 2001, p. 108, propose four psychological states which accompany the disease progression, which may fluctuate from person to person and can occur at any time. The *initial crisis state* occurs shortly after diagnosis and is manifested by emotional numbing, denial and shock. In the *transitional stage* the individual starts to seek assistance and may experience anger, guilt and self-pity. This is followed by the *acceptance stage* and usually occurs when the individual has experienced a major clinical manifestation of the disease and now becomes proactive, seeks options and adapts lifestyle. The fourth stage is referred to as the *preparatory stage* and occurs when the individual addresses the fear of dying and dependency as well as end-of-life issues.

Special considerations

- HIV infection can lead to neuro-psychiatric symptoms which may occur at any stage and be precipitated even at the onset of somatic symptoms. It is important to note that pre-existing psychiatric disorders and personality traits may be exacerbated by the onset of HIV illness.
- Psychiatric disorders may result from or may be co-morbid with HIV infection. The more common diagnoses found in association with HIV/AIDS are dementia and a spectrum of cognitive disorders, delirium, mood disorders, substance abuse, anxiety and sleep disorders. These disorders may also occur in infants, children and adolescents.
- It is well documented that neuro-psychiatric syndromes develop due to HIV/AIDS, which cannot be attributed to CNS opportunistic infections or neoplasms. It is believed that HIV invades the CNS early in the course of the infection and may cause neuronal death. The syndromes and disorders are believed to result from subcortical infection of the brain. This is evidenced by neurocognitive impairment in adults, arrest of developmental milestones in children, as well as neuropathological lesions of the brain (seen at autopsy or on scans taken). Prevalence rates published vary, but higher rates are seen in the later stages of the HIV infection.
- It is important for occupational therapists to note that subtle neuro-psychological impairment may be found in 22%–30% of patients with HIV infection who are otherwise asymptomatic. HIV-associated minor cognitive motor disorder is a less severe disorder than HIV-associated dementia, which is believed to involve neural cell dysfunction rather than cell death, and does not necessarily progress to HIV-associated dementia. Both of the disorders do, however, decrease the survival risk amongst patients with HIV infection. New-onset psychosis and AIDS mania present at the later stages of HIV disease and may often occur in association with cognitive motor impairment.
- Clinical features such as suicide, attempted suicide and suicidal ideation seem to occur during the course of the illness at a somewhat higher rate than in the general population. It is estimated that in South Africa individuals with HIV/AIDS are 36 times more likely to commit suicide (Clarke, 2003). In addition HIV appears to occur at a higher rate in persons with personality disorders categorized within cluster B, such as borderline and histrionic personality disorders. This may be ascribed to the high tendency of such persons to participate in high risk drug use and sexual behaviour.

  It is also important to note that high rates of depression (60%), dysthymia and anxiety disorders (25%) have been identified in persons seeking HIV-related mental health services, as well as high rates of co-morbid substance abuse disorders. Almost half of these patients additionally have a diagnosis of alcohol or drug dependence. These rates could be reflective of the population studied (i.e. persons seeking mental health services) but are still relevant for occupational therapy intervention because occupational therapists practising in the field of psychiatry are often based in public service settings. Community-based samples were however found to have lower rates of psychiatric disorders (e.g. depression 14%).

- On the other hand severe mental illness with chronicity may increase the risk of HIV infection due to several factors such as diminished understanding or even a misunderstanding of how HIV/AIDS is transmitted; the occurrence of survival sex (for food or shelter), increased same-sex or multiple partner sexual activity (American Journal of Psychiatry, 2000).

HIV-associated dementia

Although the prevalence of dementia is thought to be approximately 15%–20% of all AIDS patients, it declines significantly with combination antiretroviral therapy. This disorder differs from Alzheimer's disease in that it may be classified as a *subcortical dementia* and can produce a clinical triad of progressive cognitive decline, motor dysfunction and behavioural abnormalities. Symptoms commonly include psychomotor slowing, decreased speed of motor processing, impaired verbal memory and learning efficiency and later impairment of executive functions. Behavioural manifestations may vary from apathy to psychosis (American Journal of Psychiatry, 2000; McGuire, 2003).

Other psychiatric syndromes

- *Delirium* may occur in the later stages of the disease at rates of 43%–65%, and, importantly, may be caused by high dosages of certain antiretroviral drugs.
- New onset psychotic symptoms. HIV infection is considered to be one possible cause of new onset psychosis, other causes being medical or concurrent substance abuse.
- AIDS mania, which may occur co-morbidly with AIDS dementia, presents at advanced stages of the disease and sufferers generally have no family or personal history of mood disorder. It may also occur in association with cognitive-motor impairment (American Journal of Psychiatry, 2000).

Paediatric HIV/AIDS syndrome

HIV/AIDS impacts more significantly on the developing nervous system of the child, whilst certain cognitive defects occur in some infected youth. Conditions such as HIV-associated progressive encephalopathy or HIV encephalopathy have been identified and are characterized by a triad of symptoms, including impaired brain growth, progressive motor dysfunction and loss or plateau of developmental milestones. Symptoms may be similar to those of dementia in adults (American Journal of Psychiatry, 2000).

It is of particular interest to occupational therapists that although children are generally considered to be asymptomatic, several studies have shown that some cognitive and language delays occur, including receptive and expressive language deficits and visual motor deficits, without any other real signs of HIV-related disease. Rates of approximately 30% for mood disorders and 25% for attention deficit disorders have been recorded amongst affected youth, with the incidence of substance abuse in the HIV group found to be approximately 30% (American Journal of Psychiatry, 2000).

Environmental and social factors impacting upon HIV/AIDS infected persons

Although the pathogenesis and disorders associated with HIV/AIDS are of particular significance, the disorders can only be understood within a context of environmental and social factors which can impact significantly upon the 'wellness' and quality of life of those who are infected. Most significant of these factors for occupational therapy include:

Loss of self

A study conducted by Lavery et al. (2001) on the origins of the desire for euthanasia revealed that persons with HIV or AIDS did not, as initially thought, desire euthanasia because of depression, hopelessness, grief, psychological distress and avoidance of pain and suffering, but rather because of a perceived *loss of self*, which is defined as:

> a progressive diminishment of opportunity to initiate and maintain close personal relationships as well as feelings of estrangement and alienation (Lavery et al., 2001, p. 362).

This was found to occur due to a sense of disintegration which resulted from the symptoms, loss of function and an understandable loss of community.

Poverty

According to a study conducted in the USA, the majority of persons with HIV/AIDS seeking mental health services were socially and economically disadvantaged (American Journal of Psychiatry, 2000). Conditions of poverty have been found to compromise overall health outcomes, particularly in the case of children, which is certainly the case in South Africa and other developing countries. Farmer et al. (2001) maintain that the reason AIDS mortality has dropped precipitously in affluent countries is largely due to those infected having greater access to Highly Active Antiretroviral Therapy (HAART).

Additional social problems faced by most HIV/AIDS infected persons, particularly in the African context, comes in the form of large-scale poverty and unemployment. This situation robs them of the chance of eating the correct foods, practising adequate infection control and purchasing the antiretroviral drugs or other comforts that will strengthen their resistance, give quality to and prolong their lives, as well as provide them with some dignity in the final stages of the disease. As the condition of the HIV-infected individual worsens, so too does the likelihood of increased absenteeism from work and resultant decrease in productivity, ending finally in the loss of employment and depletion of employment-related medical benefits (in those countries with little or no state-funded healthcare), which adds to the vicious cycle of poverty.

According to Deane (2003, pp.10–11) a fairly new phenomenon, 'presenteeism', also occurs and refers to that stage when the individual with HIV/AIDS reaches a level where their productivity decreases considerably and, rather than being absent (where their days of absence may be capped) and ultimately losing payment for work, they 'clock in' to work but work at very low levels of productivity.

Urban versus rural living

According to the American Journal of Psychiatry (2000) rural inhabitants compared to urban dwellers reported lower perceptions of social support from family and friends, reduced access to medical and mental health care, increased loneliness, stigma and fear of disclosure of status. It is possible that similar findings in South African rural populations may occur. However a recent undergraduate study by Norman et al. (2003) on AIDS orphans indicated that the African ethic of *ubuntu*, certainly in caring for AIDS orphaned children, appears to play an important role in ensuring that these children are cared for by their communities. Simply defined, *ubuntu* means 'I am a person through other persons' (Malcome, 2003), and it engenders a very strong sense of community support amongst indigenous peoples of Southern Africa.

Socio-political factors

If governments and the political forces within governments do not adequately support the provision of the resources and infrastructure to promote aggressive preventive programmes and antiretroviral medication for those who would benefit most, this will impact negatively upon HIV-infected persons. In countries where they are available and promoted, antimicrobial therapies and combination antiretroviral treatment have shown improved treatment effectiveness, increased survival in patients and potentially less development of viral resistance (American Journal of Psychiatry, 2000). An example of the efficacy of medication given by McQuire (2003) is that effective antiretroviral treatment for individuals with AIDS Dementia Complex reduces the neurotoxicity secreted by the macrophages, thus disabling rather than killing the neurons and decreasing the incidence of dementia.

Marginalized groups

Those who are discriminated against in terms of gender, race, politics, economic status, cultural or religious or political affiliations may be particularly vulnerable to sexual or other forms of exploitation and thus also HIV infection. Such individuals often have limited or no access to health promotion information and health and social services. This would most likely also mean that such infected persons would have decreased access to treatment (Mann and Tarantola, 1998).

Education level, social status and power

Mann and Tarantola (1998) report that more than half of the cases with AIDS in Brazil have only primary level schooling, and women, who throughout the world account for 40% of infected cases, have low social status and limited power within relationships and the community. These women are then unable to protect themselves from infection (for example, by insisting on condom use).

The culmination of these factors may result in a vicious cycle ending in severe disintegration of families and support systems. Commonly one or both parents are sick for long periods of time and then may die in fairly close succession leaving possibly a grandmother to look after the children. During this process food runs out, children may stop going to school and end up begging on the streets and ultimately become street children.

Practice guidelines for occupational therapists in treating HIV/AIDS-related conditions

Introduction

The onslaught upon all the biopsychosocial systems of each HIV/AIDS survivor demands an absolutely integrated and holistic approach to treatment. The individual's level of immunity and current health status have a direct impact upon treatment at each stage of the disease process. Initially treatment programmes may be no different than for any person with, for example, a similar neurological or psychiatric problem. However as the opportunistic conditions advance, immunity reduces and co-morbid diseases and syndromes develop, the treatment programmes become more multifaceted and complex. In later stages promotive programmes for the family and caregivers and palliative programmes for the patients become necessary.

Diagnosis and assessment

Before discussing treatment guidelines it is necessary to consider briefly the contribution of the occupational therapist in terms of diagnosis and assessment, particularly as psychiatric disorders have been found to go undetected, be misdiagnosed and under-treated or inappropriately treated in primary healthcare settings (American Journal of Psychiatry, 2000).

The first task of the occupational therapist would be to do baseline screening to assess the mental status of persons with HIV/AIDS, followed up with regular ongoing assessment. By virtue of the occupational therapists' relationship with and regular contact with individuals in a variety of treatment settings, they are in a unique position to provide comprehensive input about a person's behaviour, day-to-day functioning and efficacy of coping skills. In addition the occupational therapist will be able to note subtle changes and particularly the occurrence of new or an exacerbation of existing symptomatology and will also be able to determine their ongoing and changing physical, emotional and cognitive state, which is crucial for regulating effective treatment.

The occupational therapy assessment, as proposed by Gutterman (1990), lists eight aspects that should be addressed. These include activities of daily living; past and present health status; social environment and networks available; pain or other limiting problems; time management (including fun activities); substance abuse issues and how handled; assessment of muscle strength, coordination, sensation, ambulation and cognition; work history and changes in work role since the onset of HIV/AIDS.

As certain syndromes associated with AIDS mimic psychiatric disorders, the occupational therapist will be able to identify subtle signs indicating development of psychiatric symptoms, particularly in settings for persons with primarily physical conditions. Observation of physical status and signs of neuropathy as well as response to medication and possible drug-to-drug interactions should thus also be monitored by the occupational therapist.

Careful investigation by psychiatrists, augmented by clinical observation by occupational therapists, is needed to exclude other possible causes of the clinical features noted, such as substance abuse. The contribution of the occupational therapist to making a diagnosis is thus critically important.

It should be noted that the Mini Mental Status Examination (MMSE), which is widely used by occupational therapists, has not been found to be sensitive enough to pick up early HIV-associated cognitive behaviour (Folstein et al., 1975). It is further suggested that the Pizzi Holistic Wellness Assessment, as well as the Pizzi Assessment of Productive Living, be considered, together with clinical observations, as useful assessment tools (Pizzi and Burkhardt in Crepeau et al., 2003).

Guidelines for treatment

Crossley (1997) maintains that the pursuit of health is actually the pursuit of moral personhood, as the concept of health acts as a metaphor for social control. In contrast to this the presence of disease serves to 'sully' an individual's identity in so far as it can be seen as a metaphor for lack of control, and an indicator of 'badness', 'immorality' and 'irresponsibility'. This statement should remind the occupational therapist of the importance of having a holistic, patient-centred approach to all intervention.

The fundamental underlying principles of occupational therapy intervention for individuals with HIV/AIDS are therefore:

- The facilitation of personal empowerment, autonomy and control over their lives, which will include pain and stress management (Gutterman in Pedretti and Early, 2001).
- Restoration and maintenance of occupational roles and relationships (which contribute towards maintenance of dignity and quality of life).
- Acknowledgement and accommodation of the need for mourning and of emotional and behavioural responses such as depression, anxiety, anger and guilt which occur due to the diagnosis.
- Maintenance of physical strength, endurance and mobility (Gutterman in Pedretti and Early, 2001).

Intervention must of necessity be offered through different programmes including promotive, preventive (including harm reduction), remedial and rehabilitative programmes, as well as palliative care. Promotive programmes will not be discussed due to the constraints of this chapter but are none the less an important component of any comprehensive strategy. Gutterman (1990) correctly views health education and promotion as one of three components of the occupational therapy contribution to the management of persons with HIV/AIDS. She describes the occupational therapist as acting as an agent for change by facilitating an internal and external environment conducive to such change, and providing opportunities for learning about health promoting lifestyles.

The hypothesis by Goodkin in Crossley (1997) that the HIV/AIDS progression and length of survival may be affected by a mix of psychological, psychosocial and behavioural influences such as attitude, character, disposition, interpersonal influences, coping styles and stressful life events, is relevant to occupational therapy.

The programme philosophy as described by Gutterman (1990) for daycare centres applies equally within any other occupational therapy setting in that HIV/AIDS is viewed as a chronic disease requiring medical and psychiatric attention, rehabilitation (including arts and alternative therapies), psychotherapeutic intervention, nutritional counselling and pastoral care. The following directives given for the management of a psychiatric patient with HIV/AIDS by the American Psychiatric Association (American Journal of Psychiatry, 2000) reflect the Gutterman philosophy and are, with minor adaptations, applied to occupational therapy:

1. *Establish and maintain a therapeutic alliance with the patient.* This concept is integral to occupational therapy philosophy and should be extended to include the care providers; the cornerstone of all treatment being that of psychosocial support. Self-empowerment, positive thinking and taking responsibility for control of the illness should not be underestimated and should be striven for throughout treatment (Crossley, 1997).

2. *Collaborate and coordinate care with other mental health practitioners, medical providers and caregivers.* Knowledge and understanding of treatment, particularly the interaction of medication for HIV and psychiatric disorders/syndromes, are important for the occupational therapist, as are active participation in intervention and prevention programmes offered by other team members. Occupational therapists should also collaborate with agencies/structures/non-governmental organizations within communities providing services for or relevant to the needs of individuals with HIV/AIDS.

3. *Treat all associated psychiatric disorders.* Psychotherapeutic and occupational therapy management of these patients is not seen to be different from that of patients with primarily psychiatric disorders, and treatment regimes and protocols should be implemented accordingly but with specific considerations.

4. *Facilitate adherence to overall treatment plan.* Medication compliance is considered to be critically important to prevent viral resistance from developing (Beardslay, 1998). Psycho-education, reinforcement of the need for compliance with medication regimes; observation of side effects and efficacy of drugs should be reported to the team. Bear in mind that depression and substance abuse have been shown to adversely affect compliance with complicated treatment regimes. Pizzi and Burkhardt (2003) maintain that the occupational therapist can help people gain the habits required to maintain demanding drug regimens and to help them to adapt activities to accommodate drug side effects that impact on occupational performance.

5. *Provide information about psychosocial, psychiatric and neuro-psychiatric disorders as associated with HIV.* Here the occupational therapist may augment input given by the psychiatrist and other team members. In situations where psychiatric services are not readily available, the occupational therapist may need to play a much greater educational role, offer psycho-educational programmes, do appropriate psychiatric referrals as well as ongoing psychiatric status assessments.

6. *Participate in risk and harm reduction strategies to minimize the spread of HIV.* Decreasing the risk of psychiatric patients contracting HIV/AIDS is an important aspect of care as well as decreasing the risk of such a patient infecting another person. Certain symptoms, behaviour and psychodynamic issues could predispose the individual with a psychiatric disorder to becoming infected.

The presence of certain psychiatric conditions which increase *high-risk behaviour* includes impulse control disorders, personality disorders, untreated depressions, hyper-sexuality associated with mania, psychotic disorders, mental disorders due to a general medical condition, binge alcohol drinking and drug use. High-risk behaviours which need to be carefully monitored therefore include high-risk sexual and drug use behaviour, particularly the use of mood-altering substances, as these decrease inhibitions generally, and sexual inhibitions specifically, whilst increasing impulsivity and impairing judgement.

Patients with severe mental illness may be more at risk, not only due to the symptoms and behaviours associated with their illness, but also because of poor access to healthcare, diminished ability to care for themselves and downward mobility. Survivors of sexual abuse/crimes and psychiatric patients (of all ages) are often more vulnerable and have histories of sexual abuse, which may include long-term abuse or a single episode of sexual assault.

The American Psychiatric Association (2000) recommends the compilation of a risk history and a *risk reduction strategy* and lists factors such as acute episodes of psychiatric illness, stressful or traumatic life events and the developmental stage of the person, as contributing to the need for ongoing risk appraisal. Sexual practices and drug use consequently need to be thoroughly investigated. The role of the occupational therapist would be to identify risk behaviour, as well as situations, particularly within an institutional setting (e.g. hygiene practices, overcrowding), which could increase the risk to patients themselves and others.

Prevention is undoubtedly the key component of these risk reduction strategies, which are largely of an educational nature. It should therefore make patients aware of risk behaviours, address necessary changes in behaviour and the treatment of problems which promote risk behaviour. Knowledge of risk is, however, not considered to be adequate. Ongoing counselling and support, as well as the addressing of underlying causes of risk behaviours, are needed to ensure consistent changes in behaviour and lifestyle. The occupational therapist should participate in programmes to decrease risk and should introduce and integrate comprehensive educational programmes into their interventions. The attainment of improved communication skills and assertiveness with regard to sexual behaviour (e.g. use of condoms) in order to deal effectively with abusive and violent partners, should be an aim of this intervention.

Low-risk behaviour includes activities such as sharing of toothbrushes and shaving equipment, which may be of concern to care providers, but do not as such constitute a serious risk to the patients.

Harm reduction strategies (American Journal of Psychiatry, 2000) are proposed for injection drug users, which appears to be a more realistic option than abstinence, as substance abuse undoubtedly exacerbates risk and should be carefully monitored. These strategies include methadone maintenance treatment, needle education and bleach distribution, safer sex education, legal clean needle policies and access to sterile syringes and needle exchange programmes.

> Post-exposure prophylaxis (PEP) is considered to be essential and protocols and policies should be put in place to expedite it, with counselling forming an integral component. Patients should also be made aware of safety issues and protecting themselves from opportunistic infections. The therapist should also be particularly vigilant with regard to this (Reed, 1991, pp. 368–9).

Maximize occupational, psychological, physical and social/adaptive functioning

This represents the area of maximal contribution by the occupational therapist and includes enabling patients to cope with their illness both medically and psychosocially, and particularly on an occupational performance level. Occupational therapy intervention is multifaceted, essentially holistic in nature, and to be effective needs to be patient- and community-centred and, in the African context, offered within a social model and primary healthcare context.

Occupational therapists can contribute by helping to create opportunities for self-actualization and empowerment of the individual in taking responsibility for their own health. This can be enhanced through the use of purposeful occupational therapy activity programmes which are specifically directed at counteracting weaknesses and enhancing strengths. Reed (1991) also proposes the use of creative activities, arts and drama to enhance self-concept and a sense of mastery. Where appropriate it is recommended that patients be encouraged to get involved in pressure/lobby groups.

The development of coping skills to deal with stigma, pain, fatigue, anger, anxiety and depression and disclosure of illness must be facilitated and may include intervention through group therapy (including family members/partners) cognitive behaviour therapy, stress management, role-play and social skills training. Stress management and relaxation techniques such as visualization, yoga, meditation and biofeedback are also effective to facilitate coping. Reed (1991) further stresses the need for the individual to be able to communicate concerns and plan and problem solve together with family, partners and friends.

Fatigue, pain, paralysis, reduced joint range, low endurance, sensory disturbances and muscle weakness or tone problems need to be treated according to methods and principles as applied in the conventional treatment of various performance components. Of note is that McGuire (2003) considers aggressive pain treatment to be the single most important and challenging intervention in the case of patients with HIV disease. In addition, anxiety and depression seem to be both overriding and underlying symptoms and thus also demand specific attention throughout treatment.

Gutterman (1990) mentions the use of acupuncture and relaxation as helpful in the management of HIV-related pain and, in addition, visualization and guided imagery may be used to help with anxiety and pain reduction.

Alternative and complementary healing methods may also be utilized, with care taken to ensure that such services are provided by appropriately trained practitioners, especially where these can enhance quality of life and provide some enjoyment such as aromatherapy, massage and yoga (Gutterman, 1990).

Help the patient to deal with spiritual/religious issues

Spiritual strength and religious belief can often be a source of great strength and comfort to someone with HIV/AIDS. Although the occupational therapist is not qualified to deal actively with existential, spiritual crises that may occur, these needs cannot be ignored. Sensitivity to, and acknowledgement of, the person's specific needs must be followed up and, where appropriate, referral(s) made to pastoral and other religious counselling agencies.

It should be kept in mind that conservative/fundamentalist religious dogmas may take a rigid, uncompromising stance towards HIV/AIDS, and particularly towards individuals who may be homosexual and/or sexually promiscuous, or abuse substances. Spiritual counsellors who take a rigid and conservative stance against such persons may do more harm than good for an individual in times of need. On the other hand, spiritual counsellors who are gentle, caring and sensitive may often provide the most important source of comfort for the individual in their time of need. Thus sensitivity is required in selecting experienced, mature and truly caring spiritual counsellors when seeking spiritual guidance. Often the patient/individual or family members can provide names of people who will provide such support.

Preparation for issues of disability

Issues around decreased capability and disability need to be specifically addressed. The adaptation of the work and living environment, and expectations within the workplace, form a major part of the occupational therapy contribution, also within an institutional setting. Methods of energy conservation, the application of work simplification and lifestyle adaptations, including time management, should be implemented to accommodate low levels of endurance. Work visits to advise employers on methods of maintaining maximal productivity are critical in areas where there are high levels of HIV/AIDS in the workplace. A recent survey conducted in five companies (85,000 employees) in South Africa indicated that, over a three-year period, disability claims had almost doubled as a result of HIV/AIDS-related illnesses (Deane, 2003).

In addition and where applicable, the provision of assistive devices and application of utensil/environmental adaptations, at home, work and during leisure time, may be helpful in maintaining occupational performance. Assistance with introducing the individual to support groups is integral in forming a support system when they are discharged home. Peer counselling can also assist the individual to adjust more easily.

Preparation for death and dying

When dealing with issues related to death and dying the occupational therapist should facilitate the empowerment of individuals in directing their own lives. This includes informing them of their right to make decisions about treatment and/or its termination, or even end-of-life decisions such as making a will and mending broken relationships. However the rapidity with which death may occur due to opportunistic infections within a hospital setting usually makes it difficult and sometimes impossible for the therapist to support a dying patient adequately. Cultural differences and language barriers may exacerbate this situation.

If the patient reaches a stage where aggressive and/or progressive therapy is no longer indicated therapists should be challenged to find ways of assisting the patient in experiencing quality of life and dignity in the final stages of their lives. They can act as advocates and agents between patient and family, spiritual counsellor, legal advisor, partner, spouse or significant other at that stage and time of the patient's life. It goes without saying that large doses of Tender Loving Care (TLC) are essential at this stage.

Home care and advice to significant others/family regarding resources

Family, partners, friends and care providers are often a source of comfort and support and commonly take on the burden of day-to-day care of the terminally ill patient with AIDS. It is thus important that such persons are not only well informed but also supported by the treatment team. Valuable insights may be gained by practitioners through ongoing sharing. Consideration should also be given to establishing respite care support groups and family therapy, and developing home care programmes.

If support groups are not available, occupational therapists should facilitate the establishment of such groups and ensure that the individual and family are put in touch with appropriate resources within the community, for example, feeding schemes, providers of home-based care kits (e.g. disinfectant, petroleum jelly, analgesics, etc.), child support systems and peer counsellors/HIV survivors, as well as hospice facilities.

Guidelines for inpatient psychiatric units

(Taken from the American Psychiatric Association (APA) 1996 and approved by APA Board of Trustees 15 December 1996.)

These guidelines are included as they have relevance for occupational therapists practising in institutions in both developing and developed countries.

- The guidelines emphasize the need to prevent HIV transmission (bearing in mind that high-risk behaviour such as sexual contact, needle sharing, sharing of implements, tattooing and self-mutilation may occur in psychiatric settings).
- HIV/AIDS patients should receive the same quality of care as any other patient (this should include rigorous diagnosis and treatment of psychiatric disorders).
- Patients should receive counselling on HIV-related issues, such as risk reduction measures and medication for HIV infection.
- Family members and significant others should be involved in counselling and education.
- Confidentiality must be protected so that patients will not be dissuaded from testing, treatment and behavioural counselling and disclosure.
- HIV tests should not be conducted for screening purposes.
- Patients should have a discharge plan which includes provision for ongoing medical care.
- Practitioners should apply universal precautions and be aware of how HIV/AIDS-related conditions may affect diagnosis and treatment.

Guidelines for intervention in communities

When working in District Health Services in communities with a significant prevalence of individuals with HIV/AIDS it is important to:

- Establish a list of appropriate resources, both within and outside these communities, that can be utilized to provide assistance for individuals with HIV/AIDS and caregivers who are living at home and require support.
- Form partnerships with community structures in an attempt to strategize the best interventions for the individuals who may be referred back home after treatment.
- Provide guidelines for supporting family and caregivers.
- Monitor the home situations of those individuals who have been discharged. It is possible that there may be more than one person with HIV/AIDS in the home, and such families can disintegrate rapidly when the impact of the disease is added to the ravages of poverty and unemployment. Ensuring support in the form of feeding schemes and home-based care kits can often provide huge relief for such families.
- Assist with ensuring that proper arrangements are made for people left behind, for example children and spouses/partners, in the event of the breadwinner dying.

HIV/AIDS within a legal, ethical and personal/professional perspective

Occupational therapists in the South African healthcare system are daily referred large numbers of patients who are either HIV-positive or have full-blown AIDS. The innate fear of contagion, coupled with the latex barrier of gloves, places a wedge between the patient–therapist relationship. As a result of this therapists are faced not only with making enormously difficult ethical and moral decisions but also with the pain and strain upon their own inner resources at having to watch the frequent and rapid demise of patients whom they have grown to care for over time.

The stigma and fear associated with dealing with individuals with HIV/AIDS is well known and experienced personally by many practitioners and members of the public alike. The multiplicity of ethical challenges and dilemmas this poses for therapists cannot be underestimated as, for example, many of these patients may appear relatively functional one day and within a week, as a result of some or other opportunistic infection, may become critically ill necessitating drastic downgrading or even curtailment of existing treatment programmes.

Attitudes and experiences of practitioners providing services to HIV/AIDS patients and their caregivers/partners

An extensive literature review undertaken by Barbour (1994) on the impact of working with individuals with HIV/AIDS found that judgemental attitudes existed amongst a significant number of health professionals including occupational therapists. Ethical dilemmas seem to revolve mostly around issues of fear of contagion and physical contact with the individual, discrimination, equity, access to treatment and confidentiality and are best understood against a framework of common attitudes, beliefs and emotional responses, which include:

- Fear of contagion and death, which is very real despite proof of the fragility of the virus and knowledge of prevention and precautions (Decosas, 2002; Joubert and van der Reyden, 2003).
- Prejudice against HIV-infected patients often related to sexual practices, homosexuality, high-risk behaviours and exposure to alternative, often unacceptable lifestyles (Barbour, 1994; Joubert and van der Reyden 2003).
- Belief that it was *not* unethical to refuse to treat persons with HIV/AIDS (Barbour, 1994).
- Feelings of not wanting or not choosing to work with such persons if given a choice (Barbour, 1994; Joubert and van der Reyden, 2003).
- Wanting to avoid treating infected children due to the personal pain it causes therapists (Joubert and van der Reyden, 2003).

- Despondency and sadness when patients die, particularly where a close relationship has been established, often over time (McKusick et al. in Barbour, 1994).
- Feelings of anger at parents of HIV/AIDS babies, who are perceived as being responsible for the suffering caused to their child. Also feelings of ambivalence towards some patients because they are perceived as having indirectly or even knowingly inflicted the suffering upon themselves (Joubert and van der Reyden, 2003).
- Feeling 'detached' from the patients because of mandatory precautionary measures such as gloves, gowns and, in some cases, even masks, which seems to negate the very essence of a therapeutic relationship (Joubert and van der Reyden, 2003, p. 3). As Huss in Pizzi (1990, p. 201) states:

non-touch may be just as devastating at a time when words are insufficient or cannot be processed appropriately because of disintegration of the individual.

- Being on the receiving end of negative attitudes and even discrimination by the community (Pandya, 1997).
- High stress levels and burnout, which have been found to occur in health professionals treating individuals with HIV/AIDS. McKusick et al. in Barbour (1994) noted higher levels of anxiety and a greater fear of death amongst health professionals working with AIDS patients. The findings of McKusick et al. are relevant to therapists working with large numbers of HIV-infected patients in that a health professional who acted as a 'buddy' for a number of different individuals with AIDS was more likely to develop psychiatric symptomatology such as depression than one who had to provide support to a single individual over a longer period of time. This finding also applies to care providers and family members.
- Conflicts experienced by occupational therapists who, on the one hand, have the goal of restoration of function, occupational roles and relationships and on the other hand have to find suitable goals and to provide a realistic service for someone who is terminally ill (Piemme and Bolle in Barbour, 1994; Joubert and van der Reyden, 2003).

Other stress factors identified in Joubert and van der Reyden's 2003 study are:

- Demands for HIV counselling of patients and feelings of being inadequately trained to provide such a service.
- Uncertainties around prognosis, which makes planning, treatment and goal-setting difficult.
- Having to deal with the added burden of psychiatric problems in patients who are primarily physically ill or disabled on the one hand and having to deal with physical problems in patients who may already

have primary psychiatric problems on the other. Added to this is having to deal with the devastating effect which these additional problems may have on the patients and their families.

In addition, in developing countries there is the possibility of inadequate treatment resources and policies, particularly around the provision, monitoring and cost of antiretroviral treatment, which make intervention strategies difficult or even impossible.

The legal context: the law and HIV/AIDS

The legal and ethical situation regarding HIV/AIDS is very well documented and contained in many global policies, codes, rules, regulations and guidelines. Where applicable the 'law' is written up in a Bill of Rights which may form part of the Constitution and Acts of Parliament of a particular country. Regulations, rules and codes of practice, as prescribed or recommended by government departments, professional organizations and statutory health councils, such as the Health Professions Council of South Africa, contain invaluable information.

The legal situation is in fact straightforward and essentially prohibits any discrimination against a person with HIV/AIDS. It should be kept in mind that these principles and rules apply equally to the patient and to the health practitioner who may have contracted HIV/AIDS. In addition the health practitioner is entitled to post-exposure prophylaxis (PEP) if risk of infection occurs on duty.

HIV/AIDS within an ethical context

The nature of the occupational therapist–patient relationship, the patient's problems, and the events and situations with which clinical therapists need to cope with, all challenge the traditional mode of practice. This gives rise to ethical and moral dilemmas that require a sensitive, life-affirming and professionally sound approach that is based upon unquestionable professional integrity.

The management of ethical and moral dilemmas is essentially about *ethical decision making*. The term 'ethical decision making' is at times used interchangeably with *moral reasoning*. However moral reasoning should, according to Barnitt (1993), be seen as a more philosophical enquiry about norms and values than about what is right or wrong. Seedhouse in Barnitt (1993) furthermore differentiates between ethics as related to life-and-death issues (dramatic/persisting ethics) as distinct from ethics as a day-to-day event. This is precisely the area where moral dilemmas occur in occupational therapy, as what seems to be morally right may not be ethically appropriate and vice versa.

According to Dada and McQuoid-Mason (2001), ethical decision making requires that three factors be taken into account: first, the *choices* (options) that may be selected from; second, the *consequences* of such decisions; and third, the *context or setting* of the healthcare dilemma. Seedhouse in Barnitt (1993) proposes a useful ethical grid comprising four levels to be used as a tool to improve healthcare decision making and ethical judgements. The first level deals with autonomy, respect and individual needs, the second level deals with the duties and motives of the therapist, whereas the third deals with possible consequences of such a decision and the fourth level deals with external considerations, for example legal considerations, risks and the wishes of others.

Of relevance for the appropriate management of a patient with HIV/AIDS are the principles of autonomy, beneficence, non-maleficence and justice, which merit brief discussion, as do the rules of duty to treat, informed consent, confidentiality and use of scarce resources (Dada and McQuoid-Mason, 2001).

Basic principles

The following four basic principles, as articulated by Beauchamp and Childress (in Mappes and de Grazzia, 1996), encompass the obligations of health practitioners towards people with HIV/AIDS, whilst also providing a frame of reference according to which intervention may be planned and implemented and problems may be appropriately identified, analysed and resolved.

Autonomy

Autonomy is defined by Mappes and de Grazzia (1996) as self-governance or self-determination and may also be described as non-interference by the practitioner. Applying the principle of autonomy essentially means that a person is respected as an autonomous being with the capability and freedom to decide and act, and that people are allowed to remain in control of their lives and have the right to make decisions affecting their lives and health.

Ackerman (in Mappes and de Grazzia, 1996) makes a significant point in acknowledging that inasmuch as autonomy is the desired goal, it should be kept in mind that autonomy may be compromised by several factors such as the impact of the illness on values and lifestyle, depression, anxiety, guilt and denial, as well as social and cultural constraints and lack of information. This means that the person's ability to make appropriate choices may be impeded, causing the patient to become vulnerable and unable to deliberate or perhaps even articulate life goals.

Ackerman also describes the duty of the health practitioner as helping to 'neutralise the impediments' that would hinder effective decision making. In cases where autonomy is diminished, as in the case of a seriously ill or mentally disordered individual, autonomy must be protected, respect shown and an attempt made to facilitate at least some control.

The acknowledgement of autonomy is consequently basic to the implementation of the rules of both informed consent and confidentiality.

Clinical dilemmas arise, for example, if a patient refuses treatment which would seem to be beneficial or participates in alternative treatment methods which may be questionable, or even proven to be dangerous. Conflicts can also arise between the patient's or individual's attitude towards conventional Western medical practices and traditional healers and requires sensitive handling on the part of the therapist.

Beneficence

Beneficence, which is often seen as the cornerstone of the health professional–patient relationship, essentially requires that the practitioner should do that which is in the best interests of his/her patients or, stated differently, that which will contribute to their improved health and welfare. It also implies that the practitioner should prevent the patient from coming to harm. It may, however, become problematic when what the practitioner believes to be in the best interest of the patient is not ethically appropriate or contrary to the patient or their family's wishes or not possible due to limited resources for treatment.

Non-maleficence

Non-maleficence, or not deliberately doing harm to our patients, is a fundamental principle. Barnitt (1993) warns that, for the therapist, doing no harm may more often imply not doing psychological, rather than physical, harm.

Some clinical dilemmas encountered include where the patient is left to die and food, medication or items that provide comfort are removed; or where patients do not receive treatment or receive inadequate treatment, because of a lack of resources or even governmental policy, or where treatment facilities are inadequate or non-existent.

Justice

Justice as a principle requires that social benefits and social burdens be distributed fairly; it can therefore be equated with equity. In the case of occupational therapy, this would refer to accessibility of services, distribution of equipment and materials, allocation of time and effort and practising without bias or prejudice. However, as providing equal treatment to all patients may be a practical impossibility, sensitive, compassionate prioritizing is essential.

Heart-wrenching clinical dilemmas arise because of the unavailability of medication and the use of scarce resources and medication for dying patients whilst younger, healthier patients are unable to access these resources. In addition, questions arise around whether it is in fact worth treating someone with limited life expectancy, or continuing with treatment when sudden and rapid disintegration of health may make continuation of treatment seem futile.

Basic rules of treatment

Questions frequently asked include:

* How do I select patients for treatment?
* May I refuse to treat an individual with HIV/AIDS?
* May I terminate treatment when I find out that a patient is HIV positive?
* Should I continue treating when the patient becomes terminally ill?
* What do I do when the patient is discharged but still needs treatment?

Duty to treat

The rules which regulate health practitioner practice are contained in ethical rules of Statutory Councils, Ethical Codes and the codes of practice of professional organizations, and describe the obligations and duties of such health practitioners.

A duty to treat simply means that the occupational therapist has a duty to continue to treat a patient with whom treatment has commenced and may not abandon such an individual. Treatment may consequently be terminated only under very specific circumstances, such as when patients are cured or do not require further treatment; they refuse treatment; sufficient instructions can be issued for future treatment or where the practitioner gives sufficient notice to discontinue practice, in which case referral to other agencies should be made (Dada and McQuoid-Mason, 2001).

Practitioners in private practice may refuse to treat a patient (except in an emergency), whereas therapists employed by an organization are obliged to treat patients according to their employment contract (as in a hospital), and can therefore not refuse to treat a patient except on sound clinical grounds. A diagnosis of HIV/AIDS can consequently not be a reason for refusal to treat a patient or to terminate treatment, and even if the therapist is not legally obliged to treat a patient, they still have a social responsibility to do so.

Several factors may make the implementation of this rule problematic and include situations where a patient is being discharged prematurely without consultation with the occupational therapist, and where limited resources make it impossible to continue with treatment.

Dilemmas also occur when decisions need to be made about whether to commence or complete treatment for patients who are in the terminal stages of AIDS or alternatively to spend time and effort with patients who have a better prognosis. Weighing up of therapy costs, for example transport and hospital costs, against the use of this money to pay for better diet or to pay for other related interventions which may reduce the effects of a compromised immune system or even to improve palliative home care, are very real and painful dilemmas with which the occupational therapist needs to cope.

The duty to treat may also be affected by the scope of rehabilitation, which may be severely curtailed, depending on the stage of infection.

Some experienced therapists maintain that HIV-infected patients in advanced stages do not attain optimal functional independence once they have reached a certain stage of the illness, and at times do not even pass the initial phase of rehabilitation before they reach terminal stages, but rather follow a gradual downward spiral in both performance components and performance areas. As one therapist described it, it is a process of 'one step forward and one step backwards' (Joubert and van der Reyden, 2003, p. 3)

Joubert and van der Reyden's 2003 survey also revealed that programme planning was seriously compromised in that goal setting depended on the stage of the disease process. It was also found to be very difficult to do appropriate future planning with patients and their families who were not aware of, or would not acknowledge, their HIV status.

Informed consent

Questions frequently asked:

- Should I inform the patient of his status?
- How do I explain the 'universal precautions'?
- How do I deal with issues of death and dying?
- How much do I tell my patient?

The occupational therapist may not treat a patient without that patient's consent or, in cases where the patient is unable or incapable of making such a decision, their guardian's consent. This right is accepted and acknowledged in most countries and is entrenched in common law and the Bill of Rights in South Africa and is therefore virtually inviolate. Consent is needed before any assessment or treatment may be commenced and presupposes that the patient's consent to receive/participate in treatment is based upon a substantial understanding and knowledge concerning the nature and effect of what is being consented to. This means that the patient needs to be informed of procedures and equipment to be used; the possible duration and cost of treatment; common risks involved in treatment; both negative and positive effects of treatment, as well as alternative treatment options and implications of non-compliance, which is particularly relevant in the case of the person with HIV/AIDS. The patient consequently has a right to information about his condition, a second opinion and access to information in the treatment file.

Several factors complicate the implementation of this rule when dealing with a person with HIV/AIDS who has a co-morbid psychiatric disorder, and particularly in cases where the patient may have dementia or mania; may suffer from severe depression and not be motivated to participate in any therapy; or even function at a level at which comprehension of the treatment process may be difficult or, where the patient, due to delusions, may be averse to treatment. The occupational therapist does, however, have recourse to the care provider, the medical superintendent and even the Health Ministry in certain circumstances, in cases where the patient is unable to consent to treatment. This consent does not absolve the occupational therapist from making a genuine attempt to *inform* the patient, a process which, in the case of a patient with a psychiatric disorder, may be an ongoing one.

The moral dilemma is often around how much persuasion the occupational therapist should use to ensure participation in treatment, particularly in the case of a patient who is experiencing extreme pain. Such decisions should be made on the basis of sound clinical judgement about the patient's capacity to comprehend, and made in the best interests of the patient's health. Where the patient attends occupational therapy, it can however be construed as tacit consent to treatment.

A further dilemma faced by the occupational therapist in treating the person with HIV/AIDS lies with informing them of their HIV status. Any person has the right to know their own status but equally may refuse to know their status. If the occupational therapist needs to inform the patient, however, appropriate counselling and support should be provided and treatment options reviewed.

Confidentiality

Questions frequently asked:

* Can I ask to know my patient's HIV status?
* Is the patient entitled to know my HIV status?
* In what circumstances may confidentiality be violated?

(Winston in Mappes and de Grazzia, 1996; Dada and McQuoid-Mason, 2001)

Confidentiality has formed one of the basic tenets of professional practice since the Hippocratic Oath was first written. It safeguards the integrity of the patient–therapist relationship and is inherent in the principle of autonomy. Ethical and moral conflicts arise around the issue of a patient's interests and safety versus those of a third party.

Ethical rules require the practitioner to safeguard information which ought to be kept secret, which a person would normally wish to be kept secret, or information which a particular individual wishes to keep secret. The clinician may not divulge information except where the patient has consented or where a court of law or act of parliament orders him/her to do so. However, should a third party be placed at real and serious risk by the patient, disclosure ought to be made. This third party may be other health workers, a spouse or sex partner. As a general rule, the dictum of 'protective privilege (privacy) ends where public peril begins' applies (Torasoff v Regents of the University of California, 1976).

But, as Sim (1996) correctly says, the occupational therapist needs to ensure that the person to whom the information is divulged knows the 'rules' and has a legitimate need to be informed; he also emphasizes that although not an inviolable moral requirement, confidentiality should not be sacrificed too readily, and safe custody of information should be ensured.

Confidentiality issues related to HIV/AIDS centre largely on informing colleagues and/or relatives and/or third parties about the person's status. A study undertaken for the World Health Organization in 33 countries found that the majority of these countries have either enacted laws or have policies in place to allow for such disclosure (Laurence and Gostin, 1995). Such disclosure may, however, be considered only when the patient's behaviour may cause real harm (in extreme cases) to another person's health and life, as in the case of ongoing sexual or needle-sharing relationships. As previously mentioned, a person has the right to know their HIV status; however, should such information lead to a person seriously harming themselves or others, such action should be reconsidered. Likewise, should disclosure to a third party put the person's life at risk, all risks need to be weighed up.

Disclosure by the therapist to a third party should be seen as a last resort and can be made only after other avenues have been exhausted. This, for instance, includes counselling the patient about the need for disclosure and the implications of non-disclosure and risk behaviour. Should disclosure be absolutely essential, the occupational therapist should still attempt to gain consent from the patient and make a disclosure if that attempt fails. The therapist should then inform the patient that he is ethically bound to warn other parties and that this will be done on a confidential basis.

Employing bodies and colleagues have no right to request to know the status of a colleague and the occupational therapist may not disclose such information to an employer. Employers may only request that a person's status be disclosed if this information is an essential requirement for the job. The therapist should keep in mind that legal action may be taken by the patient against the practitioner for disclosure without consent.

The Joubert and van der Reyden survey (2003) found that due to *the need for confidentiality* it is particularly difficult in cases where an HIV-positive child's parents have died and the therapist cannot reveal this to the secondary caregiver of the child, but feels concerned about the vulnerability of the caregiver to becoming infected, or where the therapist knows the patient's partner or family members are at risk of becoming infected if they do not take the necessary precautions. Confidentiality also becomes a problem during group treatment, i.e. ensuring that the patient's status is not revealed in the group. There is also the risk/problem of discussing HIV/AIDS-related issues with the patients through an interpreter.

Another common problem seems to be the fact that the doctors often do not reveal the patient's status and/or that the patient has not received post-test counselling. Although therapists have no right to know a patient's HIV status, this puts them in a difficult position because without this information they cannot easily provide guidelines to the patient on aspects that may enhance their health status.

Utilization of scarce resources

Questions frequently asked:

- Should I commence or continue treatment even without adequate resources?
- What should I do in situations where facilities are inadequate and inappropriate for care?
- Am I, as a single-handed occupational therapist, obliged to treat patients who have AIDS, when large numbers of non-infected patients also need treatment?
- Do I stop treatment when the patient becomes terminally ill in order to use time and resources for other patients?

(Dada and McQuoid-Mason, 2001)

The ethical rules of the healthcare professions cannot be compromised, even in a situation of reduced/scarce resources. Situations where resources such as medication, and even food, are stopped and blankets removed when the patient is seen to be dying, are however known to cause considerable distress amongst practitioners. The test will always be that of what the 'reasonable practitioner' would have done in similar circumstances. Dilemmas facing the therapist include the allocation of resources, as for example a wheelchair, to a person who may have only a few weeks to live; use of expensive splinting material for a splint which may, due to psychiatric symptomology, not be used; not having splinting material available to manufacture a much-needed splint.

Guidelines for therapists in coping with stress

Being continuously aware of the danger of infection, dealing with issues and stressful situations as mentioned, and on top of all that, still needing to function effectively and professionally within a framework of ethical and legal principles and constraints, are challenging to all health professionals. Incidence of burnout and compassion fatigue amongst health practitioners is well recorded and therapists often feel poorly equipped to deal with situations arising within and around the treatment of people with HIV/AIDS (see Chapter 14 for further information about compassion fatigue).

According to Folkman in Holland (2001, p. 82), there are two essential processes inherent in coping. The first is cognitive appraisal, which involves an individual in evaluating their coping resources and options in response to an event or situation perceived as potentially threatening or harmful. The appraisal poses and answers the question, 'What can I do?'. The second is situational appraisal. Proposed *coping mechanisms* for therapists to consider are as follows:

Collective decision making

This is recommended because the difficult decisions surrounding treatment and occupational therapy programmes for HIV/AIDS patients places a considerable responsibility and stress upon the therapist's shoulders. An example of such a decision is whether or not to terminate a treatment programme when the patient has seriously deteriorated. Taking unilateral decisions at times like this places even more stress upon the therapist. It is thus helpful to put a structure in place that enables an integrated and collective approach to decision making which can ensure compassionate but objective outcomes for the patient. Whatever decisions are taken should, if possible, be done in consultation with the patient. It is clear from a review of the literature that virtually no practical guidelines exist to assist occupational therapists or other health practitioners to cope with these dilemmas.

To facilitate collective decision making, it is advisable to form an 'advisory' team of consistent members from the various health disciplines who have experience in treating HIV/AIDS patients. Confidentiality requirements should, however, be respected. This advisory team should meet on a regular basis or as the need arises.

The process of decision making should depend upon careful scrutiny of the patient's expressed wishes, concerns of loved ones, current biopsychosocial and occupational level of functioning and the stage of the illness. It should be based upon compassionate and objective considerations which ultimately provide what is best for the patient, for example exchanging an active rehabilitation programme with a gentle diversional or palliative programme.

Support groups

As with the establishment of teams for collective decision making, it is important that support groups be established. These groups should act as a more informal opportunity at which therapists can share and ventilate day-to-day concerns, frustrations and needs and to offer support to one another, sometimes simply by providing an empathetic ear and caring response.

Support groups may also include compassion fatigue groups with colleagues, i.e. self-affirming groups where personal, interpersonal and spiritual strengths are acknowledged.

A set time should be dedicated, on a regular basis, for such support group meetings and this should be during work hours, preferably over lunch and tea breaks when therapists can relax. But if the need is great, these meetings should be extended after hours.

Try to make the atmosphere as pleasant and relaxed as possible; for example, serve tea and coffee and try putting on some gentle background music to create the ambience conducive to ventilation of inner concerns.

Elect a facilitator who must provide adequate time for each participant to express their concerns, and renegotiate additional time to complete this if the time available runs out.

Contact breaks (time out)

Another method of helping to reduce the stress of therapists who have prolonged and intensive contact with HIV/AIDS patients is to try to build in regular break periods wherein the therapist has breaks of a few weeks during which their patient load consists of non-infected patients. This may help relieve the stress of full-time contact and give the therapist 'time out' to de-stress.

Debriefing and counselling

Formal debriefing sessions should be built into the support system for all health-related staff to ensure that it is available on a regular basis. Therapists should not have to wait until they are 'burnt out', suffer compassion fatigue, or are severely traumatized before they have access to such a service. In situations where this service is not available, institutions should be encouraged to train specific staff to take on the role of counsellors and debriefers.

Mentorship/confidant system

A mentorship/confidant system should be established in which, for example, more experienced therapists can act as mentors for newly qualified therapists appointed in their departments. The formalization of such a system may provide a helpful support for therapists working in HIV/AIDS-loaded work environments. Mentors/confidants could:

- Provide a support system for ventilation of concerns (in the absence of, or to replace, support groups as described above).
- Monitor the therapists' need for debriefing and intervene when necessary.
- Encourage therapists to give expression to related thoughts and feelings, especially those which may be controversial in nature, for example, feelings of resentment towards the parents of AIDS babies.

'Ventilational' recreation

Creating an after-work recreational programme may provide the therapist with the opportunity to achieve catharsis. This could be in the form of participation in a physically demanding sport activity such as squash, jogging, aerobics or swimming which may help facilitate expression of pent-up emotions. Other ways of doing this could be involving oneself in creative activities such as art, music, writing or pottery.

Spiritual support

When one is constantly faced with death and dying, it is natural to interrogate, examine or turn to one's spiritual side. As occupational therapists, the concept of holism is entrenched within the philosophical fibre of our profession. This simply means that the inter-relationship between the mind, body and essentially, also, the 'soul' or spiritual side must be respected. This spiritual component includes personal belief in higher power(s), God(s), religions and a life force (Hammell, 2001). Apart from assuring our patient's access to spiritual support it also implies that therapists need to nurture their own spiritual resources as a strength in times of need.

Lewis in McColl (2000, p. 221), in an exploration of the meaning of pain, suggested that 'the existence of illness, disability and death challenges our view that the world is an orderly and good place'. It is in the process of searching for meanings to questions around spirituality that both the therapist and patient often turn to spiritual sources which may help them gain greater understanding and acceptance around related issues.

The entire concept of spirituality needs to be more intensively explored by occupational therapists, in terms of how it can offer comfort to the therapist through prayer, meditation and reading of relevant literature and religious teachings, which can also provide a source of considerable comfort to the patient with HIV/AIDS.

Ribeiro (2001, p. 68) maintains that:

> the bottom line is that to be client-centered you have to care about the person, you have to care about their life as if it were your own, and you have to hold their spirit in great respect.

It should be added to this that we also need to hold our own spirit in great respect and feed it and feed from it, as and when our professional–emotional life demands.

Conclusions

HIV/AIDS poses one of the greatest challenges that healthcare professionals have ever faced. By virtue of their holistic training and focus on human occupation, occupational therapists have the skills and abilities to make a significant and positive difference to the quality of life of individuals with HIV/AIDS throughout the progress of the disease process. This includes maintaining productivity and morale in the early stages, helping individuals to compensate for their decreasing strength and abilities in the middle stages and in the final stages providing opportunity for those with HIV/AIDS and their loved ones to face the final outcome with confidence and dignity.

Barbour (1994) maintains that health professionals working with HIV/AIDS cases become so preoccupied with the problematic aspects of the disease process that they forget the considerable rewards which can be involved when working with these individuals. Intellectual stimulation, job satisfaction at being able to help, admiration at the courage of many of the patients and developing specialized skills and abilities all help to make intervention worthwhile.

Questions

1. Discuss the ethical rules and principles which will apply in the following situation:

   You are referred an 18-year-old female who has become a paraplegic following a motor vehicle accident. Besides a large pressure sore on her lumbo-sacral area, which will not heal, she is motivated, has just completed matriculation and is keen to follow a career in journalism. You have arranged a place for her in the local college and she is progressing well with rehabilitation when she suddenly develops an HIV-related aseptic meningitis resulting in excruciating headaches, seizures, cognitive disturbances and behavioural changes including such low motivation that she refuses to get out of bed. Her doctor says she has little chance of surviving much longer than perhaps a few weeks.

2. What is the primary contribution of the occupational therapist to the treatment of the individual with HIV/AIDS?
3. Discuss three ways in which the occupational therapist can ensure that the autonomy of the individual/patient with HIV/AIDS is respected at all times.
4. Provide a critical evaluation of the possible value of using alternative therapies in treatment of individuals with HIV/AIDS.
5. Write a short essay on the importance of spirituality for individuals suffering from HIV/AIDS.
6. Discuss the implications of the physical sequelae of HIV/AIDS for occupational therapy intervention.
7. Discuss the implications of the psychiatric sequelae of HIV/AIDS for occupational therapy intervention.

Chapter 5
An occupational therapist's perspective on sexuality and psychosocial sexual rehabilitation

LOUISE FOUCHÉ

Sexuality is an integral part of being human (Couldrik, 1998a). When treating a client holistically the occupational therapist is therefore obliged to address the client's sexuality. Sexual rehabilitation (also described in literature as sexual counselling) has been described as part of the occupational therapist's role with physically disabled clients. Specific interventions with heart, spinal cord injured clients, multiple sclerosis, hip replacement, stroke and rheumatoid arthritis clients has been documented. However there is a lack of research and literature available on sexual rehabilitation in psychiatric clients.

The reason may be found in Williams and Wood's (1982) statement that working with mentally disabled children raises volatile ethical and social dilemmas. Couldrik (1998a) adds that society also has issues that are deterrents, for example cultural taboos, language, legal and ethical boundaries, as well as moral dilemmas. This is even more true for psychiatric clients where complex dynamics and numerous factors influence their sexuality, for example changes in libido, influence of diagnosis and medication, decreased inhibitions, poor social judgement and considered not being 'compos mentis'.

The question that arises is if occupational therapists are obliged to treat a client comprehensively and holistically, this applies to all clients, in all the different fields of occupational therapy, irrespective of the diagnosis. If the answer is 'yes', then what is an occupational therapist's scope in addressing the sexuality of psychiatric clients? Due to limited information on this subject, it is necessary to stimulate debate, share ideas and build up a body of knowledge and experience on the subject in an attempt to answer the above question and in order to ascertain what should be included in occupational therapy curricula.

Defining sexuality and sexual rehabilitation

Before considering treatment, it is important to have an understanding of the concepts of sexuality and sexual rehabilitation. Sexual rehabilitation should not be confused with sex therapy.

Sex therapy

The primary objective of sex therapy is to relieve the client's sexual dysfunction. Some sex therapists incorporate a broader objective that may include the improvement of a couple's communication and their general relationship, but ultimately all focus is on improving sexual dysfunction (Kaplan, 1974). Ultimately, therefore, sex therapy focuses on sexual intercourse and the experiencing of sexual satisfaction.

Focusing only on the biological aspect of sexual functioning is, however, not always satisfying for some disabled clients. Zola (1982), who has a physical disability, states that there is too strong a focus on sex as a capacity and technique that emphasizes 'one ability, one organ and one sensation' and neglects other components and skills influencing sexuality. A broader perspective is therefore required.

Sexuality

There are numerous different definitions of sexuality. Four definitions have been included here:

1. Kuczunski (in Turner et al., 1996, p. 205):

   Human sexuality is the complete attribute of every person, involving deep needs for identity, relationships, love and immortality. It is more than biologic, gender, physiologic processes, or modes of behaviour; it involves one's self-concept and self-esteem. Sexuality includes masculine and feminine self-image, expression of emotional states of being, and communication of feelings for others and encompasses everything that the individual is, thinks, feels or does during the entire lifespan. Sexual behaviour, more than any other behaviour, is intimately related to emotional and social well-being.

2. Chipouras et al. (in Evans, 1985, p. 664):

   an integration of physical, emotional, intellectual and social aspects of an individual's personality which expresses maleness and femaleness.

3. Greengroos (in Couldrik, 1998a, p. 493):

   sexuality concerns your way of life, the way you are treated, the way you react to other people and your own image of yourself as a human being.

4. Medlar and Medlar (in Yallop and Fitgerald, 1997, p. 53):

   sexuality is a basic, fundamental aspect of human behaviour. Sexuality is more than sexual behaviour: it encompasses one's feelings of femininity or masculinity and how one acts or dresses, speaks and relates to others within one's entire network of social and interpersonal relationships.'

The above definitions indicate how broad the concept of sexuality is and how it permeates every aspect of a human being. However, since the definition is so broad, it is important to stipulate which aspects may be viewed as sexuality in order to know which aspects to assess and treat. Bodenheimer et al. (2000) suggest that body image, psychosocial adjustment and interpersonal relationships form part of a client's sexuality. Evans (1987) implies that self-esteem, personal hygiene, appropriate social skills and grooming can be seen as part of sexuality. Couldrik (1998a) adds self-concept, social relationships, motivation and roles as part of sexuality. Fontaine (1991) identified intrapersonal and interpersonal factors required for satisfactory sexual functioning. The intrapersonal factors are: identifying, accepting responsibility and managing sexual and non-sexual feelings appropriately, positive self-esteem and accepting one's body. The interpersonal factors are: ability to communicate feelings, sharing intimacy and resolving conflict.

Sexual rehabilitation

Sexual rehabilitation can be defined as the treatment of relevant psychosocial and physiological aspects that influence sexuality.

Occupational therapists are not trained sex therapists and additional formal, specialized training is required (Miller, 1984). In contrast, according to Evans (1987) occupational therapists have the necessary knowledge and skills to provide sexual rehabilitation. These skills include the occupational therapist's ability to analyse the components and qualities of activities and find ways to adapt an activity or the environment to enhance performance. The therapist has the knowledge of the interrelated dynamics of the client's physiological, neurological, psychological and interpersonal relationship components that influence a client's sexuality (Evans, 1987). Fouché (2001) has incorporated some of the components and extended the list to include the following, which she views as sexual rehabilitation for psychiatric clients.

1. to execute good personal hygiene and grooming;
2. to exhibit a positive sexual self-image;
3. the ability to give and receive physical touch;
4. the ability to be intimate;
5. the ability to give and receive nurturing;
6. the ability to communicate effectively;
7. the ability to form healthy relationships;
8. the ability to channel sexual energy appropriately;
9. to understand factual information regarding sexually transmitted diseases and contraceptives;

10. to provide help concerning sexual adaptations;
11. to handle inappropriate sexual behaviour correctly.

Importance of sexual rehabilitation for all clients including psychiatric clients

According to numerous studies (Evans, 1985; Agnew et al., 1985; Kennedy, 1987; Novak and Mitchell, 1988; Couldrik, 1998b; Kingsley and Molineux, 2000) occupational therapists are in agreement that sexual rehabilitation should fall within an occupational therapy regime. Novak and Mitchell (1988, p.110) go so far as to state that:

> A therapist who advocates treatment designed to assist the patient in achieving the highest level of functioning but does not consider the interdependence of a patient's sexuality and his/her other areas of functioning in the treatment model, is not practicing from an occupational therapy perspective of holistic care.

Additional reasons for occupational therapists to provide sexual rehabilitation are briefly described below.

Occupational therapists ostensibly treat their clients holistically. However, there seems to be limited evidence of the incorporation of sexuality into models used by occupational therapists. In the Model of Human Occupation (1993) Kielhofner specifically excludes sexual expression as he is of the opinion that it cannot be viewed as a human activity (Couldrik, 1998b). However when reviewing the Model of Human Occupation roles are stipulated as part of the habituation subsystem. Being a wife or husband implies having specific tasks and sexual functioning could be incorporated.

In the model of Adaptation through Occupation (Reed in Couldrik, 1998b) sexual expression is included in the performance area on self-care. The Canadian Occupational Performance Model incorporates sexual needs into a physical component of a person (Couldrik, 1998b).

The World Health Organization (in Couldrik, 1998a) recognizes sexual expression, regardless of illness or disability, as a fundamental human right. Kitzinger (in Couldrik, 1998a) states that people who do not have sexual relationships are seen as abnormal. Northcott and Chard (2000) state that disability will not alter human needs for affection and intimacy. If disability prevents or inhibits the full expression of a person's sexuality or is of concern to the individual, then these needs should be addressed. The occupational therapist is the ideal team member to address them.

Sexuality is an integral part of people. Patients who avoid realistic acceptance of their own sexuality also fail to accept their disabilities (Weiss and Diamond in Agnew et al., 1985). Agnew et al. (1985) found that not only clients' attitudes but also the negative attitudes of professionals towards clients' sexuality are thought to play an important role in hindering a person's ability to adapt to physical disability.

There is a correlation between the sexual wellbeing of disabled people and life satisfaction (Gatens in Couldrik, 1998a). Satisfaction in sexual relationships is regarded as a component of a quality life. Sexual difficulties can have a profound influence on the wellbeing of the whole family (Christopher in Couldrik, 1998a).

In a study by Northcott and Chard (2000) clients explained that their condition affected their sexual functioning. They believed that they should have received sexual rehabilitation as a routine part of their healthcare and that they should not have had to seek this out themselves. The question is how much of a problem or concern is it for psychiatric clients?

Occupational therapists work with activities and enable people to engage in activities that have value, meaning and purpose for them. This is intrinsic to occupational therapy. Sexual expression can be classified as an activity and it is closely linked to social roles (Couldrik, 1998a) thus making it part of an occupational therapist's role.

Turner et al. (1996) make a case for first addressing sexuality and sexual needs as this area occurs on the lowest level of Maslow's hierarchy of needs. This implies that if the therapist wishes to provide effective treatment, she should address the client's physiological needs (these have the strongest drives) first, before addressing higher needs (for example increasing self-esteem) in treatment. The physiological needs encompass basic bodily drives such as the need for food, drink, air, sleep and sex.

According to the Occupational Therapy Practice Framework (2002) sexuality is seen as part of a client's activities of daily living. It is incorporated in the personal ADL where it is described as 'sexual activity' and 'care of personal device', i.e. contraceptives and sexual devices. When a broader perspective of sexuality is held, the following aspects of personal ADL also address sexuality, namely personal hygiene and grooming. On a level of instrumental ADL, caring for others and even communication devices use can be incorporated. Therefore for an occupational therapist to treat the client's ADL (both personal and instrumental) comprehensively, these aspects should be incorporated into standard assessment and treatment programmes.

It can be argued that if occupational therapists advocate holistic client care irrespective of the client population, and sexuality is considered as part of the scope of occupational therapists in the physical field, then it must form part of the occupational therapy treatment of psychiatric clients. There are additional unique reasons why sexual rehabilitation should be addressed in psychiatric clients.

According to the DSM-IV-TR™ (2000), the diagnostic criteria and clinical features of some psychiatric disorders, for example major depression and bipolar disorder, include a decrease in libido in the depressed client and an increase in the client's libido when in a manic state. These symptoms will have a direct influence on the client's sexuality and relationship with their partner. The majority of medications prescribed for psychiatric disorders have side effects that influence the client's libido and sexual performance. For example some antidepressants may inhibit erection in men and vaginal lubrication in women (Barrett, 1999). This can create a vicious cycle. Clients diagnosed with major depression experience poor libido and isolate themselves. The client may not understand the role played by the disorder and the medication, as they only experience the decreased libido, social isolation and the physical problems caused by the medication. The partner may not understand their partner's withdrawal and decreased libido and could feel that they are no longer attractive. The client's feelings of guilt and a sense of worthlessness are exacerbated and the partner feels hurt and rejected, which in turn influences their relationship.

It is important to note that in the United Kingdom sexual activity may be illegal for some patients, especially those unable to give consent, or detained under the Mental Health Act. For other patients, prohibiting sexual activity may violate their rights under Human Rights legislation.

In the case of South Africa, the Mental Health Care Act 2003: Chapter 3 Clause 14(1), which is based on the United Nations Charter of Human Rights, stipulates that therapists and nursing personnel will only be allowed to prevent or withhold psychiatric clients from intimate relationships if 'due to the mental illness the ability of the user to consent is diminished'. How the therapist will be able to distinguish between clients who can consent and those who cannot is still uncertain. However this clause indicates that there is a move to allow the clients more choice. This could create an increase in sexual activity in mental institutions, and psychiatric clients' sexual problems can be expected to increase.

It has been noted that psychologists and social workers are helping sexually abused clients to come to terms with their abuse, yet few are directly addressing issues like the increase in their personal space and poor sexual self-image which arise from the abuse. These aspects seem to have a negative influence on the clients' sexuality and relationships with others, especially with members of the opposite sex.

During her research Fouché (2001) discovered undignified and unacceptable case scenarios of psychiatric clients. For example a couple who were both suffering from chronic mental illness were separated as one of them became psychotic and was placed in a closed ward. They had no private facilities and were found having sexual intercourse through a wire fence.

From the above it can be seen that sexual rehabilitation is part of the occupational therapist's scope. Although this is the view held by the majority of therapists, few are actually incorporating it into their treatment since they feel unprepared for the task and explain that they do not have the necessary knowledge and skills. Agnew et al. (1985) and Couldrik (1998a) found that occupational therapists expressed their lack of confidence and doubt in their abilities to close the gap between theory and practice. However the more experience their therapists have, the more comfortable they become with providing sexual rehabilitation (Yallop and Fitzgerald, 1997). Therefore, although the need to address client sexuality has been realized, the way to go about it remains unclear.

A perspective on sexual rehabilitation

There are limited models or suggestions for sexual rehabilitation provided by occupational therapists. Neistadt (in Hopkins and Smith, 1993) proposes three sexual counselling competencies (namely awareness, knowledge and interpersonal skills) that occupational therapists should have in order to address sexual rehabilitation. Although these competencies are appropriate for clients with physical disabilities, it is still uncertain how some of them can be implemented with psychiatric clients. A brief overview will be given and it will be evaluated critically with regard to the implementation for psychiatric clients.

Awareness competencies

Sexuality is still viewed by many cultures as a private and sensitive matter and the occupational therapist should at all times be aware of her client's level of comfort on the subject. Both the occupational therapist's and the client's discomfort with sexuality will jeopardize the counselling. If the occupational therapist is acutely aware of her own attitudes and feelings she will be able to monitor her transparency more effectively.

Neistadt (in Hopkins and Smith, 1993) states:

> Therapists need to be aware of their own and society's attitudes towards sexuality, sex roles, sexual preferences, and disability. In addition therapists need to be aware of the emotional and physical needs of people with disabilities.

These awareness competencies of an occupational therapist can therefore be summarized as:

- The occupational therapist's beliefs, values and attitudes towards sexuality (as influenced by her upbringing, or societal, religious and cultural norms).
- The occupational therapist's comfort with her client's sexuality.
- The occupational therapist's comfort with sexual practices, preferences and views that differ from her own.
- The occupational therapist's views on sexual rehabilitation.

Occupational therapist's beliefs, values and attitudes towards sexuality

Diamond (in Yallop and Fitzgerald, 1997) states that values, beliefs and feelings are a result of the cultural and religious background of a society. Couldrik (1998a) states that sexual expression is enmeshed in cultural, social and emotional values. Occupational therapists should be aware of their own values and beliefs about sexuality and how they affect their relationship with their clients (Yallop and Fitzgerald, 1997).

Neistadt (in Hopkins and Smith, 1993) suggests that occupational therapists become aware of their personal attitudes towards sexuality by giving thought to the development of their own sexuality from infancy to young adulthood. The occupational therapist should reflect on the attitudes of those close to her and critically evaluate how their views influenced the development of her own attitudes today.

It is important for occupational therapists to be in touch with their own sexuality and the effects of their own experiences and confidence regarding the subject. Past personal sexual abuse and failed sexual relationships will impact on the occupational therapist's attitudes. The occupational therapist needs to reflect on these experiences.

Pizzi (1992) states that knowledge of cultural differences provides clues for healthcare providers to adapt to services accordingly. Pizzi views cultural issues and differences as including sexuality and gender roles. Johnson (in Pizzi, 1992) found that some black women in America have little or no voice in sexual matters such as refusing sex or demanding the use of condoms as, in their opinion, it can mean the loss of income or loss of housing and child care. These women were of the opinion that they had to do as a man says in order to please and satisfy him so that he would remain in the relationship. These are beliefs which indicate the difference in cultures. Some occupational therapists believe that these views are stereotypes of the female role rather than of the culture. In countries with many different cultural groups, such as South Africa, the occupational therapist should be aware of the different cultural views on sexuality. If she does not know, she should be sensitive towards differences and ask the client for clarification, especially regarding polygamy/monogamy, matriarchal/patriarchal systems and homosexuality.

Comfort with client's sexuality

Occupational therapists should be aware that clients still have needs for intimacy, affection and sexual intercourse and that a disability does not remove these needs. The occupational therapist should reflect on how she views her clients' sexuality in general and how it influences the way she relates to her clients. Fouché (2001) found that occupational therapists who feel comfortable with their psychiatric clients' sexuality are more likely to provide sexual rehabilitation than those who do not. Do occupational therapists feel more uncomfortable with a psychiatric client's sexuality than they would with a physically disabled client?

Comfort with differences

Occupational therapists should be aware of a broad spectrum of different sexual practices, different sexual preferences and different values of people. They should reflect on how their own views and values may cause them to be judgemental or prejudiced towards those with different views and values. Once again, this may render therapy ineffective and damage the therapeutic relationship.

Views on sexual rehabilitation

The occupational therapist should reflect on her own views concerning sexual rehabilitation with clients. Does she agree with it? What does she view as sexual rehabilitation? What does she consider to be boundaries or limits? What sexual rehabilitation goals would she be prepared to strive for in therapy? What would the occupational therapist consider to be 'off-limits' during sexual rehabilitation with psychiatric clients?

Knowledge competencies

Occupational therapists have the necessary knowledge and skills for sexual rehabilitation. They include knowledge of:

1. anatomy and physiology of sexual organs
2. sexual response cycle (four progressive phases on excitement, plateau, orgasm and resolution phase)
3. effects of disability on sexual functioning and sexuality
4. interrelated dynamics of physiological, neurological, psychological components and interpersonal relationships
5. activities.

There is literature available on how different physical disabilities affect the sexuality and sexual functioning of clients. There is, however, a lack of knowledge on the specific effects of psychiatric diagnosis on sexuality.

This should not deter the occupational therapist, however. They have knowledge of the signs, symptoms and clinical picture of different disorders and after an assessment can determine what performance components have been affected. This knowledge, combined with the knowledge of the interrelated dynamics, should give the occupational therapist a clear idea of possible problems that the client may experience. For example after an assessment the occupational therapist may find that her psychiatric client has cognitive problems, e.g. poor social judgement, and dispositional problems, e.g. poor drive. This will have a negative influence on the client's sexual functioning as social judgement and appropriate drive are needed for optimal sexual functioning.

Additionally, input and feedback from the client concerning his sexual problems are required and will aid the occupational therapist in identifying problems and setting up appropriate and individualized treatment goals.

Psychiatric diagnosis and medication have a direct influence on clients' sexuality and sexual performance abilities. However, additional secondary problems are likely to be spin-offs of the initial problem. Secondary problems that could develop include, for example, increased feelings of worthlessness, guilty feelings, increase in depression, and problems in the relationship and communication between the partners. Occupational therapists can expect that the increased libido of a bipolar client will have an impact on the relationships with their sexual partner.

Occupational therapists are also experts on activities and how to adapt them. Activities, as a medium of treatment, are an excellent means for addressing sexuality problems in a non-threatening way. For example, sexually abused clients who need a big personal space and who freeze up when touched can be included in games such as balloon volleyball where they can bump into others without it having a sexual connotation. The activities are then slowly graded where the intensity and frequency of appropriate social touch is increased in a non-threatening way. Later in the programme the significant other can be incorporated in the treatment.

Interpersonal skills

The most important element in sexual rehabilitation is the therapeutic relationship. If it is strong and comfortable, the client will be able to open up to the occupational therapist. However if the therapeutic relationship is strained, following the correct procedures painstakingly, it will not lead to effective therapeutic interventions. The occupational therapist should therefore reflect warmth and empathy, and be congruent at all times. According to McAlonan (1996) clients preferred therapists who were approachable, empathic, willing to listen, were adequately comfortable with sexuality and had sufficient knowledge to dispel myths and misconceptions about sexuality and disability. When the occupational therapist does feel uncomfortable, she should monitor the client's transparency and in limited cases it may be appropriate to verbalize her feelings to the client. However, absolute discretion is necessary. In some cases it would be preferable to refer the client to another therapist. Some clients with personality disorder may make sexual comments to shock or manipulate the occupational therapist. The occupational therapist should be aware of this and handle it accordingly.

The occupational therapist should be aware of counter-transference, which may manifest in inappropriate self-disclosures and invasive questioning by the therapist for unnecessary details (Foulder-Hughes, 1998).

Neistadt (in Hopkins and Smith, 1993) recommends the following:

• Acknowledge client's sexuality.

- Provide relevant information.
- Discuss sexual adaptations.

However these aspects relate mostly to physical clients and should be reviewed for the psychiatric client.

Acknowledge a client's sexuality

According to Barrett (1999) as people become more open about acknowledging the importance of sexuality in their lives, they seem more willing to seek help when there are problems.

The occupational therapist may acknowledge the subject by saying:

> People who have a similar diagnosis or use similar medication experience difficulties and have questions around their sexuality and sexual functioning. I have some information and will try to help you and answer your questions. If I do not have the answers to your questions I will find out or refer you to someone who could help you (adapted from Neistadt in Hopkins and Smith, 1993).

Alternatively Barrett (1999) suggests a more direct approach by asking 'Have you noticed any changes in your sex life as a result of your diagnosis?' (p. 3).

The occupational therapist must select any method with which she is comfortable, as long as the topic of sexual functioning is initiated. However it is important that the occupational therapist 'opens up' the topic for discussion and subtly indicates to the client that the subject is not taboo in therapy and that she is willing to help with problems. Clients may not respond immediately but will go away thinking about it or will wait until they have enough courage or until the therapeutic relationship is more defined to broach the subject.

In a study by McAlonan (1996) clients stressed the need to know what options are available to them during sexual rehabilitation. Occupational therapists should therefore explain the options available and then allow them to make choices.

Provide relevant information

Due to limited research and literature it is more difficult to ascertain what would be considered as relevant information for psychiatric clients. Whether clients are acute or chronic, their remaining cognitive abilities and their diagnosis will make a difference in determining relevant information. The method of providing the information may also differ for a psychiatric client. Possible methods include presenting groups with themes of 'Strengthening my marriage relationship' or 'Explaining my diagnosis to my husband/wife/partner' or 'Communicating sensitive issues' for higher-functioning clients. Didactic groups for clients and their partners on the depression, what it is, how it influences sexual performance, etc., may be presented by the doctor or nursing personnel. The multidisciplinary team could make different pamphlets available on the subject. The occupational therapist will have to use her discretion as to what is considered relevant information for each individual client.

A therapist's personality traits, body language, affect and attitude influence the client's receptiveness, confidence and amount of disclosure and level of satisfaction regarding information received. Clients prefer direct open communication where information was provided in a matter-of-fact way. The therapist's willingness to listen and answer questions is emphasized (McAlonan, 1996).

General counselling skills are valuable in sexual rehabilitation. Sometimes merely talking about the problems helps; in other words unburdening by expressing the problems to an empathic ear can be curative. The occupational therapist should at all times be aware of the clients' feelings and boundaries and must be sensitive when they become uncomfortable. Once again the importance of the therapeutic relationship is stressed, over and above the information provided.

Discussion on sexual adaptations

Because of the nature of psychiatric disorders, which include problems with cognition, disposition and affect, adaptations of a physical nature are limited. The occupational therapist may have to work more closely with the partners and explain to them how they could compensate. However, this in itself may cause a problem, since the partner is then changing role from that of an equal to more of a 'therapist/parent' situation, which is not always acceptable for the partner in a sexual relationship and may cause strain. Occupational therapists should discuss what would be considered sexual adaptations for psychiatric clients.

Assessments

There are limited assessments within the occupational therapist's role that will specifically assess clients' sexuality and sexual functioning. However, the following should form part of the assessment.

The occupational therapist should initiate the subject early on in the assessment. Once she has initiated the subject and acknowledged her client's sexuality, the client should be asked to complete the Canadian Occupational Performance Measure (Law et al., 1998). As it is unstructured and clients identify their own priorities, they will feel more comfortable listing sexual functioning problems, if of course there are problems present. If the problem is beyond the scope of an occupational therapist, the client may be referred to either a psychologist or a sex therapist. Additionally the therapist should assess the client's personal and instrumental ADL as well as the performance components as part of a standard assessment.

Woods (1984) suggests that the clients explain their current problems concerning their sexual functioning and give a brief sexual history comparing their sexual functioning before and after the onset of their disability. It is important to determine what the clients consider to be normal for them. Northcott and Chard (2000) state that 'sexuality is a unique and individual state' and therefore generalizations are inappropriate. It must be stressed that the occupational therapist cannot use her values or beliefs as the norm.

There are some questionnaires that may be filled in by clients. The mental health portfolio has two tests, namely the Golombok Rust Inventory of Sexual Satisfaction and the Golombok Rust Inventory of Marital State (Milne, 1992). There is a separate questionnaire for males and females. However, clients need to have insight in order for the questionnaires to be of value. These can therefore only be used for higher-functioning clients.

Treatment categories

Fouché (2001) identified 11 categories of sexuality that the occupational therapist could address, depending on what problems are identified in the assessment. These categories could also be assessed separately.

As mentioned previously these categories could be debated and critically evaluated.

To execute good personal hygiene and grooming

Psychiatric clients with severe disorders or chronic clients often display problems concerning their grooming and personal hygiene. Once again occupational therapists do address this aspect during the treatment of personal ADL, but explaining the relevance to the clients' sexuality and relationships is often neglected.

Neistadt (in Hopkins and Smith, 1993) suggests that one way to acknowledge the client's sexuality is by complimenting him/her on a new haircut or nail care or a particular blouse, as this is a means of letting clients know that they are still attractive and appealing as people. The occupational therapist working with psychiatric clients may also use this intervention to acknowledge their sexuality. During the research done by Fouché (2001), an occupational therapist explained how she helped a transvestite to apply make-up appropriately as part of his treatment, as it was a priority identified by the client.

To exhibit a positive sexual self-image

Self-image is the worth that a client ascribes to him/herself. Disability has a negative impact on clients' self-esteem (Novak and Mitchell, 1988). A sexual self-image is the worth they ascribe to themselves as sexual beings.

Fontaine (1991) identifies positive self-esteem and acceptance of one's body as important intrapersonal factors that contribute to a healthy sexual relationship.

Do clients view themselves as attractive people? How do they feel about themselves in the company of other sexual beings? Attractiveness does not indicate the presence of beauty, as someone who may not be physically beautiful may still view themselves as an attractive person with qualities they can share with someone in a meaningful relationship. When treating the above aspects the therapist may select non-threatening activities and then upgrade them.

Self-respect is an aspect that needs to be addressed when dealing with sexuality. This entails self-worth, attractiveness and an acceptance of self in the environment in which they live. Often self-respect is not considered with the psychiatric client. This needs to become an intrinsic experience of self, which can be discussed with the aid of the self-respect and sexuality interconnections diagram. Figure 5.1 was used successfully with street children from the Hillbrow area in Johannesburg, South Africa.

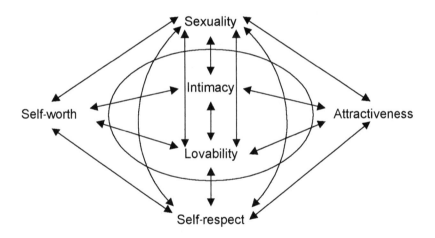

Figure 5.1 Self-respect and sexuality interactions (Alers and de Freitas, 2003, adapted from Pedretti, 2001)

The ability to give and receive physical touch

Studies done with children in children's homes have shown how important touch is to people. Another example of the importance of touch was shown in a study of the rate of development of premature babies who were stroked by nursing personnel for 15 minutes a day compared with those who were not stroked (Siegel, 1989). As being touched is such a basic human need, this does not cease due to a psychiatric disorder.

Fontaine (1991) identifies touch as an interpersonal factor that may be viewed as a means of communication within a sexual relationship. When people are not touched, it leads to a loss of intimacy that is integral in the symptoms of depression, anxiety and stress (Couldrik, 1998b).

When last have chronic psychiatric clients and geriatric clients in institutions been touched? It goes without saying that the touch given by caregivers should always be socially appropriate.

Another example is clients who suffer from tactile defensiveness. Partners are unable to understand that clients experience discomfort when touched and thus interpret this as rejection, which leads to conflict in relationships. This in turn leads to problems in their sexual relationships.

After sexual abuse the client is often alarmed by touch. This needs to be discussed and normalized, with the client explaining that it is a normal reaction to the abuse. The reaction needs to be discriminated from tactile defensiveness. The partner needs to be aware of the client's reaction and the reasons so that they can work through the problem together.

The ability to be intimate

Fontaine (1991) identified sharing intimacy as an important interpersonal factor required when forming sexual relationships. She states that establishing intimacy in a relationship conveys comfort, reassurance, support and consolation. Intimacy may be categorized into emotional and physical intimacy.

Kaplan (1974) states that sexual symptoms and sexual abandonment of schizophrenic clients serve as a defence against intimacy which guards the emergence of a psychosis. The occupational therapist should therefore be careful and not address intimacy in schizophrenic clients.

The ability to give and receive nurturing

Being nurtured is a basic human need and the most likely way to be nurtured is to be touched. Psychiatric clients, like all human beings, have a need to be nurtured, yet this need is not being addressed in institutions. Nurturing may be divided up into emotional and physical nurturing. Aspects of both giving and receiving nurturing should be evaluated. Occupational therapists can address this aspect successfully within a patient's treatment plan and by making use of non-threatening activities. It is often the small things that make people feel nurtured.

The ability to communicate

Intimacy is established through effective communication (Masters in Barrett, 1999). Occupational therapists may therefore also address effective communication as part of sexual rehabilitation.

Numerous problems exist because people find it difficult to express themselves and communicate with others. Talking about sex can be threatening, particularly when people fear that it may lead to rejection, to loss of spontaneity or to increased tension in a relationship already strained by disability (Barrett, 1999). Clients are afraid they will hurt their partners and thus keep quiet. Communicating effectively about different topics, including non-sexual and sexual issues, is raised in almost all books on enhancing sexual relationships.

As psychiatric clients experience problems communicating about everyday non-threatening subjects, more intimate and sensitive subjects are even more difficult to discuss. Their poor self-image intensifies their fears of rejection. Using role-play an occupational therapist could assist a client to verbalize how much he loves his wife and in this way address these issues.

Occupational therapists present life skills groups to clients and often include assertiveness training, yet few occupational therapists make the link to sexuality. The occupational therapist should indicate to the client that they could be assertive when the partner wants sexual intercourse and they do not. The client will then be able to refuse without feeling guilty yet still show respect, however, cultural issues also need to be considered. In addition occupational therapists may address conflict management; according to Fontaine (1991) the ability to resolve conflict is an interpersonal factor for healthy sexual relationships.

The ability to form healthy relationships

Mannion (1996) found that marriages affected by mental illness have a higher rate of divorce and separation. He also found that clients suffering from mental illness experienced feelings of social isolation, experienced less display of affection and reported sexual problems and even a complete lack of sexual relationships.

Schover and Jensen (in Barrett, 1999) identified four 'couple skills' that are important to a well-functioning relationship. These skills are:
1. *Allocating roles*: Schover and Jensen (in Barrett, 1999) describe it as:

> Flexibility in sharing tasks and functioning in ways that avoid a parent–child type of interaction between partners and fostering opportunities for private adult time away from the demands of daily routine.

Novak and Mitchell (1988) found that there were changes in clients' roles and responsibilities in the family unit which lead to insecurities and questions needing attention.
2. *Respecting boundaries*: Couples develop a fluctuating balance between intimacy and autonomy, between the need for closeness and the need for privacy. However a disability may disrupt the balance the couple had previously and this may need to be re-established.
3. *Communication styles*: The need for and importance of communication about sexual and non-sexual issues has been discussed above. Schover and Jensen (in Barrett, 1999) add that with a disability, clients can make use of four defence mechanisms that could influence their communication. They are: withdrawal, passive acceptance, projection and denial.

4. *Relationship rules*: Couples need to agree on rules in their relationship. Example of these rules could be: 'We make a commitment that our relationship will not be threatened by conflicts and that we will resolve them when this occurs'. Couples may need to be encouraged and supported in making new relationship rules after a disability.

The issue of relationships is a broad subject. The multidisciplinary team may treat this aspect together, as all have unique skills and contributions. The social worker and psychologist may make use of marital and family therapy. Intrapersonal problems may be addressed in psychotherapy, as these influence the client's ability to form healthy relationships. This goal may take years to accomplish, depending on the client's psychiatric disorder, his prognosis and insight. Some life skills training groups presented by occupational therapists also address relationship skills.

To channel sexual energy appropriately

Chronic clients may have poor social judgement and fewer inhibitions yet have normal sexual impulses. Psychiatric institutions in most countries do not have private facilities for these clients to have sexual intercourse, due to all the practical, ethical and moral problems. One of the ways that occupational therapists working with chronic clients use to overcome this problem, is to try to channel the clients' sexual energy by including physical activities in the programmes during the afternoons. This however only addresses the symptom in the short term.

To understand factual information regarding sexually transmitted diseases and contraception

All factual information regarding the client's sexuality, including the influence of their medication and diagnosis, information on sexuality transmitted diseases and contraceptives, is included in this category. Fouché (2001) initially did not consider this as part of the occupational therapists' role and was of the opinion that the nursing personnel or doctors were the appropriate multidisciplinary team members for the task. Fouché found, however, that occupational therapists working in psychiatric institutions are the team members who provide information on HIV and are also distributing condoms.

The reasons for this, as suggested by Fouché (2001), were that the clients have a closer relationship with the occupational therapists, from whom they receive daily treatment. This coincides with Novak and Mitchell's (1988) statement that clients were most comfortable discussing sexual issues with team members with whom they had a greater amount of daily contact time as there was more time for the discussion. This gave them a better opportunity to develop a more comfortable relationship, which aided in a frank and open discussion on their sexuality concerns. Evans and Asreal (in Foulder-Hughes, 1998) shared this opinion, and believe that occupational therapists were frequently the first members of the team to whom a survivor of sexual abuse entrusted the details of their experience.

Providing help concerning sexual adaptations

Although sexual adaptations are prominent in treatment of physically disabled clients, these are very limited in psychiatric clients. An occupational therapist who treats clients who have undergone sex changes helps them to compensate in subtle ways and teaches them how to sit, talk, walk, eat, etc., as a person of their new gender. The occupational therapist needs to consider what other sexual adaptations would be applicable to psychiatric clients.

Handling inappropriate sexual behaviour correctly

Although handling inappropriate sexual behaviour correctly is not directly an aspect of sexual rehabilitation that can be treated, occupational therapists should still be aware of the impact it has on their clients. The socially appropriate norm of society should be upheld and when clients show sexually inappropriate behaviour the occupational therapist should explain to them that this is not acceptable. Belittling or laughing and patronizing clients for sexually inappropriate behaviour is not professional and may reinforce unhealthy views the client has of sexuality.

Neistadt (in Hopkins and Smith, 1993) proposes that one of the possible reasons for clients to present with sexually inappropriate behaviour is precisely a means of showing their frustration at not having their sexuality acknowledged.

Additional thoughts on sexual rehabilitation

There are some thoughts that need to be mentioned and clarified concerning the occupational therapist's role in sexual rehabilitation with psychiatric clients.

Research

Although sexual rehabilitation with physically disabled clients has been described, there is limited information on the occupational therapist's role in sexual rehabilitation with psychiatric clients. Although the role of sexual rehabilitation is defined as part of occupational therapy, irrespective of the client group, there are still unique differences between physical and psychiatric clients and these need to be further researched. Additionally, there seems to be a distinct difference between acute and chronic clients, and the methods of intervention concerning sexual rehabilitation with these two client groups will differ. In order to define the differences, occupational therapists are once again encouraged to write up and publish their experiences.

Acknowledging sexuality during daily treatment

Occupational therapists are addressing some of the categories mentioned above in life skills training programmes or additional treatment, yet the majority do not extend it one step further and make the overt link to their clients' sexuality. Although some clients may make the link and generalize the information to different functional areas of their life, it cannot be expected that all clients will have the insight to make the link themselves.

When occupational therapists relate these skills to clients' sexuality, they are providing sexual rehabilitation. As sexuality is part of being human, it is not always necessary to treat it in isolation, but to ensure it is overtly acknowledged and integrated into daily treatment sessions. This may be considered as directly treating the client's functioning.

Including partners in treatment of sexual rehabilitation

It is important to remember that the majority of clients are either in a relationship or in search of a person with whom to form a relationship (Barrett, 1999). If the client is in a stable relationship, their partner must be included in a sexual rehabilitation programme (Fontaine, 1991; Edmans, 1998), irrespective of the client's sexual preference. Fouché (2001) described how an occupational therapist provided a home programme for a couple in order to address their ability to be emotionally nurturing to each other. However it worked only when the partner was also included. It is important to get permission from the client before contacting the partner.

Mannion (1996) suggests that therapists be proactive and establish a working alliance with these clients' partners. He noted that inviting a partnership also validated the spouse's contribution, which in turn enhanced the resilience of the client with mental illness.

Networking and supervision

Fouché (2001) found that occupational therapists have a great need to discuss their clients' sexuality and problems that they have experienced.

Fouché has raised numerous thought-provoking questions, which warrant serious consideration. For example, should there be facilities available for chronic clients to have sexual intercourse in privacy? When a forensic client, who committed a sexual offence, is admitted, is it necessary to address his sexual issues before his discharge? Should occupational therapists or nursing staff just hand out condoms to chronic clients, knowing they possibly do not have the insight to use them at the appropriate time to prevent spreading sexually transmitted diseases? Although there are no clear-cut answers, it is important for occupational therapists to debate these issues, and to talk to and share ideas with each other.

Due to the sensitive nature of this issue it is even more important for occupational therapists on all levels to ensure that they receive regular supervision and support when they provide this service.

Limitations for occupational therapists

Occupational therapists should recognize their limitations as occupational therapists-in-the-field and know when to refer the client. What would the occupational therapist's limitation be?

First, occupational therapists should not view sexual rehabilitation in isolation (Couldrik, 1998a), meaning that they should not focus solely on the client's sexual functioning and make that the only goal in treatment. It is an area that needs to be addressed within a wider, holistic treatment regime. It is interesting to note that Monga et al. (1998) found that the more actively clients were performing household chores, outdoor work and social functioning, the better their sexual functioning was. Occupational therapists should therefore remember that sexuality permeates every part of the client's being and realize that improving general functioning could improve sexual functioning. However, it is important not to assume that all problems will be solved when focusing only on general functioning.

Second, all sexual dysfunctions as classified by the DSM-IV-TR™ (2000), for example voyeurism and fetishism, are beyond the occupational therapists' scope. Clients who have mainly biological dysfunctions that cause sexual problems, for example premature ejaculation, impotence, orgasmic dysfunction, vaginismus, etc., should be referred.

Lastly, if the occupational therapist is so uncomfortable with the issue of sexuality that she will be untherapeutic or will cause damage, then she should refer the client to someone else.

Curricula and training

In order to stop the feeling of discomfort or incompetence in the occupational therapists with regard to sexual rehabilitation, it must be incorporated into the existing occupational therapy curricula. It was found that providing students with training improved their attitude and level of comfort concerning sexuality, as well as increasing their knowledge (Payne et al., 1988; McAlonan, 1996; Couldrik, 1998b; Hay et al., 1996; Agnew et al., 1985). The exact nature and depth of information that needs to be included in the curricula remain unclear (Agnew et al., 1985). Continued educational training should also be provided to therapists working in the field (McAlonan, 1996).

Conclusion

Sexuality is an integral part of all human beings, irrespective of their disability. Occupational therapists are obliged to address their clients' sexuality and sexual problems if they truly practise from a holistic framework. Psychiatric clients are expected to have problems in these areas due to the nature of their disabilities. As a rule of thumb, the occupational therapist therefore needs to assess and provide sexual rehabilitation. In whatever way she accomplishes it, it must be accompanied with sensitivity, within a stable therapeutic relationship, where the therapist is aware of her attitudes towards her own and her client's sexuality. It is an area of occupational therapy that needs to be researched and extended in order for occupational therapists to address the needs of their clients adequately and by so doing will improve their functioning.

Questions

1. Give your own definition of sexuality and sexual rehabilitation.
2. *Sexual rehabilitation is viewed as part of the occupational therapist's role.* Support this statement by making use of appropriate examples and arguments.
3. *Sexuality and sexual rehabilitation are as necessary for psychiatric clients as they are for clients with physical disabilities.* Express your views on this statement.
4. Describe how an occupational therapist would acknowledge her client's sexuality during treatment.
5. Briefly describe the aspects you would address when providing sexual rehabilitation to a psychiatric client.
6. Explain the limitations of occupational therapists regarding the provision of sexual rehabilitation.
7. Reflect on your attitudes, briefs and values regarding your own and your psychiatric clients' sexuality. Contemplate how this would influence your therapeutic relationship with clients.

Chapter 6
Community-based occupational therapy in psychiatry and mental health

STEPHANIE HOMER

This chapter is based on the philosophy and practice developed by the Community Rehabilitation Research and Education Programme (CORRE) of the University of the Witwatersrand, Johannesburg, together with the rehabilitation staff and people of Limpopo Province, South Africa. Throughout the chapter the occupational therapist may be seen as having the role of service developer and clinician, or service developer and educator and manager of the auxiliary staff and people carrying out the day-to-day intervention, or as the consultant on disability rights and rehabilitation for community organizations that wish to address the needs of people with disability. The role the occupational therapist takes on in practice will depend on the resources and manpower available within the health service and community in which the occupational therapist works.

The purpose of community-based rehabilitation (CBR) is to create culturally appropriate prevention and intervention services that reach the largest number of people in the most cost-effective way (Lysack and Kaufert, 1994).

Therefore in community settings the questions the therapist should ask are:

- What are the local mental health needs?
- Does the existing mental health service fulfil these needs or does it need to change?
- What type of service will benefit the most people?
- Where should the service be so that people can access it easily?
- What is the best use of the available resources?

Whilst the first steps in developing CBR may be to have the needs of those with mental disability recognized and some basic services offered at the community level, the ultimate aim is to ensure that families and communities recognize the rights of those with disability and accept the concept of equality (Mendis, 1994). Therefore the CBR service programmes should include: mobilizing the community to promote mental health and accept and integrate those with mental disability, ensuring equal access to mental health services, and transferring knowledge and skills to people with mental disabilities so that they can cope better with their daily life. Table 6.1 provides the framework for the information presented in this chapter.

Table 6.1 Components of a CBR service

Programme component	Expected outcome	Principles and approaches	Questions
Equality within the Rehabilitation Service	A rehabilitation service that is: • *Appropriate* to the common local needs • *Acceptable* to local culture and the health service provider • Equally distributed throughout the area and easily *accessible* with regard to time and transport • *Affordable* to the consumer, the community, and the health service provider	• Needs Analysis for the area • Strategic Planning for CBR • Community participation • Analysis of cost effectiveness	• Have I asked people what they need? • Am I aware of local culture and traditions? • Is there a plan for the development of CBR? • Were all the stakeholders involved in the plan? • Are people excluded from CBR due to lack of knowledge or poor coverage? • Is this the most efficient way to work?
Transfer of knowledge and skills to individuals, families and the community	• Individuals and families understand their mental health problems and have skills to cope with the problems • People in the community have skills to participate in planning and monitoring community mental health services	• Needs analysis at the family level • Education • Goal-setting • Problem-solving skills • Participation in activities	• What is important for this family? • Does the consumer/family/community feel in control? • Will change continue after I leave?

Table 6.1 contd.

Programme component	Expected outcome	Principles and approaches	Questions
Mobilize the community to promote mental health and prevent mental illness	• Ordinary people have a better understanding of mental health and illness • Community leaders support and develop mental health services • Organizations actively promote mental health and try to prevent mental illness	• Health promotion • Community participation • Leadership development • Intersectoral approach	• Has the prevalence of mental health problems changed? • Is CBR an 'agenda item'? • Is there a champion for CBR in the community? • Which organizations are involved in CBR?
Mobilize the community to accept and integrate those with mental health problems	• People with mental health problems are included in family life • People with mental health problems are included in local schools, recreation activities, places of work, and community events • People with mental health problems and their families are active participants in support groups	• Education • Activity participation • Education • Intersectoral approach • Activity participation • Group development • Leadership development	• Does the consumer feel accepted by the family? • Does the consumer feel they are free to participate in community activities? • Can the support group continue without me? • Can the support group lobby for change in the community?

What are the local mental health needs?

The success of the CBR service in any country is dependent on the appropriate assessment of needs, and a needs analysis (Department of Health, 1997a and 2000). Funding is usually based on information on the prevalence of health problems, and the problem distribution throughout the district, i.e. the medical needs. A more detailed analysis of local health needs would include an understanding of the effects of the mental health problems on the consumer, their family and community and the needs that arise from this. In addition the health service provider and the health professionals will have needs. Research results from other areas can be applied to communities as long as there is a 'near match' to the sample population and their existing health structures.

Whenever needs are identified people start to have expectations for the future. The priority need of a person with mental disability may be the love and understanding of their family and they may expect the occupational therapist to align with them against the family. The family's priority need may be for the person who is mentally disabled to contribute to the productivity of the family by looking after the home, so that others can go to work, or by earning money. Their expectation of the occupational therapist may be to ensure that the client works. The community leaders may be more concerned with protecting the community and need to confine the people with mental disabilities so that they do not endanger the property and health of others. The occupational therapist may need the client, family and community to understand the causes of mental disability and treatment and expect that this knowledge will increase compliance with treatment and acceptance by the community.

How many people require a mental health service and how do you find them?

Establishing the numbers of people requiring a service is essential for appropriate services to be planned. Research indicates that the majority (97%) of people living in a rural community know someone with mental illness (Masilela and MacLeod, 1998). Participatory Rapid (or Rural) Appraisal (PRA) mapping is an appropriate tool to help community members identify people with mental illness, especially those who are not using the mental health services. Mapping is a rapid, practical activity that most people enjoy and should be done with a variety of community groups in order to get a comprehensive map of those people who may need services. A youth group may know of young people with problems with alcohol- or school-related stress, whereas mothers attending the antenatal clinics would be more likely to recognize post-partum disorders and young children with learning problems. In urban areas it may be more appropriate for the occupational therapist to do mapping with a street or ward committee, teachers, a local church group or clinic nurses. If the occupational therapist already has access to a group of people who are disabled, e.g. a self-help group or people attending a daycare centre, mapping may still be used to find others who do not use rehabilitation services.

Mapping can also be used to identify existing service delivery points throughout the district such as state health services, disabled people's organizations and informal health services. The map of the existing services can then be compared to the areas of greatest need.

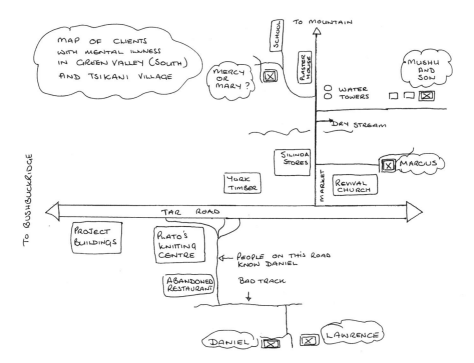

Figure 6.1 A map showing how to find clients in a rural area. This was part of a larger map drawn by people with disabilities. The people were invited to meet the therapists and attend the mapping meeting by advertising through the local church and radio station.

Mapping uses community knowledge and is a way to initiate relationships with community members. Involving community leaders such as a Ward Committee or local tribal office can be the first step in making the community aware of the needs of people with mental disability and creating political involvement in the future CBR service. The important thing to remember with mapping is that you go to the community – the community does not come to you. That way you start to understand the context of the community in which you are working.

Other ways to find people with mental disabilities are:

- Ask the local clinic sisters for a list.
- Attend the 'psychiatric clinic day' when all the people with mental illness and epilepsy come for repeat prescriptions.
- Get referrals from the District Hospital.
- Advertise a 'Meet and Greet' session over the radio (make sure you choose an easy to remember day and venue).
- Do a household survey (this may be the most inclusive way to find people but it is expensive and time-consuming).

Follow up with either a home visit or by advertising a meeting. This initial contact should be used to ensure that possible consumers and their families are aware of their rights, and have information about the CBR services, as well as to begin the process of identifying specific consumer and family needs. Such an approach increases people's access to CBR services.

How many people and what types of disabilities will you find?

Information on the prevalence and impact of disability is required to plan appropriate CBR services, especially when the service needs additional health resources or the redistribution of these resources at district level. Table 6.2 gives some figures on the prevalence of mental health problems.

Table 6.2 Prevalence of mental health problems and mental disabilities

	WHO	South Africa	Developing countries	Most prevalent problems
National	12% (2001)	3.4% nationally (CASE, 1999)	0.6–1.2% mental disability (Mendis, 1994)	Strange behaviour 0.1–0.2%, learning 0.2–0.4% and epilepsy 0.3–0.6%*
Mental health problems				
Moderate to severe mental disability (all ages)		2% in rural South Africa (Concha and Lorenzo, 1993)		Intellectual/ learning disabilities; epilepsy and alcohol-related problems (Concha and Lorenzo, 1993)
Childhood disability		Intellectual impairment 2.2%–3.3% of childhood disability (Kromberg et al., 1997)		
Adult				Schizophrenia and epilepsy (Modiba et al., 2000)

*Whilst epilepsy is a neurological condition, historically it has been treated by the psychiatric team.

Prevalence figures do not necessarily reflect the occupational therapist's caseload. The reason for the difference between prevalence and actual caseload is that those most likely to need mental health services are the people with learning disabilities or severe forms of mental illness. Their disabilities are extremely debilitating and result in them having few inner resources to cope with living without support in the community. Once on your caseload they may need services over several months or years. Some mental health problems, such as depression, alcoholism and dementia, may not be perceived as illnesses. Stress and depression may be masked by physical symptoms and not recognized by the general practitioner or clinic nurse as needing mental health services. Therefore, although prevalent, they may not be referred for occupational therapy.

The DALY (Disability Adjusted Life Years) Scale by Murray and Lopez (1994) may be used to show that people with chronic disability require a greater percentage of health resources whereas typically mental health problems rank fairly low when resources are allocated according to prevalence.

Common problems

What are the most common problems experienced by people with mental illness living in the community, and what are the communities' most common problems about living with people with mental illness?

Mental health problems impact on all areas of the person's life, and the life of their family. Difficulties may be noted in completing roles at home, work and school, or with friends and the community. People with severe mental disability often cannot hold down a job or complete regular tasks within the home. Their behaviour may be erratic and socially inappropriate, and this may result in them being ostracized by the community or by their own family. Therefore the needs of the consumer, family and community are to be considered during the needs analysis. Common needs can be identified through quantitative research, but qualitative research such as focus group discussion and PRA tools (Venn diagrams and matrix ranking) provide quick information. Occupational therapists should not assume they know the needs of the consumers. A simple PRA exercise like that reported by Petrick et al. (1999) showed that occupational therapists and consumers prioritized different needs, did not talk the same 'language' (leading to misunderstanding about priorities) and occupational therapists ignored the expressed needs of the consumers.

What are the consumers' needs?

In one rural South African area the highest-ranking problems identified by the consumers at a psychiatric clinic and their caregivers were the financial burden of paying for traditional and Western healthcare (95%), the difficult behaviour of the client (85% of caregivers), disruption of daily routine (including income generation of caregivers) and conflict within the family (Masilela and MacLeod, 1998). The majority of caregivers identify difficult behaviour as aggression, verbal abuse, lack of cooperation, roaming the streets and not heeding the advice of the family. Caregivers and many clients in rural African communities did not know the cause of the illness (Masilela and MacLeod, 1998). The economic and social burden on the family is fourfold: loss of income and roles of the person with illness, loss of potential income and increase in role responsibility of the major caregiver, increase in medical care costs, e.g. travel to clinics, traditional healer charges, and loss of social support in the community due to beliefs about the cause and spread of mental illness.

Families would like help with:

A cure	32.5%
Financial assistance or grant	17.5%
Transport to hospital/clinic	15%
Advice on handling	15%

Sadly, only 10 per cent of caregivers reported that they got help from health personnel (Masilela et al., 1996); they were more likely to receive advice from community members (Masilela and MacLeod, 1998).

What are the needs of the community?

Work with the broader community is not seen as a traditional role of the occupational therapist but it is essential in order to promote mental health and integrate those with mental disability into the community in which they live. Mental disability is identified if the behaviour of the person is outside the acceptable *social* behaviour norms for that community; therefore needs may reflect local culture and local knowledge of health. Communities have to deal with inappropriate behaviour at community gatherings, also damage to property, aggression and assault (Masilela et al., 1996). Possible reasons for such extreme behaviour are that the early signs of illness are not recognized, there is poor treatment compliance, or traditional interventions are tried first. Traditional African beliefs link the signs and symptoms of mental disability with witchcraft (often associated with the belief that it is caused by someone jealous of you), or the wrath of the ancestors (because you have done something wrong or immoral), or with a professional calling. Hallucinations may be interpreted as the ancestors calling the person to become a traditional healer or that the person is possessed by the Holy Spirit and should become a church prophet. They may be sent for training in these skills. Ordinary people have very little knowledge of Western medicine. The treatment of choice is usually a traditional healer (Freeman, 1992; CASE, 1995) who is an expert in herbal medicine, interpreting the spirits of the ancestors, or the will of the gods/God. Use of herbalists and spiritual healers, and consultation with the dead, are not confined to African cultures. Many people in developed countries seek help from revivalist churches, alternative therapies (herbal remedies, vitamin supplements, acupuncture), mystics and fortune-tellers.

Limited research has been done on the needs of the broader community. Educating the public about the causes and types of illness and how to behave towards people with mental disability have been identified as appropriate ways to increase early detection of disability and acceptance within the community. Greater visibility of the mental health services was requested, as were recognition of traditional healers and the development of local centres for people with mental disability. Community leaders accepted that they had a role to play in meeting each of these needs. Ordinary people recognized that they could offer social or emotional support and financial support (often through donations of goods) to families affected by mental disability (Masilela et al., 1996; Modiba et al., 2000).

Some community groups need more help than others, specifically communities that are predominantly indigenous, poor, have a high prevalence of chronic medical disease or are exposed to a high level of stress through violence or disasters (WHO, 2001b).

Service provider needs

Service providers need to develop and follow national policies for mental health, use technology appropriate for the primary care level and provide cost-effective services. To run an appropriate CBR service and access resources effectively occupational therapists have to be aware of policy documents and use these to motivate for changes in local service delivery. However, 40% of countries do not have a mental health policy (WHO, 2001b). Lack of policy and standards results in inefficient health programmes. In South Africa this is clearly illustrated in official policy documents. Mental illness and disability are identified as priority national health programmes and the development of community mental health services is a specific goal (Department of Health, 1997a), but policy documents on rehabilitation at clinic level (Department of Health, 2000) do not mention services for people with mental health problems. Small wonder, then, that CBR services are difficult to establish in many countries.

Even when policies are in place a situational analysis is essential for planning and budgeting services (WHO, 2001b). This should cover the needs analysis, as well as an analysis of the resources and funding available, other health providers in the area, where services are offered (coverage) and what services are used or rejected by the consumers (WHO, 2001b). Many countries cannot afford specialist mental health programmes at primary healthcare level so the philosophy of CBR is to look at the common needs of all people with disability and develop programmes to help everyone (Mendis, 1994). Occupational therapists, therefore, have mixed caseloads and services for those with mental disabilities are unlikely to be prioritized.

Understanding how the local community functions can be vital for the success of CBR, even at the individual and family level. All communities are rich in resources that may help and support the client, their family and the occupational therapist. It is important to build up a network of contacts directly and indirectly related to health. Also there is a variety of power structures which drive community projects, provide access to funds and bestow recognition or support for health projects, or on an individual health worker. It is important to identify these structures and to work with them. Mapping may tell you what structures are present and where they meet and PRA tools such as Venn diagrams and matrix ranking can be used to find out more about the activities, power and influence of community structures.

A good analysis of needs and situation will provide the occupational therapist with a greater awareness of local and national politics and consumer needs. It will make the community and consumers aware of the CBR service, and will provide the occupational therapist with a number of useful contacts in the community. Throughout the process consumers, community members and health service staff will develop expectations about the future CBR service. Great care should be taken to ensure that everybody understands that needs will be prioritized, not all of the expressed needs will be met in the short term, and that solutions should be realistic in terms of technology, personnel and funds. Once the analysis is complete it should become part of the community profile document maintained within the department, and the service providers, consumers and community should be informed of the results. This formal community profile is a useful document for the District Information System.

Appropriate service programmes to address needs

An appropriate CBR service would include the following:

- mobilizing the community to be active participants in mental health
- education about mental health and disability
- information about how to access local health resources
- the development of healthy lifestyles for clients and the broader community
- early detection of people with mental disabilities
- training in activities of daily living
- training in handling difficult behaviour
- access to finance.

Programmes should follow national policy and incorporate the principles of equity, appropriate technology, community participation and multisectoral interaction (WHO, 1978). As each district has different CBR service needs the services in one district will differ from those in a neighbouring district, and the service in one country may differ from those of its neighbours. It is essential for each district to identify priority unmet needs – the gap between what is available and what is needed – and plan how to meet these needs. All service programmes should be monitored and evaluated (WHO, 2001b).

Mobilizing the community to participate in the CBR service

Community knowledge and skills are essential components of successful CBR programmes (Mendis, 1994) and the importance of community participation cannot be emphasized enough. Participation should include being part of planning and monitoring the CBR service, promoting mental health and the prevention of mental disability within their own family or organization, and accepting the participation of people with mental disability in community organizations and events. Mobilizing the community to be active participants in CBR will take time and is often one of the most frustrating aspects of CBR. The broader community may not expect to be actively involved in CBR. Community leaders and organizations and families of those with mental disability may be resistant to participate because the occupational therapist is the expert paid to deal with the mental health problems. They may have very limited expectations of what the CBR service can provide – particularly if they have seen projects started but not finished by other workers. Finally, many communities have had little education or opportunity to develop leadership skills and simply do not know what to do. This is particularly true of people living in poor areas or developing countries.

The first steps to mobilize the community are:

- health promotion about mental health and mental disability
- intersectoral collaboration with existing community organizations
- establishing a small core of people who will act as champions for the rights of people with disabilities
- establishing a support group for people with mental disability.

Health promotion and prevention of mental disability within the community

In order for people to take responsiblility for their own mental health they need information about health, a healthy lifestyle, the causes of mental disability, and the early signs of illness. Education is often the first step in the process of developing acceptance of people with mental disability. Target groups may be teachers, women's groups, youth groups and informal health service providers, as well as those directly affected by mental disability. Knowledge has to be translated into terms and concepts easily understood by lay people, and the occupational therapist must refrain from using medical jargon. Health promotion should not merely be knowledge-based, but should provide people with the opportunity to live a healthy lifestyle, help others in stressful situations, or help the early detection and referral of those who are ill. It is this activity participation that differentiates the role of the occupational therapist from that of the nurse or health educator in health promotion.

Promotion of health and healthy lifestyle

This has three components: a healthy activity profile (balanced activity profile); a healthy diet; and the prevention of disability.

Balanced activity profile

Few people are aware of the importance of activities for a balanced, healthy lifestyle. The occupational therapist may provide information about activity clocks and the need to balance leisure activities with work and personal care in order to reduce stress. Restful sleep is induced by using relaxation techniques.

Eating to promote health and prevent disability

Appropriate occupational therapy activities include planning healthy meals, meal preparation, budgeting for purchasing healthy food, growing food gardens, keeping chickens and finding free sources of healthy food by harvesting the countryside.

Deficits in a number of nutrients including vitamins B_1, B_6 and B_{12}, folic acid, vitamin C, zinc, iron and manganese are associated with mental symptoms and poor learning (Davies and Stewart, 1987). Boosting the diet of pregnant women may prevent congenital intellectual disabilities, and improving the protein, vitamin and mineral diet of young children may counteract the effects of malnutrition on learning in school-aged children living in poor areas. A vitamin B-rich diet may prevent illness due to stress in adolescents and adults. Many people with mental illness also suffer from nutritional deficits due to poor eating habits, e.g. they may go for several days without eating or they may eat only one type of food. Their health education should cover information about healthy eating habits and a balanced diet to prevent weight loss and improve mental function. Examples of food that should be included to promote mental health are wholewheat bread, peas and beans, lentils, soya and legumes, bananas, avocados, mangos, nuts and seeds, dairy produce and eggs (vitamin B_{12}), green vegetables (broccoli, cauliflower, parsley, cabbage, green pepper), and potatoes (Davies and Stewart, 1987).

Preventing disability through infection and intoxication

Measles and malaria are two preventable diseases that can cause mental retardation and specific learning deficits. Occupational therapists should inform communities about these causes and how to prevent them. This would include education on the Expanded Programme on Immunization (Mendis, 1994), checking the Road to Health charts to see if children have been immunized, and promoting the use of mosquito nets, chemical sprays or traditional methods such as burning dung to prevent malaria.

Alcoholism and addiction are linked to an increase in stress or head injury due to violence and traffic accidents, and increase the risk of learning problems in the child if the mother consumes alcohol during pregnancy. Teenage pregnancy, truancy and drug use are common in poverty-stricken areas as the young people there have very limited choices about recreational activities. Occupational therapists need to work with schools and youth groups to develop appropriate healthy replacement activities such as sport and recreation.

Knowledge of mental illness or disability

Information on recognizing mental disability and the wide range of causes as well as discussions on rights, acceptance and integration are appropriate topics for the wider community as well as families affected by mental disability. Occupational therapists are good at developing education sessions that require active participation such as short role-plays depicting the problems faced by consumers and their families. Such education sessions are useful starting points for discussion on how each member of the community can help themselves, or nearby families in stressful situations, as well as helping people with mental disabilities. Leaflets at clinics, schools, libraries or community centres or talk shows on the local radio could be used to spread information about the CBR programme.

Intersectoral collaboration with existing community organizations

Mobilizing a community to ensure that the rights of people with disability are upheld means intersectoral collaboration. The role of the therapist is, first, to ensure that community organizations and government departments other than health are aware of the rights of people with disabilities. Second, the therapist needs to work with these agencies to identify what practical contributions they can make to the CBR programme, and third the occupational therapist must establish a method of maintaining contact and discussing ideas. The fourth step is to ensure the public is aware of their work.

As the rights of disabled people include acceptable health services, and integration into schools, places of work and community activities, the key stakeholders are community leaders and groups, disabled people's organizations, and government departments of Social Services, Education, Sport and Recreation, Labour, and Housing.

Community leaders and groups

In some communities it is essential to contact local leaders to gain permission to work in the community, as well as some guarantee of safety. These leaders will also inform the community of the activities of the occupational therapist and give the community permission to interact with the occupational therapist.

Community social groups often form around sport, religion, music and dance, drama, funerals, celebrations, self-improvement, making food and earning or saving money. These groups may be willing to help the occupational therapist to understand the local community, include people with disabilities into their group, or pass on their knowledge of groups to people with disabilities.

Disabled people's organizations (DPOs)

There are a number of consumer-based non-governmental organizations (NGOs) offering support services in the field of mental health. They can provide leaflets about the organization, arrange talks about mental health and the work of the organization, and offer intervention such as home care, counselling, support groups and work opportunities through sheltered workshops and self-help groups. Offices are mainly in the metropolitan areas, but workers are deployed throughout the provinces. Unfortunately few consumers know about these organizations so the occupational therapist should know which NGOs operate in the district or country in order to increase awareness and access to these organizations (DPSA, 2001).

Social services

Occupational therapists should be aware that neglect can be a very real issue for people with mental disabilities and people who are not adequately cared for in the community should be referred to social services (Department of Health, 1997b and 2000). They may be neglected, isolated or abused by their family, have no family and need support to care for their own needs. Social workers help resolve family conflicts and may provide temporary funds for financial relief. Social services can also be approached for funding protective and sheltered workshops for people with mental disabilities or for funds to set up such small income-generating projects, e.g. sewing and woodwork groups.

Health services

In many countries medication is usually the only intervention offered at the local clinic or health centre, although the advent of community service for doctors and occupational therapists has seen a growing number of 'visiting days' for doctors and occupational therapists. If the primary healthcare (PHC) nurse at the clinic is to be the access point to rehabilitation services a referral system needs to be developed to ensure that those who are both acutely ill and chronically ill are referred to the rehabilitation team as well as to the psychiatric ward. This means the PHC nurse must be informed about what mental health service is offered and who can benefit – even better if she is involved in developing ideas for service delivery.

It should be remembered that many PHC nurses fear people with mental illness (Homer and Sehayek, 1995) due to their cultural beliefs and lack of training in psychiatry. Clients are often brought to the clinic in a confused, aggressive or violent state and may be so psychotic they are totally unaware that they are ill and they refuse admission to a psychiatric ward. Therefore the early detection of the onset of illness or the deterioration of an illness should be a primary focus and the PHC nurse should be taught some basic handling skills. People on medication for chronic mental illness or epilepsy usually attend the clinic on a monthly basis and the nurse is expected to complete a brief assessment of their mental status. It is a good idea to ask a responsible adult in the family to report any change in behaviour to the clinic as people with poor memory, judgement or insight into their illness may report that they are well when they are getting worse. Referral to the district hospital may be essential for the diagnosis or to adjust medical treatment of those with mental illness or epilepsy (Mendis, 1994).

Clinics are frequently chosen as occupational therapy outreach service points so accessibility needs to be carefully considered:

- Are they evenly distributed throughout the district or are some areas better off than others?
- Are they easily accessible on foot and by public transport?
- Is the occupational therapy service provided at times that suit the community or times that suit the occupational therapist?
- Is the community aware of the occupational therapy service and what it offers?

Education

There are two components to work on: access to the education system, and curriculum content. Access to education may be a right for children and adolescents with mental disabilities but in many areas there are no facilities, or local school teachers are unaware of what is available or how to access it. Discussions with the education department should be around referrals, provision of educational resources for children with intellectual disabilities, and ways to help teachers cope with slow learners in the classroom.

If information on mental health is included as a permanent part of the school curriculum, it will ensure equitable distribution of knowledge. Occupational therapists can teach teachers how to tell if someone has a health problem, the dangers of drug and alcohol use, and how to recognize signs of stress related to school, home life and traumatic events, and where children can go for help, e.g. Child Line, social workers and nurses. In addition, as the health of the nation has been shown to depend on the literacy of its mothers, Adult Based Education and Training (ABET) should ensure that its literacy training covers mental health issues and access to mental health resources for adults.

The occupational therapist may also persuade head teachers to open up the school premises for after-hours recreation activities for children and adults.

Sport and recreation

The Department of Sport and Recreation (South Africa) is involved in building recreational facilities such as playgrounds, promoting play and recreational activities at pre-schools and primary schools, as well as supporting sport for adults. Occupational therapists should help them develop playgrounds for centres for children with disabilities and help youth groups access funding to develop local sports groups.

Labour

The Department of Labour is a good resource for training courses for micro-enterprises. They may supply either funds or trainers for projects such as making kitchen units, small bread-making projects and creative handwork such as batiks. Self-help groups need to be advised on how to access these resources, and supported through the lengthy process. It is important to check about termination of employment with all clients and liaise with the social worker and the Department of Labour about unfair dismissal from employment due to mental disability and difficulties obtaining unemployment benefits or a disability pension from employers.

Housing

Whilst many people with mental disabilities live with their families, some wish to live alone and need to be helped with access to state housing schemes (Pretorius, 1998). This usually means liaising with local councillors. In South Africa the government's low-cost housing scheme now allows new houses to be built in existing homesteads. This means that people with mental illness can have their own house within their family homestead or neighbourhood rather than face the stress of relocating to a new area and losing their social support systems.

Informal health service providers

Existing support systems for people with problems can be quite varied. These are often useful support systems to refer people in stressful situations, such as the main caregiver. Examples include: a good listener with whom people can discuss their problems, the local priest, a village elder, someone with standing (often a person with a higher level of education) in the community, and of course, the traditional healer. Informal service providers should be informed about the CBR services and given education on mental health and disability so that a referral system can be set up. Practical advice on handling specific behaviours is usually appreciated and it is hoped that by improving the knowledge of people working in the informal health services the service they render will improve (WHO, 2001b).

An intersectoral approach to CBR may enhance the viability of CBR projects and fulfil the need to make the 'best use of available resources'. It is often surprising how many services may exist in an area but, due to a lack of networking, organizations are often unaware of one another and may even duplicate the services offered.

Establishing a small core of people who will act as champions for the rights of people with disability

For many countries occupational therapists are a 'luxury rather than a right' (Henley and Twible, 2001, p. 1) and community work in Africa is often dependent on a single district post, often held by expatriate occupational therapists working a fixed time contract (Voluntary Service Overseas model), or by newly qualified occupational therapists doing a year's community service (South African model). Personnel rotate frequently and re-advertised posts may not be filled immediately. This can quickly lead to each occupational therapist 'reinventing the wheel', or starting new projects that collapse when they leave. To ensure the sustainability of any CBR project it is important to find people in the community who will help CBR projects to continue even when there is no occupational therapist.

Such champions of CBR may include:

- community leaders working for the mental health needs of their community
- people trained in disability issues who will stay in the community and work with the community to continue the process of identifying needs, changing attitudes and basic rehabilitation services
- consumers and their families who are able to support each other and lobby for their rights within the community.

Getting community leaders working for the mental health needs of their community means involving the community in the planning, standard-setting and monitoring of rehabilitation services. The first step may be to involve the community through the District Council. Whilst this is a limited perspective of community participation, it is a starting point. Some communities have local CBR or health committees of consumers, community and health workers. This is more in line with the policy that CBR services should be 'provided in partnership with people with disabilities and their caregivers' (Department of Health, 1997b and 2000). The occupational therapist, who may provide training on leadership, running meetings and strategic planning, should support such committees.

It is assumed that well-supervised community workers (Henley and Twible, 2001) can help the majority of people with disability and that this is a cost-effective use of limited resources. Current international practice in CBR consists of community workers involved in day-to-day intervention, supervisors (people with further training) monitoring their work, and therapists acting as programme managers developing overall service plans, and managing the CBR programme (Mendis 1994; Thorburn, 2000; Henley and Twible, 2001).

Occupational therapists may be instrumental in establishing training for community workers. Such training ranges from training volunteers to help individual clients or small groups in specific activities to training paid auxiliary workers, e.g. Occupational therapy assistants or community rehabilitation workers. To ensure success and sustainability training should comply with national policy and standards, or in the absence of this guidelines are available from the World Health Organization (WHO) or the local training centre for occupational therapists. Ad hoc training can lead to unrealistic expectations from the health service provider, community workers and consumers.

Establishing support groups that involve service consumers and their families is an important role for the community-based occupational therapist and as support groups occur naturally in all communities, the concept is usually accepted. To begin, consider the merits of a separate group for people with mental disabilities rather than inclusion into a group of mixed disabilities, or integration into existing community groups. People at the creative ability level of participation may be accepted within an existing group, e.g. a choir, but those at lower levels of creative ability are less likely to be accepted or able to make a valued contribution to the group without assistance (see Chapter 1). In addition, they may have different needs from people with physical disability, so a separate support group may be more appropriate.

The practicalities of organizing these groups and developing their independence can be lengthy due to the inherent problems of mental disability. People with mental disorders may be socially isolated as they are suspicious of people, very anxious in social situations and have poor conversation skills. Due to the stigma of mental illness they may have little opportunity to practise social skills with family, friends and the community. Even clients attending a clinic over many years may not know the names of others attending on the same day. Problems with memory and task completion means that they may not remember the dates or place of the meeting or may get side-tracked when making their way to the meeting. Low motivation and energy may also affect attendance.

A social support group creates the opportunity to gain acceptance, learn about mental illness and ways to cope, and develop friendships. Groups often start at a very simple level before the participants are ready to see themselves as part of a group with a purpose. Simple activities such as asking the participants to introduce themselves to the others attending the clinic, and to say something about themselves, the problems they are having, and ways in which they try to cope, whilst sharing light refreshments is one way of starting. The therapist can inform people of community events, e.g. a football match, and help them to participate in some way as this is an important component of disability equity (DPSA, 2001).

Caregivers can also benefit from a support group that creates the opportunity for them to share the problems of caring, learn about how others cope and learn ways to reduce stress. Caregivers' groups and social support groups may grow into consumer groups active in mental health rights, but it may take several years to move from an occupational therapy-directed to a client-controlled group. The groups should be actively involved in disability issues, at the very least by participating in awareness-raising campaigns e.g. International Day of the Disabled (Department of Health 1997b, 2000). At the highest level of participation they should be fighting for their rights by lobbying local organizations and councillors.

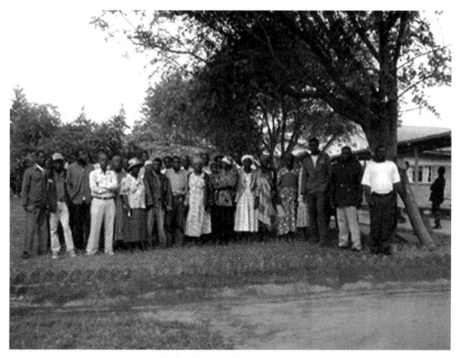

Figure 6.2 The Sizanani support group started with people sharing oranges and soft drinks when attending the clinic. They are now active in helping the people to attend the clinic regularly, visit those who do not attend the clinic, and give help and advice to the community about mental illness and disability rights.

An appropriate and accessible service for the consumer and family

Regular home visits are essential CBR practice in order for the occupational therapist to understand the client in the context of their home and community, as well as to mobilize the family to participate in the intervention process. The initial meeting usually involves providing information about the CBR service and helping the client and family establish their problems and needs. This is an important step in establishing a relationship between the occupational therapist and the family, and creating empowerment for the client and family.

Some families may show little interest in the occupational therapist or therapy; this lack of interest must be understood in the context of their society and past experience. Articulating problems and needs to an unknown therapist is difficult when your culture seeks to protect the family name and reputation from strangers. Many cultures also believe that interacting with those who are ill spreads mental illness. Families are therefore understandably reticent about social contact and it may take several visits before the family will trust the occupational therapist enough to give an accurate history and discuss problems.

Consider what happens to the family before they came into contact with the CBR service. Families may try alternative or informal healers first.

These may be very successful in dealing with stress-related signs and symptoms, anxiety disorders and mild depression, but not with the severely mentally ill (unless the disorder is due to a toxic psychosis). A variety of healers may be tried before the family accepts that the disability persists despite the intervention of the healer. For the majority of rural Africans the next port of call will be the local clinic and district hospital. At this point people with epilepsy are frequently 'cured' through the use of anti-epileptics and those with psychosis may have their violent behaviour and hallucinations controlled by anti-psychotics. However occupational performance may remain impaired due to changes in their cognitive abilities, energy levels and motivation. Clinics have little to offer those with intellectual disabilities. By now the family may have exhausted their belief system of cure through the traditional healer, nurse and doctor, and will be in a cycle of learned helplessness – no matter what they try nothing works. Why then should they believe an occupational therapist (a relatively unknown type of healer) who says that things will get better? Their belief in your ability will develop only when they see change in behaviour in their family.

Even if the family agrees to intervention, their expectation is that the occupational therapist will be the agent of change. After all, it is their experience that the traditional healer, clinic nurse or doctor will provide the cure. On the other hand the occupational therapist's expectation is that the family will continue with therapy whilst she is not there. This dichotomy of beliefs can lead to poor intervention. Occupational therapists also need to consider whether the family can cope with the additional stress of being the agent of change. Families simply may not have the time and energy to carry out intervention, especially if the burden of care is coupled with the burden of poverty. Low nutritional intake means that families will have low energy levels and much of this energy is expended in the hours of heavy labour required to provide basic needs such as water, food and fuel.

The family may expect change to be rapid, like the effects of the medicine provided at the clinic or healer, whereas the occupational therapist may expect change over several weeks as learning skills takes time. Therefore it is important to select the first activity/intervention together to ensure interest and commitment to the process. A successful first activity is essential for motivation to continue with therapy.

Mobilizing the family to promote mental health and participation in family and community life

Rehabilitation in the home is a way to mobilize the family to become active participants in CBR. Families need knowledge about the illness, its cause and prognosis as this helps with the process of acceptance. They need to know the rights of disabled people and information about how to access services such as medicine, grants, housing, rehabilitation, appropriate schools and support agencies. Apart from increasing their knowledge, they also need to be taught how to help the person with mental health problems participate in family and community life, this could involve living a 'healthy lifestyle', better communication and social skills, household management and income generation, or stimulating early development for young children (Mendis, 1994).

Many of the people with mental disability living in the community are functioning at the creative ability level of presentation or the early stages of participation (see Chapter 1). They find it difficult to do routine activities at home because they are forgetful, or they have low energy levels or low motivation, or poor planning. Insight may be poor and many perceive themselves as needing less assistance in daily activities than the caregivers actually give them (Masilela and MacLeod, 1998). A CBR programme of home visits to improve independence skills can decrease the burden of care on the caregiver and enable both client and caregiver to be more economically productive. Gains in independence create hope for the future and this can lead to change in attitudes in both the client and family members.

Improving participation in family life requires a three-pronged approach: the training in structuring a daily activity routine appropriate to their level of creative participation, handling difficult behaviour and adequate, appropriate medication.

Daily routines and habits

Doing things for themselves and taking part in activities at home are important in skills development and prevent the client from ruminating on their disorder. Therefore families need to learn how to structure the day. This should start simply and the occupational therapist should be knowledgeable of the local and family norms. Together an activity should be selected that conforms to the client's interests and level of creative participation. Commonly requested activities are daily washing, wearing clean clothes, making beds and cleaning the room or helping in the yard. Then, depending on the level, the family may tell the client what to do, watch him and give appropriate encouragement; share the task with the client; or divide the task into steps and supervise the client doing one part of it.

Families should be taught the principles of rewards and shaping behaviour and how to implement a reward system. It is best if the behaviour is modelled for them by the occupational therapist and then practised in front of the occupational therapist. With the guidance of the occupational therapist a programme can be built up to the daily implementation of one activity, through to a half-day and finally a full day of structured activities. Practical projects such as food gardens provide for a variety of needs and aims. Participation promotes correct energy expenditure, builds physical fitness, increases motivation to participate in other activities, improves self-esteem by having an end product (even digging a patch of

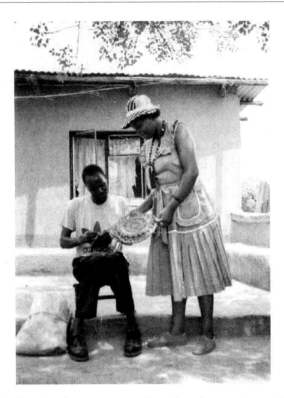

Figure 6.3 Doing handcrafts is an accepted work and recreation activity in many cultures. By learning to weave sisal mats this client earned a little money and his relationships with his family began to improve as he contributed to the household wealth.

ground over can be satisfying) and by being involved in an activity recognized and valued by the family and community. The food to be produced should be selected for the nutritional needs of the family so as to promote a healthy diet. Finally, if enough food is produced, it can be sold to create income. A vegetable garden maybe in the homestead area, or part of a community garden (allotment). A garden at home may bring the family together. It is also a good project to build with the Local Agricultural Officer and The Food Gardens Foundation provides simple newsletters, posters and cheap seeds for a small annual fee.

Families also need to be taught how to help the client participate appropriately in social and recreational activities at home or in the community. In some families such interaction is discouraged or the client's attempts may be ridiculed. Clients may also avoid the stress of interaction with the family because it is always negative. The occupational therapist can help the family see the 'cause and effect' of these negative interactions and help them develop more appropriate responses. This may be more effective once the family has learnt how to shape and reward concrete behaviour such as getting the client to wash on a regular basis. Start with simple social activities: sharing a meal, listening to the radio or TV together, sitting in the same room or going for a walk. Community activities can be introduced once the client has had success at home. To begin with the client will be a spectator rather than a participant in activities. Suitable activities may be visiting nearby family or friends, going to the shops, attending church or a sports event.

Handling difficult behaviour

Apart from building good habits, families need to be aware of activities and stressors that make the illness worse for their family. These may include their behaviour towards the client, specific activities or topics of conversation, unexpected occurrences, e.g. a visitor, family celebrations, or the effects of alcohol. The occupational therapist should help them identify which stressors should be avoided, and how to predict and prevent the effects of those stressors that cannot be avoided.

If you work in the community you will at some point have to help a client with aggressive behaviour and some general guidelines are given below:

1. Always be prepared for the possibility of aggression:

- Find out as much as possible about each client before meeting them – especially anger triggers.
- Work outside, or if you work in the house make sure that you are closer to the door than the client and can leave the room easily if necessary.
- Check there is someone who can help close by – family or neighbours – before you start work.
- Explain why you are there, so the client understands what is happening.
- Build up a relationship with the client first, family second.

2. If the client is known to be aggressive:

- Help the family identify 'cause, effect and reinforcement' and correct their behaviour where necessary.
- Always talk calmly and quietly to the client.
- Ensure the client is taking medication regularly. If they are not, then give health education about medication and encourage them to go to the clinic.

3. If the patient then becomes threatening:

- Talk calmly and quietly.
- Avoid sudden movements as they may think they are being attacked.
- Inform the client that their behaviour is not acceptable.
- Reassure them about who you are and why you are there and what is really happening.
- Try to involve them in an activity that reduces adrenaline and takes them away from the stressor, e.g. suggest a walk.

4. If the situation is dangerous:

• Explain that you are going to leave but that you will return when they are feeling better.
• Make sure the family or neighbours know the client's state of mind and why you are leaving.
• Help the family get help if the client needs restraining. This may mean calling in the local police.
• Make a firm appointment to see the family again.

5. Afterwards:

• Reflect on what triggered the behaviour and how it was handled. This should be done with colleagues, the family and the client.

Medication

Medication is not usually the role of the occupational therapist but in community work it is vital that medication compliance checked during home visits. Mendis (1994) identifies the provision of medication for mental illness as an important second-level prevention programme in CBR. Medication checks are best done in the client's own home and this is a useful role for the Community Health Worker (CHW), Occupational Therapy Assistant or Community Rehabilitation Worker (CRW).

People with mental illness will have difficulty attending clinics for repeat prescriptions (Modiba et al., 2000), taking daily medication and reporting on their illness accurately. Poor attendance and compliance may be because they do not understand the instructions about taking the medication, or they forget to take it, or they do not want to take it because of the side effects or lack of insight into their illness, or they start to feel well so they stop taking the medication. Poor attendance or hoarding of medication leads to under-medication, poor control of symptoms and probable decline in ability to care for themselves, and/or total relapse. One outcome of reduced medication is that clients may experience florid symptomatology. If the client is aggressive, then the family becomes afraid of precipitating the aggression by trying to get them to hospital or to the clinic. Health education for both client and family can help them cope with the aggressive behaviour and access medicine. Overmedication (taking more tablets than necessary) results in a decline in ability to take care of themselves, periods of no medication (if the patient waits the full month to return for medication), or increase in medication provision (if the client returns to the clinic earlier than expected for repeat medication). Masilela and MacLeod (1998) report that only 12.55% of caregivers supervise taking medication.

Simple and cost-effective remedies for this situation include:

• ensuring that an appropriate family member attends the clinic with the patient to report back on their illness
• teaching the client and family the importance of medication

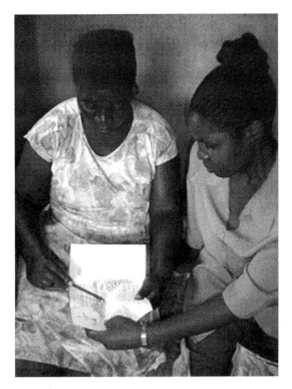

Figure 6.4 Teaching the family to count the client's medication to check whether it is being taken correctly.

- teaching the family how to count the medicine to ensure it is taken correctly
- keeping medication in a safe place (away from children) and where it will be seen every day, e.g. with their toothbrush. This will help them to remember to take the medicine.

It must be emphasized that this is a continuous education process.

Overcoming poverty by increasing access to money

Many people with mental disabilities are unable to work on the open labour market. Those who return to work may find that they cannot cope with the same pressure of work or the same type of job, or fear that they will have relapses. Mental disability exacerbates the poverty cycle, and the financial burden of care is often cited as an overriding problem for both clients and caregivers. There are a number of options that can be explored with the family:

- social assistance
- income generation at home or within self-help groups
- sheltered or protective workshops.

Whilst the issue of 'welfare handouts' versus 'empowerment' remains controversial – with even organizations such as Disabled People South Africa (DPSA, 2001) rejecting 'handouts' in one sentence and then calling for greater access to social grants in the next – occupational therapists have an important role in educating people about grants available and how to access them (Pretorius, 1998; Frieg and Hendry, 2002). There is consistent evidence that people with disabilities do not have easy access to grants, particularly those living on farms or in isolated rural areas (Concha and Lorenzo, 1993; Modiba et al., 2000). Grants may cause problems within the family; e.g. the grant is spent on alcohol or drugs, or given away by the grant holder, or the family has control of the grant and uses it for themselves and not the grant holder, so the occupational therapist also should discuss control of money within the family.

What will I leave behind?

A CBR programme is judged on its 'relevance, effectiveness, sustainability and impact' (UNDP, 1993 in Zhao and Kwok, 1997, p. 2).

In terms of *relevance* it is essential that consumers speak for themselves (DPSA, 2001) and that community and consumers are not only 'heard' but are also active participants in the development of the service (Lysack and Kaufert, 1994). Relevance also has to apply on an individual basis. For example, if you work with individuals, is your priority changing their level of function or improving their immediate financial status?

Effective programmes are based on sound research, hence the need to keep up to date once graduated. Effective programmes also have to comply with the principles of *equality and efficiency* and answer the questions: 'Where should the service be to provide the easiest access for the consumers?' 'Is the service equal throughout the district/province?' and 'Is this the *most* efficient way?' For example, if an occupational therapy outreach service is provided to identify people who need rehabilitation but then the clients are expected to travel to the hospital for the service, are you really providing an accessible service? Are auxiliary staff as effective as therapists at providing social groups for people with mental illness? Is it better to work with individual cases or develop groups?

Indicators of *impact* include change in participation of people with disability in school, work and social activities, change in income, work or educational status, and change in attitudes in the person with the disability, their family or the community in which they live (Zhao and Kwok, 2000). Thus CBR seeks to alter the community as well as the individual.

Sustainability is about what one person or one project can realistically achieve, e.g. should you work only with those who have mental health problems or should you work on preventing mental health problems in the community, perhaps by starting an activity centre for the young people? When starting in a new area you need to identify what you will have achieved and what you will leave behind that will continue to benefit the community when you go. Activities should be selected based on their relevance to the common mental health needs of the community as well as whether they are affordable. Both the referral system and access to social grants should be so well developed that they would run without the direct intervention of the occupational therapist. The other area to develop is that of champions for CBR. If you are the first occupational therapist in an area, then most of your work for the first year may well be taken up with networking and establishing priorities and systems, i.e. developing service delivery systems rather than individual client intervention. The transition from hands-on occupational therapist to service developer can be difficult. Many community occupational therapists feel overwhelmed by the needs of the community and may over-commit themselves to a wide number of projects or committees. As a consequence they may find that they either cannot fulfil the roles adequately or burn out trying to do so. By using intersectoral approaches the occupational therapist endeavours to increase the chances of sustainability.

Conclusion

This chapter has looked at how to build up a community service based on the needs of the people in that community in order to ensure that people with disabilities are given 'maximum opportunity to become an equal and active member of the community' (Henley and Twible, 2001, p. 2). Key factors affecting CBR are that too few people are trained for CBR, stakeholder groups are not involved in the CBR process and policy makers show little interest in CBR (Mendis, 1994). CBR services therefore need careful planning to ensure that the needs of people with disability are met despite turnover in staff and to ensure that the succession of occupational therapists can adapt quickly to their new role, and work stresses are minimized, which in turn should encourage occupational therapists to remain in community service. It is hoped that innovative postgraduate CBR programmes will produce a generation of *experienced* occupational therapists committed and skilled in community work.

Questions

1. What questions should be asked to determine whether the rehabilitation service is appropriate for people with mental illness living in the community?
2. If you are starting a new community service, how can you find people with mental health problems?
3. What would an appropriate CBR service include?
4. Why might families find it difficult to comply with home programmes?
5. How can you judge whether a CBR service is appropriate?

Chapter 7
Auxiliary staff in the field of psychiatry: requirements, functions and supervision

DAIN VAN DER REYDEN

For the purposes of this chapter, the author has used 'auxiliary staff' or 'auxiliaries' as generic terms for both the occupational therapy auxiliary and the occupational therapy technician categories of staff.

Occupational therapy assistants are currently trained in several countries, notably the United States, Britain, Canada and South Africa. Historically, in South Africa, occupational therapy departments in psychiatric institutions have made extensive use of support staff. Initially, these staff members were allocated from the nursing establishment on a rotation or on a relatively permanent basis. They were often assistant nurses who demonstrated interest in craft or other activities. During the 1960s and 1970s, staff with trade or technical qualifications were often employed to run workshops for patients.

The situation differs in other parts of the world, according to the staff structure and policics of the country. Often auxiliary staff are not available, or not trained to assist in the occupational therapy intervention. South Africa has been proactive in the training of occupational therapy auxiliary staff to assist with the intervention programmes in psychiatric rehabilitation facilities for people with mental illnesses, and their services are considered to be vital.

From the 1960s to the 1980s, professional nurses were frequently allocated to organize and manage areas such as the industrial contract area and recreational activities, in the absence of a qualified occupational therapist. For many years, psychiatric institutions ran very productive workshops and handcraft areas, producing high-quality products, without the aid of an occupational therapist. The staff allocated to these areas were usually called 'therapy' nurses. They provided a variety of constructive and recreational activities with the main aim of occupying, training and stimulating patients. It must be acknowledged that many newly qualified occupational therapists benefited from the vast experience of these 'therapy' nurses and technicians.

174

As a result of the increase in the numbers of occupational therapists and the formalization of training for auxiliary categories (support staff), occupational therapy departments are now better staffed. Staff numbers are, however, rarely adequate to provide the needed service, especially in medium- and long-term units.

The need for auxiliary staff also does not seem to have decreased with the increase in numbers of qualified occupational therapists. In fact, the opposite seems to be the case, largely due to the extension of occupational therapy services into new areas of practice, the opening of new departments, specialization within the profession and demand for occupational therapy services in the private sector and different levels of healthcare provision.

The role of the occupational therapist, particularly within institutions, is often that of manager, planner and organizer of programmes and services for entire populations of patients. Occupational therapists therefore currently make extensive use of auxiliary staff to implement many aspects of direct service provision within the psychosocial field of practice. The primary healthcare approach, as now implemented in most countries, presents exciting challenges to the occupational therapist, as well as auxiliary staff, and demands that comprehensive mental health and psychiatric services be provided at community level.

There has been a substantive shift in attitude and approach towards auxiliary staff, who are currently accepted as valued members of the profession, with a specific role and contribution which is certainly not inferior, but rather complementary, to that of the graduate occupational therapist.

Current situation

In the United Kingdom the health system incorporates occupational therapy assistants (OTAs) and rehabilitation assistants, as well as technical instructors, all of which assist occupational therapists.

The South African health system makes provision for a category of mid-level workers, which includes the OTA who has completed a one-year certificate course; the occupational therapy technician (OTT) who has completed a two-year diploma course, and the community rehabilitation worker (CRW) who has completed two years of training.

Occupational therapy auxiliaries were trained to function mainly within institutional settings, whilst community rehabilitation workers are trained to practise within a community setting. In South Africa the present trend is for the profession to train only one category, that of technician, who will have advanced occupational therapy auxiliary-specific skills, as well as extensive community development and community-based rehabilitation skills, and who will be able to function effectively in both institutional and community settings.

Ethical and legal context

Auxiliary staff must comply with the professional requirements of the country in which they practise, such as registration, annual payment of fees, ethical rules and other professional conduct requirements.

Registration of occupational therapy auxiliaries

Occupational therapy auxiliaries need to register with a licensing body or similar health professions council in order to practise and need to comply with similar rules and regulations to those that govern the occupational therapist. Most countries determine that occupational therapy auxiliaries must practise under the supervision of an occupational therapist, and may not establish a private practice or work independently of an occupational therapist.

The occupational therapist is obliged to provide an appropriate level of supervision and, importantly, retain professional responsibility and liability for treatment implemented by occupational therapy auxiliaries under her supervision. Legally, 'supervision' is defined as having control as to the manner in which such person/s does their work (telling them what to do and how to do it) (Dada and McQuoid-Mason, 2001). A supervisor is furthermore defined as one who ensures that the tasks assigned to others are performed correctly and efficiently (American Occupational Therapy Association, 1989).

The responsibilities of the occupational therapy auxiliary include the following:

- Conducting oneself in accordance with the ethical principles, rules and guidelines of the profession and statutory licensing body, treating patients and care providers without any bias with regard to nationality, socio-economic status, religious affiliation, politics, personal preferences or personal gain. This essentially means placing the interest of the patient above all else and demonstrating the highest level of professional integrity at all times.
- Accepting and practising within a supervisory relationship, which would include effectively and efficiently executing the prescription of the occupational therapist, implementing protocols as indicated, and demonstrating loyalty to the profession and employing body.
- Maintaining professional registration and actively participating in continuing professional development activities where and as required by the licensing authority and performing only those tasks which s/he has been trained to do or has gained sufficient experience to do.

Additionally, it is expected that the auxiliary will exercise the degree of competence and care which could reasonably be expected from an auxiliary with that level of training and experience.

Responsibility of the employing body

The appointment of a registered occupational therapist or other suitably qualified health practitioner to provide and ensure ongoing supervision remains the responsibility of the employing body. The author, however, believes that both the occupational therapist and the auxiliaries involved need to motivate for ongoing supervision.

Responsibilities of the supervising occupational therapist

The occupational therapist retains overall responsibility for services provided and is vicariously liable for actions of auxiliaries, as well as overall quality assurance. It is thus essential that the occupational therapist accepts the supervisory management function as an integral part of her role. The time spent on supervision should be offset by the time gained by auxiliary staff coping more efficiently with tasks delegated to them, and the service offered.

The occupational therapist should provide adequate supervision and management of services provided by auxiliaries, whilst providing appropriate referrals, prescriptions and protocols for implementation, and delegating effectively. The occupational therapist should not expect the auxiliaries to perform any acts for which they have not been adequately trained, or do not have the experience and skills to do, and should furthermore facilitate continuing professional development and ongoing training.

In situations where the supervising therapist is employed to supervise and is not the service-providing therapist, the author believes that this therapist must of necessity accept responsibility, not only for supervision, but also for organizing, supervising and developing the service at that centre.

These duties will therefore include an evaluation of the institution or centre, which could consist of an extensive visit, possibly a survey, as well as discussions with all staff concerned, in order to determine real needs and ascertain policy. This would be followed by planning and organizing the service which could realistically be offered, considering staff and facilities available.

It would be important to determine the role of the auxiliary staff in the provision of the service, to prevent exploitation, which means that the supervisor should obtain a job description for the particular staff member, or if not available, draw up such a job description. The supervisor should furthermore ensure that management is well informed and in agreement with the role of the staff member.

Communication channels should be established between auxiliary staff and other departments and between the occupational therapist and auxiliary staff, and so should lines of authority, as problems may arise if auxiliary staff take instructions from the supervising occupational therapist which may be contrary to, or not supported by, other staff, such as professional nurses in the ward. The occupational therapist should therefore anticipate possible difficulties and communicate regularly with wards and management to keep inevitable misunderstandings to a minimum. All changes, plans and special programmes should also be discussed with all involved.

Tasks and functions of auxiliary staff and other practical considerations

The appointment of auxiliary staff enables the occupational therapist to spend a greater part of the day in direct service provision and, together with auxiliary staff, carry greater patient loads. It enables the occupational therapist to establish programmes for large numbers of patients, which can be implemented by auxiliary staff, and to develop and provide a variety of services within a variety of settings. Auxiliary staff can therefore assist the occupational therapist to establish a more effective and efficient service and will contribute to the development and maintenance of occupational therapy services at institutions, clinics or centres, which includes the development of community outreach programmes.

The functions and tasks of auxiliary staff are defined largely by principles and guidelines as contained in the rules of registration and the ethical rules which apply to all health professionals, the health needs of the community and, importantly, the scope of practice of the profession.

Guiding principles

The *occupational therapy assistant* is trained to work according to the *prescription* of the occupational therapist, so her main contribution lies within the *implementation* phase of intervention.

The *occupational therapy technician*, on the other hand, has either specialized activity skills, a trade qualification, advanced occupational therapy auxiliary skills and/or training in community rehabilitation and development. Such a person therefore is able to work within prescribed protocols of intervention, for example for the treatment of a person with schizophrenia, and may implement these based on assessment findings.

Occupational therapy auxiliaries are trained to deal with the non-complicated, routine, normally medium- to long-term, 'standard' type of cases. Any client with multiple handicaps or diagnosis, who is treatment-resistant or has an unusual clinical picture, would generally not be treated without direct occupational therapy intervention. The occupational therapist retains the responsibility to plan, institute and terminate interventions and programmes. The auxiliary staff therefore assist the occupational therapist with those aspects of treatment and departmental organization which do not require constant and/or direct intervention, or all the theoretical, knowledge, skill and expertise of the occupational therapist.

Tasks which may be undertaken by auxiliary staff

The novice occupational therapy auxiliary should be able to cope effectively with the following:

- General observation of patient and reporting back to the occupational therapist.
- Conducting interviews to obtain background information.
- Preparing treatment sessions to be conducted by the occupational therapist.
- Planning of activities suitable for treatment as requested by the occupational therapist.
- Executing aspects of treatment as prescribed or delegated by the occupational therapist.
- Supervising individuals or groups involved in task-centred activities and conducting task-centred groups.
- Assisting with organization of programmes or events; for example, literacy training, sports days, concerts and outings.
- Management of standard performance area training programmes such as home management training, leisure programmes or income generation.
- Assisting the occupational therapist to overcome barriers of communication with people from different language or cultural groups.
- Recommending activities to the occupational therapist for particular areas of treatment and/or patients, for example, for certain cultural groups.
- Counselling care-providers on the use of basic procedures; for example, the handling of an aggressive client.
- Assisting with development of new areas of treatment, such as a tuck shop, beauty parlour, or obstacle course.
- Manufacturing basic equipment and assistive devices in the physical field.
- Record keeping of patients' progress.
- Assisting with departmental administrative tasks; for example, obtaining quotations, answering the telephone, doing statistics, also maintaining equipment and stock control, compilation of requests for supply of materials/tools/equipment and departmental care, such as general neatness and care of area.
- Maintaining general safety of patients by applying basic safety precautionary measures and ensuring the compliance of safety.

The occupational therapy auxiliary with the necessary training in community rehabilitation and development, who works within a community setting, will be able to:

- Enter such a community appropriately and be able to negotiate with relevant structures.
- Screen the community for persons with disability.

- Conduct a basic assessment through observation of performance of everyday activities.
- Select appropriate protocols of interventions with supervision of an occupational therapist (or suitably qualified health practitioner).
- Implement protocols.
- Establish projects within the community setting, such as income-generation or leisure programmes.

Experience within the occupational therapy department, the quality of guidance and supervision received from the occupational therapist and the attitude and enthusiasm of each staff member will, together with their own basic training, largely determine the quality and extent of the contribution made by auxiliary staff.

Limitations of practice

Auxiliary staff practice is limited by training, experience and regulations. The two major limitations, as mentioned, are that the occupational therapy auxiliaries may not work for their own account (that is, establish a private practice) and are obliged to work under the supervision of a qualified occupational therapist. The occupational therapist is responsible for referring patients for treatment.

Most current training does not equip the student and entry grade occupational therapy auxiliary to do the following *without the supervision of the occupational therapist*:

- Carry out treatment without referral from an occupational therapist.
- Make an occupational therapy diagnosis, do in-depth assessments, use specialized or standardized occupational therapy tests, or select patients for occupational therapy. Depending on the setting, clients may be identified by the occupational therapy auxiliary as requiring occupational therapy.
- Plan or modify remedial or rehabilitation programmes without input from the occupational therapist, or adapt or grade activities for rehabilitation without consultation. Selection can be made on the basis of extensive activity knowledge.
- Use specialized techniques for which the occupational therapist is specifically trained and which require knowledge of basic clinical sciences, and/or clinical conditions and extensive occupational therapy theory. This includes: group therapy (particularly socio-emotional group work); creative arts therapy; sensory integration; design of splints; selection and grading of neuro-developmental techniques; final fitting of pressure garments and splints; design of specific assistive devices; and planning treatment using therapeutic apparatus.
- Attend ward rounds or clinics in place of the occupational therapist.
- Formally evaluate clients' progress (continuous reporting is, however, essential).

- Write in a client's hospital file (it is essential, however, for them to write in the occupational therapy department file).
- Plan discharge.
- Give interpretative information to clients, patients or care-providers, except for routine cases.
- Organize an occupational therapy service or make decisions regarding departmental policy. The occupational therapy auxiliaries should, however, be actively involved in planning, decision making and review of programmes.
- Occupational therapy student evaluation. Auxiliaries may, however, help in the supervision of students.

The service components listed, although representative of the South African situation, correspond closely to the guidelines for the supervision of assigned occupational therapy components as articulated by the Canadian Association for Occupational Therapists (2003).

It should be remembered that experience adds to level of skill and knowledge and should therefore go hand in hand with increased responsibility. The occupational therapy auxiliary is able to assist with most aspects of patient and departmental management with the supervision and guidance of the occupational therapist, and should be actively encouraged to do so.

Some guidelines for selecting auxiliary staff

Formal selection procedures will probably be in place in most organizations. Should this not be the case, appropriate protocols should be established and detailed records kept. It is imperative that staff be selected with great care, particularly in the field of psychiatry and mental health. Personality traits, life experiences and emotional maturity will largely determine successful functioning. The following characteristics have been found to be advantageous:

- Flexibility and emotional stability, genuine concern for the welfare of others, and preferably a sense of humour.
- Ability to demonstrate effective coping skills in terms of problematic or stressful situations.
- An understanding and acceptance of the norms and expectations of the department or area, and being prepared to work under the supervision of the occupational therapist.
- Sound interpersonal relationships and the ability to work with others, as well as an understanding of the need to be part of a team and the department and to be prepared to be loyal to the department and institution/centre.
- Eagerness to learn, being practically inclined and demonstrating common sense.
- Honesty and integrity (which should be confirmed by referees).

- Ability to verbalize how they see their role in the department, and indicate the skills and abilities they could bring to the department.

Appointing an older person who has already developed considerable interpersonal and other coping skills is often very successful. On the other hand, a younger person who has not yet developed fixed ideas and habits could also make a major contribution.

It has been found to be of value for appropriate selection to provide a thorough orientation to both the profession and the department. The use of a questionnaire to indicate interests, prior knowledge and skills, as well as a practical demonstration of the ability to handle patients (e.g. teaching patient to do an activity) has been found to provide valuable information to inform selection.

It is obviously of great benefit to appoint qualified and registered auxiliary staff. Such persons are better able to interpret and implement prescriptions and guidelines, have extensive skills and are able to render a more efficient service. Importantly, training also equips staff with the appropriate attitudes and values for patient care.

Training of auxiliary staff

Training, which is currently offered in several countries, is of shorter duration with fewer fieldwork requirements, but shares common knowledge and skills with occupational therapy training, whereas the graduate training focuses more heavily on theory, evaluation, management, research (Sands in Crepeau et al., 2003) and service development, the training of the occupational therapy auxiliary focuses on direct service delivery.

Training needs to support both everyday practice and changing practice to ensure the effectiveness of service provision (Ham and Fenech, 2002). Training should preferably be formal, leading to a recognized qualification and registration with the professional regulatory body, and may also take the form of continuing professional education.

All staff, even formally trained auxiliary staff, require *in-service education* before they are able to contribute maximally, particularly if such persons have practised in a different field or area of practice. The content of such training should be adapted to the background of the person involved and to the needs of the occupational therapy service.

Some guidelines for in-service training

The occupational therapist needs to give all new appointees a comprehensive orientation to the occupational therapy department, outline the role and functions of auxiliary staff within the department and clarify professional, ethical and conduct requirements. In-service training may be didactic, practical and/or experiential and may include the following components.

Regular meetings should be held with auxiliary staff to update them and to obtain feedback. Informal discussions and formal lectures form an essential part of all in-service training. Auxiliary staff should be kept informed of new developments and be directed to reading matter which will enrich their working experience and improve skills and knowledge.

Demonstrations to and by auxiliaries to their peer group may be included, as well as discussions of cases treated by both occupational therapists and auxiliaries and practical activity skills development sessions.

Visits to other centres should be arranged and encouraged, as well as rotation of auxiliaries between different departments or institutions. This should however be for a minimum period of four weeks to ensure attainment of skills. It should be kept in mind that auxiliaries should be able to cope with all fields of professional practice. Competence should thus be maintained.

Auxiliary staff should be included in meetings and planning exercises and should, as mentioned, be encouraged to participate in, and contribute to, all departmental matters. Special projects and responsibilities should be allocated to ensure high levels of motivation, learning and achievement and to counteract burnout.

The occupational therapist/occupational therapy auxiliary supervisory relationship: context and practical guidelines

Supervision must be seen as a process in which two or more people participate in a joint effort to promote, establish, maintain and/or elevate levels of performance and service, with one person identified as having ultimate responsibility for the quality of service (Canadian Association of Occupational Therapists, 2003). The supervisor is responsible for setting, encouraging and evaluating the standards of work performed by the supervisee (American Journal of Occupational Therapy, 2002).

Quality supervision is therefore a mutual undertaking which serves to promote development and growth; assures appropriate utilization of training and potential; provides guidance, encouragement and support; fosters respect and encourages innovation. It also allows different individuals to work towards common goals within a supportive and rewarding relationship (American Occupational Therapy Association, 1999).

This supervisory relationship, which can at times be fraught with uncertainty and also conflict, remains one of the occupational therapist's most rewarding responsibilities and provides a vehicle for the fulfilment of the management functions of planning, organizing, teaching and controlling.

It should be kept in mind that the basis of an effective supervisory relationship is a partnership and must thus be pursued enthusiastically by both occupational therapists and their auxiliaries. In this way the supervisory relationship becomes not only an enriching experience for all staff concerned, but ultimately benefits patients and their care providers. The slogan of the 2000 Occupational Therapy Association of South Africa

(OTASA) Support Staff Congress in South Africa expressed it beautifully. It read, 'Together we do it best!'

The context within which the supervisory relationship will need to be established

An understanding of the contextual framework within which supervisors and the auxiliary staff need to function is essential for the development of the supervisory relationship, as well as the occupational therapy service. Factors relevant to this framework are discussed below.

Clinical experience has shown that the challenges facing the 'new' occupational therapy supervisor are often significantly increased by limited training in, and experience of, supervising, as well a possible lack of supervisory skills, and cultural and age differences between the occupational therapist and auxiliary staff where these occur.

Procedures and programmes which staff have developed, or have been implemented for extended periods of time, as well as entrenched routines, may make it difficult later to implement change and introduce new ideas.

Auxiliary staff who have functioned in positions of increased authority and autonomy in the absence of an occupational therapist may find it difficult later to function within a supervisory relationship and the controls which of necessity follow. This may also go together with resistive and testing-out behaviour on the part of the auxiliary staff.

At times, excessive administrative and patient loads make it difficult for the occupational therapist to find time to supervise effectively.

The occupational therapist also needs to cope with the professional dilemma, particularly in large psychiatric institutions, of often not being able to find adequate time to fulfil both direct and indirect service roles. Working with skilled, highly motivated and caring auxiliary staff who are effectively implementing therapeutic programmes will however compensate largely for many of the apparent stressors.

In order for the occupational therapist to better understand the context within which auxiliary staff often find themselves, it is necessary to discuss briefly those circumstances which have been observed by the author to impact on the establishment of the supervisory relationship from the auxiliary staff point of view. It should be remembered that auxiliary staff usually provide the stable staff contingent within the occupational therapy department, as they tend to remain whilst occupational therapists tend to move on.

A situation may include having to deal with occupational therapists who have limited supervisory skill and/or being newly qualified, have limited clinical experience. The auxiliary may also have to deal with situations where the occupational therapist may remain at the institution/centre for a year or less and then leave, with a replacement only being appointed three to six months later. In the meantime, auxiliary staff take on additional responsibilities and run the department, only to be 'relieved' of these responsibilities when another occupational therapist is appointed – a situation which causes high levels of frustration and also confusion.

A common frustration is that of little or no opportunity for career path development and promotion. The tasks done by the auxiliary staff are often repetitive and can be very monotonous. Such staff are furthermore disempowered by rules and regulations which force them to work under supervision and leave little scope for decision making and innovation; a situation which is exacerbated by 'autocratic' handling by the supervising occupational therapist.

The auxiliary staff may experience their job as being of low status, with little acknowledgement from other team members, and have voiced feelings of not being fully integrated into the profession of occupational therapy.

Staff who work with long-term, severely ill, psychiatric cases, showing little progress, in environments which are often not conducive to job satisfaction, may experience burnout and decreased levels of motivation. This may be exacerbated by the development of a comfort zone and 'culture of passivity' where the occupational therapist is expected to rescue and remedy situations.

The nature of the supervisory relationship

Factors which determine the nature of the supervisory relationship

(Taken from van der Reyden, in Conlan and Nott, 2000.)
First, the competency level of the occupational therapy auxiliary will largely determine the type and frequency of supervision required. Competency is usually related to experience and may vary from that of a student to entry level (0–3 years), intermediate (3 years plus) or an advanced level where the auxiliary demonstrates increased levels of skill and knowledge, has undergone additional training and is able to deal with greater responsibility. Essentially, the greater the competence and proficiency, the more limited the supervision required; supervision cannot however ever be discontinued.

Second is the nature of the programme or type of intervention. The basic principles here are: the more acute the client, or the more complex the client population or the intervention, the greater the need for direct, on-site supervision; and the less modification/adaptation needed to the programme or intervention, the less close supervision is required. This means that remedial programmes will of necessity require closer supervision than maintenance programmes.

Types of supervision

(Taken from van der Reyden and Holland, in Conlan and Nott, 2000.)

- Direct on-site supervision. This type of supervision implies person-to-person contact, working within one site, and is characterized by ongoing contact. Direct on-site supervision can be provided as close supervision, with direct daily contact at the place of work.

- Routine supervision implies direct contact, at least every two weeks, at the place of work, with interim supervision by means of the telephone or written directions.
- General supervision implies direct contact on a monthly basis (minimally) with supervision available as needed.

Direct contact for each of routine and general supervision implies face-to-face contact for at least a three-hour period.

Principles and practical guidelines for effective supervision

The principles and guidelines below indicate components from each of the management functions and are presented in the form of practical suggestions aimed at facilitating the supervisory process. Eight principles have been identified by the author and from the input of colleagues. These are considered essential for effective supervision:

1. development of an appropriate mindset
2. effective planning
3. establishment of a supervisory structure
4. effective delegation and referral
5. effective and efficient communication
6. focus on personal development and job satisfaction of supervisees
7. establishing an ongoing training programme on both a professional and personal level
8. establishing a monitoring programme.

Development of an appropriate mindset

In order to develop the appropriate mindset, occupational therapists need to accept that auxiliaries are part of the profession, are their partners, fellow team members and the co-providers of professional services. Furthermore, they must accept that supervision is part of the duties of the occupational therapist, and that time must be allocated and set aside for supervision. Good supervision is as important as good clinical work and can be extremely rewarding.

Effective planning

Effective short-term, long-term and contingency planning is essential and can be facilitated by establishing priorities for the service and for supervision and identifying conditions needed to meet these objectives.

Drawing up a plan of action together with supervisees, clearly indicating the 'what', 'when', 'where', 'how' and 'by whom' for all tasks, functions and events, as well as establishing procedures for tasks and routine events and compiling user-friendly procedure files, will assist efficient planning.

Drawing up checklists for steps/tasks for all special events or activities and then using these checklists to allocate tasks ensures efficiency and facilitates effective monitoring. It is important to allocate a responsible person for each task and to record this.

Anticipating both positive and negative outcomes, or possible problems, such as a downpour, and drawing up of contingency plans to cope with possible and remotely possible occurrences, may avert disasters and ensure ongoing services.

Establishment of a supervisory structure

Structure needs to be introduced to counter excessive flexibility and create a framework for effective supervision. Such a structure may be established by having regular meetings, which may be held on a weekly or monthly basis and which will include inter-hospital or similar kinds of meetings. Other practical ideas include daily or weekly reminders of events and tasks, drawing up weekly, monthly or annual programmes together and publicizing these, as well as drawing up an annual plan for review of all activities and allocating specific times for this on the calendar.

It is important to conduct individual, group and departmental goal-setting sessions with auxiliaries, as this helps to focus energy and maintain motivation. 'Minimum' direct supervision opportunities for each auxiliary, depending on training and experience, should be established and fitted into the occupational therapy schedule. This may, for example, include weekly attendance by the occupational therapist of treatment sessions conducted by an auxiliary, a two-hour weekly visit to the area in which the auxiliary is based, or attendance by auxiliaries at sessions conducted by occupational therapists.

Feedback sessions to auxiliaries on sessions attended, as well as feedback from auxiliaries on patients and sessions conducted, should be formally scheduled and strictly adhered to.

Individual staff interviews need to be done six-monthly, or as prescribed by the employing body, and need to be used to review goals, plans and progress in terms of key performance areas. Written reports and self-appraisals need to be done regularly, especially after special events and to record incidents. Regular peer evaluations may be utilized effectively. Care should be taken to ensure that these are objective, fair and well controlled by the occupational therapist, and, importantly, agreed to by all concerned.

Supervision checklists drawn up together and completed, for example after special events, will help to ensure that staff members have fulfilled their obligations. Remember to praise accomplishments where appropriate.

Daily 'flash' meetings are often useful; these very short meetings are held to keep in touch, do a quick update, gauge the work climate and anticipate incidents.

Effective delegation and referral

Effective delegation is needed to ensure effective and efficient performance. It requires the occupational therapist to 'hand over', to 'let go' and
also to hold the person to whom a task has been delegated accountable.
The occupational therapist is therefore responsible for ensuring service
competence. Delegation will be more effective when time is allocated for
proper referral or delegation, tasks are fully demonstrated and the auxiliary is allowed to 'practise' with supervision. It is often useful to 'do the
task together'.

After doing a practice session, auxiliaries should be allowed to do tasks
without close supervision. Their knowledge of the tasks and performance
requirements should, however, be checked prior to the session.

It is important to monitor staff; difficulties should be confronted and a
plan put in action to remedy the situation. How and when monitoring
will take place should be negotiated between occupational therapist and
auxiliaries. It is always better to train rather than 'rescue', as little stands
to be gained by any of the parties when the occupational therapist steps
in and takes over. The only exception here would be when a patient is
placed at risk.

Referrals and prescriptions should clearly describe those aspects in
which the auxiliary staff are not adequately trained or experienced to
make decisions. Relevant background details, aims, main principles, content of programme and, particularly, precautions, must be specified.
Referrals should preferably be discussed, the observations and feedback
needed identified and time made available for feedback and future planning for each case/group. The auxiliary should assist in the selection of
activities to fit the prescribed principles.

Effective and efficient communication

It goes without saying that a good supervisor needs to communicate well,
but effective communication does require time and considerable commitment. To avoid communication difficulties which tend to occur, the
supervisor needs to establish an effective system of communication for
each setting/area and set clear expectations and outcomes in terms of
communication. This will include orientation of all staff to the department, hospital or clinic, its policies, plans and procedures.

Documents which set out the vision, mission and programmes should
be drawn up and made freely available to staff for use as reference material. An effective network should be established within the occupational
therapy department and between sectors; daily journals, e-mails and special notice boards may be useful.

All referrals or prescriptions for treatment should be absolutely clear.
The occupational therapist must ensure that they are properly understood and that they can be implemented. These referrals and
prescriptions should preferably be in writing and must be recorded.

The occupational therapist should report back regularly on meetings attended, on plans and developments and issues of general interest (e.g. management decisions, new appointments, visitors, etc.).

It is important to develop good listening skills – auxiliaries should be allowed time to communicate, and genuine two-way communication should be facilitated at all times. This means getting feedback on efforts to communicate, following up on suggestions, negotiating rather than prescribing and consulting continuously, even if it does take more time. Having an open door policy will promote communication, but limitations have to be set in terms of time and the availability of the supervisor.

The supervisor needs to be sensitive when dealing with staff issues, always keeping in mind that sincere interest, absolute fairness, respect and confidentiality help to build relationships characterized by trust. Give praise where it is due. Encourage initiative and give staff opportunities to share ideas with peers and other staff and encourage reflection on performance behaviour.

Focus on personal development and job satisfaction of supervisees

The facilitation of personal growth, empowerment and development of professional competency and personal skills of staff are considered to be essential within an effective supervisory relationship. This principle is easily applied, constitutes a very rewarding aspect of the supervisory process and can be facilitated in several ways, such as ensuring that staff have the necessary skills and knowledge to perform tasks allocated to them, and are aware of the 'bigger picture' and their unique contribution to it. It is essential for all staff to attain a sense of mastery and service competency. It is beneficial to create opportunities for development and promotion by building on strengths and developing expertise, also by revitalizing programmes to offer new challenges to staff.

Empowerment will be enhanced by setting goals together, maximal involvement in decision making and taking on specific responsibilities; also by establishing projects to develop skills and teaching each other. Such projects will also counteract burnout and introduce opportunities for professional growth.

Other measures include improving working conditions and the physical work environment, as well as endeavouring, where possible, to establish a better post structure and, if not possible, to motivate and arrange for more informal 'benefits'.

Being supportive, taking a personal interest in staff and creating an atmosphere of care and trust will increase feelings of personal worth which may be further enhanced by arranging events such as birthday clubs, competitions and a reward system, giving recognition for and rewarding effort, commitment and achievement.

Establishing a staff incident file and keeping it up to date are essential for staff development and should include factual notes of both positive and negative incidents.

Establishing an ongoing training programme on both a professional and personal level

Ongoing training needs to be facilitated by supervision and may take the form of formal education, continuing education, self-directed study and informal personal growth activities. It should always enhance reflection of practice and clinical reasoning.

On a *professional level*, training opportunities may include regular in-service training sessions, attendance of short courses offered on an internal basis or through other organizations. These may be both formal and informal and may be directed at personal development and/or attainment of practice skills. It may also include the upgrading of modules completed during basic occupational therapy auxiliary training, for example in paediatrics or psychiatry, or in the form of additional modules which were not part of basic training (e.g. community development and community rehabilitation) but are required for effective practice at the current site of work. It is furthermore necessary to provide information on and encouragement for further study, particularly with a view to laddering into the degree course, or for the attainment of continuing professional development points.

Establishing special projects, for which staff take responsibility, will enable them to develop special skills such as developing an income-generating project. Involvement in research projects undertaken in the department and facilitation of involvement in and increasing awareness of what is happening in the profession and the professional association, such as attendance of professional congresses and workshops, should be encouraged.

On a *personal level*, training should address practical life skills, such as time and stress management, as well as financial management skills which have often been identified as a special area for input. It should also address ways of increasing autonomy and control, counteracting burnout and should include specific ways in which to acknowledge personal and interpersonal strengths and achievements. An example is the introduction of a fun system called 'spook' (ghost), where an unknown colleague (to the person) shows special care, gives small anonymous gifts or praise to a fellow employee. Such a system would need to be organized by the supervising therapist to include all staff.

Establishing a monitoring programme

The occupational therapist should make staff aware and demonstrate that monitoring is a positive and necessary function, which provides much-needed performance feedback, opportunities for growth and recognition for both supervisors and auxiliaries. It must be seen to be a process integral to growth and development, and which is completely impartial.

The occupational therapist should be knowledgeable about clinical governance procedures and take responsibility for introducing and monitoring such programmes.

Monitoring systems should be planned in conjunction with all staff and procedures and time frames negotiated and agreed upon. Required outcomes in key performance areas should be identified, as well as how to deal with errors, omissions and needs and how to ensure that the plan is implemented. Monitoring should include at minimum a six-monthly general review of all programmes and activities.

Conclusion

Major developments have taken place in the occupational therapy profession during the past 25 years. We have witnessed the introduction of a cadre of staff which, even during the 1960s, was not a consideration. The content, duration and approach to training, the sharing of tasks and roles, the development of effective relationships within occupational therapy settings and appreciation of the contribution of support staff, have changed and developed considerably in many countries. These practitioners are accepted as highly valued members of our profession and essential to effective service provision, especially in the field of mental health and psychiatry.

Although occupational therapists at times still grapple with the dilemmas inherent in the supervisory relationship for which they have to take responsibility, as part of the legal and ethical requirements which govern practice, experience has shown that working together with auxiliaries is both personally rewarding and professionally enriching.

Questions

1. Considering the guiding principles for the allocation of tasks to auxiliaries, describe the role of the occupational therapy auxiliary in terms of assessment, treatment planning and implementation.
2. As an occupational therapist, you are required to establish an effective communication system within your department. How would you practically go about doing this?
3. Discuss the possible dilemmas within the occupational therapist–occupational therapy auxiliary relationship, clearly identifying the factors that impact on this relationship.
4. Discuss the aspects you would cover in an induction programme for newly appointed auxiliaries at the institution where you are employed.
5. Describe the responsibilities of the supervising occupational therapist with regard to continuing professional development of auxiliaries and indicate at least five different suitable activities which may be provided.

Chapter 8
Rehabilitation of the mentally ill in long-term institutionalization

ERLA VENTER AND KOBIE ZIETSMAN

The authors acknowledge that institutionalization relates to people in a care or hospital-type setting. Therefore the term 'patient' is used in this chapter.

Occupational therapy in a long-term institution can be compared to the art of growing bonsai. These little trees are planted in small containers and need constant nurturing in order to survive and eventually become works of art. In the same way the art of rendering an occupational therapy service in this field requires the occupational therapist to carefully nurture therapeutic skills.

In chronic psychiatry the therapeutic process may stretch over many years and some therapeutic goals may take a very long time to reach. Rehabilitation in this field of therapy is determined by the restrictions imposed by chronic psychiatric illness. Theories come and go, and different treatment models are developed, adopted and discarded.

Bonsai artists use different methods and change the style of their trees – but commitment and loving care are the deciding factors that will keep their trees alive and well. The thoughts expressed by the authors of this chapter have developed over years of tending their 'bonsais' while adhering to the core philosophy of occupational therapy that has purposeful activity at its roots.

The stigma of mental illness

Over the past 30 years the focus in chronic mental health care has been shifting steadily to community care and away from lifelong hospital care (Haug and Rossler, 1999). However, the reintegration of the mentally ill patient into the community is complicated by society's negative perception of mental illness, and professionals involved in this field are inconvenienced by the stigma attached to mental illness. It complicates the already difficult work. A common rationalization used by professionals is to equate mental illness with physical illnesses such as diabetes. It seems unfair that people tend to be sympathetic to the physical disorder yet shy away from the mental disorder.

The stigma attached to mental illness is, however, the result of strong emotions experienced in response to the behaviour of mentally ill people. Wishing away the stigma of mental illness – no matter how fervently – will not take it away. Occupational therapists in this field have to confront this as a reality. They need to explore, confront and deal with it as part of the occupational therapy strategy for reintegrating our patients into the community. It is essential to be honest with yourself and acknowledge your own uncertainties and misgivings before trying to facilitate change in those who are in need.

'Stigma' is defined simply as: 'a distinguishing mark of social disgrace' (Collins English Dictionary, 1979). The 'marks' of mental illness are deviations from normal behaviour that are difficult to comprehend, tolerate or accept. They tend to trigger strong emotional responses from those around the mentally ill person – fear, confusion, humiliation, anger, disappointment and frustration, to name just a few. At times terrifying crimes are committed by mentally ill people, such as that described below, and this feeds the community's fear, mistrust and lack of acceptance of all mentally ill people. The media capitalizes on this and the stigma is increased by shocking news reports and sensational movies that portray inaccurate clinical pictures.

Reducing the stigma of mental illness

Case study

While a man was psychotic he believed his family was endangered by evil forces and the only way to save them would be to kill his best friend.

Now that he is well again, he seems to his occupational therapist to be a soft-spoken, gentle man with a love of literature and nature – a man

. . . who needs to be helped to discover his new reality, and to assume the responsibility of the new significances in his new existence' (Du Toit, 1991, p. 18).

The occupational therapist has to establish a therapeutic relationship with this man and walk a therapeutic path with him in the confines of the institutional environment.

The therapeutic process has no news value and nothing will be written about him again. The horror and fear of his deed will remain in the minds of the public, but the guilt, sadness and loneliness of the patient and his family become the therapeutic challenge of the occupational therapist and the rest of the multidisciplinary team.

Occupational therapists can try to alleviate the stigma of mental illness faced by this and other patients in many ways:

A start would be to try to understand the full impact of the stigma on the situation of our mentally ill patient. It not only affects his reintegration into the community, but also his potential for gaining insight into his condition, in that it causes him to resist deep emotional insight.

The public has been conditioned to reject mental illness by negative emotional responses to the behaviour of mentally ill people. When the patient finds himself suffering from this 'despicable' illness, he uses his defence mechanisms to protect himself – he rationalizes, minimizes, denies, projects, etc. Treatment has to start at the origin of the problem, which is emotional. Occupational therapists need to build a caring, accepting and empowering relationship with the patient. Du Toit quotes Buber as follows:

> What do we expect when we are in despair and yet go to a man? Surely a presence by means of which we are told that nevertheless there is meaning (Du Toit, 1991, p. 18).

The patient and his significant others need to be supported and guided towards insight and acceptance of the condition through the strength of the therapeutic relationship. Psycho-education plays an important part, but can work effectively only if the resistance of those concerned has been sufficiently dispelled. Unfortunately, a perfect recipe for this intervention cannot be provided, but occupational therapists need to keep this in mind when planning each individual's treatment, using all the different treatment modalities at their disposal.

The stigma of mental illness can be addressed only by creating and utilizing opportunities for positive, corrective emotional experiences for the patient and his significant others. The patient needs to be affirmed for who he is in spite of the symptoms of his illness.

The family needs to be affirmed for the role they play, supported in the trauma they experience, and guided in the adjustment they need to make.

Every activity in which the occupational therapist involves a patient has scope for affirmation in the form of recognition of their efforts and achievement; acknowledgement of their emotional responses; and respect for the value of their ideas.

Through every activity a patient engages in, he presents himself, and it is that 'self' that needs to be affirmed.

The concept of institutionalization

For the purpose of this discussion, the concept of institutionalization entails the care, treatment and rehabilitation of chronic patients in hospitals or rehabilitation centres for long periods of time and in some cases permanently.

Tessa Durham (Durham in Creek, 1990) suggests that frustration in institutional care develops as a result of adherence to the medical model that defines treatment as outlined in Figure 8.1.

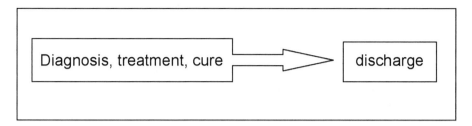

Figure 8.1 Medical model definition of treatment (Durham in Creek, 1990).

Adherence to this approach in long-stay psychiatric establishments leads to frustration and a sense of failure when the 'cure' and discharge never come. Institutional care therefore implies an extended treatment phase with, in most cases, no hope of eventual discharge.

The effects of institutionalization

Long-term institutionalization comprises two main components: the receivers of the care, and the caregivers.

Receivers of care

Bettelheim (Bettelheim in Barton, 1976) used the term 'psychological institutionalism' to describe the detachment, isolation, automaton-like rigidity, passive adjustment and general impoverishment of personality that they noted in emotionally disturbed children living in institutions. Barton uses the term 'institutionalization' to denote the syndrome of submissiveness, apathy and loss of individuality encountered in many patients who had been in a mental hospital for some time.

However, Barton prefers to use the term 'institutional neurosis' for this syndrome 'because it promotes the syndrome to the category of a disease rather than a process' (Barton, 1976, p. 1). He would like the psychiatric team to understand, approach and deal with it in the same way as other diseases. The passivity of the condition adjusts the individual to the demands of reality in the institution, but hampers or may prevent his return and adjustment to life outside.

The clinical features of institutional neurosis, as defined by Barton (1976), consist of the following symptoms: apathy, lack of initiative, loss of interest (more marked in things not immediately personal or present), submissiveness and sometimes no expression of feelings of resentment at harsh or unfair orders. Furthermore, there is a lack of interest in the future and an apparent inability to make practicable plans for it. There is a deterioration in personal and toilet habits and standards generally, as well as a loss of individuality and a resigned acceptance that things will go on as they are – unchanging, inevitably and indefinitely.

These symptoms are being recognized as features of a separate disorder, different from the one that was responsible for bringing the patient into hospital. It is produced by the way in which people are cared for in mental institutions and long-term psychiatric wards. Barton (1976) gives supporting evidence for his theory by stating that a similar set of symptoms is sometimes found in people in such institutions as prisoner-of-war camps, refugee camps, orphanages, tuberculosis sanatoria, prisons and convents. The causes of institutionalization, according to Barton are:

- loss of contact with the outside world
- enforced idleness
- authoritarian medical and nursing staff
- loss of personal friends, possessions and personal events
- medication
- ward atmosphere
- loss of prospects outside the hospital.

These factors should be seen as artificial divisions of an overall picture. They all contribute to the totality of institutionalization. Improvement of one of the factors should not be expected to bring about a magical recovery of the syndrome as a whole. Although Barton described this in 1976, this is still true for people in long-term institutions as described above. The emphasis these days is also rather on de-institutionalization.

The caregivers

This brings us to the subject of the caregivers. The treatment of the effects of institutionalization should take place on a total team basis. The attitude, approach and handling principles of all team members should blend into a comprehensive therapeutic climate that will counteract the development of institutional neurosis. Webber (1995) refers to McGee and Menolascino (1991), who identified the four postures people adopt when interacting with patients:

1. The Authoritarian Posture
2. The Cold Posture
3. The Over-protective Posture
4. The Posture of Solidarity.

The Authoritarian Posture

This can be equated to what Barton (1976) refers to as bossiness of staff and it automatically places the patient in a submissive role. The message that the patient receives from his caregiver is that he is incapable of making choices at any level. The patient feels alienated from himself and others and can take little part in his own destiny – he is devoid of responsibility. This posture tells us a lot about the caregiver's attitude or value base – which may be a need or desire to dominate or control others.

The Cold Posture

This posture is when the patient is alienated from others and feels unworthy of human contact. He can become emotionally fragmented if his needs are ignored and he is not involved in dialogue with others. Self-esteem is poor and this may lead to frustration, anger or, at worst, total passivity. The Cold Posture is demeaning and can lead to dependence or an unhealthy, fragmented independence.

The Over-protective Posture

This is a caring posture that leads to dependence. The individual is rarely given the opportunity to make a choice and thus to develop. This posture may also lead to unhealthy passivity. The attitude evident in this caregiver is a need to gain or maintain control over others. By smothering the patient, the caregiver is demeaning him.

The Posture of Solidarity

Use of this posture epitomizes awareness and responsibility. The message this caregiver sends to the patient is that he has the right to be valued unconditionally. This caregiver is often able to establish a bond with previously rejected and oppressed individuals – patients who complied for fear of punishment now cooperate because of a sense of solidarity.

The caregiver needs to look inward and appreciate his own value base: 'What is it in my own psychological make-up that causes me to smother or dominate a patient?' The caregivers must recognize the need for flexibility and maturity in themselves. It is essential to keep in mind that patients only gain value when addressed in a value-giving language.

It is imperative that occupational therapists and the entire multidisciplinary team should continuously evaluate their own 'posture' in terms of the thoughts expressed above. The question could be posed: are we truly empowering our institutionalized patients?

Loss of contact with the outside world

Patients should have regular access to the outside world through newspapers, magazines, the radio and television. News discussions and quizzes should take place on a regular basis. Visits to parks, resorts and shopping centres can also play an important role in keeping patients in contact with the outside world. This is an important role of the occupational therapist.

The occupational therapist can bring the outside world into the hospital by implementing a balanced activity programme, which is coordinated to resemble events in the outside world. Throughout the year, the entertainment programme should aim to resemble seasonal activities outside, for example, athletics during the athletics season, soccer practice during the corresponding season and celebrating national holidays and festivities. Inter-hospital sports competitions provide an excellent opportunity for practising social and domestic entertainment skills. For example, patients can be involved in preparing a meal for visitors and assist in other organizational tasks. When sports events take place, special care should be taken to provide appropriate sports attire. A real uniform often helps develop team spirit and personal pride.

Service organizations and volunteers can bring the outside world into the hospital. They can visit individuals or groups of patients, take them on outings or organize social events.

Enforced idleness

Occupational therapy can also counteract the problem of enforced idleness. Special care should, however, be taken to cater for the needs and tastes of patients to involve them optimally in balanced activity programmes. Factors that should be taken into consideration include age, culture, level of intelligence and level of creative ability. All spheres of activity should be included.

The long-term psychiatric patient has a unique problem in maintaining self-esteem, which in itself contributes towards institutionalization. Self-esteem increases when there is greater congruence between the self and the ideal self. To combat the negative effects of institutionalization and give purpose and dignity to patients, the occupational therapist should pay attention to encouraging and supporting patients in purposeful activity. The occupational therapist should never demand or order a patient to participate.

Programmes for large numbers of institutionalized patients

Health establishments providing services for mental healthcare users are required to provide care, treatment and rehabilitation. Rehabilitation is defined by the South African Mental Health Care Act (2002, p. 6) as a 'process that facilitates an individual attaining an optimal level of independent functioning'. This definition implies that the caregiver must have a sound knowledge of different levels of functioning.

The occupational therapist responsible for developing programmes for large numbers of institutionalized patients must develop processes and procedures that can be implemented by occupational therapy assistants and nursing staff. Large numbers can range from 500 to 1,000 patients. The definition of rehabilitation gives clear guidelines for the process. It indicates that there should be a balanced programme that enables patients on different levels of functioning to participate actively. The rehabilitation process based on levels of functioning does not necessarily follow the medical model where 'cure' and 'discharge' are the expected outcome, but instead has a goal of increase of functional participation in daily life.

Assessment

All the members of the multidisciplinary team should do independent admission assessments. A minimum period of four weeks gives the occupational therapy staff time to observe the patient in different situations. It also gives the patient time to adapt to a new environment. During this period the assessment and testing can be done by involving the patient in different functional situations. The final assessment is presented at a multidisciplinary case presentation meeting.

The results of the assessment: can be entered on Axis V of the DSM-IV-TR™ (American Psychiatric Association, 2000) (see section below on the multidisciplinary team); can help in grouping patients of the same functional level together; and can indicate strengths and weaknesses that need individual attention within the large group situation.

The assessment form

Because the occupational therapist relies to a large extent on the observations made by auxiliary occupational therapy staff, it is advisable to design an assessment form containing all the relevant aspects to be assessed and a short description of the observation that might be noted. An example of one aspect could be the following:

Cognitive abilities – normal concentration span

Concentration	*Good*	*Fair*	*Poor*
	25–30 min	15–25 min	0–15 min

Regular supervision is necessary to ensure that supplementary staff understand all the concepts of the assessment. They must, for example, understand clearly the difference between a hallucination and a delusion.

Test battery

One of the exciting developments in mental health care is the development of standardized tests that enable caregivers to perform objective assessments. These should be done by the occupational therapist. It is advisable to develop a test battery to complement the assessment form. A proposed test battery is listed below:

• Adaptive Behaviour Assessment System (ABAS) (Patti et al., 2000). The ABAS consists of 239 questions to determine a person's ability to adapt in the community.

- Folstein's Mini-Mental State Examination (MMSE) (Folstein et al., 1975). A screening test for dementia. Some health workers mention that they can also detect depression through this test.
- Cognitive Assessment of Minnesota (CAM) (Rustad et al., 1993). The CAM establishes cognitive levels of performance. It is useful to establish, for example, whether a claim made by a patient that he wants to undertake university studies is a part of his delusional thoughts, or whether he actually has the potential to undertake these studies. It is reassuring to occupational therapists to establish objectively when this type of thought is clearly a delusion.

Standardized memory tests are also available.

Levels of activity participation

Du Toit (1991) provided occupational therapists with a very accurate tool to establish a patient's level of functioning. This forms the baseline from where to start the rehabilitation process (see Chapter 1).

The model shown in Figure 8.2 reflects du Toit's levels of Creative Ability. The wide baseline for care and treatment reflects the great effort that is needed from caregivers at a level of Tone. As the patient's functioning improves, the burden of care becomes less. The rehabilitation effort, on the other hand, will be very limited on a level of Tone but will increase as the patient's functioning improves. The middle diamond of the overlapping triangles reflects the functional levels of the patient population found in these facilities.

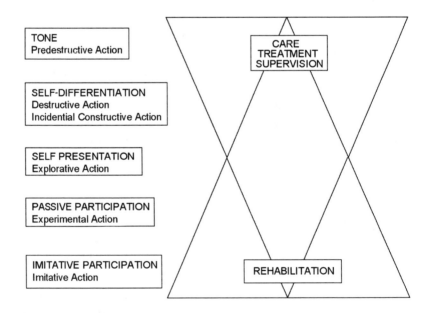

Figure 8.2 A model of care, treatment and rehabilitation required based on du Toit's levels of Creative Ability.

When developing the different aspects of programmes, the levels of activity participation must form a golden thread through the whole process.

The multidisciplinary team

It is advisable that the team meets once a week. Case presentations must be done and after the different disciplines have presented their assessments, a DSM-IV-TR™ or ICD-10 diagnosis should be made. The team should formulate an individualized biopsychosocial plan of action.

Rehabilitation objectives

Based on the biopsychosocial plan of action, the different disciplines must formulate rehabilitation objectives. The occupational therapist must deal with individual rehabilitation objectives within the large group scenario. At this stage there is a need for a generic programme that can accommodate different levels of functioning, so that individual rehabilitation objectives are incorporated in large group objectives.

The generic rehabilitation programme

The generic programme must give the caregivers the scope to enter any rehabilitation objective, whether for an individual or large group related

Table 8.1 An example of a generic rehabilitation programme

WARD:							
GROUP:							
Time	Monday	Tuesday	Wednesday	Thursday	Friday	Saturday	Sunday
07h00–09h00			SELF-CARE ACTIVITIES • Bathing • Washing • Dressing • Dental care • Eating/Breakfast				
09h00–10h00			LIFE SKILLS • Making • Folding linen own bed • Grooming (Handcare/ nailcare/footcare/Vaseline • Cleaning locker				
SPIRITUAL ORIENTATION AND PHYSICAL EXERCISES							
10h00–10h30	TEA	TEA	TEA	TEA	TEA	TEA	TEA
10h30–11h45	Work	Education	Physical Sport	Work	Life Skills	Physical	Spiritual
11h45–14h00	LUNCH	LUNCH	LUNCH	LUNCH	LUNCH	LUNCH	LUNCH
14h00–15h30	Recreation	Social	Education	Spiritual	Social	Recreation	Social
15h30–16h00	SUPPER	SUPPER	SUPPER	SUPPER	SUPPER	SUPPER	SUPPER
16h00–20h00	INSTRUCTED SOCIAL AND RECREATION Watching TV Playing games Listening to radio Intermingling Reading						

to the programme. This programme must yet again allow for active participation on different levels. This programme is developed in conjunction with nursing staff because nursing and occupational therapy must implement the programmes as a team.

The following generic headings represent all activities related to contact with the outside world:

1. life skills training
2. physical activities
3. spiritual activities
4. work or stimulation activities
5. recreational activities
6. social activities
7. educational activities.

Each heading should appear at least once per week on the programme whilst life skills training will appear on a daily basis.

The implementation of the generic rehabilitation programme

It is the responsibility of the occupational therapist to develop areas and activities under each of the seven headings given in the previous section. Some activities will take place in the occupational therapy department whilst other will take place on the ward or sports ground. The occupational therapy department should cater for all levels of patients and should be an extension of the ward programme. An example can be food preparation in the kitchen in the occupational therapy department. All special areas must be programmed on a weekly basis to ensure optimal utilization. These areas should represent the outside world.

The auxiliary staff use the generic programme to plan specific activities on a weekly basis. It is important to give staff and patients opportunities to choose which activities they prefer. The institutionalized patient is often deprived of the opportunity to make choices. In order to make it possible for staff to choose activities, under each heading the occupational therapist must develop a list of all activities, equipment and materials available at that specific facility. For example:

Work and stimulation activities
- Gardening
  - flowers
  - food

- Needlework
  - embroidery
  - knitting
  - crochet
  - rugmaking

- candlemaking
- shoe repairs
- leather work
- woodwork
- adapted paper technology (APT) (making low-cost furniture from cardboard, paper and flour glue)
- furniture cleaning
- paper making
- domestic activities
  - cooking
  - laundry

- multisensory stimulation for low functioning patients

In-service training will be needed whenever a new activity is introduced and an activity analysis must be done to determine how activity presentation is modified to enable patients on different levels to participate actively.

Specialized areas additional to the generic programme

It is a challenge for the occupational therapist to develop work-related activities in facilities with large numbers of patients functioning on a level of self-presentation and lower.

The work-related activities mentioned previously have been introduced very successfully at the Randfontein Care Centre, near Johannesburg in South Africa. The success depends on careful structuring and planning by the occupational therapist.

- coffee shop
- kitchen
- boutique
- recreation centre
- barber shop
- sport areas
- library
- food gardens
- independent living area.

The Adaptive Behaviour Assessment System (ABAS) (2000) can be of value to plan a pre-discharge programme.

As mentioned before, the ABAS (2000) asks questions concerning a person's ability to adapt in the community. When a patient scores low on certain questions, the occupational therapist must consider the relevance of this skill in terms of the situation where the patient will be placed.

An instruction to the supplementary staff may read as follows:

Follow the normal generic programme, for example – Life Skills Training and plan laundry as a chosen activity. Observe the patients functioning and answer the relevant questions.

Rehabilitation objectives

A patient is placed in a group of patients at the same functional level. The biopsychosocial plan of action is based on individual problems yet the rehabilitation must happen within a group setting.

The next process needed is to incorporate individual rehabilitation objectives in a group setting. This process must yet again allow the auxiliary staff to formulate individual rehabilitation objectives within the group setting.

A rehabilitation objectives guide is formulated using the seven headings of the generic programme. The caregiver chooses an appropriate objective from the key and enters it on a form under the identified heading.

An example is the following:

Educational activities

Orientation for place

- Identify the areas of daily living, e.g. bed, toilet and bathroom in the ward
- Find the way to the above areas
- Identify surrounding areas of the facility, e.g. tuck shop, phone, sports fields, dining room, etc.
- Find the way to the above areas
- Identify the name of the facility
- Identify the name of the local town or city
- Identify important community places, e.g. shops, library, clinic, post office, police station, etc.

These objectives are formulated in a graded fashion starting with the easiest objective. This allows yet again for different levels of function. The chosen objective provides the caregiver with the activity for a group of patients who share the same rehabilitation objective.

The form that is used to enter the rehabilitation objectives is used simultaneously as a progress report. An evaluation score key is added and each rehabilitation objective is scored regularly.

Evaluation Score Key

    1 = Independently
    2 = With supervision
    3 = With some assistance
    4 = With a lot of assistance
    5 = Totally dependent

The occupational therapy process in large group settings

The challenge for the occupational therapist working in large group settings is to develop procedures to enable auxiliary staff to do rehabilitation with large numbers of patients. The occupational therapist must, however, be intimately involved in the occupational therapy process to ensure that the service remains relevant.

It can be difficult 'to let go' if an occupational therapist prefers the hands-on approach. It is, however, very rewarding to observe a group of 50 low-level patients actively involved in a work-related activity.

Issues related to discharge from health establishments

When a chronic patient's condition has stabilized sufficiently to permit discharge from hospital, a decision needs to be made about his future: Can he survive independently or does he need to be placed in a supportive environment? A number of placement options are available to the patient.

Factors to consider:

- the level of functioning of the patient (functional and creative ability level)
- the socio-economic situation of the family
- the emotional climate in the family resulting from the effects of stigma or other emotional trauma.

There is no single, clear-cut set of directions to follow in the process of reintegrating the patient into the community. The occupational therapist has a vitally important role to play and can contribute in a number of ways:

- The therapeutic relationship with the patient provides a sound basis for decision making and support of the patient and family. In a trusting relationship the information gathered can be considered reliable and guidance and support more readily accepted.
- Assessment of functioning with attention to strengths and weaknesses/ challenges determines the degree of independence or need for further care. It is not the level of functioning alone that will determine a placement. A relatively low-functioning person can be accommodated in a supportive family environment and vice versa.
- An understanding of the family situation determines the amount and nature of support and guidance needed. Emotional support and education about the illness and functional implications, e.g. the negative effects of schizophrenia, can be of great value in one case and might meet with a lot of resistance in the next. The reason for the

resistance will have to be explored with the help of members of the multidisciplinary team, because it might be indicative of problems that will jeopardize the integration of the patient back into the family.

- Knowledge of long-term placement settings, their criteria for admission and management style is essential. Religious orientation, cultural factors such as diet, style of communication and discipline, to name but a few, can cause a placement of a patient to succeed or fail.
- Teamwork is of the essence – social workers, psychologists and occupational therapists have a wonderful opportunity to complement each other's services.

The occupational therapist's knowledge of the patient's level of functioning and his skills acquired in the course of his rehabilitation can contribute greatly to his reintegration into his home or other placement. The family can be helped to access the strengths of the patient and involve him in the running of the home in a realistic way instead of regarding him as a burden. The therapist who understands the origin and nature of the stigma of mental illness will not be a threat to the family but will involve and support them as team members in this important phase of the therapeutic process.

For many patients a family placement is not an option and a halfway house can be considered. In a house like this the ex-patients live together as a substitute family group with professional and volunteer support. Close networking between community nurses, occupational therapists, volunteers and the patient group is essential. Professionals can learn a lot from the way chronically mentally ill people support each other and deal with the stigma of their condition. A real scenario is as follows:

When asked whether they felt safe in their halfway house, which was situated in a low socio-economic part of town, a patient commented with a laconic smile: 'They are scared of us because we are crazy!'

People with mental illness have a wonderfully practical way of assessing each other's needs and balancing life between independence and accepting help.

A large proportion of chronic patients need to be placed in long-term rehabilitation centres due to lack of family support or a level of functioning that is insufficient for the semi-independent existence in a halfway house. This results in them having to live in large numbers in institutions. This poses another challenge to the occupational therapist and the other members of the team.

Conclusion

The 'magic' of occupational therapy is observed when practical situations are structured and planned in such a way that a person with a functional problem can experience success. The essence of rehabilitation lies in the experiencing of task satisfaction whatever the patient's level of functional ability might be.

Questions

1. Describe the clinical features of institutional neurosis as defined by Barton.
2. Give a definition of rehabilitation and discuss how this will influence the planning of programmes for the long-term mentally ill.
3. Name and discuss the four postures of caregivers interacting with patients.
4. Name the seven aspects that represent a well-balanced rehabilitation programme.

Chapter 9
Vocational rehabilitation in psychiatry and mental health

LYNDSEY SWART

Work is an essential part of our lives. Not only do we spend a large proportion of our waking hours engaged in work activities, but work is our means of earning a livelihood. It also gives us a sense of personal identity and social contribution. Healthcare professionals generally agree that work has therapeutic value and is fundamental to a person's sense of wellbeing. Despite these widely accepted benefits of work, people with severe or long-term psychosocial disabilities have traditionally been excluded from the workplace. Numerous studies have shown that regardless of intelligence level, educational background, previous training or previous work history, employment rates for people with psychosocial disabilities remain dismally low (Marshak et al., 1990; Xie et al., 1997; Wilson et al., 1999). Based on their study of 1,000 cases, Marshak et al. (1990) concluded that people with psychosocial disabilities were only half as likely to achieve positive vocational outcomes as people with physical disabilities.

There is, however, cogent evidence that people with psychosocial disabilities can and should work. Various studies reveal that with proper interventions and support, the majority of people with psychosocial disabilities are able to function in various levels of competitive employment (Desisto et al., 1995 a and b; Grinfeld, 1997; Harding, 1997). There is furthermore a considerable body of research to demonstrate that people with severe and enduring psychosocial disabilities benefit in general from work (Riddell, 2002). Successful employment is associated with reduced hospital admissions (Bond, 1992), increased social interaction with friends, reliable use of medication (Kuldau and Dirks, 1977) and increased quality of life (Arns and Linney, 1993). In fact, Hill (1995) proposes that for people with psychosocial disabilities, one does not get better in order to work, but one works in order to get better.

The underlying principles and practices of occupational therapy lend themselves well to vocational or work rehabilitation. The philosophical base of occupational therapy requires a *holistic* approach to the client and the use of *meaningful and purposeful activity* as the fundamental treatment tools. In vocational rehabilitation, the same principles apply: comprehensive, holistic assessment of the client, analysis of the job and work environment, and the use of work tasks, work activities and reasonable accommodations to assist the client in fulfilling the essential job requirements. 'Work is at the heart of the philosophy and practice of occupational therapy. In its broadest sense, work, as productive activity is the concern in almost all therapy' (Jacobs, 1985, p. ix).

The effect of psychosocial disability on ability to work

The impact of symptomatology and diagnosis

Studies on the effect of psychiatric symptomatology (which refers to abnormalities in moods, thoughts and behaviours resulting from the mental illness) and diagnosis on a person's ability to work has produced mixed findings. While some researchers have found psychiatric symptomatology and diagnosis to be a poor predictor of vocational outcome (Anthony, 1994; Rogers et al., 1997; Xie et al., 1997), others have found diagnosis and symptomatology to have a significant bearing on the ability to secure and retain employment (Marshak et al., 1990; Jacobs et al., 1992; Arns and Linney, 1993). These latter studies generally predict better vocational outcomes for people with mood disorders and personality disorders, and poorer vocational outcomes for people with schizophrenia.

For the occupational therapist working in a vocational rehabilitation setting, vocational planning decisions should never be based on a client's diagnosis or presenting symptoms alone, but should be the culmination of a comprehensive vocational assessment.

Common work-related limitations in people with psychosocial disability

Functional limitations caused by psychosocial disabilities may vary greatly from individual to individual and depend upon the diagnosis, chronicity of the condition, medication being used, and social, environmental and personal factors. In some instances a person with a psychosocial illness is able to work with little or no restriction. In other instances, they may experience significant and even debilitating limitations. Some of the more common workplace limitations that people with psychosocial disabilities have are described by Mancuso (1990) as follows:

- Difficulty in screening out environmental stimuli, such as sounds, sights or smells, which interferes with the person's ability to focus on work tasks.
- Inability to sustain concentration. This often manifests in restlessness, shortened attention span, distractibility and difficulty in remembering verbal instructions.

- Lack of stamina. Common problems include difficulty in working a full day and drowsiness caused by medication.
- Difficulty in handling time pressures and multiple tasks. The person may have difficulty managing assignments, setting priorities or meeting deadlines.
- Difficulty in interacting with others. Getting along with co-workers, fitting in with the workplace culture, relating to superiors, relating to subordinates, reading social cues.
- Difficulty in handling negative feedback. This includes difficulty in understanding and interpreting criticism, knowing what to do to improve and initiating the necessary changes.
- Difficulty in responding to changes at work, for example, new rules, new job duties or a new co-worker.

Other problems can include:

- Cognitive impairments, including difficulty in organizing thought processes, problems with abstract thought, visual-perceptual problems, poor insight, difficulty in making decisions, difficulty in planning, problems with judgement, difficulties with logical reasoning and problem solving.
- Excessive absenteeism due to periods of psychiatric illness, which may be aggravated by workplace stress or by the episodic nature of many mental illnesses.
- Motivational problems, which seriously impair the person's will to even try to work.

The episodic nature of mental illness

Most mental illnesses tend to be episodic in nature, causing sufferers to go through periods of relative wellness followed by periods of increased symptoms and functional deterioration. While these periodic 'ups' and 'downs' are frequently predictable and preventable, they may also occur without warning and for no apparent reason, which can severely disrupt a person's work ability and work attendance in the long term.

One of the more common triggers of psychiatric symptoms is stress. The work environment, with its various rules, regulations, customs and demands, is frequently a source of significant stress for workers. In workers with psychosocial disabilities, this situation sometimes becomes a negative spiral of increasing stress and symptoms, which can eventually severely impair the worker's ability to hold a job.

Predictors of employment success

Extensive research has been conducted on the predictors of employment success in persons with psychosocial disability. In a review of the literature, Tsang et al. (2000) found the following:

Premorbid functioning, and particularly previous work history, to be the most consistent and reliable predictor of employment success. Clients who had worked before were more likely to secure and retain employment. The better their previous work history, the greater their chances of employment success.

Social skill or social functioning level was also found to be a strong and consistent predictor of vocational outcome. Tsang et al. (2000) point out the importance of social skills that allow individuals to develop supportive social networks, cope with day-to-day stresses and find and hold a job.

Cognitive functioning was found to be a significant predictor of good employment outcome. Clients with cognitive impairments, especially impairment in attention span, were found to have poorer employment outcomes.

Family relationships. It is widely accepted that families play an essential role in support and care for discharged patients with mental illness. Tsang et al. (2000) conclude that those clients who have supportive families are more likely to adjust to the demands of the world of work and experience employment success than those who do not have family support.

By assessing significant predictors of employment success, the occupational therapist is able to predict more accurately the employment and placement potential of their clients with mental illness. This information enables them to select the best vocational rehabilitation strategy for each client, and to tailor their interventions optimally to suit their client's individual needs (Tsang et al., 2000).

Employment barriers facing people with psychiatric disabilities

People with psychosocial disabilities face a multitude of barriers when seeking employment. It is important that the occupational therapist be aware of these barriers, and take them into consideration during the vocational rehabilitation process.

External barriers

Job availability

Economic downturns and recession disproportionately impact individuals with disabilities and particularly those with severe psychosocial disability (Noble et al., 1997).

Prejudicial attitudes and misconceptions

The barriers caused by being categorized as 'mentally ill' can be overwhelming. Prejudicial attitudes can be harboured by families, employers, fellow workers, rehabilitation professionals and psychosocially disabled people themselves. Examples of typical misconceptions about psychosocially disabled people include: they tend to be violent, they tend to act irrationally, they are unable to tolerate stress, they have impaired intellectual abilities, they are unreliable and they require full-time supervision.

Limitations in vocational rehabilitation facilities

Common problems with vocational rehabilitation facilities include:

- Programmes tend to be time-limited and provide no ongoing support for the client. This way of functioning is entirely contrary to the reality of severe psychosocial disabilities, which tend to be episodic in nature and fluctuate over time in terms of severity and impact (Noble et al, 1997).
- Poor integration of medical and vocational rehabilitation services. When there is poor or no communication between acute psychiatric rehabilitation professionals and vocational rehabilitation professionals, the gains made in acute psychiatric rehabilitation are often diminished or lost. Services are also often unnecessarily replicated, which is costly and time-consuming for all involved.
- Many insurance schemes tend to put their energies and resources into determining eligibility for compensation as opposed to rehabilitating people to return to work. Comprehensive vocational rehabilitation programmes thus frequently lack qualified staff and resources.
- Many financial backers of vocational rehabilitation programmes tend to use the number of job placements as a primary measure of the effectiveness and efficiency of the programme, and award funds accordingly. With the traditionally low placement experience of people with psychosocial disabilities, it becomes apparent why many vocational rehabilitation programmes for this sector are inadequately funded.
- Vocational rehabilitation professionals are frequently not skilled in the special needs of people with psychosocial disabilities. These professionals often unwittingly reinforce stigma through their interactions with clients by holding faulty ideas about the nature of disability, by perpetuating negative stereotypes by expecting clients to conform to dictated treatment and dependency roles and by casting clients inappropriately into unskilled jobs (Garske and Stewart, 1999).

Disability benefits often provide a disincentive to work

Many income replacement benefits contain a clause stipulating that if the recipient earns even a nominal income, the benefit will be discontinued. Such benefits serve to discourage a person with a disability from returning to work.

Internal barriers

The effects of the psychiatric disability

Severe psychosocial disability often interferes with a person's functioning in their everyday activities. Functional limitations may differ from person to person, depending on the type and severity of the disability. Some examples of the most common functional limitations are discussed later in this chapter.

The effects of the stigma of mental illness

Despite great advances in our understanding of mental illness over the past few decades, our society still has difficulty in accepting and dealing with people living with psychosocial disabilities. Misunderstanding about the nature and the cause of mental illness causes people to react with fear, shame, guilt and embarrassment. For people with psychosocial disabilities, these reactions tend to aggravate feelings of inadequacy, poor self-esteem, rejection and loneliness. This frequently results in people with psychosocial disabilities being denied full participation in family life, normal social activities and productive employment (Garske and Stewart, 1999).

The vocational rehabilitation process

Vocational rehabilitation is a truly inter-professional practice, straddling the vastly different worlds of medicine/rehabilitation and work. Medical and rehabilitation professionals working in this field must develop an appreciation for the philosophies, practices and culture of the workplace, in order to function effectively. Depending on the country and the specific context in which the vocational rehabilitation service is offered, the occupational therapist may find him- or herself working with a broad range of other professions such as occupational health doctors, occupational health nurses, physiotherapists, social workers, ergonomists, employers (e.g. line managers, human resource officers and health and safety officers), trade union officials, attorneys, advocates, teachers, vocational counsellors, industrial (occupational) psychologists, educational psychologists and administrators.

The vocational rehabilitation process comprises the following services: (ILO, 1985):

1. Vocational assessment: obtaining a clear picture of the person with disability's remaining physical, mental and vocational abilities and possibilities.
2. Vocational counselling: advising the person with disability accordingly in the light of vocational training and employment possibilities.
3. Work preparation and training: providing any necessary reconditioning, toning or formal vocational training or re-training
4. Selective placement: assisting the person with disabilities to find suitable work.
5. Follow-up: until resettlement is achieved.

For people with psychosocial disabilities, vocational rehabilitation programmes may be offered in a variety of settings including hospital-based, employer-based, specialized vocational rehabilitation facilities, training centres, sheltered workshops, community centres or case managed in multiple different settings. Depending on the setting in which he or she works, the occupational therapist may be involved in any one or more of the basic five services. Interaction with other persons providing services to the client, and coordination of the various medical and rehabilitation services being provided remains essential throughout the vocational rehabilitation process.

Vocational assessment

The vocational assessment encompasses 1) intake (or initial) interview, 2) general medical (psychiatric) examination, and 3) evaluation (Jacobs, 1993).

Initial interview

Occupational therapists may perform the initial interview, which usually entails communication with the client and, if possible, members of their family and other relevant role-players. The purpose of the initial interview is to:

- Initiate a therapeutic relationship with the client.
- Gather information on the client's education/training backgrounds, psychiatric history, other relevant medical history, current treatment and current functional status (including functional problems).
- Clarify the client's motivations, objectives and needs in enrolling for the vocational assessment.
- Make relevant observations regarding the client's behaviour, verbal and non-verbal communication, interaction with others and attitude towards the occupational therapist and the interview process.

Medical examination

While occupational therapists do not perform the general *medical examination* themselves, they always require this information to ascertain the psychiatric diagnosis and to establish any precautions or treatment issues that may be relevant to a particular client. It is thus essential that the occupational therapist obtain a report from the examining medical practitioner – usually a psychiatrist.

Evaluation

The *evaluation* component of the vocational assessment lends itself well to occupational therapy concepts, knowledge and skill. The following performance components should be included in the vocational evaluation of people with psychosocial disabilities (adapted from Randall, 2002):

1. Work motivation
- Perception of disability in relation to work
- Responsibility and maturity
- Short- and long-term goals
- Level of interest and effort
- Level of energy and drive
- Motivating and demotivating factors

    - Intrinsic (personal)
    - Extrinsic (environmental/ social)

2. Work endurance
- Current activity profile/time routines
- Attendance, punctuality and time-keeping
- Self-discipline
- Stress coping skills and psychological stamina/endurance
- Symptom management skills and treatment compliance
- Nature and degree of side-effects

3. Basic work habits
- In relation to the human environment

    - Self-awareness, social sensitivity and social appropriateness
    - Attendance and punctuality
    - Communication skills (both verbal and non-verbal)
    - Attitude towards others at different levels (managers, subordinates, peers)
    - Teamwork skills
    - Conflict resolution skills

- In relation to work tasks

    - Task concept (see Chapter 1)
    - Task-related concentration (span and quality)
    - Working memory
    - Instruction interpretation (written, verbal and visual instructions)
    - Judgement, decision making and problem-solving skills
    - Self-checking and error correction
    - Use of materials and tools

- Work-related skills and knowledge

    - Education/vocational qualifications
    - Occupation and occupational level
    - Breadth and depth of prior work experience
    - Job-seeking skills

4. Productivity
- Work speed
- Quality of output

- Initiative
- Productivity under pressure
- Consistency of performance

Techniques of evaluation

Botterbusch (1982) categorizes work evaluations into four techniques:
1) Psychological measurements; 2) Work samples; 3) Work simulation
(situational assessment) and 4) On-the-job evaluations.

1. Psychological measurements

These are standardized measurements, which imply a degree of uniformity
in administration and scoring. A comparison is generally possible with a
normative group. Psychological measurements can often be used as a starting point in the vocational evaluation process, to help develop a profile of
the client. They are also useful in substantiating other evaluation data
(Buys, 1993). Examples of psychological measurements include general
intelligence, interest, abilities, aptitudes, achievement, behaviours and attitudes. While many psychological measurements require specialized training
and are administered by qualified psychologists and psychometrists, there
is a number of self-report questionnaires, inventories and checklists that
can be administered by occupational therapists in the psychosocial setting.
Examples of these measurements are presented in Table 9.1.

Occupational therapists making use of psychological measurements
should be aware that such measurements usually involve a degree of
measurement error, by both the observer and the subjects. Instructions
may be misunderstood or forgotten. The subjects may wish to make a particular impression and may deliberately bias their responses. Fatigue,
language barriers and motivation can also significantly affect their
responses. Psychological tests should therefore be interpreted with great
caution, and should always be used in conjunction with other evaluation
techniques.

2. Work samples

Rosenberg (1973, p. 55) defines a work sample as 'a well-defined *work
activity* involving tasks, materials and tools which are identical or similar
to those in an actual job or cluster of jobs'. Work samples are generally
performed according to time standards, which indicate the client's ability
to complete the task in an acceptable time frame. Work samples have the
advantage of resembling actual work. They allow the occupational therapist to observe basic work habits, motivation and productivity as well as
the specific skills required by a particular work sample.

There are many excellent commercially available work samples that
cover a diverse range of work-related tasks and activities. Examples of
commercially available work samples include the *Valpar* range of products, and the *TOWER* system, both of which were developed in the USA.
Commercially available work samples are, however, generally costly to

Table 9.1 Psychological measurements that can be used by occupational therapists

Category	Name of test	Author	Date
Stress, emotion and life events	The Hospital Anxiety and Depression Scale	Zigmond and Snaith	1983
	General Health Questionnaire	Goldberg and Williams	1988
	Perceived Stress Scale	Cohen et al.	1983
Coping	COPE	Carver et al.	1989
Social support	Short Form Social Support Questionnaire	Sarason et al.	1987
	Significant others scale	Power and Champion	1988
Causal and control beliefs	Self-efficacy measurement		
	(a) Multidimensional Health Locus of Control Scale	Wallston et al.	1978
	(b) Recovery Locus of Control Scale	Partridge and Johnston	1989
Individual and demographic differences	Courtauld Emotional Control Scale	Watson and Greer	1983
	Positive and Negative Affect Schedule	Watson et al.	1988
	Rosenberg Self Esteem Scale	Rosenberg	1989
	Life Orientation Test	Scheier and Carver	1985

Compiled from: Johnston et al., 1995.

acquire and sometimes may not meet the evaluation needs for a particular client or work setting. In these instances, occupational therapists are able to develop their own non-standardized work samples by taking work tasks and work activities directly out of the industry or their client's workplace. Performance standards against which the client is measured should be obtained from the industry or the client's employer.

3. Work simulation

Work simulation involves placing the person into a realistic *work situation* where environmental, interpersonal, task, tool and other such demands are met. Work simulation can be set up in the vocational rehabilitation facility, or on-site at the workplace. During work simulation, variables such as work speed, level of supervision and stress factors can be altered systematically so that the client's ability to deal with each situation can be assessed. A good understanding of the process of job analysis is necessary in order to set up a meaningful job simulation.

4. On-the-job evaluation

The client is evaluated on-site in a competitive work situation. All the criteria of the job and the work environment are therefore taken into consideration. Performance standards and behavioural norms should be evaluated in accordance with the culture, standards and norms of that particular company or industry. It is recommended that the occupational therapist involve employees from the company with appropriate expertise to assist in the evaluation, particularly when the job is of a skilled nature. On-the-job evaluation is usually appropriate towards the end of the vocational rehabilitation process, when the client displays a high degree of work readiness. A comprehensive, clear, written agreement between the occupational therapist and the employer is essential. Such an agreement should cover the purpose of the evaluation; the roles played by each party; the manner in which the client will be evaluated; the criteria on which the evaluation will be based and the roles and duties of each party following the assessment.

5. Interpreting standardized work evaluation tests

In order to interpret the evaluation data correctly, the occupational therapist needs to understand the reliability, validity and the performance basis (Jacobs, 1991) of the standardized evaluation tests used:

- Reliability – a reliable test ensures that the results are consistent and stable from one measurement to the next.
- Validity – a valid test measures that which it is designed to measure.
- Performance basis

  - Norm-referenced tests – these tests compare an individual's performance to that of a standardized population sample. The individual's performance is thus compared to the performance of a norm group.
  - Criterion-referenced tests – these tests provide information regarding the individual's ability to perform specific behaviours, skills or activities. The individual's performance is thus evaluated against pre-established performance criteria. Because it carries no population bias, criterion-referenced testing is generally preferred in vocational rehabilitation settings, as an individual's performance is compared with pre-established industrial standards, rather than the norms of a specific group of people.

Vocational evaluation is a continuous and ongoing process that takes place throughout the vocational rehabilitation process. Following the initial evaluation, the client's progress is constantly evaluated and monitored to determine work readiness, placement suitability and the need for reasonable accommodations. Ongoing evaluation is particularly important in the case of people with psychosocial disabilities. Due to the effects of their medication, environmental stresses and fluctuations in their condition, their work performance can change significantly from one day to the next. An effective vocational rehabilitation programme should closely monitor these changes and attempt to identify any work-related factors that could be precipitating psychiatric symptoms.

Vocational counselling

The International Labour Organization (ILO, 1981, p. 58) defines vocational counselling as:

> assistance to individuals in developing a career or vocational plan. It involves helping the individual in clarifying his values, establishing vocational goals, identifying alternatives, formulating and implementing a career plan and periodically reviewing and revising such a plan on the basis of new information, goals and progress made.

Vocational counselling is usually performed during one-to-one counselling sessions with the client, but may involve meetings of the various role-players involved in the client's rehabilitation. The client requires basic skills in decision making, planning, logical reasoning and judgement in order to participate actively in the vocational counselling process. The occupational therapist may be required to perform vocational counseling. The role of the vocational counsellor is to:

- Clearly understand the client's vocational interests, needs and goals, and determine how realistic his or her job goals are.
- Provide the client with honest and practical feedback on their performance in the vocational evaluation. The client should understand how their impairment limits their ability to work, and what kinds of accommodations they may require in the workplace.
- Provide information on suitable and realistic opportunities for training, education and work.
- Assist the client to develop a career plan, consisting of short- and long-term goals, in the light of the above information. It is essential that the vocational counsellor obtain input from the appropriate members of the rehabilitation team regarding the career plan.

Although the vocational counsellor gives guidance and feedback to the client during the development of their career plan, it is very important that occupational choice remains ultimately the decision of the client. Vocational counsellors should avoid imposing their opinions on the client.

Work preparation and training

The vocational assessment and counselling phases identify the client's current position on their personal vocational spectrum, as well as their long-term objectives and goals. The path to those long-term objectives and goals constitutes the work preparation and training phase.

For clients with psychosocial disabilities, there are five main types of intervention that can be used in the work preparation and training phase: 1) pre-vocational interventions; 2) work hardening programmes; 3) transitional work programmes; 4) case management; and 5) formal training.

Pre-vocational interventions

These programmes deal with the treatment of cognitive and psychosocial performance components such as attention span, planning skills, interpersonal skills, time management skills and coping skills. Group work can be used very effectively in treating these performance components.

Work hardening programmes

Defined by the Commission on Accreditation of Rehabilitation Facilities (1991) as programmes which are interdisciplinary in nature, and which make use of conditioning tasks that are graded to progressively improve the biomechanical, neuromuscular, cardiovascular/metabolic and psychosocial functions of the person in conjunction with real or simulated work activities. Work hardening provides a transition between acute care and return-to-work while addressing the issues of productivity, safety, physical tolerance and worker behaviour. Work hardening is a highly structured, goal-oriented, individualized treatment programme designed to maximize the person's ability to return to work. Work hardening programmes are invaluable in building up self-esteem and confidence, and in consolidating work habits in clients with psychosocial disabilities. They are, however, very labour-intensive and as a result, can be costly. They are probably best and most cost-effectively provided in specialized vocational rehabilitation facilities that have established programmes covering a wide range of work activities. They could also be provided on a case management basis, making use of various facilities and services in the community.

Transitional work programmes (TWPs)

Like work hardening, TWPs are individualized programmes that facilitate an impaired worker's gradual transition from disability to modified work to the eventual vocational objective (Shrey and Lacerte, 1997). Unlike work hardening, TWPs are work-site based, and the worker receives remuneration while participating in the programme. TWPs hold numerous advantages for those clients who are already employed, including early return to work, reduced duration of illness and disability, reduced illness and disability costs, increased employer involvement and accountability, reduced work disruptions, enhanced morale (the employee feels valued by the employer), and protection of the employability of the worker. The other great advantage of TWPs is that realistic environmental factors including the physical environment, company culture, work ethic and labour influences are factored into the rehabilitation programme. For people with psychosocial disabilities, these environmental influences are frequently a source of considerable stress, and can significantly interfere with the person's ability to perform their job. Depending on the degree of infrastructure within a particular company, the role of the occupational therapist in TWPs can range from taking prime responsibility for developing and implementing a TWP, to case management of a particular client, to delivering a specific on-site service to a client, for example, training in stress management techniques or implementing reasonable accommodations.

Case management

Case management is a proactive, integrated and coordinated process that assesses impaired workers' needs; plans, negotiates, implements and coordinates services; and evaluates services to determine outcome characteristics (National Coalition of Associations for the Advancement of Case Management, 1993, quoted by Hursh, 1997). The case manager is typically a rehabilitation professional, and often an occupational therapist. The role of the case manager is described by Hursh (1997) as follows:

- understanding the client's disability needs
- determining readiness for return-to-work planning
- developing individualized disability case management plans
- negotiating, implementing and coordinating internal and external services and service providers
- monitoring quality and quantity of service delivery
- documenting and evaluating service delivery and outcome characteristics.

Case managers may work directly for the state, an insurance company or a private rehabilitation provider. They could also be private practitioners who have expertise in rehabilitation methods and procedures, medical and healthcare services, service costs and claims adjudication procedures (Hursh, 1997).

Formal training or retraining

Clients may enrol in formal vocational training programmes at universities, colleges, schools, training centres and special training institutions, as part of their vocational rehabilitation programme. The role of the occupational therapist in this instance would be to help the client select an appropriate course of training, assist with the application and enrolment process, and help the client to identify the need for, and request, reasonable accommodations where appropriate. Once the client has commenced their training, the occupational therapist should provide supportive follow-up on a regular basis. Following formal training or retraining, most clients re-enter the vocational rehabilitation facility for placement services.

Selective placement

The International Labour Organization (1981, p. 52) defines selective placement as:

> the process aimed at placing disabled people in employment suited to their age, experience, qualifications and physical and mental capacities. It should make use of all the normal resettlement services and provisions, in the light of the known and carefully assessed needs of each disabled person. This is the final stage of rehabilitation and includes three distinct processes: (1) knowing the worker; (2) knowing the job; and (3) matching the worker to the job.

In some developed countries, for example the USA, specially trained placement officers are used to perform the vocational placement function. Many countries, however, do not require staff to have specific qualifications, and the occupational therapist may frequently find him- or herself entrusted with this responsibility.

Placement options

Depending on their work abilities and potential, clients may be placed in one of the following three categories of employment: 1) sheltered employment; 2) supported employment; 3) competitive employment.

Sheltered employment

Sheltered employment generally refers to extended employment provided under special conditions (e.g. in a sheltered workshop or at home) to people with disabilities who, because of the nature and severity of their disability, are unable to perform a job under ordinary competitive working conditions (ILO, 1981). Sheltered employment may be provided by the state, but more often it is provided by private establishments, usually run by voluntary associations or as cooperatives or, more rarely, as genuine commercial enterprises (Visier, 1998). Sheltered employment environments may vary depending on the country, the nature of the sheltered employment structure, the degree of disability and whether the employer is party to a collective agreement. In most sheltered employment environments, the workers are considered clients or trainees and the management approach is primarily supportive in nature. In other sheltered employment environments, workers enjoy quasi-employee status, with some therapeutic support. A small minority of sheltered employment environments afford workers full employee status, with equal rights and obligations (Visier, 1998).

There is a number of disadvantages of sheltered employment, including segregation from the employment mainstream; lack of (or inadequate) remuneration; and hindrance of personal and vocational development. Sheltered employment, and particularly that which does not offer the individual full employee status, should only be used as a placement choice when the person with disability is clearly and unequivocally incapable of meeting the demands of competitive or supported employment with or without reasonable accommodations.

Supported employment

Supported employment is a way of enabling people who need additional assistance to obtain and develop their careers in real jobs, so that they can enjoy the social and economic benefits of employment. Support is provided on an individual basis to both employer and employee for as long as it is required (O'Bryan et al., 2000). Support is provided by either a *job coach* or a *natural support*. A job coach is usually a professional or para-professional who provides on-the-job support and advocacy services to the worker and helps them achieve independence in the employment setting. The job coach is expected to reduce their presence at the job site over time, as the client becomes better adjusted and more independent. The role of a job coach is ideal for the certified occupational therapy assistant (Jacobs, 1993). A natural support entails utilizing appropriate personnel within the person with disability's work environment to provide ongoing support, training and instruction. Several studies have indicated the advantage of natural supports over job coaches, in that the presence of a job coach may inhibit interaction between the worker with a disability and co-workers and supervisors (Storey and Horner, 1991; Kilsby and Beyers, 1996; Banks et al., 2001).

Riddell (2002) quotes a number of studies from the United Kingdom, the United States and Canada which indicate that supported employment is effective for participants, improving their financial situation and enhancing their sense of wellbeing and social integration. Supported employment has also demonstrated success in opening pathways to competitive employment for people with severe and persistent mental illness (Lehman, 1995; Bond et al., 1997).

Competitive employment

Competitive employment is normal, mainstream employment, where the employee performs work under similar conditions to all other workers, and accepts the same performance standards, regulations and remuneration system. Competitive employment can be performed with or without reasonable accommodations.

The placement process

Placement involves the following phases: 1) Knowing the worker/client; 2) Knowing the job; 3) Matching the worker and the job; 4) Effecting the placement.

Knowing the worker

The information obtained in the assessment phase is used to draw up a profile of the client, including their interests, aptitudes, strengths, limitations, potential and precautions. It is important that as far as possible, these factors are objectively measured using valid and reliable measurement tools.

Knowing the job

This entails drawing up a job profile, which contains a list of the essential job functions and an analysis of the physical and psychosocial demands required by the job. The job profile should be presented in such a way that the job demands can be easily compared with the worker profile. For example, performance components such as concentration, ability to follow written instructions, ability to work independently and physical strength, could be listed on both the job profile and the worker profile. A job analysis is usually performed in order to get the information for the job profile. The International Labour Organization (1981, p. 40) defines job analysis as:

> systematic and detailed information about a job. It must indicate what the worker does, how he does it, why he does it, and what skill is involved in doing it. In addition to the physical and mental requirements and working conditions, the analysis may also include facts about tools used, machines operated and special skill required in the job and how this is acquired.

With their well-developed skills in task analysis, the role of job analysis falls easily within the occupational therapist's professional scope of practice.

Matching the worker and the job

The worker profile is compared with the job profile to determine whether the client is able to perform the essential requirements of the job. Where the client's abilities do not match the job requirements, the occupational therapist should investigate the possibility of bridging this gap through rehabilitation, skills training or reasonable accommodations. It is also important that the occupational therapist consider the long-term effects of the psychiatric disability when assessing a client's suitability for a particular job. The importance of a good person–job match for people with psychosocial disorders is expressed in various studies. Harding et al. (1987) point out that psychiatric symptoms can be reduced if there is a good match between the client and the environmental demands. It is also important that there is ongoing re-evaluation for the client–job match, particularly in view of the changing nature of many psychiatric illnesses (Strauss et al., 1985).

Effecting the placement

Effecting a placement entails helping the client to get a job, and making the job secure for the client. This involves four main functions: 1) job search support and 2) training in job-seeking skills; 3) job induction; and 4) evaluation for, and implementation of, reasonable accommodations.

1. Job search support

Within the vocational rehabilitation literature, job search support has been identified as one of the services likely to lead to a successful placement outcome (Riddell, 2002). Of the various methods of job hunting, networking using both the client and the placement officer's resources has been identified as being the most effective job search strategy (Burns, 1987; Riddell, 2000).

The role of the occupational therapist in helping the client to find a job is generally as follows:

• Establish a job register of job information sources.
• Help the client to identify and develop their own personal resources, especially amongst employed people, e.g. friends, family and former employers.
• Advise the client on community job information resources, e.g. private employment agencies, specialized employment agencies for people with disabilities, and state employment agencies.
• Help the client to plan and implement a personal job search campaign.

Job clubs, where groups of people with disabilities get together on a regular basis to support each other and share job leads and job search information, have also proved to be effective. The occupational therapist could act as a non-directive facilitator to these group meetings.

2. Training in job-seeking skills

Clients may need training in completing job application forms and preparing a curriculum vitae (CV), or résumé. They should be taught to present themselves as positively as possible, with an emphasis on their strengths and skills and how these relate to their ability to perform the essential job requirements. Clients should acquire a sound understanding of any legislation that protects their rights as a job seeker with a disability. They should also receive guidance in dealing with 'difficult' issues, such as gaps in their employment history due to hospitalization and psychiatric treatment. Because most job application forms follow a similar format, it is suggested that the client carry a correctly completed sample application form with them during their job search, so that all their details are readily at hand. For clients who have never worked before, or who have a poor work history, a *functional* CV is often a good idea. A functional CV stresses a person's functions, achievements and capabilities (as they relate to a particular job) rather than their employment history.

Clients should also be properly prepared for the job interview. The occupational therapist usually gives guidance in:

- Knowledge of any legislation that may affect the client as a disabled interviewee, including the employer's duties and responsibilities and employee's rights. The client should also be advised on what action to take if they feel they have been unfairly discriminated against by a prospective employer.
- Preparation before an interview. This includes the planning involved in arriving at the interview punctually and with all the necessary documentation and information.
- Appearance and mannerisms.
- Verbal techniques, including what information to give and what information to ask.
- Dealing with difficult questions, for example gaps in employment history, little education or too many short-term jobs.
- Acquiring basic information about the companies applied to and the specific job being applied for. This information can usually be obtained from the company public relations officer, the employment agency or the company prospectus.
- Requesting the need for reasonable accommodation in the interview process, if necessary. For example, a client who experiences afternoon fatigue due to the effects of medication may request a morning interview.

Techniques used in interview training usually include counselling, discussion and role-play, the latter being an effective means of allowing clients to practice newly learned skills. Videotaping the role-play process is a good way of helping the client to identify their problem areas, but should be used with caution, so as not to break down a client's self-esteem.

3. Job induction

Job induction is the process of facilitating the (re)introduction of a person with disability to employment by minimizing potential difficulties and/or offering special assistance where required. Occupational therapists who are involved in job induction usually perform the following functions:

- Serve as an intermediary between the personnel manager, the supervisor and the client, particularly in the case of clients with severe disabilities.
- Arrange for on-the-job training.
- Assist in the formal orientation process.
- Provide disability sensitization and awareness training to co-workers, supervisors and subordinates where necessary.

- Evaluate the need for reasonable accommodations and facilitate the implementation thereof, where necessary.

4. Evaluation for, and implementation of, reasonable accommodations

Many countries have special legislation or regulations which give people with disabilities the right to reasonable accommodation in the workplace. A reasonable accommodation is any change to a job or to the work environment that enables a qualified individual with a disability to perform the essential requirements of the job and to enjoy equal employment opportunities. What is reasonable will depend on the facts and the circumstances of a particular situation, and could include considerations such as the overall financial resources of the employer, the nature and the cost of the accommodation, the type of operation of the business, health and safety issues, interference in the operation of the business and disruption of a collective agreement. Reasonable accommodation does not require lowering of performance standards or removing essential functions of the individual's job. The primary criterion for determining whether an accommodation is reasonable is how effective the accommodation is in enabling the person to perform essential job functions.

Reasonable accommodations can be provided in all phases of the employment process, including recruitment, selection and training; in the working environment; in grievance procedures; in the performance management process and in employee benefits and conditions of service. Reasonable accommodation can be requested by the person with the disability, or on their behalf by a family member, friend, health professional (occupational therapist) or other representative.

The provision of reasonable accommodations should be based on a systemic, problem-solving approach, which uses the client's experiences and recommendations as a starting point. The accommodation process should begin with identification of a performance problem, then apply task analysis and client assessment to further define the problem. Several potential solutions should be identified, with the final choice being based primarily on how effectively the accommodation allows the individual to perform the essential job requirements. Cost-effectiveness, convenience and business-related factors can also be taken into consideration when making a decision as to which reasonable accommodation to use.

Reasonable accommodation is always conducted on a case-by-case basis with input from the person with the disability. Examples of reasonable accommodations commonly used for people with psychiatric disabilities are (The Center for Psychiatric Rehabilitation, Boston University, 1998; The South African Federal Council on Disability, 1999):

- Restructuring jobs – having minor, non-essential job duties eliminated; dividing large assignments into smaller tasks and steps.
- Flexible scheduling – changing the start or the end of the work day to accommodate side effects of medication; working part-time; taking

more frequent breaks; taking time off for therapy appointments; working from home.

- Flexible leave – being able to use sick leave for mental health reasons; taking extended leave without pay due to hospitalization.
- Specialized equipment and assistive devices – receiving daily instructions via e-mail instead of verbally; allowing employee to play soothing music using a cassette player and a headset; allowing employee to tape-record meetings and discussions.
- Modifying work sites – installing wall partitions around work stations to minimize visual and auditory distractions; increase natural lighting.
- Providing a job coach, mentor or natural support – provides support, training and advocacy on the job.
- Accommodations in training – allowing extra time to learn new job tasks; allowing employee to tape training sessions.

Follow-up

Follow-up is the control function of vocational rehabilitation services. It measures how effectively the programme objectives have been achieved, provides ongoing support to the client and endeavours to correct any problems that may have arisen. The importance of *ongoing support* for workers with psychosocial disabilities has been well documented in the literature (Hill, 1995; Noble et al., 1997; Ahrens et al., 1999).

Employer intervention strategies: the occupational therapist as a disability management consultant

Occupational therapists with expertise in vocational rehabilitation are increasingly moving into corporate and industrial work settings as consultants to employers on issues of disability equity and disability management. Apart from the traditional rehabilitation services described in this chapter, these therapists are also performing the following functions:

- Conducting sensitization and awareness training sessions on disability and disability issues.
- Advising employers on the practical implementation of applicable disability legislation, regulations and good practice.
- Advising employers on the management of employees with disabilities in the various phases of employment, including: recruitment and selection; training; in the normal work environment; performance management; grievance procedures; dismissal and the fair provision of employee benefits.
- Advising employers on reasonable accommodation-related issues.

In order to perform these specialized roles, occupational therapists have to acquire a basic understanding of the world of work, including corporate and industrial culture; human resources management; financial management; labour relations and marketing. Other specialized knowledge and skills required by the occupational therapist include: a sound understanding of industrial disability management; disability benefit and disability insurance structures; legislation affecting employees with disabilities; case management skills; and knowledge of relevant community resources.

Summary

Vocational rehabilitation offers an exciting and rewarding field of practice to occupational therapists working in the field of psychiatry and mental health. As one of the final stages in the rehabilitation process, the aim of vocational rehabilitation is to optimally (re)integrate the individual with a disability into society and, wherever possible, remunerative employment. Because vocational rehabilitation spans the corporate/industrial sector as well as the medical/rehabilitative sector, the occupational therapist has the opportunity to work with a wide variety of people and professions. In order to do this successfully, the therapist needs to acquire new skills and expertise in industrial disability management. The challenge for many schools of occupational therapy is to develop appropriate undergraduate and postgraduate training programmes that will empower their graduates to move out of the clinics and into the workplace. For it is in the workplace and in society that true integration of people with psychosocial disabilities can really occur.

Questions

1. Describe the ways in which psychosocial disabilities can limit a person's ability to function in competitive employment.
2. Describe the main barriers to employment commonly experienced by people with psychosocial disabilities.
3. Describe the five stages of the vocational rehabilitation process.
4. Name and describe four techniques of evaluation used by occupational therapists in evaluating people with psychosocial disabilities.
5. Name and describe five types of intervention that can be used in preparing people with psychosocial disabilities to enter or return to the workplace.
6. Name the four phases of selective placement, and describe the occupational therapist's role in each phase.

Chapter 10
Psychiatric occupational therapy in the corporate, insurance and medicolegal sectors

LEE RANDALL

Occupational therapy is not a prominent profession outside of health, rehabilitation and education circles. One reason is that the profession is relatively small and not very well marketed or publicized in broader society. It is sometimes confused with other professions, such as occupational health and industrial psychology. Finally, those who need occupational therapy at some point in their lives form a minority group within the population.

Thus, occupational therapists stepping out of the health sector and into the corporate, insurance and medicolegal sectors may be strangers in a strange land. They must be adept at explaining what occupational therapists do and how they do it. A psychiatrically oriented occupational therapist has an even harder time, as social perceptions of the profession focus largely on hands-on physical rehabilitation, therapy for learning disabled children, or domiciliary and geriatric work. Employers, managers, trade unions, attorneys and insurance companies can be surprised to discover the depth of our mental health training and skills and may confuse occupational therapists' expertise with that of psychologists and psychiatrists.

For all of these reasons, there are particular prerequisites for providing effective corporate, insurance and medicolegal services. This chapter spells out what these services entail, and suggests what an occupational therapist should consider prior to taking on such work. Each of the three sectors could justify a chapter in itself, so this is an introduction to the key concepts rather than an in-depth presentation of what is required to work in each setting. Other chapters in this book, particularly those on clinical reasoning, vocational rehabilitation and occupational therapy in forensic psychiatric settings, will overlap in certain respects with the information contained in this chapter. The chapter refers to the South African legal system but will be relevant in many respects to procedures in other countries.

Reasons for referrals to occupational therapy

When an occupational therapist is asked to perform corporate, insurance or medicolegal work, it is frequently in the capacity of an expert advisor/consultant/evaluator, and less frequently in the capacity of a therapist. Typical referrals in the former category, specific to the psychiatric field, include the following:

- A request from an employer to assess an employee's work capacity with regard to a specific high-level job, after some time off work with a stress-related illness.
- A request from a company's occupational health doctor to assess what sorts of reasonable accommodations the company may need to make for an employee recently diagnosed with bipolar affective disorder.
- A request from a trade union to help evaluate the level of sensitivity and respect shown to employees who have psychiatric problems such as job-related post-traumatic stress disorder.
- A request from a claims assessor at a disability insurance company to perform a functional capacity evaluation of someone who has been out the workplace for some time, to assess his suitability for a vocational rehabilitation and return-to-work programme.
- A request from a risk manager in a disability management consultancy to perform a work capacity evaluation of an employee who has started taking excessive amounts of sick leave for mental health reasons, and is not coping with his/her usual job duties – this is sometimes called *pre-claims screening* or *early intervention*.
- A request from an attorney to evaluate someone who has physical injuries and psychosocial problems after a car accident, and to write up a medicolegal report. The occupational therapist will recommend and cost those therapeutic and rehabilitative interventions, types of special equipment, and human and financial assistance needed to restore the person as closely as possible to pre-accident levels of functioning and independence. This may include, for example, assistive devices, adapted clothing, supported living options or home modifications, attendant care, household assistance, vehicle modifications or special transport allowances, vocational rehabilitation or other forms of occupational therapy, retraining or job realignment and workplace accommodations. In addition to producing a written document, the occupational therapist may need to provide expert oral testimony in court.
- A request from the court system to act in an advisory capacity and evaluate reports produced by two occupational therapists in a civil claim, where their recommendations differ widely and they cannot reach agreement as to the claimant's needs.
- A request from a commissioner at the Council for Conciliation, Mediation and Arbitration (CCMA) to assist with a hearing between an employer and a psychiatrically disabled employee, to establish whether

unfair discrimination occurred and what reasonable accommodations the employer could be obliged to offer the employee

Being able to predict return-to-work prospects and evaluate work capacity is crucial in the insurance and corporate fields, where occupational therapists' main roles are to comment on and intervene in relation to work-related functioning. This requires one to develop professional judgement with regard to the likelihood of someone resuming work, with or without rehabilitation/treatment.

In the medicolegal field, work capacity is important but functional capacity in relation to a variety of productive but unpaid activities is equally essential and a focus of the occupational therapist's attention. The growing role of occupational therapists in this regard is beginning to be reflected in the international literature.

> Changes in the law regarding compensation for loss of capacity to perform household services has led to increased demand for occupational therapists' assessment skills to determine the impact of impairment upon individuals' abilities to perform unpaid labour such as housekeeping, child care or yard work and the cost of replacing this labour. Judges now require detailed information on functional abilities. Individuals such as entrepreneurs or farm wives, whose work is multi-dimensional, can benefit from the occupational therapist's ability to analyse and describe their jobs and relate this to their past, present and potential function. It is a positive sign that occasionally both sides in a dispute will agree to share the cost of an occupational therapy assessment and analysis of costs of future care (Kennedy, 1997a).

Within the corporate, insurance and medicolegal sectors, typical reasons for referrals for therapy include the following:

- a request from an employer to provide stress management therapy sessions to a group of middle managers
- a request from a disability insurance company to implement a vocational rehabilitation programme for a policyholder who has been off work with depression and has been receiving disability benefits for some time
- a request from an employee to assist him/her with job-related coping issues, due to psychiatric symptoms and medication side-effects impairing his/her work capacity
- a request from an attorney to provide therapy for a successful claimant in a civil case, where part of the compensation payout was earmarked for occupational therapy.

The therapeutic role may also take on the form of case management, where an occupational therapist is briefed to follow up an employee/claimant over the longer term, helping to resolve day-to-day functional difficulties and promoting maximal independence and participation.

Professional experience and exposure required for corporate, insurance and medicolegal work

Many occupational therapists feel ill-equipped to enter corporate, insurance and medicolegal territory, especially when they have been trained largely in healthcare settings, have client-centred orientations and are used to the back-up of a multidisciplinary team. Newly qualified therapists would be wise to stay away from this kind of work until later in their careers, and those wishing to take it on should find themselves a mentor with suitable experience to groom them.

Before launching into corporate or insurance work, occupational therapists need to develop a solid appreciation for the role of occupational therapy in different settings and to be familiar with the highest ethical principles of practice. They need to appreciate the difference between 'patients' and 'clients' or 'customers'. They need to go beyond a 'hospital mentality'. A certain amount of work experience, life experience and business savvy is useful, prior to taking on the extra challenges of working in these sectors.

Employers become frustrated with occupational therapists who do not appreciate business realities, have naive or utopian expectations (like seeing the workplace as some sort of proxy rehabilitation centre), flout basic occupational health and safety regulations, or advise courses of action that would contravene labour legislation and industrial relations principles. To avoid falling into these traps, occupational therapists should seek exposure to the following, prior to taking on corporate or insurance work:

- a range of real-life work settings, with different work methods, work tools, work equipment and workplace cultures
- prevailing employment practices and labour legislation (including any codes of good practice attached to such legislation)
- the spectrum of equipment, devices and forms of financial and human assistance which are realistically available, and which can maximize the work capacity of employees with impairments and activity restrictions.

The occupational therapist entering the medicolegal field needs to have all of the above prerequisite areas of familiarity, and in addition should have been exposed to:

- a range of community realities (from impoverished to well-to-do communities)
- the spectrum of interventions, equipment, devices and forms of financial and human assistance which are realistically available, and which can restore claimants' functioning as closely as possible to premorbid levels in the work sphere, personal management sphere and leisure sphere. This includes, very importantly, the approximate costs and lifespans of equipment, and the costs, frequency and duration of interventions and forms of assistance.

Preliminary work

Prior to plunging in and performing a piece of corporate, insurance or medicolegal work, the following preliminary steps should be undertaken:

- Screen the referral to check its appropriateness – this includes clarifying what questions need to be answered, and whether an occupational therapist is best placed to answer these. It may also involve checking specific aspects of the request and whether one feels confident to handle all aspects. For instance, an occupational therapist with limited psychiatric experience or interest may refer cases with a significant psychiatric component to colleagues with this speciality focus.
- Where an evaluation of an individual is required, ensure that the 'customer' or referring party understands the occupational therapy evaluation process – including its holistic and in-depth nature and practicalities such as the length of time it typically takes and what items must be brought to the examination. Practical arrangements can be made either via the referral agent, or directly with the client/employee/claimant/plaintiff who is to be examined. Confirm in writing details such as when and where examinations, meetings, work visits or home visits will take place. It is often a good idea to re-confirm appointments telephonically two to five days in advance.
- Agree on what 'product' is required – e.g.: a functional capacity evaluation or work capacity evaluation report, job analysis, workplace review or medicolegal report. Negotiate deadlines, ensuring that these can be realistically met and allowing some contingency time for unexpected events. There could be difficulties with obtaining collateral information or with contacting other professionals involved in the matter, delays in obtaining quotes for unusual pieces of equipment, or delays resulting from internal problems such as sick leave, equipment failure or interruption of services. Deadlines are particularly crucial in relation to medicolegal work, where strict laws govern the timeframe within which professional opinions must be made available. It is important to note that at least 15 court days before the trial, attorneys must give notification that they intend to call particular witnesses, and at least ten days before trial they must make their witnesses' expert opinions available to the other side.
- Negotiate and finalize billing arrangements with the referring party and/or client – this includes details such as the therapist's hourly rate, what services and items will be charged for, and whether a surcharge will be applied if work must be performed on an urgent or after-hours basis. Cancellation fees, in the event of a no-show by the examinee, may also need to be agreed upon. To prevent disagreements and unanticipated financial shortfalls it is best to provide referrers with written payment terms and conditions and to secure their written agreement to these terms prior to performing any work.

- Secure background documentation well in advance of the examination or meeting and delay these events, if necessary, so that relevant information has been viewed prior to their taking place. Review all information provided, noting whether unusual arrangements may need to be made. For example, if an examinee is not likely to be able to provide a clear account of him/herself, arrange for a family member or other informant to be available. If an examinee is a wheelchair user, arrange for wheelchair access. An interpreter may need to be organized. Any additional costs associated with such arrangements may need to be negotiated with the referring party.
- When the client/claimant/plaintiff/employee is present for an examination, prior to actually commencing it is wise to clarify the relationship between the therapist and the party who requested the examination. Most often, the therapist will in effect be an independent contractor with no formal ties to the latter, but the person being examined will sometimes misunderstand this. At best, this could lead to inappropriate requests (for instance, to pass on a change of address to the insurance company/attorney); at worst, it could lead to the examinee doubting the objectivity of the therapist or venting emotions at the occupational therapist which should ideally be directed at the referring party.

Professional self-presentation and standards of behaviour

Occupational therapists venturing outside of the health, rehabilitation and education sectors serve as ambassadors for the profession and must fulfil the highest standards of objectivity and professionalism. They need to be acutely sensitive to the particular context in which they are working at the time, including the cultural, organizational and legal nuances and principles shaping that context. This sensitivity will reflect in their general communication style and choice of terminology, in their clothing and dress style, and in their adherence to norms relating to timekeeping, general behaviour towards others, manner of using facilities, manner of running their own practices and billing for their services, and so on.

In the corporate setting

Occupational therapists in a corporate setting must show an appreciation of the difficulties both employers and employees face, must be aware of relevant legislation and employment practices, and must grasp the realities of the particular business and type of job which is under scrutiny. They must be able to differentiate clearly between illness and disability and between work settings and rehabilitation settings. Occupational therapists need to be familiar with relevant labour legislation of their own country, such as the Employment Equity Act, Labour Relations Act, Basic

Conditions of Employment Act, and Compensation for Occupational Injuries and Diseases Act. Arising out of this legislation, they should know and understand terms such as *employee* versus *contractor, disability equity, reasonable accommodations* and *unjustifiable hardship, anti-discrimination* and *affirmative action*. They should grasp the particular legal definition of disability which is contained in the Employment Equity Act. They should also have an appreciation of broader economic and labour market issues, particularly those impacting upon the particular industry and company with which they are involved. They should be super-sensitive to the concept that 'time is money', and the need for businesses to show high levels of productivity and a healthy bottom line.

In the insurance setting

Occupational therapists performing insurance work must show sensitivity to the purpose and limitations of a range of insurance products, particularly disability insurance policies and income replacement policies. This requires a basic understanding of how insurance policies define concepts such as *temporary* and *permanent* disability and *partial* and *total* disability, as well as familiarity with terms such as *lump sum payments, monthly benefits* and *top-up benefits*. They must be aware of the vested interests of different parties, especially those of the insurance company and those of policyholders and their families, but also those of employers. They need an accurate grasp of the role of various stakeholders, including brokers, policyholders/claimants, claims assessors, chief medical officers employed by insurance companies, and external health professionals such as general practitioners and medical specialists consulted by claimants. They must follow legal and ethical requirements with regard to releasing information derived from their professional examinations of claimants, and must be aware of the broader protective mechanisms available to insurance consumers, including the ombudsman for life assurance. Due to reportedly high levels of fraudulent or spurious disability insurance claims, and the possibility that large financial incentives may lead claimants to distort their symptoms, they need to be vigilant for signs of symptom exaggeration and inconsistencies in the information presented to them. They should, if in any doubt, gather sufficient collateral evidence to satisfy themselves that they have reached a full and fair understanding of the claimant's situation.

In general, therapists should be aware that insurance work requires them to step aside from a client-centred 'advocate' or therapeutic role, into an evaluator role which recognizes the 'greater good'. This does not mean abandoning their client handling skills, such as establishing rapport and validating the individual's worth unconditionally during the examination. For those who feel ambivalent about having to go beyond the considerations of the individual claimant, it may help to focus on the fact that broader society needs to have workable insurance products which pay out on legitimate claims only.

In the medicolegal setting

Occupational therapists in a medicolegal setting need to present themselves in a way which shows appreciation of their particular role in serving the ends of justice – for instance, as an expert witness or as an advisor to a court or a mediating body. It is crucial that they avoid being 'hired guns' (i.e. being overly influenced and having their expertise exploited by one side in a dispute). They need to reach an objective opinion regardless of which legal team has hired them. They need a grasp of basic legal language, including terms such as *plaintiff* and defendant, *general damages, documentary evidence, discovery, loss of earnings, loss of amenities of life, undertakings, possibility versus probability, pleadings, summons, apportionment* and *contingency*. Certain Latin terms may also need to be understood and used, both in report-writing and in terms of general business dealings between the therapist's practice/facility and the instructing attorneys. These include terms such as *curator ad litem* and *curator bonis* and the term *domicilium citandi et executandi*. It is essential to have a sound basic legal textbook or dictionary available.

Medicolegal occupational therapists also need to grasp the roles and vested interests of a large variety of stakeholders including attorneys and advocates for the plaintiff and for the defendant, claimants and their families, claims handlers, compensation systems (such as the Road Accident Fund), and fellow expert witnesses from their own and other disciplines. Even more so than in the insurance sector, they need to understand what is sometimes termed 'compensationitis' (i.e. the tendency for people who have submitted compensation claims to consciously or unconsciously exaggerate their symptoms, in the hope of maximizing their compensation payouts).

Common to all three settings

In all three settings, occupational therapists must ensure that they do the most thorough examination that is possible and appropriate under the circumstances. Leaving out relevant functional assessments will weaken the base of information from which they draw their professional conclusions, and could reflect adversely on their credibility (particularly in medicolegal settings).

Having formed final opinions, occupational therapists must be prepared to outline clearly their professional reasoning process and their conclusions in writing (and potentially also orally – for instance, when required to testify in court, or when invited to present their conclusions to managers or human resources officers). Where possible, they need to use non-confusing terminology which can be understood by someone from outside of the profession. They must report on *all* aspects of any examinations they undertook – if a particular assessment tool did not yield a valid and useable score (for instance, if the examinee was not able to complete it, or if his/her responses were clearly not in keeping with reality), this must be explained. They must be willing to defend their professional opinions to a variety of audiences – including non-health professionals such as employers, managers, human resources officers, claims assessors, attorneys and judges, as well as (at times) to fellow occupational therapists and other health professionals.

This means that occupational therapists' professional reasoning must be sound and well substantiated, and that it should meet the 'reasonable person' standard – i.e. they should not expound weird or wonderful ideas, paint an unrealistic picture, or make outrageously extravagant or conservative recommendations. As already noted, they should not be influenced by anyone in particular and should reach as objective an opinion as possible, regardless of the consequences of expressing this opinion. They should take special care never to step outside of their scope of professional expertise or to encroach on another professional's domain, but should be willing to defer to other experts' opinions whenever this is appropriate.

Occupational therapy assessments and reports that are produced for the purpose of going on to provide treatment or rehabilitation often focus on clients' assets and downplay their impairments. This is in keeping with a rehabilitation philosophy (Kennedy, 1997b). In relation to corporate, insurance and medicolegal work it is important to pay equal attention to both assets and limitations:

> The client must be viewed based on what their future is likely to be and not necessarily what is hoped for. Adequate consideration must be given to the possibility of a less than optimal scenario (Kennedy, 1997b).

Finally, when performing corporate, insurance and medicolegal work the occupational therapist should guard against having too many confusing or conflicting 'multiple relationships'. This means, for instance, that they should *not* examine clients/claimants/plaintiffs whom they know on a personal level, and they should keep social interactions with referring parties such as employers, claims assessors and attorneys to a restricted level (lest their professional opinions are too influenced by their friendships with these people).

Written communication

Skill in producing written communications is paramount in all of these fields of work. Typically, occupational therapists will be asked to provide an in-depth report documenting their examinations and findings and providing conclusions and recommendations. Such a report may be centred on an individual (such as a particular employee, claimant or plaintiff), or may be more general in scope (for instance, dealing with a company's level of accessibility for employees with disabilities).

Contents of reports

The specific content will vary from situation to situation, but all reports should clearly identify the author, his/her qualifications, his/her contact details and the date on which the report was produced. Where the report concerns a specific individual, personal particulars of that individual should be presented in the first section of the report, followed by assessment and referral information (such as the date and place of the assessment, the referrer's name, the purpose of the examination, the names of people who accompanied the examinee, the language(s) in which the examination took place, and any relevant scheme names, policy/claim/case numbers and reference numbers (including that given by the occupational therapy facility/practice)).

For the remainder of the above type of report, as well as for other kinds of reports, the exact content will be dictated by the questions which need to be answered and which led to an occupational therapist being called

Table 10.1 List of contents for reports

Corporate reports	Insurance reports	Medicolegal reports
Employee particulars	Claimant particulars	Plaintiff particulars
Employer and job details	Insurance details: *Insured occupation*	Claim details: •Date of injury
Assessment information: •Purpose •Date(s) and venue(s) •Methods	•Employer •Fund name •Policy number •Referrer	•Referrer •Case/claim no.
Background information	Assessment information: •Purpose	Assessment information: •Purpose
Summary of professional findings and opinions	•Date(s) and venue(s) •Methods	•Date(s) and venue(s) •Methods
Conclusions and recommendations	Background information	Background information
	Assessment findings: •Physical function •Psychosocial function •Occupational performance	Assessment findings: •Physical function •Psychosocial function •Occupational performance
	Conclusion and recommendations	Conclusion and recommendations, with a focus on: •Loss of amenities •Loss of work capacity •Special equipment and assistance required

in. Bear in mind that it is often a waste of space to regurgitate or replicate lengthy passages from other documents – these can simply be referred to, and the main points summarized as needed.

Length of reports

A full report may run from a few pages, in the case of a straightforward insurance referral or after a brief intervention with a particular employee in a workplace, to 50 or 60 pages in the case of a large or complicated medicolegal claim. It may be helpful to obtain a clear brief from the 'customer', e.g., an employer, claims assessor or attorney, so as to know the depth of information required and approximately how long a report is expected from the occupational therapist.

Time frame for producing reports

In many cases, the referring party for corporate, insurance and medicolegal work would like the report by yesterday! While this is clearly not possible, and quality should not be compromised for the sake of producing a report as fast as possible, a good general guideline to follow is to produce reports within two to three weeks. This helps ensure that the information does not became stale, and at the same time speeds up the time frame within which any recommendations made can be acted upon. This includes, for example, the author's recommendations for what should happen with a particular employee in the workplace, or for what types of further medicolegal examinations should be booked for a particular plaintiff. In the insurance sector, timely provision of the occupational therapy report is appreciated because it is often a key element used by the claims assessment team in making decisions regarding a disability claim. Delays in receiving reports may well cause insurance companies to stop paying disability benefits to the claimant, pending the report's arrival – which is sure to elicit an angry telephone call from the claimant concerned!

Report formatting

It can be very useful to have a standard template or layout to guide report-writing, knowing that this can be modified and tailor-made as needed for particular pieces of work. Page numbers and section references are required, along with a clear system of numbering to clarify the importance, sequence and interrelation of portions of the text, e.g., 1.2, 1.3, 1.3.1. This is particularly true in the medicolegal setting, as without these easy pointers much ambiguity and confusion can result. Headers and footers are extremely useful and can contain information such as the author's name and professional designation, client's name and date of the report.

Writing style

Occupational therapists writing reports for the corporate, insurance and medicolegal worlds should bear the following writing style guidelines in mind:

- Reports should be set out clearly and succinctly. They should be broken up with appropriate headings and numbered as necessary, including page numbering, formatted in a way which is reader-friendly and coherent, and contain references and substantiating information as required.
- Longer reports can benefit from the addition of a list of contents and an executive summary.
- The concluding section of a report should not contain new information, but should draw together all the threads from earlier sections in the report, make sense of them and, if appropriate, present a set of recommendations.
- Additional information can be added in the form of appendices and attachments, in the interests of keeping the main body of the report clear and concise.
- Proofreading, spell-checking and grammar-checking methods should be employed to ensure that the final product is as free from errors as possible.
- Particular care should be taken when checking dates, names and highly pertinent details (for instance, policy numbers, case reference numbers, job titles, dates of accidents, dates of birth and/or identity numbers, and full names of individuals).

Writing for the reader

The occupational therapist must have a very clear sense of for whom the report is being prepared. This is to ensure that the style is appropriate and to ensure that the content does not contravene any ethical or legal principle. For instance, a report containing in-depth information on an employee's psychiatric difficulties would not be released to a line manager, but could potentially be released to an occupational health practitioner within the company (who is bound by the Hippocratic Oath and will not breach the employee's confidentiality and privacy rights). In the insurance field, occupational therapists would be wise to make it clear to claimants – *prior* to evaluating them – that the full findings will be presented in the report and made available to the relevant claims assessor. In the medicolegal field, plaintiffs and their families need to be made aware that the occupational therapy report may, in effect, become publicly available through the process of the court case. This is particularly relevant when the report makes mention of highly personal information, such as information relating to bladder and bowel functioning and sexual functioning.

Submitting reports

Prior to writing the report, the occupational therapist should have established to whom it should be forwarded, and how (in person, by post, by legal courier, etc.). In some cases, the same report will go to more than one destination, while in other cases two or more versions of the report will be produced for different readers (as when a therapist provides a more medically-oriented report for a company occupational health nurse, and a strictly job-oriented report for the line manager).

The occupational therapist should carefully consider the pros and cons of forwarding reports by facsimile and e-mail, as these methods are potentially much less secure than mail (general or registered), courier or hand-delivery. Due to their speed and convenience, facsimiles and e-mails are often the preferred choice for the person who has requested the report, but the therapist/author must also strive to minimize the risks of anything going wrong. For instance, facsimiles can be intercepted or may inadvertently be sent to the wrong destination if an incorrect or out-of-date fax number is used. E-mailed documents, unless in a write-protected or read-only format, can be altered without the author's knowledge and may also be intercepted and read by people other than the intended reader. Some therapists have a firm policy of not forwarding documents via these routes, and will provide hard copies only of their reports. These considerations are less important for reports which are generic in nature, and more important for reports which contain highly personal information, such as details of psychiatric episodes, pertaining to a particular individual.

Retaining reports and other information

Exact hard copies of all reports relating to individuals (whether employees, claimants, plaintiffs or clients) should be retained by the therapist (or by the facility in which the therapist is employed) for a period of ten years. They should be kept inside the relevant client file along with supporting documents such as letters of instruction and background medical/psychiatric information. It is important that information is not destroyed – for instance, it is best to keep rough interview notes, raw data, original questionnaire and assessment forms, etc., in the file. Particularly in the medicolegal field, throwing away such information can be seen as an attempt to 'sanitize the file', and may call into question the credibility and substantiation of the final report.

Occupational therapists should store information using a filing system or reference system which makes it easy to retrieve. In relation to corporate and insurance work, even what may appear to be a one-off involvement (for example, a single request to perform a work capacity evaluation, or a single intervention with a particular employee) can lead to further work in the future. In the medicolegal field, it is usual for an initial piece of work (such as an examination and compilation of a medicolegal report) to be followed, sometimes months or even years later, by other work (dealt with below).

Thus, occupational therapists performing corporate, insurance or medicolegal work must be prepared at any time to field enquiries, requests for further work, or even referrals for complete reassessments. In the case of multi-therapist facilities, the principal therapist or chief therapist will have to handle queries which relate to cases where the therapist originally involved is no longer working at the facility.

It is useful to have information easily accessible, both because this contributes to an impressive professional image and because it saves time. For example, being able to lay hands on a file when a phone call comes in may allow the therapist to handle a telephonic enquiry immediately, rather than having to retrieve the file and make a call back. For space reasons, however, it may be necessary to archive older files in a separate storage area, possibly even off-site.

Even more recent files may be archived with some confidence, if the likelihood of further work is minimal – for instance, in the case of medicolegal referrals, where the case has been fully settled. An accurate reference system should guide the therapist immediately as to where the file can be found.

Whatever storage systems are utilized, these should allow for confidentiality. They should be located in a lockable room away from public access and should be relatively fireproof – such as metal, rather than wooden, filing cabinets.

In most practices nowadays, some sort of storage system will also allow for an electronic version of the report to be kept on computer disks, CDs, etc. It is not recommended that electronic versions be kept on the hard drive of a computer which could be accessed by an unauthorized person. Disks and CDs must be clearly labelled and also stored in a lock-up, fireproof place, such as a safe. It is good practice, in addition, to make back-up copies which will be stored somewhere separate.

Provision of duplicate copies of reports

If reasonable requests are received for duplicate copies, from legitimate sources and with the necessary permissions granted by the claimant/client, the therapist should make duplicate copies available. However, stringent controls are needed to ensure that reports are not released inappropriately. Occupational therapists working in the corporate, insurance and medicolegal sectors should familiarize themselves with the Data Protection Act, which spells out confidentiality principles and how and when to release information correctly.

Particular considerations for carrying out home visits and work visits

Corporate, insurance and medicolegal work have in common the possible need to conduct home visits and work visits. In both cases, the visiting occupational therapists should remember that they are entering another's territory, and should adhere to the appropriate etiquette. They should also bear in mind a number of safety considerations and practical realities.

Home visits

Home visits can yield very valuable information and clarify the therapist's understanding of the circumstances in which a client/claimant/plaintiff/ employee finds himself or herself. On the other hand, they can present the most challenging and difficult-to-structure of all assessment environments, which may affect the quality of one's findings, level of concentration of the examinee, and validity of test results. They may require the therapist to venture into unknown and potentially dangerous areas, and may result in the occupational therapist being alone in an unfamiliar setting with an unpredictable subject who may or may not welcome the examination process and may or may not understand the therapist's role. For instance, the occupational therapist may bear the brunt of the person's displeasure with the insurance company, employer or compensation system. Home visits may also subject the therapist to all sorts of emotional strategies and influences (including, for example, being offered a three-course meal or a gift!), and can be difficult to fit into a normal booking schedule due to uncertainty about the travel time required and how long the visit itself will take. Finally, occupational therapists may find themselves unsure of how to behave in the homes of people who are culturally very different from themselves, and may inadvertently make social *faux pas* – such as eating with their left hands in the home of a devout Hindu or Muslim family, or sitting down in the presence of elderly relatives, when cultural norms for that family require younger people to stand until invited to be seated.

Being well prepared for home visits will increase the occupational therapist's confidence, efficiency and effectiveness. This means having at hand all the assessment tools and materials one might need (within the limits of what can be transported!) and being armed with thorough directions to the home – with, if possible, an advance description of the sort of setting it will offer for the examination. Having some means of communication such as a mobile phone or a phonecard is important, so that the occupational therapist can contact his/her office and/or the clients in the event of vehicle breakdown or other delay.

Work visits

Many of the same considerations pertain as for home visits, but with greater formality and possibly more severe professional consequences if things go wrong. When setting up a work visit it is important to establish who the 'host' of the visit will be, for instance, a line manager, a human resources officer or an occupational health nurse. This will usually be someone reasonably senior. A work visit can seldom be set up merely by communicating with the relevant employee/claimant/plaintiff. The purpose of the visit needs to be spelt out clearly in advance, and requests for any particular facilities such as a private interview room, or a quiet testing area, should be presented upfront. Requirements particular to the job site should be dealt with, such as whether there is a dress code or whether safety clothing will be supplied by the company or by the visiting therapist, arranging of security clearances, and so on. Work hours must be taken into account too – it would generally be inappropriate to schedule a work visit for knocking-off time, shift change-overs, lunch-breaks, etc.

On arriving at the workplace, the occupational therapist should introduce himself or herself to the host and briefly reiterate the purpose of the visit. If the therapist has brought equipment (ranging from a tape measure and stopwatch through to a video camera) for the visit, this equipment may need to be presented for security clearance. During the visit, the occupational therapist must take in broader issues to do with the workplace and general work environment and industry, but must at the same time stay focused and tailor his/her activities to fulfil the main purpose of the visit. It is important not to overstay one's welcome or to take up too much of the valuable time of someone who has job requirements to meet and is in effect doing you a favour by allowing for a work visit.

On an interpersonal level, it is best to be equally polite, friendly and respectful to everyone encountered, regardless of their rank within the company. It is generally best not to be drawn in terms of one's professional opinion, discreetly commenting that a period of digestion and going over the findings of the work visit (and possibly also other findings, such as those of an individual examination) is necessary prior to an opinion being formed.

Particular considerations for serving as an expert witness and testifying in court

Occupational therapists entering the medicolegal field take on the role of expert witnesses within their domain of expertise. They become a part of the greater medicolegal team, consisting of attorneys and advocates and that mix of medical and allied health professionals that is relevant to the case. Besides their own examinations of plaintiffs, they may need to participate in pre-trial work such as:

- meetings of experts
- pre-trial conferences between the opposing teams

- drafting a minute reporting on areas of agreement and disagreement between themselves and other experts, particularly occupational therapy experts appointed by the other side, but potentially also other experts such as industrial psychologists, clinical psychologists and psychiatrists.

These are all measures designed to narrow the issues in dispute, thus helping to curtail the duration of trials, facilitate settlements and contain costs. Having agreed to act as an expert witness in a particular case, the occupational therapist must make all efforts to attend scheduled events of this nature, but can request timely warnings from the instructing solicitor. Time incurred on all of these activities is logged and billed for in the usual way.

In all of this work, occupational therapists must bear in mind that their main purpose is to support the role of the court, which is to award fair damages. In awarding compensation, the court attempts to restore the injured party to their pre-injured state, *not* to enrich them. As ordinary witnesses are barred from expressing opinions, expert witnesses occupy a privileged position in being asked for their professional opinion – it is crucial not to abuse this privilege in any way. What gives them the right to express their opinion is the authority vested in them by virtue of their specialized training and experience. Occupational therapists who overstep their qualified authority may be barred from any further court work, or at least fail to secure any further medicolegal referrals.

When oral testimony is required in court, occupational therapists need to bear in mind the laws relating to the giving of evidence. While space does not allow these to be spelt out in full here, broadly this means sticking to established facts and professional opinions which are based on the best available information, and staying away from mere hearsay and lay opinion.

Both in their written formulation of cases and in their oral presentation of evidence, occupational therapists need to untangle complex issues – such as being able to differentiate the functional impact of the injuries/events in question, from the functional impact of any pre-existing conditions.

They also need to develop the ability to explain what qualifies them to express a professional opinion (this includes not only their formal qualifications, but also the types of work experience they have gained over the course of their careers), and to handle cross-examination on the witness stand.

Some of the most important principles to bear in mind are the following:

- Thorough preparation prior to the trial date is crucial. The occupational therapist should be deeply familiar with his/her own report and recommendations, and have a sound grasp of other experts' opinions where these have a bearing on an occupational therapy perspective.
- When taking the witness stand, communication should be directed at the judge, not the questioning or cross-examining lawyer. Having a

highlighted copy of your own report, possibly with 'evidential notes' written in the margins to guide the giving of oral evidence, will avoid the need to fumble through a long report.

- Lay language should be used, rather than specialized professional terminology. Where professional terms or concepts specific to occupational therapy are used, these may need to be clarified through the use of lay language paraphrasing, giving of examples or drawing of analogies, or even through physical demonstrations.
- Value-laden statements should be avoided, along with flowery language and the provision of superfluous information. Specific language is preferable to global or overly general statements.
- Weaknesses in one's professional arguments should be acknowledged openly. It is also far better to say 'I don't know' or 'I am not sure', than to guess at something, or to express an opinion which cannot be substantiated. Dogmatism should be avoided and opinions should not be seen as carved in stone – they may need to be amended if new information comes to light.
- Absolute words like 'never' and 'always', should be avoided, and a positive, definite opinion should be expressed only where there is supporting evidence for this. At the same time one should not come across as hedging too much, i.e. being reluctant to express a final opinion at all. Where opinions are based on literature, statistics, etc., the sources of this information may need to be quoted.
- Legal practitioners may use particular trick questions and trial tactics, designed to undermine the credibility of expert witnesses. Familiarity with these tactics and an ability to remain emotionally neutral will be tremendously helpful in court.
- Attempts to pick apart one's expert report should be met in a calm and reasoned manner rather than with anger or defensiveness.
- The credibility, character and qualifications of fellow expert witnesses should not be called into question, although differing opinions may be expressed and substantiated if the matter under discussion is within the occupational therapist's scope of expertise.

Administrative infrastructure

The occupational therapist offering corporate, insurance and medicolegal services requires a sound administrative infrastructure, fixed consulting rooms which have a professional appearance, clear long-term contact details and good communications technology, such as voicemail, fax and e-mail capabilities. Written documents need to be produced to a high standard, preferably using up-to-date word processing software and any other relevant software such as spreadsheets or graphics software and printed out in strong black ink on good quality white paper.

Administrative staff are virtually a necessity for the therapist who focuses predominantly on these avenues of work, to handle the level of filing, correspondence, billing, report-generation and other clerical functions involved. These staff also serve to provide continuity when the occupational therapist is away on home visits, work visits, attending meetings or testifying in court. Anticipated absences and periods of unavailability (for instance, trips overseas) need to be communicated in advance to major referrers and clients – to allow alternative plans to be made if, for instance, a trial or crucial meeting will occur while the occupational therapist is away. If appointments need to be cancelled from the occupational therapist's side, this must be done professionally and courteously, with due regard for issues such as costs and inconvenience and making all attempts to minimize the latter. For instance, medicolegal appointments may have been booked long in advance and timed very specifically – particularly for clients who live in rural areas and may need to travel to a city to access several medicolegal experts from different disciplines, sometimes from both 'sides', within a short timeframe. It may be appropriate for the occupational therapist to cover wasted costs or at least write off some of his/her own charges, if a claimant/plaintiff/client is significantly inconvenienced.

Conclusion

Corporate, insurance and medicolegal work are amongst the more challenging roles which can be taken on by an occupational therapist. Together with the challenge can go a high level of job satisfaction, particularly for the therapist who desires intellectual stimulation. It can be immensely pleasing to find oneself able to defend one's professional opinion in a court of law, before a layperson such as an employer, or before a public defender such as the ombudsman for life assurance, with confidence and in a way which leads to a fair outcome. In some ways this type of work is thus the 'gold standard' of professional competence and judgement, and it places occupational therapy in a position of prominence in sectors where not many occupational therapists are seen.

Questions

1. Give six instances when an occupational therapist may be called on to act as an expert advisor/consultant/evaluator in the corporate, insurance or medicolegal sectors.
2. Describe four ways in which an occupational therapist may play a therapeutic role in the corporate, insurance or medicolegal sectors.
3. Discuss the general prerequisites for working in these sectors.
4. Outline the type of preliminary work which may be required when accepting a corporate, insurance or medicolegal referral.

5. Briefly describe the principles of professional self-presentation and the standards of behaviour required of an occupational therapist in these sectors.
6. Discuss the features of written communications which are produced in the course of rendering corporate, insurance and medicolegal occupational therapy services.
7. Describe the possible pitfalls associated with conducting home visits and work visits, and how best to address these.
8. Mention three types of pre-trial work and court work in which an occupational therapist may become involved, when working in the medicolegal sector.
9. Highlight the most important features of the administrative infrastructure required in an occupational therapy practice which offers corporate, insurance and medicolegal services.

Useful websites relating to labour legislation and medicolegal work

South African Department of Labour: www.labour.gov.za/docs/legislation
The Expert Witness Institute (United Kingdom): www.ewi.org.uk
The Society of Expert Witnesses (United Kingdom): www.sew.org.uk
The Academy of Experts (United Kingdom): www.academy-experts.org.uk
The Expert Witness Newsletter (Canada): www.economica.ca
The Expert Witness Network (USA): www.witness.net.html

Chapter 11
Forensic psychiatry and occupational therapy

MICHELLE MOORE

Forensic psychiatry deals with mental disorders as related to legal principles. The word 'forensic' (from the Latin word *forum*) means 'belonging to, or suitable for, the court or public discussion' (Kaplan and Sadock, 1998). It can thus be defined as interaction of psychiatry and the law (Fairhead in Crouch and Alers, 1997).

Relevant legislation

It is essential that occupational therapists familiarize themselves with relevant acts for the particular country they work in, and update themselves regularly on changes to legislation that may affect them. Acts of relevance in the United Kingdom are the Mental Health Act 1983, Criminal Procedure and Investigations Act 1996, the Human Rights Act 1998 and the Criminal Justice Act 2003. In South Africa, The Mental Health Care Act No. 17 of 2002, the Criminal Procedure Act No. 51 of 1977 and the Correctional Services Act No. 111 of 1998 are applicable.

Criminal laws and acts deal with the capacity of the accused to understand proceedings as well as the mental illness or mental defect and criminal responsibility. If the court finds that the accused is not capable of understanding the proceedings, the court shall direct that the accused be detained in a psychiatric hospital. Where the accused is directed to such a hospital, the accused may, if he is capable of understanding the proceedings so far as to make a proper defence, be tried and prosecuted for the offence. If the court finds that the accused was not criminally responsible due to mental illness he can be found not guilty or directed to be detained in a psychiatric hospital or a prison. The accused's capacity to appreciate the wrongfulness of the act can lead to diminished responsibility and will be taken into account with sentencing.

Psychiatric hospitals may admit, care for, treat and rehabilitate forensic patients, mentally ill prisoners and persons referred by court for psychiatric observation. Maximum security wards are provided for mentally ill prisoners. These wards provide not only for observation cases, but also for mentally ill offenders who have been acquitted, prisoners who become mentally ill while serving a sentence and mentally ill patients who cannot be managed in a general psychiatric ward due to danger to themselves and others.

Observation cases

Observation cases are accused patients who are referred for assessment which will be undertaken by a multidisciplinary team to determine their mental state. The observation is done over a period of 30 days, after which a registered psychiatrist or clinical psychologist will write and submit a comprehensive report taking into consideration the findings of the multidisciplinary team. The report should contain information on the competence of the accused to stand trial and his criminal responsibility.

The *multidisciplinary team* responsible for the assessments includes the following professionals:

- psychiatrist
- psychiatric registrar
- clinical psychologist
- occupational therapist
- social worker
- nursing personnel.

Additionally, the observation unit may also make use of a jurist and a neurologist to share their expertise. The psychiatrist may refer the accused to a neurologist for special tests such as electroencephalogram (EEG), magnetic resonance image (MRI) scans or computerized axial tomography (CAT) scans in order to detect possible organic problems that may have led to the strange behaviour. His presence on the team is optional, but can be significant in the interpretation of the tests done.

Physical examinations of the head, eyes, ears, nose, throat, the respiratory system and the genito-urinary system help to determine problems/injuries that may lead to permanent disabilities or other psychiatric disorders such as depression and dementia.

As in other areas of occupational therapy, activity is used during evaluation. By involving the accused in an activity, several areas of functioning can be assessed and possible simulation can be detected. The occupational therapy report is often the key for the psychiatrist to determine the mental state of the accused, as it is much more difficult to simulate behaviour when engrossed in an activity.

Simulation, also known as malingering, is characterized by the voluntary production and presentation of false or grossly exaggerated physical or psychological symptoms and is presented by the accused in an attempt to:

- avoid difficult situations, responsibilities or punishment
- receive compensation, free hospital board and room
- retaliate when he feels guilty or suffers financial loss, legal penalty or job loss.

For the occupational therapist to conduct a comprehensive assessment, it is necessary for her to familiarize herself with the following details of every client:

- facts about the alleged offence
- the act and section under which the accused stands trial
- previous charges against the accused
- stressors that might have led to the alleged offence.

The occupational therapy evaluation process can consist of the following:

- observing the accused on a daily basis in the work, leisure and social activities structured in the unit
- evaluating him/her in specifically structured groups with 4–6 members as well as in individual activities if necessary
- each individual's responses are recorded specifically and to the point
- at the end of the 30-day period, the occupational therapist uses the information to write the report
- reports are presented to the multi-professional team for discussion.

Aspects to be evaluated:

- Current functioning in terms of:

  - Behaviour
  - Personality
  - Motivation
  - Appearance

- Cognitive functioning in terms of:

  - Thought processes
  - Memory
  - Concentration
  - Distractibility
  - Intellectual functioning
  - Following of instructions
  - Judgement

- Affective functioning in terms of:

  - Range of emotions experienced
  - Appropriateness of emotions
  - Pathological emotions present

- Interpersonal relationships in terms of:

  - Eye contact
  - Verbal and non-verbal expression
  - Casual interaction
  - Self-assertion
  - Leadership skills
  - Difference in behaviour in different situations.

Although these specify the 'negative' signs that may indicate pathology, the positive signs should also be noted in order to write a comprehensive report at the end of the 30-day period. All notes have to be very specific and describe any prominent traits to assist the occupational therapist in writing the final report. Thorough assessment of the factors above is essential to assist the multidisciplinary team in determining the capacity of the accused to stand trial and his/her criminal responsibility. *Please note that it is important to take these factors into account in structured as well as unstructured activities and in both group and individual settings.*

Prior to completing the final report, a full team discussion is convened to scrutinize all reports written and make one of the following decisions:

- Arrange a special case conference.
- Collect more information.
- Extend the observation period.

Extension of the observation period is permitted only if approved by the court.

In severe cases where there is a possibility of life imprisonment, a panel of psychiatrists is appointed. A maximum of three psychiatrists should serve on the panel: one hospital psychiatrist appointed by the head of the health establishment, a private psychiatrist and, optionally, a psychiatrist of the accused's choice.

Usually the psychiatrist is called as an expert witness, but other team members or healthcare practitioners may be requested to support the court in their decisions.

An accused found to be unfit to stand trial due to a mental illness/diagnosis, might be referred to a health establishment/psychiatric unit and managed as a mentally ill patient. For an accused found to be fit to stand trial, but his/her responsibility at the time of the offence is in question, three possibilities remain (Fairhead in Crouch and Alers, 1997):

1. Fully responsible: Trial proceeds.

2. Not responsible due to mental illness: Referred to a health establishment/psychiatric unit.
3. Diminished responsibility on the basis of mental illness: influences the sentencing.

Admission as patients

When the accused is found not capable of understanding court proceedings and not responsible, he is admitted as a patient.

Movement of patients in the hospital system

Initially the patient has limited privileges and security in the ward is strict. Movements of patients are monitored closely and treatment mainly takes place in the secure ward. As the patients' conditions improve, they move to a semi-secure or medium-secure ward with more privileges and then to an open ward from where they may participate in work-related or project-centred activities before finally moving back into the community. No set time frame for movement between the above-mentioned wards can be set, as movement depends entirely upon the individual's charge, the rehabilitation process and his/her progress on medication and feedback on returning from therapeutic leave periods.

The multidisciplinary team

Consistent and cohesive teamwork is essential in the treatment of the patients as all policies and procedures are governed by law. The patient population includes people from all walks of life. Different ages, cultures, diagnosis, level of education as well as different offences can be found and should be taken into account by all team members when assessing and treating these patients.

The following professionals form part of the multidisciplinary team:

- Psychiatrist (also referred to as the consultant)
  Determines the diagnosis, advises the team on changes to medication and dosages.

- Psychiatric registrar
  Performs the physical examinations, prescribes medication and monitors behaviour.

- Psychologist
  Performs psychotherapy on request and treats the state patient accordingly.

- Social worker
  Maintains the contact with the community, mainly the family, and does

investigations into home circumstances before therapeutic leave or discharge.

- Occupational therapist
Mainly responsible for the planning and coordination of the daily activities of the patients. In some cases work assessment to determine the possibility for work or disability grants lies with the occupational therapist.

- Occupational therapy auxiliary (not available in all settings)
Responsible for supervision of patients in work-related or product-centred activities and performing group activities to enhance skills for activities of daily living.

- Advocate (not always an active member of the team, rather acts as consultant on the law)
Advises on the legal aspects regarding management, leave and discharge of patients.

- Nursing personnel
They are responsible for the day-to-day management of the activities in the wards and the administration of the medication as prescribed.

Therapeutic leave

The head of the establishment usually requests therapeutic leave on the recommendations of the multidisciplinary team. The team may consider therapeutic leave when the patient's psychiatric condition seems stable and the home circumstances are favourable and supportive.

Periodic review

A report on the health status of the patient should be submitted six months after commencement of the treatment and then every 12 months thereafter.

Discharge

The multidisciplinary team may recommend the discharge of the patient if the decision is unanimous. The head of the health establishment may apply for the discharge of the patient on the recommendations of the team and a written report by the psychiatrist. Recommendations and applications are submitted to the Attorney General. If the offence is extremely violent, e.g. murder, the application and all written reports from the relevant multidisciplinary team must be submitted to a judge in chambers.

The role of the occupational therapist

The role of the occupational therapist is to ensure that the patients admitted engage optimally in activities in the health establishment or psychiatric hospital. Coordinating a well-balanced programme in the various stages of rehabilitation lies mainly in the hands of the occupational therapist and the nursing personnel. Occupational therapy support staff can play a vital role in the treatment programmes of long-term forensic patients.

As previously mentioned, the forensic patient moves from a secure ward, to a medium-secure ward and finally to an open ward before moving into the community. The occupational therapist is usually one of the team members who remains the same through the different stages and is able to develop a valuable and trusting relationship with the patient.

The occupational therapy assessment

It is recommended that patients be evaluated within two weeks of arrival to determine the aims for the patient in the specific ward. The main focus in the secure ward is to provide a full assessment to plan the treatment of the patient effectively. The assessment can be done through an interview with the patient, observation in a structured or unstructured environment and participation in activities from different activity spheres. Information obtained from the assessments made in the observation unit/ward should be verified as changes may have occurred. It is essential to take into account that a large number of forensic patients experience problems with substance abuse and therefore thorough assessment of behaviour and interpersonal relationships is indicated. Poor emotional insight is a general problem with these patients. Using assessments to determine the level of creative participation to divide the patients into smaller groups is recommended as the large number of patients can be overwhelming at times. Due to the long periods of stay and the movement of the forensic patient through the different wards, ongoing assessment and treatment are recommended.

The occupational therapy programme

It is essential that the occupational therapist take into account the different cultures, ages, etc., when compiling programmes for the patients, as differences may lead to unsatisfied and frustrated patients. The long periods of stay can lead to institutionalization. The main causes of institutionalization, according to Barton (1976) are:

- loss of contact with the outside world
- enforced idleness
- authoritarian medical and nursing staff

- loss of personal friends, possessions and personal events
- medication
- ward atmosphere
- loss of prospects outside the hospital.

The occupational therapist should strive to include stimulating activities in the programme, taking into consideration cultural differences in the population. The overall aim should be to improve, as far as possible, and maintain the functioning levels of the patients through structured and unstructured activities with the underlying aim of preventing/diminishing institutionalization to ensure the successful reintegration of patients into the community.

A balanced daily programme should include activities of:

Personal management

This implies that the patients are directly involved in the ward and the ward routine, as certain essential tasks are allocated, e.g. dining room assistant responsible for setting the tables before each meal. The selection of patient for ward duties can be linked to good behaviour and can be used as motivation for moving on to the next ward. When focusing on self-care activities it is again very important to take into account the differences in culture, religion, etc., and the methods used, e.g. in some cultures and religions it is customary to grow the nail on the small finger of the left hand.

Leisure

The available space and privileges of patients should be taken into account when choosing leisure activities. The following can be considered:

- table activities such as board games
- sporting events or activities, such as soccer games between selected teams with supporters for each group
- activities involving music, e.g. dances, manufacturing of musical instruments and forming a band
- structured recreation activities such as concerts where the patients can use own initiative for performance, e.g. gum boot dances, singing or performing
- more passive activities such as watching television and reading should be monitored closely to prevent patients from withdrawing from active participation.

Work/education

Due to the length of stay, it is recommended that patients be involved in work-related activities. This enables the occupational therapist to make recommendations on the patient's return to the original workplace, entry into the work environment after discharge or applications for disability grants. The success of sub-contract work is due to the fact that large numbers of patients can be treated and observed and it can be utilized for patients from all walks of life. These activities can be graded to fit different functioning levels of the patient population. Work activities provide structure and a sense of belonging that enhances self-image. They can act as external motivators, especially if work performance is connected to wages. Educational opportunities for patients should be explored to give them the opportunity to improve themselves and be more prepared for the open market possibilities after discharge.

As the patients move from the initial admission ward to the more open ward, the focus of treatment may differ. The balanced daily programme as mentioned can include most of the specific aims, but can also be introduced in smaller groups or individually if possible.

Secure wards

The main aim of the programme in the secure ward can be seen as orientation and it gives the personnel the opportunity to become acquainted with the patients. The occupational therapist's main focus will be to assess the patients, before implementing a balanced activity programme.

The following can be considered as focus areas:

- Psychomotor activation/channelling aggression through activity participation e.g. motor activities.
- Improving awareness of self, others and the environment (especially if patient is still psychotic).
- Orientation to time, place and situation.
- Stimulation of other cognitive abilities, like insight, concentration and memory.
- Stimulation of appropriate emotional responses.
- Teaching of new skills to improve leisure time use. (Preferably the patient should be able to continue these activities after discharge, therefore take into consideration the financial position and environment at home.)

Medium-secure wards

Patients in the medium-secure wards are granted more privileges which are usually in the form of ground parole. Parole is graded as follows (Fairhead in Crouch and Alers, 1997):

- supervised (accompanied at all times, less than an hour)
- limited (send to run errands on the grounds or between wards, only a hour or two)

- occupational therapy parole (attend structured activities at the department or sub-contract work in a structured work area)
- unlimited parole (mostly applicable during weekends and during the week when not involved in specific rehabilitation activities).

Although the aims mentioned under the secure wards are still applicable in the medium-secure wards, the focus gradually shifts, with the emphasis now on taking more responsibility. The patients gradually get more involved in the rehabilitation process to prepare them for reintegration into the community. At this stage therapeutic leave assessments by the team may commence.

More specific aims are:

- Improving intellectual and emotional insight into the offence, medication and mental illness by involving them in specific educational groups on the various topics.
- Improving self-care or self-presentation through specific group activities focusing on education and skills training, e.g. personal hygiene group.
- Improving general work abilities through product-centred activities, e.g. manufacturing leather articles or participating in sub-contract work.
- Improving life skills.

It is important to remember that these patients still need a lot of support in decision making and the responsibility will gradually shift. Opportunities for practising skills should be created through role-play, making use of everyday examples in structured activities or the work area or creating opportunities with structured activities as described in the daily programme or organized outings.

Open wards

In open wards, the idea is to give the patients more responsibility in order to prepare them to engage in the community during therapeutic leave periods and discharge. Patients are now allowed to leave the ward freely, although it is still expected that they will abide by hospital rules and regulations.

More specific aims will be:

- Intensive life skills training: The patients get the chance to practise skills obtained in the medium-secure wards by going for outings, attending educational classes outside the health establishment or receiving therapeutic leave.

    The life skills training programme includes the following:

    - communication skills
    - conflict and criticism handling skills

- problem-solving skills
- money handling skills (budget, new prize trends)
- work-related skills (job seeking, application for a job, writing of a curriculum vitae, interviews, etc.)

• Recreation: The responsibility of arranging sports events, religious events, etc., is given to the patients. They form their own groups or committees and the occupational therapist mainly acts as advisor.
• Specific work skills: Although it is not always possible to practise specific work skills in the hospital, work simulation to an extent should be made possible. The possibility of practising specific work skills during the therapeutic leave periods should be explored.

Community

Although it is recommended that patients be allowed to practise skills in rehabilitation centres or the community after discharge, these types of centres are not readily available. The possibility of skill development in specific work spheres needs to be developed. The continuation of rehabilitation is important to prevent relapse, but empowerment of the community to handle forensic patients is essential. The gap between health centre rehabilitation and community should be covered to ensure effective and lasting rehabilitation of such patients. The following can be recommended:

• community education
• infrastructure changes in the community
• structured referral systems after discharge (Fairhead in Crouch and Alers, 1997)
• halfway houses
• day centres
• community social centres
• sheltered workshops
• protective workshops
• outpatient clinics
• support groups.

General safety measures

All personnel should at all times be aware of the possible 'danger' when working with forensic clients. As the diagnosis and extent of mental illness has not yet been determined during the observation period, no activities or assessments should be conducted without the presence of professional wardens or guards. The following measures can be suggested when working with the forensic patients, especially while in the secure and medium-secure wards:

- Always structure the room so that the therapist is closest to the door.
- Conduct assessments and treatment in the presence of other personnel.
- Do not wear jewellery or ties around the neck.
- Never take keys into the treatment area (if stolen, they can be used as weapons or a way to escape).
- Never interview patients without the knowledge of other personnel.
- Report life threats to the whole team as soon as possible.
- Care should be taken when choosing activities and materials during assessment and treatment, as possible weapons can be manufactured from the most unlikely materials.
- Ensure that all materials and equipment are counted at the beginning of the session and that everthing is checked and verified as returned at the end of the session.

Conclusion

The treatment of the forensic patient can be closely connected to the views of Mary Reilly (Occupational Behaviour Model, Reed and Sanderson, 1999). She proposed that occupational therapy should activate the residual forces of the individual and equip him with the abilities to perform his expected roles and responsibilities in the community. As described in the treatment programme the patient should be given responsibility and become an active member of his treatment team, with the therapist as the facilitator.

Occupational behaviour and performance alone is not enough, however. A structured daily programme is suggested for each step in the rehabilitation process. This gives the patients the opportunity not only to obtain information, but also to practise the life skills connected with it.

In South Africa in particular, the high crime rate, the impact of HIV/AIDS on mental illness and the poor community/family education and infrastructures are definitely points of concern in forensic psychiatry. In other countries these particular factors may assume less importance, but other factors relevant to the society concerned will come into play.

Case study

The court sent a 35-year-old Tswana-speaking male for a 30-day observation period. It was directed that he be evaluated under section 77 and section 78 of the Criminal Procedure Act, 1977 (Act No. 51 of 1977) as applicable in South Africa. He was charged with attempted murder.

The following background information could be verified:

- According to the family:
  - Stepbrother suffers from mental illness (from his father's previous marriage)

- – Maternal aunt suffered from postnatal depression
- – A relative died in a psychiatric hospital several years ago, diagnosis not known

- Social behaviour of client:

  - – No substance abuse
  - – No previous offences
  - – Not very religious, does not go to church often
  - – Was raised by older sisters, both parents worked away from home

- Personal history:

  - – Enuresis up to the age of 14 years
  - – Passed grade 12, repeated grades 3, 4 and 12
  - – Did not complete his training to become a teacher, only the first two years

- Employment record:

  - – Employee benefit organization for six years as a clerk
  - – Commenced work as a senior administrative officer at the Department of Labour and was still employed at the time of the offence, trial and 30-day observation period.

- Other information:

  - – Planning to separate from his wife (arranged marriage)
  - – Ten-year-old daughter from a previous marriage
  - – Eight-year-old son in the current marriage
  - – Dependent on salary from his occupation

- Relevant psychiatric history, personality traits and behaviour of the patient:

  - – A known patient with bipolar mood disorder, previous admissions at three different mental health care centres.
  - – During the interviews, he was paranoid towards his family and the family doctor, as he stated that they are conspiring against him. The client was psychotic during the first interview.
  - – His supervisor at the Department of Labour stated that he suddenly became hysterical at work and cried a lot.
  - – His colleagues stated that he started complaining of insomnia, he was scared to answer the phone and requested that they escort him home. Then suddenly about a week after these complaints, he took the afternoon off and did not return to work for the rest of the week. They were then informed of his arrest.

    The investigating officer explained that he was arrested for attempted murder. He tried to run down a policeman with his motor vehicle. During investigations he had pressure of speech, was disorientated and confused.

The family doctor stated that the relapses are due to the observatus not complying with the taking of medication, and a lot of stress at home, he feels inferior to his wife, who earns more and needs to travel a lot.

His wife stated that he sometimes refuses to take his medication. He does not qualify for free medication, and he refuses to buy it.

Questions relating to the case study

1. Explain the roles and responsibilities of the occupational therapist in the observation unit with regard to the case study described.
2. Making the assumption that this client will be found not responsible due to mental illness and referred to a health establishment as forensic patient, answer the following questions:

   a) What other options could the court have taken?
   b) Explain the roles and responsibilities of the occupational therapist in the secure/medium-secure/open wards.
   c) Discuss the importance of preparing the patient to return to his original workplace.
   d) Discuss the roles of the team members in ensuring the successful reintegration into the community.

3. Choose specific life skills that you should take into consideration when compiling the treatment programme and explain why.

PART THREE
CHILDREN AND ADOLESCENTS

Chapter 12
Occupational therapy intervention with children with psychosocial disorders

ROSEMARY CROUCH AND VIVYAN ALERS

The discipline of child psychiatry has changed in focus over the past few years and gains have been made in the social and economic approach to the treatment of the child. 'Developmental psychopathology, still a young science, is making it possible for clinicians to make more informed judgements about the future course of the disorder and the influences upon it that need to be assessed' (Rutter and Taylor, 2002, pp. xii–xiii).

In some countries, including South Africa, occupational therapy in the field of mental health must be seen to be a priority because of the prevalence of children who have been abused emotionally, physically or sexually, and because of the many children who are brought up in impoverished and violent circumstances.

> Physical abuse, neglect and psychological abuse have considerable psychological importance, because these experiences happen as part of ongoing relationships that are expected to be protective and nurturing (Emery and Lauma-Billings in Rutter and Taylor, 2002).

Impairment of psychosocial functioning is by far the largest group of disorders in children and therefore in this chapter emphasis is placed on these disorders. The focus will be on the child within the community, but mention will be made of the treatment of children within a day-hospital and inpatient setting. Child psychiatric units differ according to the treatment approach of the team, but wherever the child with a mental health problem is treated, the occupational therapist is considered a vital member of the multidisciplinary team.

Pumariega (in Rutter and Taylor, 2002) advocates that a full interdisciplinary team should be involved in all procedures and protocols related to the treatment of the child with a psychosocial disorder.

> Plans of care should be individualized to the needs of the child and family, including attention to the cultural issues and should follow the child continuously through all levels of care, being amended as needed' (p. 2856).

This is indeed ideal, but in many countries throughout the world where resources are sparse, it is not possible.

The occupational therapist working with children with psychosocial disorders should have experience of children, psychological maturity and a good knowledge of the models, philosophies, frames of reference and theories of the profession so that the children can be treated in a holistic, all-encompassing manner. A sound knowledge of child development, conscious evasions and unconscious defences is also required.

Psychiatric disorders impact on children's ability to function at their potential in the psychosocial environment, and with the appropriate background of experience and training the occupational therapist is able to assess the degree to which such functioning is impaired (Angold in Rutter, 2000).

The psychosocial disorders of childhood are not defined in this chapter. Please refer to the following literature for the description of conditions:

- The DSM-IV-TR™ (American Psychiatric Association, 2000)
- Kaplan and Sadock (2000) *Comprehensive Textbook of Psychiatry*, 7th edition
- Rutter and Taylor (2002) *Child and Adolescent Psychiatry*, 4th edition
- The ICD-10 (WHO, 1992).

It is important to note that there is no clear distinction in the literature between some of the childhood disorders and adult disorders such as depression, schizophrenia and obsessive-compulsive disorder. Some differences exist in the definition of childhood disorders between the DSM-IV-TR™ (American Psychiatric Association, 2000) and the ICD-10 (WHO, 1992) (e.g. obsessive-compulsive disorder and post-traumatic stress disorder are under anxiety disorders in the DSM-IV, but not in the ICD-10).

Attachment theory: a critical domain of concern

The resurgence of attachment theory has become the trend in fieldwork over the past few years when considering styles of attachment of individuals with mental health problems. Attachment theory was developed by Bowlby during the 1950s when he became aware of the problems children experienced when separated from their parents during the Second World War. Attachment behaviour is activated when a child seeks proximity to their caregiver because he/she is lost, frightened, hungry, injured or at risk of injury, and needing comfort. All higher primates come with the capacity for attachment inbuilt. It is a biological survival mechanism. Children develop different attachment patterns with different carers but the style of the attachment between the child and their main carer will become the child's 'internal working model' (Bowlby, 1988) and form the template for future relationships.

Stern (1985) describes the process of attachment as a process of affective attunement. This is the interpersonal exchange of affect that occurs between the mother/caregiver and the baby. This relates to the 'dance' of nuances, sounds, touch and interaction between the mother and the baby that relates to the underlying feeling states. These vitality affects help infants to regulate and integrate their feeling states, which leads to an early development of a sense of self. The infant is biologically programmed for survival, with the limbic system operating the survival instincts, including the traumatic stress reflexes of fight, flight and freeze.

Perry (1995) has shown how the limbic system of children develops in relation to the interaction between the caregiver and the infant. The limbic system includes the hippocampus and amygdala regions, which are integral to information processing from the body to the cerebral cortex. The amygdala processes and stores emotions and reactions to emotionally charged events, including implicit memory, which is the core of somatic memory. It registers the emotional significance of events.

The amygdala plays a role when 'flashbacks' occur. The hippocampus works as the data processor of sequential personal experience. This is the seat of explicit memory and requires language as a component. The hippocampus matures within the second year of the child's development. Thus the developmental milestones of an infant should be considered not only with regard to their sensorimotor development, but also to their emotional stability development, or attachment stability.

The experiences of early infant life have a far-reaching effect on the emotional and social being of the child in later life. The attachment patterns that children develop through their experiences of how early care needs are met, have a lasting effect on their later attachment patterns in life, and thus on their interactions in society (Holmes in Bannister and Huntington, 2002).

There are three main styles of attachment in children. Where the mother/carer is inconsistently reliable an *insecure ambivalent* attachment style prevails. A *secure* attachment style develops when a carer is consistently reliable. When the mother/carer is consistently unreliable an *insecure avoidant* attachment style develops. Attachment styles are carried over into adulthood and thus these correspond with the child attachment categories. In adulthood attachment relationships occur in marriage and within the subsequent families. The *preoccupied* style of attachment relates to the inconsistently reliable relationship, and *secure* attachment corresponds with consistently reliable relationships. An adult will exhibit a *dismissive* attachment style in their relationships when their attachment style is consistently unreliable, see Figure 12.1.

Patterns of disorganized attachment result in the individual having an extreme lack of development of the ability to convey intentions and emotions through language as well as to differentiate self from non-self. Attachments can become disorganized when the caretaker is also a source of fear. Attachment behaviour is activated when the child is frightened: he

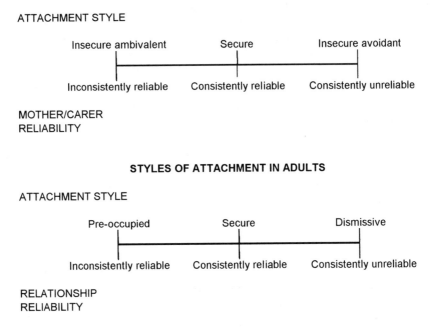

Figure 12.1 Styles of attachment (Chimera, 2003).

or she will seek proximity to the attachment figure. If the attachment figure is also the source of the fear, the child is faced with an unsolvable paradox and their coping mechanisms are overwhelmed. This results in a disorganized attachment style. With *disorganized* attachment patterns the child lacks the attunement and mirroring, thus impulse regulation is impaired and confused feelings occur. A higher level of psychiatric problems may be present, especially those associated with anxiety (Holmes in Bannister and Huntington, 2002). These problems continue into adulthood. Thus in the light of the context that the child with a psychiatric disability presents him/herself it is important to take into account the effect of the attachment patterns on the psychiatric illness. There is a high correlation between *disorganized* attachment and severe child psychiatric conditions.

The importance of attachment behaviour relates to the child's social, emotional and behavioural development, and thus *disorganized* attachment behaviour may be a predisposing factor for mental health problems. The Diagnostic Statistical Manual IV (DSM-IV) (American Psychiatric Association, 1994) and the International Codes of Disease 10 (ICD-10) (World Health Organization, 1992) describe attachment disorders as *inhibited* (failure to interact) and *disinhibited* (indiscriminate sociability). The implications of the repeated change of primary caregivers or the persistent disregard of the child's emotional and physical needs (comfort, stimulation and affection) are manifold when considering present-day political and social climate in many troubled regions of the world. Many children have been separated from their primary carers due to abuse, war, displacement, natural disasters, illness or death and poverty. The HIV/ AIDS pandemic has left many children infected, affected or orphaned with a resultant vulnerability to disorganized attachment styles.

The implications of understanding attachment theory for the occupational therapist lies in the importance of a consistent, trustworthy therapeutic relationship to model, and for the child to experience, secure attachment patterns. *The therapist in effect becomes the secure base.* When the learning disabled child displays behavioural problems, the occupational therapist needs to consider the underlying reasons related to their attachment styles. Problems exhibited by children with *disorganized* attachment behaviour can include the following:

- Social behaviour – superficially charming, little eye contact, poor peer relationships, fighting to gain control over situations.
- Emotional behaviour – indiscriminately affectionate with strangers, grandiosity, inappropriately demanding or clingy, lack of affection for carers, resentment, rage, anger and violence, opposition, blaming of others, poor impulse control, restlessness, holding present carers responsible for past hurts, coercive, obvious lying, manipulative lying, early sexual activity, stealing, preoccupation with violence including cruelty to animals, destructiveness and self harm.
- Developmental behaviour – lack of cause and effect thinking, abnormal eating patterns, lack of conscience or moral sensibilities and self neglect.
- Occupational behaviour – risky behaviour, the play occupation is disrupted (age-appropriate play does not occur), sensation seeking.

For further information on Attachment Theory, see Howe (1995), Hughes (1997), Cassidy and Shaver (1999), and Solomon and Siegel (2003).

The occupational therapist's role in child psychiatry and mental health

In many countries occupational therapists are involved at a primary healthcare level and they work alongside social workers, nurses and teachers in the field. Lougher intimates that Wilcock (1998a) provides an excellent framework for occupational therapists working in the community (Lougher in Creek, 2002, p.409). It is seldom that the child is seen individually in this setting. They are seen either with the family or in groups with other children.

In the developed world and some other countries the typical multidisciplinary team still exists in hospitals and clinics where the psychiatrist, child psychologist, occupational therapist, speech and hearing therapist and psychiatric nurse work hand in hand. As stated by Kaplan and Sadock (2000, p. 2848) 'The case of a child having to be separated from the parents or care-giver, to be given appropriate treatment, often has to be made.' This is usually when the child is at risk of being a danger to self or others, i.e. in a psychotic state. The primary focus of residential treatment is to create a therapeutic living environment that contains the child safely. During hospitalization the intervention by the whole multidisciplinary team can take place before the child returns home.

The role of the occupational therapist in this environment will vary depending on:

• the overall policy of the unit
• the orientation of the multidisciplinary team and the treatment approach
• the facilities available in the unit.

The role of the occupational therapist should encompass:

• A complete assessment of all physical and psychosocial aspects of the child including strengths and resources. This assessment will contribute significantly to the team diagnosis and focus of intervention.
• With the team, formally involving the child and family in developing a plan of intervention encouraging the family's participation and motivating them to become part of the treatment process (Kaplan and Sadock, 2000).
• Demonstrating and evaluating the adaptive functioning and social interactive skills of the child.
• Structuring opportunities for the child to develop more satisfying relationships by releasing and sublimating emotional drives.
• Modelling a consistent trustworthy therapeutic relationship to enable the child to experience secure attachment patterns.
• Treating specific problems such as concentration and memory, perceptual and learning difficulties where necessary, but this should not be the main focus of intervention.

Kaplan and Sadock (2000, p. 2853) state that

Occupational therapy contributes substantially to the treatment program by being less confrontational and focusing on strengths.'

They also say:

For an inpatient or residential treatment centre to be effective in the treatment of the child or adolescent, it must have a full range of therapeutic modalities – occupational therapy, group therapy, family therapy and school programmes, and include therapeutic psychopharmacology' (Kaplan and Sadock, 2000, p. 2852).

Equipped with a clearly defined frame of reference, and an understanding of appropriate general principles, occupational therapists can exercise flexibility, variation and imagination when designing and implementing therapeutic approaches to the treatment of the child (Clancy and Clark, 1990).

The assessment

It is usually helpful to be able to assess children's styles of social interaction and ways of talking in several contrasting situations, for example with the rest of the family, during occupational therapy structured tasks and from school reports (Rutter and Taylor, 2002).

Assessment and evaluation of the individual child or group of children should:

- precede therapy
- be repeated at least once throughout the intervention process; and
- conclude the therapy process – 'wrapping it up' (Clancy and Clark, 1990).

Included in the assessment should be the following:

- an assessment of the child/children's psychological and physiological development
- an assessment of the child/children's ability to express emotions and general behaviour
- an awareness of the child/children's living environment. 'Children in temporary accommodation feel very vulnerable and treatment should not be too challenging' (Lougher in Creek, 2000, p. 409)
- an understanding of the protection systems of the country for the child/children and knowledge of any child protection systems in place
- 'the level of co-operation and support of carers' (Lougher in Creek, 2002, p. 409).

Before the occupational therapist can assess or evaluate a child, a careful and sensitive contact must be made with the child in a manner which is least threatening. A mother figure may need to be present, but in certain cases this is not desirable. A supportive relationship between the occupational therapist and child/children is essential.

It is important to familiarize the child or children with the area in which the occupational therapist is working and the tasks that she will be using for the assessment. The following approach is intended as a guideline, but bear in mind that in some circumstances time pressure requires the occupational therapist to assess the child/children more expeditiously. This is important in poor socio-economic environments where there is great pressure of work with few professional services available, and also in the private sector where payment could be difficult for parents.

First session. The child/children is shown around the playroom and given the opportunity to play and explore. Neutral activities such as drawing, painting or games may be suggested. Boundaries need to be set for the child to give security and safety to the therapeutic relationship. The development of a trusting relationship is essential.

Second session. Again the child/children may be encouraged to explore and may be offered plasticine, papier mâché or clay for play. This is followed by an opportunity for free play. This should include verbal or non-verbal interaction with the child.

The approach should be non-directive and the child/children should be encouraged to express themselves freely and discover the limits of the assessment venue. The length of the sessions depends on the children's tolerance, but normally ranges from 30 minutes to an hour.

It is important to interview, or have an informal discussion with, the caregiver or mother/parent, since the information given will provide collateral information which will aid in the assessment. It is necessary to be sensitive when asking painful questions.

Observation of behaviour is the central focus of the diagnostic interview: 'All clinicians associated with the child should make a point of keeping in mind a checklist of the behavioural areas outlined below, so that the child's behaviour can be compared across the various settings or "stimulus conditions" provided by the clinic' (Rutter and Taylor, 2002, p. 45).

Rutter and Taylor (2002) give guidelines on the central focus of observations to be made by the multidisciplinary team of the behavioural areas of children, so that a comparison can be made between team members. These are as follows:

- separation responses
- physical appearance, which includes abilities of dressing, hairstyle
- motor behaviour, i.e. restlessness, fidgeting, distraction, potentially injurious behaviour
- form of speech such as stuttering, low-volume muttering, pressure of speech
- content of speech and any abnormalities
- social interaction including verbal and non-verbal communication
- affective behaviour, such as shyness, sullenness, signs of depression, smiling and laughing
- developmental level.

(Rutter and Taylor, 2002, p. 45)

Inclusion of the child's self-reports is extremely important in the initial interview with the child (except in the case of attention deficit disorder). It must also be kept in mind that although there has been little cross-cultural research in psychopathology there are indications that there are differences in patterns of presentation with children from different cultural backgrounds as well as differences in appropriate parental behaviour (Rutter and Taylor, 2002).

Observations by the occupational therapist

When working as a member of a diagnostic or treatment team, or single-handed at grass-roots level in the community, the occupational therapist must become an expert in observational skills. An 'activity observation guide' and a 'social behaviour observation guide' can be found in Parham and Fazio (1997).

Observation is a systemized, disciplined activity and the occupational therapist must make considered decisions based on observations of behaviour. No interpretations may be made on the basis of past experiences, expectations or assumptions (Clancy and Clark, 1990).

Table 12.1 is a quick guide for the use of the Model of Creative Ability (du Toit, 1991) to place a child on their creative participation level so that appropriate activity selection can be made. In this way the selection of activities motivates participation. It is a far better guide than using age-appropriate/developmentally appropriate activities, especially with children who are psychiatrically ill, or those that are depressed and demotivated (see Chapter 1).

Table 12.1 V du Toit Model of Creative Ability applied to paediatrics (Barnard, 2003)

Motivation level	Action level	Key components
Tone	Pre-destructive	• Birth to ± 5 months. • Movements are irregular and uncoordinated. • Survival responses for needs to be met by the caregiver. • Dependent on caregiver.
Self-differentiation	Destructive	• ± 5 months to ± 9 months. • Sensory experiences are the primary activity focus (feeling, rubbing, chewing, biting, tasting, looking). • Child throws, tears and pulls at objects. • Starts to recognize parents, smile responses. • Communication is mostly receptive.
Self-differentiation	Incidental	• 10 months to ± 2 years old • Aware of self as an entity (separate from mother and environment). • Interaction is short-lived (1 step) and outcomes are unplanned and immediate. • Objects are manipulated more (holding, placing or rubbing) but no tool handling or skill. • Repetitive movements. • Communication is limited. Responds to 'known' people. Limited expressive vocabulary, one-word sentences.

Table 12.1 contd.

Motivation level	Action level	Key components
Self-presentation	Explorative	• ± 2 years to ± 5 years old. • Starts to control interaction with environment. • Materials are explored to determine their properties. • Products still largely unplanned but with step-by-step approach 4–5 step product can be successfully made. No norms of quality/speed. • Develops a task concept and tool manipulation is explored and tested. • Development of basic concepts occurs. • Explores social boundaries. Seeks approval from others. Communication now two-way but more for the child's benefit (egocentric). Does not fully understand situations, and oblivious to the subtleties of body language and innuendo. • Fantasy play and role-modelling are enjoyed.
Passive participation	Experimental	• School-going child (nursery and primary). • Interaction is product-centred with a consolidated task concept but external motivation/stimulation still required. Step or sequence prompting occasionally required. • Tool handling more product-centred and practice leads to some levels of skill. • Product evaluation is a need of the child, but negative evaluation is not well accepted. • Active learning, but not self-directed. Does not like to participate in unfamiliar situations. More comfortable in familiar situations and sequences previously experienced. Practise. • Relationships are less dependent and more self-maintained. Development of peer acceptance and norming is a focus, but selected peer groups may vary frequently.
Imitative	Imitative	• Early adolescence. • Task participation is product-centred and self-fulfilment-orientated, but initiative still limited. • Experienced at a variety of tool and material handling.

Table 12.1 contd.

Motivation level	Action level	Key components
Imitative	Imitative	• Works well from a model and evaluation of performance becomes comparative instead of quality-centred. • Socially conforming. Tries to imitate (be identical to) the peer group in all spheres of life. Susceptible to peer pressure. • Behaviour is acceptable/appropriate to most situations.

It must be remembered that the child does not exist in a vacuum. The observations look at the intrinsic aspects of the child, the effects of the family and others and the greater community in which they live. In other words, a child lives in a matrix within the community and these dimensions of the matrix need to be considered when observing the child and the parents/caregivers.

The tacit dimensions of the child's behaviour are much more significant than that which is explicitly observed, i.e. the meaning of the

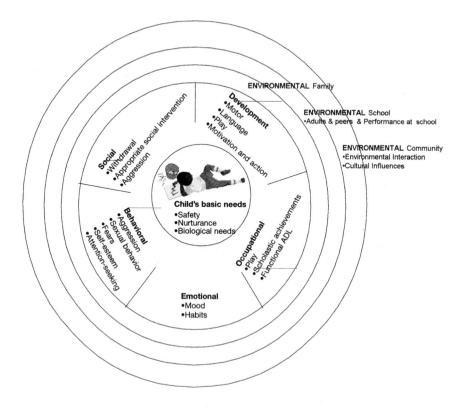

Figure 12.2 Dimensions of the community matrix to take into account when observing a child.

behaviour is more significant. The child needs to be observed in relation to his/her developmental, occupational, emotional, behavioural and social abilities. Collateral information is also necessary from the parents/caregivers. This may include whether eneuresis is present, and the child's behaviour in other situatioins, e.g. school, home or at friends. Some examples are given in Figure 12.2 under these headings. Their assets (abilities) and their challenges (disabilities) need to be assessed.

Whilst the child is involved in play and other activities such as games, the occupational therapist can carefully observe the following:

- Behaviour
  Observe the child's response to the occupational therapist and the new situation. Observe behaviour which will denote symptoms of stress and anxiety such as fears, phobias, separation anxiety, 'clowning', 'baby talk', poor self-esteem, tics, self-destructive or attention-seeking behaviour and tantrums, hypochondriacal or psychosomatic symptoms, tactile defensiveness and hyper-vigilance.

- Conduct
  Does the child lie, steal, fight, bully, disobey instructions, act aggressively, start fires, destroy toys and articles, or quarrel frequently? What is the child's response to teasing?

- Motor behaviour
  Is the child hyperactive or underactive? Does he or she display involuntary movements, poor coordination, or poor posture and tone? Is the child clumsy and apt to break things? Note the child's posture relating this to self-esteem.

- Attention span
  What is the level of the child's concentration? Is he/she distractible or preoccupied? Is there daydreaming? Is there dissociation? Is the child able to listen and carry out tasks?

- Play
  What type of play does the child tend to indulge in? Is play destructive or constructive? How age-appropriate is it? What is the child's choice of playthings and/or people and other children? Is playfulness evident? (Parham and Fazio, 1997)

- Language
  What is the content of speech and how age-appropriate is it? Is there stuttering, articulation errors or pressure of speech? Is receptive and expressive input and output intact? Is swearing present?

- Activities
  How does the child participate in creative activities and drawing activities? Does the child have the ability to complete projects? Is there

frustration tolerance? Is there a consolidated task concept? Is there apathy, withdrawal, negativism towards self, impulsiveness?

- Habitual manipulations
  Are habits such as thumb sucking, nail biting, body rocking, head banging and hair pulling present? Are there any other self-injurious behaviours?

- Sexual behaviour
  Are any of the following present: seductiveness, masturbation, homosexual tendencies or conflicts about sexual identity, inappropriate sexual behaviour towards others?

- Mood
  Is the child anxious, depressed, elated, preoccupied, apathetic, hostile or displaying feelings of guilt? Does the child have mood swings?

- Relationships with other children
  Is the child demonstrative and affectionate? Is this behaviour appropriate? Does the child keep eye-contact? Are they aware of peers, and who is the choice of playmate? Is the child 'scapegoated' by peers or disliked? Does the child take a submissive or leadership role? Is the child selfish or does he display solitary play? Does he/she spoil others' play?

- Relationships with adults
  When in the presence of adults does the child show a preference for certain adults and choose a particular adult for a particular need? Does he/she avoid talking to, or interacting with, an adult? Is the child cooperative, compliant, indifferent, dependent or independent?

This information greatly contributes towards continuous assessment. Other assessments which may be carried out by the occupational therapist, include:

- gross and fine motor skills
- perceptual motor skills
- sensory integrative function.

It must be stressed, however, that there is a tendency for occupational therapists to carry out only the above three assessments, when the focus of attention is actually the psychosocial disorder. The intervention for the child, as a result of the assessment, would be inadequate and would not contribute to the multidisciplinary diagnoses and plan of intervention, as described by Rutter and Taylor (2002).

Occupational therapy intervention

Occupational therapy intervention will depend on the nature of the child/children's psychosocial disorder as well as the overall plan of the multidisciplinary team.

It is very important for the occupational therapists to use the same therapeutic approach and handling strategies as the rest of the team. Should there be any opinion for a different approach the occupational therapists must discuss this openly and assertively with the team members. It is important for the occupational therapist to contribute her own ideas, modifications and observations to the team so as not to be counter-therapeutic in any way. This is vital for the successful treatment of the child. To this end, a good understanding of the uniqueness of the child is vital and the therapeutic relationship with the child is the deciding factor in the success or failure of therapy (Clancy and Clark, 1990).

Assessment should include observation of the coping style of the child. Coping styles are the way in which the child selects certain strategies to manage situations that are perceived as threatening or challenging. Coping styles are depicted on a continuum as consistently effective, situationally effective and minimally effective. Effectiveness relates to coping efforts that are appropriate for the situations and the developmental age of the child and whether they are used successfully to achieve the desired results. In the psychiatrically disordered child coping mechanisms are usually erratic, applied in a trial-and-error manner, and tend to be rigidly repetitious, with the child repeating the same coping mechanisms despite the difference in the situation (Kramer and Hinojosa, 1999).

When working in the community setting it is imperative to discuss the child's strengths and challenges (weaknesses) with the caregivers, and to help them accept the child as a person within the family. Often the child is rejected, ridiculed and belittled – thus exacerbating the psychiatric illness. Also, traditional beliefs need to be taken into account, e.g. bewitchment, and the affect on the child.

Principles of treatment for children with psychosocial and mental health problems

- The occupational therapist must develop a warm, friendly relationship with the child, and establish good rapport as soon as possible (Clancy and Clark, 1990). Trust and safety within the relationship is important.
- The child must be accepted as a unique individual and should be helped to see him/herself as someone worthwhile (Axline, 1989). Self-affirmation leads to self-worth.
- The child should be allowed to express both positive and negative emotions. Never try to block negative emotions because they seem to be undesirable. There should be a relationship of permissiveness within certain boundaries, so that the child feels free to express these feelings.
- The child should be encouraged to develop from dependence to independence in therapy, and have some opportunity to solve problems and make choices.

- Discipline, in the form of setting boundaries, needs to be consistent. Boundaries of what is allowed or not allowed in the play room give the child security, and channelizes the discipline to the behaviour and not to the child's self esteem per se; i.e. the behaviour is not acceptable but the child is accepted. Positive reinforcement is far better than negative reinforcement and can be done in many creative ways. For example, every week or month the child can make a 'try again train'. The engine and each carriage are drawn on a separate sheet of cardboard. The engine is used for the first week or month and then a carriage is used for each following week or month. The carriages are then joined to the engine to form the train. A number of 'stickers' (paper cutouts or appropriate objects) are used to fill in the picture of the engine, each sticker being a reward for good behaviour. The concept of the 'try again train' means that the positive reinforcement for positive behaviour is encouraged and the 'mistakes' in behaviour are *overlooked* in favour of 'try again'.

  Behaviour recording charts are a concrete way of explaining to the child the abstract concept of behaviour change and can be designed for short- or long-term use. There are many innovative ways of creating a behaviour recording chart (Case Smith, 2001).

  The therapist establishes only those limitations that are necessary to anchor the therapy in the world of reality and to make the child aware of her responsibility in the relationship (Axline, 1989).

- Therapy should provide opportunities for adventure, surprise and mastery. The occupational therapist should help prevent the child from developing 'learned helplessness' by offering the appropriate 'scaffolding' to successful execution of the task. The child needs support and encouragement for the initiation and the persistence in the task to obtain a feeling of mastery. This mastery needs to be intrinsic and not only for the external reinforcement (Case Smith, 2001). Mastery and success lead to an increase in self-esteem and self-worth.

Gary Landreth (1991) proposes the following basic concepts in relating to children. Children are not miniature adults, but are people worthy of respect. They are resilient and have an inherent tendency towards growth and maturity. They are capable of positive self-direction. Children's natural language is play and they have the right to take the therapeutic experience where they need it to be.

The occupational therapy environment

Whether in a community setting, such as a clinic or in the local school, or in a hospital or private practice setting, the occupational therapy environment should provide a normal play setting for the child. As play is the main medium of treatment, there must be provision for developmental play, imaginative and imitative play (dressing up, etc.), social play (house-house, etc.) and creative and expressive play.

Play therapy is an intensive form of psychotherapy with children, which is usually carried out by a child psychologist or psychiatrist who has received specific training in this technique. Many occupational therapists worldwide have received postgraduate training in play therapy and often assist with play therapy. Play therapy activities are described in detail in Oaklander (1988), Axline (1989) and Barnes (1996).

Play as therapy

In occupational therapy, the treatment of children with psychiatric disorders of any kind is usually through the medium of play. As stated by Kaplan and Sadock (2000, p. 2791), 'Play has a central place in the treatment of children and is a natural means of child communication.' Kaplan and Sadock also intimate that play has an important role in the development of the child by encouraging motor development, socialization, the development of imagination, the integration of emotions and the development of autonomy.

'Playfulness' is determined by three elements: intrinsic motivation, internal control and the freedom to suspend reality (Parham, 1997). 'Intrinsic motivation' is that which provides the momentum for the engagement in the activity, and not the external reward as such. 'Internal control' relates to the child being in charge of the actions and part of the outcomes. 'Freedom to suspend reality' relates to the child's choice of how close to fantasy or reality the play unfolds. The Test of Playfulness (ToP) is documented in Parham and Fazio (1997).

In play the process of the play (doing) is the priority, not the product (outcome). The 'how it is done' relates to the quality of the play interaction, and this is the important aspect that needs to be observed.

> Because play is process rather than product driven, it is not bound by the predictability generally characteristic of self care and work' (Parham and Fazio, 1997, p. 52).

Play activities vary greatly and there is no 'correct' way to play. The process of play should engender fun, exploration, experimentation, variety, mastery and fantasy. It is important to differentiate fantasy and reality overtly with the psychiatrically ill child, as sometimes these tend to merge and the boundaries are not clear-cut. The intrinsic motivation to play is not always appropriate with these children and they need to have play modelled for them. When a child is withdrawn or reticent to engage in a play activity, the occupational therapist can play with the appropriate toys, while asking the child questions and talking about what is being done to arouse the child's curiosity, until the child eventually comes to participate. Watching play in this instance is a passive motivation which can be changed from an extrinsic to an intrinsic source of motivation. This is effective with the anxious child or in the initial stages of the therapeutic relationship.

The different types of play develop as the child grows older. These include sensorimotor, imaginary, constructional and game play. They may overlap as children frequently combine forms of play (Kramer and Hinojosa, 1999). It is important for the occupational therapist to choose the type of play that predominates at the child's chronological age and downgrade it to the child's abilities. Case Smith (2001) describes the chronological stages of play and ability in detail from birth to ten years. Case Smith incorporates sensorimotor, cognitive and psychosocial components in all types of play. From birth to two years the play occupation is exploratory and social. At age 2–5 years three types of play predominate: dramatic (symbolic) play, constructive play and physical play. From 6–10 years children enjoy imaginative play and games and organized play develops. Games with rules encompass physical and social play.

Play should encourage spontaneity at all times to keep the child engaged in the play activity. The play activity can be set up by the occupational therapist where the specific play scene is relating to the problems encountered by the child. This is useful for specific problem areas like fear of the dark, sibling rivalry. Puppets, dolls or soft animals can be used effectively for this. Free play is when the child plays with whatever he/she chooses, with little interference from the occupational therapist. This is used for observation purposes. Children with psychiatric illnesses often lack spontaneity and thus the ability to play; they can also be destructive, or flit from one activity to another without completing the previous activity.

A child-centred approach should be used when treating children, but this does not mean that the child has free rein to play. The play needs to be directed through the child, by the child, but the occupational therapist provides the 'scaffolding' to enhance the play experience to make it meaningful and purposeful. For example, the attention deficit hyperactive disordered child does not gain the feedback from purposeful play and the completion of a play activity as they are continually distracted by outside stimuli. The occupational therapist 'scaffolds' for them to remain engaged in the activity of choice until an element of completion and mastery is attained. This then would impact on their feedback for self-esteem and task satisfaction.

Correctly used and selected play activities help the child to reach their maximum physical, mental (emotional and intellectual), social and educational potential. Therefore the choice and presentation of the play activities are important skills for occupational therapists to develop. Choice of play activity depends on the child's age, stage of development, therapeutic needs, abilities, interests and socio-economic and cultural background. The child's 'play language' is also important as this will help engage the child in the play activity. This is especially true of teenagers.

Individual treatment is often difficult at grass-roots level, but is sometimes required when a child requires additional time to establish a more supportive relationship with the occupational therapist or problems such as autism and poor concentration exist. However, the trend in occupational therapy today is to treat children in groups. Not only is it cost- and time-effective but it is clear that having other children present during play often brings out feelings and attitudes which would not show up in an individual session.

Radebe (2004) describes how in the community setting in South Africa, as traditional game called 'Tok-tok' or 'Talk-talk' is used in the Ekopholeni Mental Health Centre – Sinakelwe Crisis Centre. This is a traditional game used by children in groups, which assists debriefing after any significant event. Radebe adapted this game for therapeutic use. In this game, a number of local stones are collected for use and presented to the child. Each stone represents a family member or friend in their life. One stone represents self. The child arranges the stones and chooses which family member each one represents. The self-stone is then used to knock (Tok-tok) on any other stone to start a conversation with that stone (person represented). All the stones have a chance to participate in the conversation. The child is thus able to tell their narrative story through the conversations of the stones. This can be effectively used for assessments, especially regarding pertinent incidences that may have influenced the child's life. Many children find it difficult to talk about traumatic experiences in their life, especially when they have been exposed to questioning from multiple sources, but by engaging the child in this game, information may be obtained in a non-threatening manner.

Group therapy

Most children with psychosocial and mental disorders have a history of poor socialization and the occupational therapy environment is traditionally one of the most important areas for encouraging a child to give up maladaptive behaviour patterns and to learn more appropriate and acceptable social behaviour. Group sessions are recommended for most children and have the following advantages:

- They provide opportunities for modelling on other children with different (better) behaviour patterns through group pressure.
- They encourage identification with the peer group and stimulation of age-appropriate behaviour and activities.
- Group therapy sessions dilute the therapeutic relationship with the occupational therapist where there could be a problem.
- The other children in the group provide feedback.

(See also chapter 13.) Within the accepting atmosphere of a closed group the child has the opportunity to explore his problems in a non-threatening way and may become aware of or gain insight into feelings and motivations. The activities used within the group can have a cathartic effect, which allows the child to work through feelings, which he/she can then accept, abandon and/or internalize. It is very important to put language to the feelings with accurate labelling. (See chapter 14.)

Successful group activities include:

- puppetry
- model-making in clay and play-dough
- collages on specific topics such as fires, stealing and super-heroes
- adapted psychodrama and role-play
- painting a combined picture of a subject such as a zoo.

Selecting children for a group may not be possible in the community but where possible the following should be borne in mind:

- Choose children of a similar developmental age to encourage age-appropriate identification and activity.
- Choose children with *dissimilar problems and assets* to provide a variety of models and complementary behaviour, and to reduce reinforcement of maladaptive behaviour.
- Do not include children with widely differing abilities in the same group.
- To comply with normal grouping patterns, plan mixed groups before the age of six and single-sex groups over the age of six.

Equipment and materials

The following suggestions of equipment and materials are made for a well-prepared occupational therapy intervention:

Puppets and dolls. Hand puppets are the most suitable and should be made of rubber or plastic. Characters represented should be parents, grandparents, the doctor, policemen, the devil, dragon or dinosaur and various animals. Dolls should also be made from durable materials and the adult dolls should be at least six inches tall. There should be family members consisting of a pair of sexed male and female figures and three children such as a boy, girl and baby. All the dolls should have removable garments and be unbreakable. Play equipment for these dolls should be a pram, crib/baby sleeping place, feeding bottles, etc.

The sandpit. This should be big enough for the child to climb into or on a large low table, with curved edges to prevent cuts. In the rural community, ordinary sand or river sand can be used. Clean, dry sand should be used and buckets/pails and spades provided. Always cover the sandpit after use to prevent contamination by animals such as cats and a box of salt can be poured onto the sand to help sterilise it. Articles that can be used as building materials are also useful to have in the sand box, e.g. ice cream sticks, feathers, plastic people figures, pebbles, shells, plastic toy soldiers.

Blocks. One set of multiple-unit wooden (or styrofoam) blocks is useful. Also, large covered foam blocks can be used for obstacles or for throwing/hitting and building.

Paints and other art materials. As many different types of art materials as possible should be available. Clay (natural or processed) and plasticine or play-dough, crayons of all sizes, pots of paint and all sizes of paint-brushes should be available. They should be on shelves where they are easily accessible to the children.

The dressing-up corner should provide traditional clothes for the child to dress up in. Be sure you provide clothes that are traditionally accept-able, e.g. headscarves, long or short dresses, high-heels and flat thongs, ball gowns and nightdress, etc.

Trains, cars, guns and toy soldiers. Wooden trains, all sizes of cars and trucks, boats that float, an aeroplane and helicopter should be available. Soldiers should be in camouflage and fairly modern.

Other equipment could include telephones, percussion instruments, balls, a toy hammer and hammering knock-out bench and large packing boxes or crates and sheets/material for making houses. (See chapter 14 regarding use of scarves.) A small punch bag with a variable hanging height is also necessary.

Sensory integration equipment should be provided according to the guidelines given in chapter 15.

Children with specific difficulties

Behavioural, conduct and oppositional disorders

This is the largest group of disorders in the field of psychosocial disorders and psychiatry. Earls and Mezzacappa (in Rutter and Taylor, 2002) state that 'Conduct disorder constitutes a constellation of antisocial and aggres-sive behaviour that may become prominent in early childhood and persist through adolescence, even into adulthood.' It can be prevented if early presentation is treated. The training of caregivers and the child in anger management, assertiveness and problem-solving skills will provide psy-chosocial intervention. This is the priority in occupational therapy. Occupational therapists may also be involved in preventative programmes for conduct or antisocial disorders. These may be school-based social skills training and home-based parent training (Offord and Benett in Rutter and Taylor, 2002).

Children with these disorders tend to be of average, or slightly below average, intelligence and have disorganized attachment patterns and there are often serious problems in the family. These children often show unacceptable behaviour with repetitive and persistent patterns of behav-iour in which the basic rights of others or major age-appropriate societal norms or rules are violated.

Children with conduct disorders may have little empathy and concern for others and have difficulties in adjusting to the group of children. They are often associated with early onset of sexual behaviour, drug-taking, drinking and smoking. Some are particularly vulnerable to stress and tend to be hyperactive. A small percentage are excessively withdrawn. Generally they tend to be aggressive and exhibit acting-out behaviour. There is usually significant impairment in social, academic or occupational functioning. This impairment can be mild, moderate or severe and is more prevalent in males.

Oppositional Defiant Disorder is described in the DSM-IV-TR (American Psychiatric Association, 2000, p. 100) as:

> A recurrent pattern of negative, defiant, disobedient and hostile behaviour towards authority figures that persists for at least six months. It is commonly associated with mood and other psychiatric disorders.

The prevalence of these disorders has increased over the past decade and is higher in urban areas than rural areas.

It is important that the occupational therapist takes note of the social factors that usually accompany a child with these types of disorder. These factors are:

- poor family functioning
- familial aggregation of drug and alcohol abuse
- psychiatric problems in the family
- marital discord
- poor parenting
- in many cases, a low socio-economic and impoverished rural or urban environment
- in some cases a highly privileged, spoilt and disturbed environment
- disorganized attachment patterns.

Aims of intervention

- Early intervention – prevention is better than cure.
- For the school-age child, parenting training, social skills training aimed at improving peer relationships, the child's ability to comply with demand from authority figures and improvement of academic skills.
- Psycho-educational for parents and child on conflict resolution and anger management.

Aims of occupational therapy

- The learning of socially appropriate behaviour.
- Changing of maladaptive behaviour patterns.
- In some cases relief of anxiety.

Group treatment is the preferred therapy for children with conduct disorders.

Treatment principles

Handling

- A directive, firm but understanding approach is needed.
- A supportive relationship should be developed. Time and patience are required for this.
- Limits of behaviour must be set in terms of the child leaving the treatment area, destructive behaviour and harm to other children. An attack on the occupational therapist must be stopped immediately (Axline, 1989).
- Consistency on the part of the occupational therapist must be maintained as this gives the child a sense of security.
- Tantrums must be dealt with in a calm, matter-of-fact way and a reward given to reinforce good behaviour when the child has gained control. Restraining the child from behind with a firm hold is favoured by some occupational therapists, but this must be used with caution as it may trigger flashbacks of a traumatic event.
- The team frequently institutes a behaviour modification programme, and this is often based on a reward system.

Requirement of activities

- Activities must be age-appropriate, short-term and interesting.
- They should involve the child in a wide range of motor activity.
- They should be flop-proof, and have a good end product that encourages a task concept.
- Although the destruction of toys and materials is discouraged, the toys should be tough and should they break by mistake there should be no consequences. This will minimize the guilt feelings on the part of the child.

Structuring the treatment environment

For these children, the treatment environment, including groups, should be well structured and controlled. An unstructured environment is frightening and disorganizing for the child.

Emotional disorders

Depression in children

In a child with a dysthymic disorder the mood may be irritable and cranky rather than depressed. Often they suffer from poor appetite or overeating, insomnia or hypersomnia, low energy or fatigue, low self-esteem, poor concentration and decision making, hopelessness, low interest and self-criticism (Kaplan and Sadock, 2000).

These symptoms often result in impaired school performance and social interaction. These children may show learning disabilities rather than depression.

Major depression is also found in children and suicide is the fourth leading cause of death in children between the ages of 10 and 15 (Rutter and Taylor, 2002).

The core symptoms of a major depressive episode are the same for children and adults.

Symptoms commonly found in children with major depression include:

- lack of smiling
- apathy towards play
- lack of involvement in all activities
- becoming tearful and irritable easily
- destructive with activities and towards self, others and property
- physical complaints
- physical aggression
- deterioration of school performance
- avoidance of peers
- irritability, fighting and arguments
- exacerbation of anxiety symptoms
- school refusal.

(Kaplan and Sadock 2000)

Anxiety disorders in children

'Anxiety disorders in children cause suffering and impairment' (Klein and Pine in Rutter and Taylor, 2002). Anxiety disorders found in children include phobic disorder, separation anxiety, reactive attachment disorder, social phobia, generalized anxiety disorder, obsessive-compulsive disorders and panic disorder.

Obsessive-compulsive disorders are now more common in children, and the occupational therapist must be aware of the combination of rituals and obsessions during treatment. These may centre on 'contamination concerns, danger to self and others, symmetry and moral issues, washing, checking, repeating – until the child experiences a feeling of getting it "just right"' (Klein and Pine in Rutter and Taylor, 2002, p. 573).

In recent years progress has been made in the treatment of these disorders by mental health professionals, with a wide range of effective therapies. Intervention approaches include family education, education of school teachers, cognitive behavioural therapy and medication.

Aims of treatment

- To relieve anxiety through the use of play activities, physical exercise and relaxation and by giving the child a chance to express fears and guilt.
- To establish a secure relationship through which the child can talk freely about self and problems.

- To raise self-esteem through achievement and mastery.
- Ultimately, to influence a change in the child's personality.
- To treat specific difficulties such as concentration or a perceptual-motor disorder.

Handling principles

- Take a few sessions to gain the child's confidence and use an indirect approach to the child.
- Use play as the medium for building up a relationship.
- Do not ask the child direct questions about anything related to the presenting problem at first.
- Acknowledge the child's obvious fears and suggest that it is all right to have these fears (normalize them).
- Be consistent and constant in your approach.
- Do not hurry the child. Allow him/her to take his/her time, relax and gain equilibrium (Axline, 1989).

Requirements of activities

Play activities should be in keeping with the developmental level of the child. They should be simple, flop-proof with a high possibility of success. Activities such a painting and cooking, which will receive acclaim from others, are most successful. The child should be able to keep the finished product.

Structuring the treatment environment

The atmosphere must be relaxed and the child must be given freedom and minimal limits. However, do not frighten the child by giving them too little structure. A consistent and supportive atmosphere is required. A wide range of play activities must be available and any frightening toys removed.

Very often the occupational therapist is required to initiate treatment on an individual basis, but groups should be introduced at the first opportunity.

Psychotic disorders

Children with psychotic disorders are frequently found in impoverished urban environments, usually in the developing world but also in the big cities of the developed world. Often the psychosis is related to substance abuse, such as glue sniffing and petrol or benzene sniffing, amongst homeless street children. It is a serious problem in South Africa. Schizophrenia, autism and chronic depression can also cause psychosis, but children with these conditions are found in all strata of society and are in the minority.

All of these children need dedicated and patient handling by the multi-disciplinary team and generally form only one really good relationship with a selected team member. Hospitalization is usually required for treatment.

Aims of treatment
- To stimulate contact with reality, other children and to promote communication.
- To stimulate intellectual development.
- To stimulate emotional response and emotional contact with others.
- To attempt to try to develop latent potential.

Handling principles
- Try to form a warm and trusting relationship with the child. There may be no response at first but persevere.
- Be quietly directive in your approach to make the child aware of reality.
- Be consistent and constant in approach.

Requirements of play activities
Play activities should bring the child into contact with other children and not isolate him in any way. They should be simple and promote the use of senses such as touch and smell (play-dough and biscuit dough). The end product is usually of little consequence. Physical contact with play activities will help reinforce reality.

Structuring the play environment
- These children should always be treated individually at first, and be gradually introduced to a small, homogeneous group.
- The environment must be well structured and organized. These children do not progress in a permissive atmosphere.
- Stimulating materials such as bright posters and loud music should be kept to a minimum as they distract and often overwhelm the child. Soft and soothing music is highly recommended.

Resettlement and reassessment

The occupational therapist working in the community or in a hospital setting has a vitally important role to play in the resettlement of the child after treatment. Reassessment is an important part of this process.
The multidisciplinary team takes into account the suggestions from the occupational therapist and the other professionals, and a strategy is planned. Often children receive ongoing therapy from the occupational therapist for a period of time.

Conclusion

Child psychiatry is a fast-developing and fascinating area in which the occupational therapist can make an important contribution to the team approach to the treatment of the child. In many parts of the world, particularly in developing countries, there are many abused and neglected children who desperately need the services of occupational therapists, particularly at grass roots level. Occupational therapists are particularly versatile in their approach to intervention as they are expertly trained and capable of adapting the environment to the needs of the child. Even in privileged society, where there are many disturbed children, the occupational therapist is able to expertly provide an appropriate treatment environment in which to treat the child holistically.

The upsurge of occupational therapists dealing with children with psychosocial problems has brought about a tendency for them to dwell only on the motor-perceptual and learning difficulties of the child at the expense of the major psychosocial/emotional needs. This needs urgent attention worldwide.

Questions

1. What is the general purpose of occupational therapy in the field of child psychiatry and mental health?
2. Discuss the interaction the occupational therapist should have with the multidisciplinary team in the field of child psychiatry and mental health.
3. Discuss the approach to assessment of the child with a conduct disorder.
4. What are the basic principles of treatment for any child with a psychiatric disorder?
5. How would you structure the treatment environment for the child with an anxiety disorder?
6. Discuss the limitations in handling a child with a conduct or oppositional disorder.
7. Give examples of the type of play activities that are suitable for the occupational therapist to use in the field of child psychiatry.
8. Explain attachment theory and its relevance to the occupational therapy intervention of children with psychiatric disorders.

Chapter 13
Interdisciplinary group therapy with children

MARITA RADEMEYER AND DEIDRE NIEHAUS

Interdisciplinary group therapy is a method of treatment developed to address simultaneously children's developmental and psychosocial difficulties that would otherwise require psychotherapy as well as occupational therapy. Children who show multiple developmental and social or emotional difficulties, and who do not have access to or do not benefit optimally from separate individual therapies, may benefit from interdisciplinary group therapy. Suitable candidates for group therapy are placed in groups of four, with an occupational therapist and psychologist who act as co-therapists. The therapists plan and execute therapy in accordance with the content-process model of group therapy (developed by the authors). This type of therapy is recommended for any therapeutic setting where there is an interdisciplinary approach to therapy for children, e.g. a private practice or hospital setting.

Interdisciplinary group therapy was developed in an effort to address the needs of children with multiple difficulties, by overcoming the following limitations of individual therapy:

1. Children with multiple difficulties are often placed in two or more individual therapies, which involve time and cost factors. In the public sector resources are often limited, so that a child may not have the opportunity to undergo more than one therapy.
2. Children often find it difficult to adjust to the different therapy contexts. Psychotherapy differs from other therapies, as it is mostly unstructured. The psychotherapist does not necessarily plan the content of the session beforehand or impose her own agenda on the client, but works with what the client is ready to present. Children are expected to take responsibility for their own therapy. Occupational therapy, on the other hand, is more structured and directive. When children undergo both occupational therapy and psychotherapy, they

sometimes become passive in psychotherapy or demand less structure in occupational therapy.

3) Children who undergo individual therapy quite often show improvement in therapy, but the improvement does not always generalize to the school or home environment. In a one-to-one situation the child is able to apply his newly acquired skills. However, when the child is not in the supportive and accepting context of therapy, he may not be able to do so.

The aims of group therapy

Group therapy aims to treat primary or secondary developmental as well as psychosocial difficulties simultaneously. When a child shows a developmental lag, secondary emotional and/or social difficulties quite often develop. A child with poorly developed gross motor skills would not be able to take part freely in peer group activities such as ball playing. Such a child may withdraw socially, and have fewer opportunities to develop social skills. The child may also become aggressive or defiant. A child with perceptual difficulties may struggle to cope in the classroom and may be aware that his performance does not compare favourably with that of other children. Emotional difficulties such as low self-esteem, lack of confidence, anxiety or aggression and acting-out behaviour may develop. In these examples a primary developmental lag has led to a secondary psychosocial difficulty.

A primary psychosocial difficulty could also lead to secondary developmental difficulties. A child who has been severely traumatized is trying to make sense of his experiential world, and may not engage in activities that stimulate development. A child from a dysfunctional family may not have adults around who create appropriate opportunities for growth. A child who is very anxious may withdraw from interaction or be shunned by other children. A child who is aggressive may be rejected by peers and excluded from play activities that would stimulate development.

The content-process model of group therapy

The content-process model of group therapy was developed as a way to implement the therapeutic principles of occupational therapy and psychological treatment simultaneously. The 'content' of the group session refers to the actual activities that take place. These are planned in advance by the occupational therapist in accordance with occupational therapy practice. The activity is chosen to fit with the child's difficulty, his developmental phase and group level.

The 'process' of the group session refers to all the interactions and behaviours that take place in the group (i.e. the observable aspects), as well as the thoughts, experiences and feelings of group members (i.e. internal aspects). The process of the group will be influenced by, amongst other factors:

- the personal histories and experiences of the group members as well as therapists
- the temperament, personality aspects, behavioural patterns, etc., of members
- the phase of development of the group
- the input of the therapists
- the activities chosen for the session.

The occupational therapist uses the group content to address developmental goals and the group process is used to facilitate emotional healing and social growth. A group of six-year-old children whose fine motor skills need to be developed may be asked to make puppets, involving cutting and drawing (content). When the puppets have been completed, they may be encouraged to stage a puppet show, which creates opportunities for expressing children's current concerns and promoting interpersonal problem solving (process).

Indications for and against group therapy

Interdisciplinary group therapy shows encouraging results in the treatment of:

- problematic peer group functioning
- lack of generalization of skills after completing individual therapy
- learning difficulties which include developmental as well as psychosocial components
- developmental difficulties with secondary psychosocial components
- psychosocial difficulties with secondary developmental components.

The occupational therapist should carefully consider the following cases for group therapy:

- children who show sensorimotor integration difficulties which require mostly hands-on therapy
- children from severely dysfunctional families, where a family therapy intervention is priority
- children with severe behavioural problems or very poor concentration.

It is important that the occupational therapist prioritizes in cases such as these, bearing in mind that group therapy is never a substitute for individual therapy.

Structuring the group

Assessment procedures

Potential group members are usually referred to either an occupational therapist or a psychologist, depending on the presenting problems. If either professional feels that an interdisciplinary approach is required, then, in consultation with the parents or caregiver, it is recommended that the child is assessed by both the occupational therapist and psychologist.

Assessments by the occupational therapist and the psychologist will include the following aspects:

* sensory integration
* gross motor functioning
* fine motor functioning
* visual perceptual functioning
* work habits (if appropriate)
* emotional functioning
* social functioning
* cognitive functioning
* family functioning.

Additional aspects may include: educational functioning and neuro-psychological functioning.

After the assessment, if both developmental and socio-emotional difficulties are present, the child may be included in an interdisciplinary group. Upon inclusion in a group it is important to have information regarding the child's developmental functioning as well as socio-emotional functioning. The occupational therapist and psychologist will discuss the child's functioning in depth to establish the child's strengths and difficulties. In practice it is useful to make a working summary of assessment results for each child, outlining the areas of difficulty and treatment aims. This summary is important in making the group placement and in guiding the planning of therapy.

Selecting candidates for an interdisciplinary group

The authors have found that to deal with both content and process optimally, it is important not to have more than four children in a group. This means that a ratio of two children per therapist is maintained. If more children are included, it becomes more difficult to address the socio-emotional needs of all the children.

The following factors should be considered when selecting group members:

* The children should be on similar levels of development with similar or associated developmental problems. The therapist would use the

working summaries of potential candidates for comparison and selection. John (see Table 13.1) would benefit from being in a group with other children whose fine motor skills are being addressed.

Table 13.1 John – working summary

Areas of difficulty	Aims of treatment
Fine motor skills	To improve shoulder stability, strengthen muscles of the hand and facilitate correct pencil grip
Internal distractibility	To improve time spent on task and establish self-regulation of concentration
Social withdrawal	To establish contact with other children through learning age-appropriate games, and teach self-assertiveness skills to improve conflict management
Parental guidance	To give parental guidance to help create opportunities for John to socialize Medical assessment of concentration functions

- Children should be able to speak the same language.
- There should not be more than a 12-month chronological age difference between group members.
- The children should be on the same level of creative ability (De Witt, 1994).
- School-age children should preferably be of the same sex.

Avoid the following situations in a group:

- Two children from the same family.
- Two children who act out aggressively.
- Two very hyperactive children.

Treatment

The treatment environment

Interdisciplinary group therapy is best carried out in an area with space for:

- a table where the group members as well as therapists can be seated for table top-activities
- an informal area with cushions arranged in a circle, for discussions and games
- standard occupational therapy equipment for treatment of motor and perceptual difficulties.

Children respond well to predictability in the therapeutic environment, and it is therefore important for the therapist not to effect major changes in the therapy room without warning the group members. Children also enjoy having group work displayed in the therapy room, as it feeds into a sense of group identity as well as instilling pride in their work.

It is important to adhere to structuring principles in accordance with the children's diagnoses, for instance keeping dangerous equipment out of reach of impulsive children, and keeping the environment as free from distractions as possible for the child who battles to concentrate.

Content

The content of the group refers to the activities chosen by the therapists to stimulate sensorimotor development, structured in accordance with the children's psycho-social needs.

Planning the content

The content or activities for each group are planned according to the accepted occupational therapy practice. Activities are chosen to address the treatment goals as set out in the working summary.

The activities are presented in three parts in every session:

1. *Warm-up exercise.* A favourite activity amongst children is sitting in a circle, passing a ball of wool to each other. Each child holds on to his end of the wool so that a pattern resembling a spider's web is created. At the outset of group therapy this exercise is used to help the children to initiate contact and remember names. In later stages it is used to give each child a chance to bring emotional issues to the table, and other warm-ups may be used. A teddy or doll may be appropriate to talk to about the past week. For example, each child may be encouraged to tell Teddy one good thing and one bad thing that happened during the week, which would facilitate discussion.
2. *Main activity.* The activity is aimed at improving developmental skills while addressing socio-emotional issues. In John's group, the therapists help the children to cut and paste a 'snakes and ladders' board (fine motor skills), which is then used as an age-appropriate play activity to help John and his fellow group members practise turn-taking and impulse control (social skills). The activity is graded according to the children's ability and progress in therapy.
3. *Relaxation or winding down.* These could include listening to relaxing music, playing a memory game, talking about the next session or taking turns swinging in a hammock. John's group enjoys throwing a ball through a hoop as a winding-down activity.

Requirements of the activities

In group therapy each child's activities should have an effect on others. The therapist would, for instance, put out two pairs of scissors for cutting activities (to develop fine motor skills) so that children have to take turns and manage possible conflict (developing social skills). When building a puzzle to address visual perceptual skills, the group would build one puzzle, each child receiving a number of pieces. In this way the members have to cooperate and share so as to complete the puzzle.

The activity should fit with the group phase. In the first phase of the group it is important that emotional content not be too threatening, whereas in later phases it is important that socio-emotional issues be addressed. In the termination phase, where children are preparing to leave the group, more individualised activities are more appropriate.

Presentation of activities

Activities are presented taking into consideration the following points:

1. The phase of development of the group. In the first phase children may need more instruction and reassurance whereas in later phases the group may express their own ideas for activities.
2. Children's individual needs. An anxious child may need more structure and predictability while an aggressive child may need more overt limit-setting.

Process

The therapists use process to facilitate psychosocial healing and growth. This is achieved as the therapist helps to create a therapeutic culture, or healing space. It is important for the therapist to establish the norms of respect, acceptance, support, sharing, caring, sensitivity to the needs of others and being congruent. This is done by:

- Communicating respect for and acceptance of the group members, by making eye contact with a child, touching appropriately (hands or shoulders at the outset of group therapy), keeping her head on the level of the child's and facing the child when interacting with the child. Remember that the therapists model behaviour, which children will copy.
- Regarding everything the child says as important and reacting to it by listening carefully and clarifying meaning, if necessary. Validate the child's opinions and feelings (Early, 2002).
- Reinforcing appropriate behaviour, for instance, giving credit to a child who is speaking honestly: 'Thank you John, for telling us how you feel.'
- Teaching children through stories, games or directly. The therapists may each have a puppet, and stage a conversation about giving friends

a turn. If judged as not too threatening, the therapist may say to a child, 'Please give John a chance to finish what he is saying; then he will know that you are listening.'

The therapists facilitate the process by:

- allowing the children to express themselves verbally or non-verbally
- helping them to develop insight into their own behaviour
- maintaining an emotionally safe environment (where the child feels accepted and valued).

The therapeutic factors in group therapy

Based on the work of Yalom (1985) the following therapeutic factors are important in group therapy.

Instilling hope

If a child has the expectation that he is going to receive help in a group, he will respond more favourably to therapy. The therapists help to create this hope by communicating their optimism about achieving a favourable outcome in therapy to clients and their parents. Examples of what the therapists would say are as follows: 'The group can help to make life easier for you at school and home. We know that you have lots of things to teach the other children and that you will also learn from them.' This creates positive expectations and sets the tone for the therapeutic culture.

Universality

When selecting group members, the therapists ensure that the children who experience similar difficulties are placed in the same group. When the child comes into the group, he discovers that there are other children who battle with the same issues that he does. The child's feelings of inferiority, alienation and often rejection are alleviated and spontaneous improvement may even take place at the outset of therapy.

Imparting information

The therapists and group members discuss why the children come for therapy, as well as their treatment. The child's problems are discussed in concrete terms. For instance, a child with a gross motor problem can master his difficulties more effectively when he understands that his muscles need to work better and that therapy can help him with this, rather than having a generalized sense (as children often do) of being incapable.

Similarly a child who is aggressive may be offered the explanation that he has difficulty in telling people how he feels – so he shows them, but then gets into trouble. This explanation can help the child to perceive his difficulties as more manageable. The child learns not to think of himself as bad or unacceptable, but as a child with a specific problem, which can be addressed.

The flow of information does not only take place between therapist and child, but also between the group members. Children share ideas and help each other to solve problems. 'When my brother takes my toys, I tickle him. You should try that too!'

Altruism

Altruistic behaviour in the group helps a child to break the habit of self-absorption with his own problems. When a child reaches out to someone, it can:

- serve to strengthen self-esteem
- enhance relationships by teaching the child to give as well as receive
- create the expectation that if the child can help others, someone will be able to help him.

Altruism is facilitated by reinforcement: 'Thank you for giving Sam a turn', by modelling: 'How can I help you?', and by structuring activities in such a way that children can only succeed by helping each other, for example painting each other's faces.

Development of socializing skills

One of the goals of therapy is to help children widen their behavioural repertoire. This means that children learn new ways of behaving and interacting and do not always rely on old and stereotypical patterns. For instance, in helping a child learn self-assertive behaviour, the therapist may ask the group: 'What else can Peter do when he is bullied at school?' Group members may offer, 'Tell a teacher, run away, hit back', whereupon group members may discuss options and practise different behaviours.

Children are made aware in the group of how their behaviour affects other people, which can lead to more socially acceptable behaviour. For instance, the group may be asked: 'How do you feel when Sandy swears?' 'How else can she show that she is angry?'

Imitative behaviour

Children learn functional as well as dysfunctional behaviour patterns by imitating others. In therapy, the imitation of functional behaviour patterns is encouraged. Children may imitate the therapist and other group members. Children may imitate as a way of making contact with other children, as well as acquiring new behaviour patterns.

Interpersonal learning

Interpersonal learning is the process by which children learn about themselves and the world of relationships. The therapy context can function as a small, safe social world in which children can experiment with behaviours, gain self-knowledge and learn the rules of social interaction. The therapists encourage this process by creating opportunities for fantasy play (where, for instance, the shy child can be a fire-breathing dragon) as well as rule-based play and interactions (where for instance the impulsive child has to wait his turn in a card game). Children can thus assume different roles and learn to problem solve in relationships.

Cohesion

In the honeymoon phase of the development of the group, the group is characterized by 'pseudo-cohesion' (Oaklander, 1999). Children are anxious to fit in with the group and show that they are competent. They try to establish cohesion through shared interests (dinosaurs, skateboards, etc.) or shared dislikes (we all hate scary movies). True cohesion only manifests in the group:

- after the group has gone through a stage of conflict
- when the children have established and accepted different roles in the group
- when members have shared of themselves and shown vulnerability.

True cohesion gives the child a sense of acceptance and affiliation, or belonging with a group of people, which is very affirming to the child. This also feeds into greater self-acceptance.

Catharsis

Catharsis can be a way for the child to let off steam, relieve tension or express himself. He may express his feelings about past events or about his experiences in the group (Yalom, 1985). It is, however, important that the cathartic experience be used by the therapist as a learning experience for the group. Questions such as the following can be useful. 'You saw how angry/sad Harry was today. Have you ever felt like this? What makes *you* feel this angry/sad? What do you do to handle your anger?'

Handling principles

To facilitate process, the therapists have to keep a number of principles in mind:

- Therapy should aim to create a healing space. This is achieved by maintaining and communicating respect and acceptance of the child. It is only within such an atmosphere that the child will feel safe.
- Safety and containment are important to create trust between the therapist and the children, and to avoid the children feeling vulnerable in front of their peers.
- The therapists should aim to make matters that occur in the group overt.

Group members will bring important matters to group therapy, but may not be able to verbalize effectively. The therapist can open issues up for discussion by asking questions such as: 'Tom looks sad today. I wonder if something has happened?' Or 'Sam, I see that you are finding it difficult to take turns. Does this also happen when you are at school?' Unwanted behaviour should not be ignored, as this may lead to the behaviour being extinguished only in the group, and not necessarily in other situations, but rather opened up for discussion and problem solving. 'Can the group think of another word that Edith can use to show that she is angry, other than swearing?' 'Yes! Boom is a great word!'

- The therapists should try not to react to the child's behaviour in ways that most other people in the environment would react. Giving the child 'more of the same' (Keeney, 1983) will not change the child's behaviour, and might even perpetuate the problem. An example is the hyperactive child. He hears more often than not 'sit still, settle down, finish your work, keep quiet, etc.'. The therapist may react to such a child by saying, 'I see that you have a lot of energy, and that you have sharp eyes that miss nothing in this room. Can you think of ways we can use these qualities of yours to make your life easier at school?'

Reflection

Reflection (Rogers, 1977) is a comment passed by the therapist on a) what the child is doing, for instance, 'I see that you are finding it difficult to get started today' or 'I notice that you are quiet today', or b) what the child may be feeling, for example, 'This seems to make you angry. Can you tell us about it?'

Reflection can help the child develop insight into their feelings and behaviour and can facilitate problem solving.

Meta-commentary

Meta-commentary is another way of facilitating process (Beyers and Vorster, 1991). Therapists may comment on a member's behaviour or on a happening in the group. Therapists may make a general comment, may speak to the other therapist in the presence of group members or may make use of a puppet. The puppet may then 'say': 'I see that the group is working beautifully today!' or the therapists may speak about a conflict in the group while the members 'eavesdrop'. Meta-commentary is a way of addressing socio-emotional issues in the group without confronting a member, thus making the intervention less threatening.

Questions

Children often do not respond to 'why' questions. Using questions such as 'can you tell me more?' or 'and then?' often elicits more information. A therapist can also facilitate the conversation by repeating the gist of what the child has said in question form, for instance, 'My teacher shouted at me today.' 'Your teacher *shouted* at you?' Circular questioning (Beyers and Vorster, 1991) can also be used. The therapist may direct a question about one member to the group in general or to another child, for instance, 'Mary, how do you think John felt when his teacher shouted at him?' This serves to promote children's understanding of each other and facilitates group discussion. Children may also project their own feelings when answering on behalf of each other.

Non-verbal techniques

Children may not always be able to verbalize their experiences or feelings and the therapists should allow for non-verbal expression. The therapists may make use of props such as a feelings chart (different facial expressions are drawn and the child can point to the face that expresses what he is feeling), dolls or puppets (to enable the child to play a scene out instead of telling about it, for example, 'Can you use the dolls to show us what happened on the playground today?') or drawing materials, 'Can you draw a picture of the bad dream you had last night?'

Phases in the development of a group

Groups tend to develop in phases (Oaklander, 1999). Differences may occur between groups in terms of the length of these phases. Characteristics of one phase may also be found in other phases.

Honeymoon phase

During the first phase of group development, the honeymoon phase, therapy is new and novel. Interaction between group members tends to be more 'social', in other words, discussions tend to centre on age-related interests (games, toys, TV shows, etc.) rather than socio-emotional issues. Children tend to project an image of coping, of being 'OK', and group members tend to avoid conflict. They are usually very cooperative and rarely challenge the therapist. During this phase the occupational therapist needs to structure activities that will stimulate the interest and development of group members and get group participation going, but will also allow for the shift of the group process from social to therapeutic. The therapists also have to start establishing therapeutic norms.

The conflict phase

During the conflict phase the group process becomes more prominent. Children start becoming more congruent and social and emotional problems begin to manifest as children now not only discuss 'safe' topics, but also emotionally loaded issues. During the conflict phase children start challenging each other and the therapist as they sort out their roles in the group. The conflict phase is probably the most difficult phase for the therapist to deal with, but also the phase in which important interpersonal learning takes place. During the conflict phase children need to experiment with new behaviour patterns and the emphasis is on their emotional and social difficulties.

The followings aspects are important during this phase:

- Activities are still selected to stimulate development and address treatment goals, but the occupational therapist should take care that the activity does not inhibit the development of process.
- Very often the children test the limits of therapy and they test the leadership of the therapists. It is important that the therapists handle the conflict constructively and do not try to eliminate conflict by over-structuring or over-disciplining.
- It is also important that the therapists do not become involved in power struggles with group members.
- It is important to discuss limits in therapy with the members to ensure emotional safety. This should be done as soon as the first signs of conflict start appearing. The therapist can start the discussion by saying: 'We have to have rules in this group to make sure that the group works well. Who can think of a rule?'

The integration phase

The integration phase follows the conflict phase. During this stage the children start implementing new skills and behaviour patterns effectively. They show altruism towards one another and cohesion develops, based on mutual acceptance. During the integration phase, the skills acquired in the group generalize to situations at home and school.

The termination phase

The termination phase is the last phase of therapy, but is as important as the earlier phases. The therapist should acknowledge that children experience the termination of therapy as a loss. Therapy should be terminated over a period of at least six weeks. It is important that the termination of therapy be made concrete, so that children can understand the time concept. The therapists may do this by putting six blocks in a bottle. Each week the group members must remove one block and count the remaining blocks so that they can keep track of the number of sessions left.

With older children, a calendar is useful. Every week the countdown to the last session takes place, and each member gets to draw a small picture on the calendar. Children have the opportunity to discuss their feelings about termination. The therapists ask questions such as 'What will you miss most about the group? What will you remember most fondly?' At the last session a special activity may be chosen to end off the process. It is also important to discuss with the child which other relationships or contexts, apart from therapy, can fulfil some of the child's needs that were met in therapy. 'Where else or with whom can you speak about how angry you get?'

Teamwork

Working closely in a team with other professionals has many advantages for the therapist. On a professional level, the therapists learn from other professionals so as to broaden their knowledge base as well as their therapeutic skills. On a personal level, having someone as a sounding board helps in dealing with difficult cases, provides a strong support base and helps to broaden one's horizons.

The therapists not only work with each other and the group members, but also connect with other important people in the child's world. The success of therapy depends on a good working relationship between therapists and the parents of the child in therapy. A parent who feels disempowered, uninformed or negative about therapy may jeopardize the child's progress in therapy. It is important that a parent is informed about specific goals in therapy and kept up to date with the child's progress. Regular feedback and emotional support for parents are crucial.

Contact with the child's teacher is also important. The teacher sees the child every day and can give important information about the child's functioning in class as well social situations, which can help guide therapy. She can also give feedback on the child's progress.

Conclusion

Interdisciplinary group therapy is a way of treating developmental and psychosocial difficulties simultaneously. It is a holistic treatment that is useful in addressing primary and secondary difficulties that might usually require individual occupational therapy as well as psychological interventions. This form of therapy is particularly useful where professional resources are struggling to keep up with the growing demand for therapy. It is also valuable because it recreates class and family contexts, which makes therapy reality-based and facilitates the generalization of new skills.

Questions

1. Discuss the importance of the multidisciplinary approach to group therapy.
2. Discuss the selection of candidates for an interdisciplinary group.

3. Describe the four stages of group development.
4. How are therapeutic aims formulated for an interdisciplinary group?
5. What activities would you choose to present in a group with four seven-year-olds, where the therapeutic aims are to address fine motor skills and concentration functions?
6. How could the psychologist and occupational therapist complement each other professionally?

Chapter 14
Trauma and its effects on children, adolescents and adults: the progression from a victim to a survivor to a thriver

VIVYAN ALERS AND ROMY ANCER

In this chapter, the word 'patient' refers to people in hospital, 'client' refers to people in the community, and 'individual' refers to all people.

'I can see my life being different now, because I can play again.'

(Quote from an abused child after six months of occupational therapy.)

The resilience of the human spirit in the face of traumatic experiences cannot be underestimated. Occupational therapy has a contribution to make to break the perpetuation of violence and trauma through the generations and to prevent the resultant mental health problems. This is especially true when considering the recent move of Occupational Therapy from the Medical Model to the Occupational Model and the change to Restorative Justice. Children are the nation's future as today's children are tomorrow's adults, and tomorrow's adults are the livelihood of their country.

Trauma has a powerful impact on healthy growth and development. As occupational therapists we are at the forefront of developing therapeutic relationships with traumatized children, adolescents and adults. Occupational therapists are afforded the opportunity to contribute positively to development and to provide a new, meaningful, self-affirming experience that is stable and allows safety and containment; this in turn allows traumatized people to participate optimally in activities of daily living.

If we aim to work holistically as occupational therapists and we ignore the imposed problems of trauma that exist in our society today, just focusing on the presenting problems, we are not following the true philosophy of occupational therapy. How often do occupational therapists treat a child's perceptual problems and overlook the emotional problems and their sources, or an adolescent's drug addiction without addressing his sexual abuse? When rehabilitating a person who is a trauma survivor, are we truly holistic and addressing the underlying core issues? For instance, in the case of a paraplegic from a gunshot wound, do we look at their emotional anger at the perpetrator who caused the disability, or their anger at society, or is his functional physical disability only addressed in occupational therapy? Do we address the vicarious trauma (secondary trauma from witnessing violence) of the alcoholic policeman, or do we just focus on treating the alcoholism? Often these aspects are not addressed directly in therapy and only the superficial presenting problem is treated. Therefore as professionals who pride ourselves on working holistically, we have a responsibility to address these underlying needs. In paediatric occupational therapy there is a trend towards 'early intervention' to remediate and prevent developmental delay. However there is a significant lack of occupational therapists remediating and preventing developmental delay in trauma survivors. Also, occupational therapists need to take cognisance of the effects of functional or dysfunctional attachment patterns of the child (see also chapter 12).

Trauma is almost unavoidable in today's world. Traumatic experiences are interpreted differently by each individual; hence the adaptive response and interpretation of the experience is unique to each person and varies in severity. It is often mistakenly thought that the individual who was directly involved in the trauma is the only one affected, yet the effects of the trauma are far reaching. Others who are included in vicarious trauma are the caregivers, relatives, those who witnessed the trauma and those who hear about it. Traumatic events vary, e.g. being bullied at school, divorce, death of a loved one, or being a witness or survivor of a rape. The severity of the reaction to the same traumatic event varies with each individual.

Definitions of trauma

There are a number of definitions of trauma, a few of which are given below:

ICD-10 (World Health Organization, 1992, 1994) The exposure to an exceptional mental or physical stressor that is either brief or prolonged.

DSM-IV-TR™ (American Psychiatric Association, 2000) An individual who has witnessed or experienced or was confronted with an event that involved actual or threatened death, serious injury or the threat to the physical integrity of self or others. The individual's physical response involved fear, helplessness or horror.

Terr (Terr in Hudgins, 2002) Trauma is a (external) blow or series of blows rendering the person temporarily helpless and breaking past ordinary coping and defensive operations.

Traumatology Institute (Jones, 2002) An individual who has been exposed to an event or events which may be either situational or developmental in nature as a result of which that individual's coping abilities are rendered dysfunctional and at least one of the following have been present:

- An element of fatalism
- An irrevocable conclusion
- Usual coping abilities are severely impaired.

The Traumatology Institute definition is the most comprehensive. The DSM-IV-TR™ (American Psychiatric Association, 2000) definition does not differentiate between trauma and post-traumatic stress disorder (PTSD) as not all people who experience a traumatic event go on to develop PTSD. Hudgins (2002, p.10) prefers Terr's definition, as it is 'inclusive and based on how the person actually experienced a traumatic situation'.

Types of trauma

Trauma can be classified in different ways according to how the trauma is experienced.

Primary or direct trauma – this is when an individual is directly involved in the trauma, e.g. car accident, hijacking, war.
Secondary trauma – this is when the trauma is directly related to the primary trauma, e.g. a rape survivor having to appear in court.
Vicarious trauma – this is trauma as a result of hearing or being exposed to other people's trauma, e.g. journalists, those involved in the justice system, caregivers, health professionals.

Trauma can be *single, multiple or complex* in nature. A single trauma is sudden, unexpected and over after the incident, e.g. death of a sibling. Multiple trauma is when a individual is exposed to more than one trauma over a period of time, e.g. an adolescent suffers the divorce of his parents and violence in a club. Complex trauma is a prolonged repeated traumatic event, e.g. domestic violence, spousal battering. In complex cases a relationship often exists between the victim and the individual who causes the trauma, e.g. the spouse who inflicts the trauma. The victim is usually under the control of the perpetrator and often feels powerless to escape, e.g. a wife who is being physically and sexually abused by her husband and has no financial means to leave and file for divorce.

In addition to types of trauma there are also *types of victims*. The primary victim is the individual directly affected by the incident. The secondary or indirect victim is an individual who has any contact with the trauma. An individual can be both a primary and a secondary victim, e.g. someone who was involved in the events of 11 September 2001 in the United States, and who witnessed people dying around them. A more acceptable term for a victim is a 'survivor of trauma'.

Phases of trauma

As occupational therapists dealing with survivors of trauma, we need to understand that trauma can have three phases. Although these phases have time frames attributed to them, they should not be regarded as set in stone. The occupational therapist should be more aware of the behaviour of the individual than the time frame. Recovery will often not be a linear, straightforward process but rather characterized by progress and setbacks. Movement between the phases is also normal. During these phases the traumatized individual will display functional problems regarding their coping mechanisms in all spheres of daily living. The desired outcome, however, is the individual returning to their previous optimal level of functioning.

The phases are:

- Impact phase
- Recoil phase
- Reorganization/recovery phase.

Impact phase

The Impact phase can last for anything from the first few seconds following a trauma to three days afterwards. The individual will probably experience:

- shock
- numbness
- disorientation
- confusion
- irrational and disorganized thought pattern
- numerous emotions or appear emotionally blank or calm
- a need for guidance and assurance
- helplessness and regression to former stages of development.

All these symptoms are normal reactions to abnormal situations. When severe stress occurs the individual's protective mechanisms come into play to shut down emotional, physical or intellectual awareness. This is to protect the individual from becoming too overwhelmed.

In this phase a type of parental support or psychological holding is needed where the occupational therapist is calm, provides structure for the individual in order to allow the individual to feel safe and secure. It may be wise at this stage to provide practical assistance such as help with reporting to the police and contacting relatives, having mobile phones and credit cards stopped, etc. Do not force the individual to tell their story at this point. However, if they need to talk, allow them that freedom.

Recoil phase

The reality of what has happened starts to affect the individual. The individual may start to show feelings of anger, sadness and guilt. Post-traumatic stress symptoms may start to develop.

The individual may begin to remember facts that they left out or forgot in the previous phase.

A nurturing, comforting and supportive stance is necessary here. Active listening skills are vital at this stage. It is important to work with the individual to help them with time planning and stress management in order to resume the normal routines of daily living. It is also important to be aware of the individual's state of mind and be vigilant for risk factors associated with the development of PTSD.

Reorganization/recovery phase

The individual starts to integrate the trauma as part of their life. They will start 're-entering' life and start functioning optimally again. It is important for the occupational therapist to remember that the trauma will not be forgotten but the memories will eventually become easier to deal with and become part of the individual's life history.

What trauma survivors need

Traumatized people have special needs no matter what phase of trauma. These needs are:

Safety

Often in a traumatic situation the individual's safety is compromised. Therefore as an occupational therapist it is important in all your actions to make them feel safe and to be aware of their needs. Safety is often the primary issue affecting a traumatized individual. They will consistently be seeking safety. Safety is in fact on the lowest level of Maslow's hierarchy of needs (Maslow, 1987) and movement to higher needs would be hindered or rendered impossible if safety needs were not met first.

Respect for boundaries

In a traumatic situation, boundaries tend to evaporate and the individual must be made aware that their needs matter, their boundaries are respected and their boundaries will not be invaded or invalidated.

Knowing they can leave if they want to

It is of prime importance that the individual is not made to feel trapped or constrained in any way.

Structured sessions need to be provided. External structures, such as quiet, calm surroundings with no interruptions help the individual develop an internal structure. This will enhance the therapeutic relationship.

Victims' rights

Victims have a right to be treated with fairness, respect for dignity and privacy. Victims have a right to know that their stories will not be silenced. They have a right to offer and receive information.

They have a right to reparation – that is to be placed back in the position they were in before the incident. This comprises restitution, compensation and rehabilitation.

Victims also have a right to justice – to know that the crime will be addressed and justice applied.

They have a right to non-recurrence – to know that there are organizations in society or the state that are enforcing non-recurrence.

Victims have a right to protection and assistance.

The neurological impact of trauma

The effects of trauma on the brain are manifold. The *limbic system* (or midbrain) is a complex, integrated system and is the seat of survival instincts and reflexes, including stress reflexes of fight, flight and freeze. The limbic system regulates emotional experience and expression and, to some extent, the ability to control impulses. It is also involved in the basic drives of sex, aggression, hunger and thirst. The parts of the limbic system most directly involved in trauma memory are the *amygdala* and *hippocampus*.

The amygdala is involved in implicit memory, motivated behaviour and emotional significance of events. It is involved in the processing and storing of emotions and reactions to emotionally charged events. When an individual experiences a flashback, the amygdala is activated and does not have a concept of sequential time; the event seems to be happening in the 'here and now' and so retraumatization can occur.

The hippocampus is the data processor of sequential personal experience and is involved in explicit memory. When traumatic stress is excessive, the amygdala is unable to send impulses through the hippocampus to the frontal cortex for processing and meaning making. The traumatic memory 'is stuck' in the midbrain.

The *cortex* performs sensory and motor functions and regulates higher cognitive and emotional functions. *Broca's area* (in the left frontal cortex) is involved in expressive speech. When traumatic stress is excessive this area cannot be accessed, thus no words are available to process the trauma. This has significant implications for therapy. By accessing the midbrain function directly, action methods, projective techniques and guided imagery are effective in aiding the trauma survivor to process the trauma material, get it unstuck from within the midbrain, and move it into the frontal cortex in which accurate labelling about what has happened can occur (Hudgins, 2002).

Signs and symptoms of trauma

There are a number of signs and symptoms that people experience when faced with trauma. The assessment of the occupational therapist is likely to find physical, cognitive, emotional and behavioural signs. These signs and symptoms vary according to the individual.

Physical signs

- aches and pains such as headaches, backaches and stomach aches
- sudden sweating and/or heart palpitations
- changes in sleeping patterns, appetite and interest in sex
- constipation or diarrhoea
- easily startled by noises or unexpected touch, tactile defensiveness
- lowered immunity
- increase or decrease in appetite.

Cognitive signs

- poor problem solving and decision making
- confusion
- disorientation
- poor concentration
- poor memory
- nightmares.

Emotional signs

- shock and disbelief
- fear and anxiety
- grief, disorientation and denial
- hyper-vigilance
- irritability
- emotional lability
- intrusive thoughts
- increased need to control everyday experiences
- minimizing the experience
- avoiding anything that is associated with the trauma
- isolating oneself
- emotional numbing
- difficulty trusting
- self-blame or survivor guilt
- shame
- diminished interest in activities that were once pleasurable
- resurfacing of past traumatic experiences
- loss of the sense of order or fairness in the world, with the expectation of doom and fear for the future.

Behavioural signs

- substance abuse
- excessive checking and securing, e.g. of doors and windows
- anger outbursts
- crying all the time or for no apparent reason
- social withdrawal
- suspiciousness
- increased or decreased food intake.

It is important to stress that these reactions are often *normal reactions to abnormal events* and this needs to be conveyed to clients in a warm, caring and sensitive way. All clients who have gone through a trauma will experience some of the above symptoms. It is important to realize that these symptoms do not necessarily indicate psychopathology, yet as mental health professionals we need to be aware of the risk factors for the development of post-traumatic stress disorder (PTSD). These are not limited to, but can include:

- prior exposure to adverse life events
- previous history of abuse
- significant losses
- close proximity to the event
- prolonged and extended exposure to danger
- pre-trauma anxiety and depression and other mental health problems
- chronic medical conditions
- substance abuse
- lack of social support
- accompanying physical injuries to the event.

Referral to a clinical psychologist or psychiatrist is very important in such cases.

Normal reaction to abnormal events

People who have been traumatized need to feel safe both physically and emotionally. Their boundaries need to be respected, and they need to have an understanding that they can leave if they so wish. Respect for their individual space needs to be overt and they should be asked if they want to be alone or have physical touch. If touch is not wanted, this request must be confirmed and strictly adhered to. The traumatized individual needs to feel accepted, not judged. They need to be able to talk, and it is their right to have the opportunity to do so in a place that they perceive as emotionally and physically safe. Their feelings are of utmost importance and they need to have an empathetic individual to listen to them attentively. It is also the small aspects that make an individual feel more emotionally or physically comfortable and make a large impact on the individual after a traumatic experience.

Models related to trauma

The Sinani/KwaZulu-Natal Programme for Survivors of Violence model

This model describes the cycle of violence and the belief that peace is possible. The cycle of violence emphasizes that the exposure to violence leads to extreme helplessness, fear and anger. Often these feelings are repressed, especially when there is a veil of secrecy surrounding the violence. When the anger is repressed, one of three things may happen. First, the anger may develop inside the individual, and turn into hatred and the

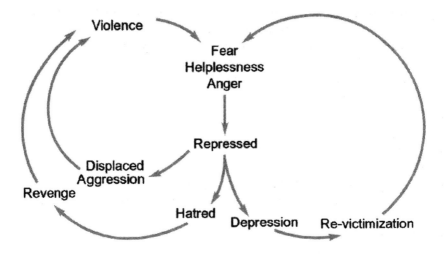

Figure 14.1 Cycle of violence (Sinani/KwaZulu-Natal Programme for Survivors of Violence).

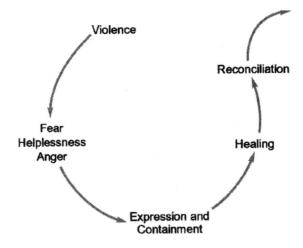

Figure 14.2 Cycle of peace (Sinani/KwaZulu-Natal Programme for Survivors of Violence).

desire for revenge. This is common when an individual's dignity is damaged or where close family members have been attacked or killed. The cycle of violence then continues. Second, the anger may be displaced onto others, for example in the form of domestic violence or sexual violence. Third, we know that repressed anger may cause depression. The individual may become depressed, withdrawn and even self-blaming. There are theories that hypothesize that this individual may then become a further target of violence, and so be repeatedly re-victimized.

Conversely, it is possible for the victim of trauma to make a journey to peace. If an individual's fear, helplessness and anger are expressed and contained in a safe relationship, then an outcome of peace is possible. Through a process of describing the trauma in detail, and also the feelings around the incident, the individual is able to work through the emotional conflicts of guilt, fear and anger. Thus healing and reconciliation can occur.

Trauma debriefing model/4-leg model

Trauma debriefing is a directive, proactive process. It is a structured procedure to engage people in talking about the experiences that traumatized them in a way that is helpful to them. The four parts of the process are:

1) Retelling the story. The purpose of this is to allow a cognitive formulation of the experience. Retelling is a means of helping the individual to remember the experience differently and not to try to forget it. This is done by reviewing the facts, verbalizing thoughts that occurred during and after the incident and verbalizing feelings during and since the incident.
2) Normalizing the symptoms. This is the process of reassuring the individual that the symptoms they are experiencing are a normal reaction to an abnormal situation. This is of utmost importance in helping the individual to understand their reactions.
3) Reframing. Reframing helps the individual regain control of their thoughts, and to see the situation from a different perspective. People often feel that they were inadequate at the time of the trauma and will question what they did or did not do.
4) Encouraging mastery. The purpose of this is to help restore the individual's coping capacity and to reduce a dysfunctional response to trauma. By encouraging mastery, the therapist helps the individual to address a traumatic situation from a position of coping rather than helplessness and to consciously recognize their own strengths and coping mechanisms. This process leaves them empowered.

The Sinani/KwaZulu-Natal Programme for Survivors of Violence (2003) has adapted this model in their community pamphlets distributed to educate and spread the word that communities can break the cycle of violence. This programme emphasizes that the most important aspect of healing is to have a supportive family and friends who will listen, support and deal sensitively with the traumatic experiences. Important points are:

1) Normalize it. Point out that the reaction is normal and usually gets better over time.
2) Talk about it. Trauma may be released from the body and mind by talking to a trusted person. Support them to talk it through when they are ready to do so. Children may be helped to draw pictures of the traumatic event. Another projective technique for children to describe the traumatic event is to use the 'tok-tok' (talk-talk) method described in chapter 12, occupational therapy intervention with children with psychosocial disorders. Never force an individual to talk about the experience, rather explain that there is a listening space for them when they are ready. When retelling the story watch for whether the past or present tense is used. If it is in the present tense, it can be re-traumatizing. Keep the individual in the 'here and now' and the story in the past tense.
3) Deal with anger. Give the individual space to talk about their anger because their anger is justified. When enough space is given and the anger is acknowledged as righteous anger, they will finally choose not to take revenge.
4) Deal with guilt. Give the individual space to talk about their guilt then point out that it was not their fault. ('No shame, no blame.' was a saying that developed out of a Therapeutic Spiral Model workshop conducted in a community setting in South Africa during 2001.)
5) Find ways of coping. Help them work out ways of coping with the event and the memories and determine what is most helpful to them when they are upset. Help structure their time and encourage physical exercise.

Therapeutic Spiral Model™

The Therapeutic Spiral Model (TSM) is an action method used to treat people suffering from post-traumatic stress disorder (PTSD) around the world (Hudgins et al., 2000; Hudgins, 2002). This model is well suited to occupational therapists as it is 'action in the here and now' and uses a creative art projection technique depicting the individual's roles. TSM is a clinical system of change used with individuals, families, groups and communities. The introduction and application of the Therapeutic Spiral Model in the community setting in South Africa during 2001 was the catalyst for the community application in the United States during 2002, called the 'Action Against Trauma training program'. Backed by research in neurobiology and trauma (van der Kolk, 1994; van der Kolk and Fisler, 1995; van der Kolk et al., 1996; van der Kolk et al., 2001; Sykes Wylie, 2004), the Therapeutic Spiral Model™ is a proven method of working with trauma survivors.

TSM has been applied successfully to a wide range of psychiatric and mental health problems in a) people who have experienced severe trauma from racial, sexual, emotional, psychological, physical and ritual abuse; b) refugees who have experienced political or religious persecution, including displacement, imprisonment and torture; c) survivors of war from religious, ethnic and political causes; d) people who have suffered trauma in childhood or as adults; e) survivors of accidents, catastrophes or war who experience guilt. Additionally, TSM has been shown to prevent secondary PTSD and to restore community resilience after national and international episodes of violence, and can be adapted to prevent compassion fatigue in Health Professionals.

While postgraduate training is necessary for international accreditation in TSM, individual action structures can be easily learned and immediately transferred into many practice settings with trauma survivors. The following is a short synopsis of the constructs, concepts and experiential interventions of the Therapeutic Spiral Model™. (See Hudgins, 2002 and www.therapeuticspiral.org for further information.)

Basic premise

Experiential methods are the treatment of choice for people who have experienced trauma. The Therapeutic Spiral Model is such a method of clinical change. TSM has a clinical, step-by-step structure that guides the safe application of experiential interventions with trauma survivors. In this way TSM prevents triggered feelings, uncontrolled regression and re-traumatization with action methods and trauma. This model is based on the three strands of the spiral: building *energy*, providing *experience* and *making meaning* of the experience. The work moves from the periphery to the core – thus spiralling down into deeper levels of awareness, balanced by moving back up as needed in order to build and test inner strengths and support. *Safety* and *containment* are key components of TSM.

Core principles and techniques are:

- creating safety through clinical intervention
- reinforcing personal strengths and rebuilding community resilience
- ensuring conscious choice before exploring any trauma issues
- a clinical map: The Trauma Survivor's Intrapsychic Role Atom (TSIRA) (Toscani and Hudgins in Hudgins, 2002, p. 74). This is concretized as a 'soul portrait'/art project that is completed over a number of sessions. Occupational therapists are able to use this effectively in the 'doing and becoming' of the individual, and can use this as a medium for discussion, action and change. The development of the TSIRA must be meaningful for the individual, and relate to their needs in the 'here and now'
- use of the documented experiential interventions (Hudgins, 2002)
- flexibility and adaptability to many populations and cultures.

The TSM has 'client-friendly constructs that explain internal, self organization for trauma survivors, clear clinical action structures for safe experiential practice with trauma survivors, and advanced action intervention modules for containment, expression, repair and integration of unprocessed trauma material' (Hudgins, 2002 p. 3).

An example of a client-friendly construct, 'Trauma Bubbles', draws on visual imagery to help communicate experiences that often have no words.

Trauma bubbles are encapsulated spheres of active psychological awareness that contain unprocessed experiences. These experiences are dissociated and split off from conscious awareness. Like bubbles, they can be popped unexpectedly, pouring images, sensations, sounds, smells and tastes into awareness without words (Hudgins, 2002, p. 21).

When the TSM is used, it is also important to realize that individuals on an action level of experimentation (du Toit, 1991) will understand the abstract concepts as they have a consolidated task concept. When TSM is used with individuals on an explorative level of action, the abstract concepts need to be concretized and explained in a manner that they understand and has meaning for them. For example, in the example given below, children like to wear the scarves, or find toys easier to relate to than scarves.

Practice example

TSM works from the premise that people cannot look at or address their traumatic experiences unless they are resourced in body, mind and spirit in order to prevent re-traumatization. There are 'Six Structures for Safety' for experiential practice, two of which are described here (Cox, 2002).

The first TSM action structure for safety with trauma survivors marks an *observing ego* role in the session. The group members walk into a room that contains a circle of chairs, a pile of scarves and individual cards with symbols on them (e.g. animal pictures, bird pictures, various abstract portraits. These cards are commercially available, or can be made for the specific purpose.) People are asked to pick one or more cards that represent 'the part of you that can witness your experiences in the here and now and find new meaning for the future'. As they do this, they find a partner or a small group and share the meaning of their observing ego card that they chose.

The second TSM action structure concretizes what *containment* means in a vivid physical and visual manner to connect with the non-verbal, emotional centres of the brain. Coloured scarves are used to form a *circle of group strengths* on the floor (toys and coloured pieces of paper can also be used). These scarves represent all aspects of life through their textures, patterns and colours, and connect people through their personal (inner), interpersonal (outer) and transpersonal/spiritual (upper) strengths as they verbally acknowledge their strengths when each person puts them down to form a circle on the floor. It is important to realize that transpersonal strengths may be religious, non-religious or ancestral beliefs. The circle that is created represents a *container* to 'hold' the experiences and emotions within the group. It establishes a 'safe' place to work through experiences in 'the here and now'. Inside the circle represents the action space. Outside represents the observing space. This helps 'put psychological boundaries and narrative labels on present experiencing' (Hudgins, 2002, p. 43).

This model has been used effectively in South Africa in individual treatment sessions with individuals from all walks of life and in groups in the community with elders, adolescents and children.

To concretize the use of the scarves for younger children and adolescents a 'fashion show' was enacted to show their strengths. This was great fun and built self-esteem in the process. When a young teenager, who had been taken away from her biological parents due to abuse, used her scarves, she built a house with the furniture and her scarves, making the house a safe place for her to be able to talk about her experiences, play 'house-house' with a secure adult (occupational therapist modelling a secure attachment style) who used the therapeutic premise of Yalom's 'corrective recapitulation of the primary family' (Yalom, 1985).

The TSM has also been used with *children* to improve their self-worth and self-esteem. Children commonly believe

That somehow they deserved the ill treatment they received from their parents, that somehow they were just too bad, too sexy or too stupid. Therefore the parents had no choice but to abuse them. Professional healers need to be very careful here about the attributions of blame to the abusers (Chimera in Bannister, 2002, p. 179).

Chimera describes a journey along a 'Yellow Brick Road' which is a journey of healing and reconciliation. In this journey she uses animal cards to depict the child's strengths, and 'healthy self'. Fears can also be concretized through animal or insect cards (snake, tiger, spider). With children, 'fear can be transformed into righteous anger. Often children feel angry but also believe that they are not entitled to their anger' (Chimera in Bannister, 2002, p. 181). TSM constructs help the child realize their strengths and coping mechanisms.

Drago-Drama is an effective action method with adolescents. It is an archetypal form of sociodrama/psychodrama for exploring personal dragons and the treasures that they guard. Drago-drama is 'a quest experience in which an individual or group of "Seekers" encounter their dragon (a life obstacle) to reclaim their Jewel of Great Worth (a life victory or goal)' (Cossa in Bannister, 2002, p. 139). A short synopsis is that in a village a dragon steals each person's Jewel of Great Worth. The individuals need to earn three gifts before they can embark on the quest to recover their Jewel of Great Worth. These are: The Shield Of Self-Confidence (personal, interpersonal, transpersonal strengths), The Wand of Whimsy (humour and the observing ego) and the Cloak of Courage (a narration of an actual act of courage). 'Courage is the ability to act in spite of our fears' (Cossa in Bannister, 2002, p. 145). The quest then continues through many life obstacles until the Jewel of Great Worth is reclaimed. Teenagers relate to this type of action as it is creative, expressive and fun.

In a 'youth at risk' group in Ivory Park, a male individual's girlfriend had died of HIV/AIDS. Her parents had custody of their child, and the father of the child was not allowed visiting rights. There were complex cultural issues involved in the reasons for this, one being that the father needed to respect the girlfriend's parents and thus could not 'make demands to older people'. When concretizing his strengths, being able to role-play an interaction to externalize his righteous anger about the situation, and an opportunity for him to discuss with his girlfriend in the 'here and now', he was able to view the situation from a different perspective (by using the observing ego card) and consider his rights as a father. He immediately depicted his strengths on his TSIRA soul portrait, (which was a cake box) and asked if he could keep his personal strength scarf which had emerged from the drama, for the following week. This personal strength was 'a good-enough father'. The support from the group was truly tangible and later resulted in the father of the child approaching the girlfriend's parents for visitation rights in a culturally acceptable manner.

In a group setting within the community in Ivory Park (informal settlement) an elder (senior citizen) whose shack had been burnt down to the ground felt such anger and self-pity that she was immobilized. When she was able to realize that she still possessed her personal, interpersonal and transpersonal strengths, she was able to talk about her feelings and to concretize her righteous anger to be able to address it effectively. She was also able to accept support from the group in a dignified manner, and later commented that the group had made her want to live again. 'Belief in yourself' was the theme that emerged and was often commented on in subsequent sessions. The group became known as the 'Iphelisweni Group', meaning 'Healing Group' in Zulu.

Over the past 20 years of development of the Therapeutic Spiral Model, evaluation and research has shown treatment effectiveness across populations. Client and therapist self-report measures showed an 89 per cent improvement in trauma symptoms after a three-day TSM application. A single-case design with a client diagnosed with PTSD demonstrated a decrease in dissociation over a series of three individual therapy sessions (Hudgins et al., 2000). An eight-day experiential programme of education, training and self-care for people affected by the 2001 terrorist attacks in the USA found significant decreases in post-traumatic stress anxiety and depression one year after 11 September 2001 (Saury, 2003).

Occupational therapy intervention

Occupational therapists have specific qualities that are advantageous when working with traumatized people. The occupational therapist's thorough knowledge about assessment, observation and integration of information gained from the individual can lead to a truly holistic treatment plan. However the occupational therapist *needs to be emotionally secure* within herself, confident and unbiased when dealing with trauma survivors. Introspection of self values, beliefs and morals need to be validated continually to enable the occupational therapist to be resilient yet empathetic towards the trauma survivor. Specific and regular self-care activities (e.g. exercise, relaxation, meditation, massage, time alone) need to be carried out by the occupational therapist to prevent compassion fatigue and to be available to model a secure and stable therapeutic relationship. The realization of the occupational therapist's own strengths through the use of the scarves is also a worthwhile self-affirming activity.

The therapeutic relationship is of utmost importance and must be built on *trust and emotional safety. Confidentiality* needs to be overtly stated and discussed to encourage safety of disclosures. Honesty and openness are key ingredients within the therapeutic relationship, and when disclosures need to be followed up or shared with the therapeutic team the individual needs to be informed of this. Confidentiality within a group setting needs to be concretized through a ritual at the end of the session, e.g. the group forms a circle facing inwards and each person crosses their arms in front of them (representing care of self) to hold another person's hand on either side (representing a connection to others). To focus on confidentiality the group members say their names whilst in this position. The Therapeutic Spiral Model also describes the 'thumb-thing', which is the connection of the right hands within a circle holding the thumb of the person on the right in the palmar grasp of the hand so that the whole forms a circle of hands. In African culture, the left hand must be placed on the right forearm to show that a weapon is not being held in this hand. This is also a form of respect. These rituals represent protecting both oneself and others by the connections of the hands. Then a contract comment about confidentiality can be stated, with each group member stating their name and thus agreeing with the confidentiality contract.

With trauma survivors, *boundaries* are of the utmost importance. Often trauma survivors do not respect or acknowledge boundaries, and need to have boundaries modelled by the occupational therapist. Boundaries relate to what behaviour is acceptable and not acceptable in a given situation, and the therapeutic relationship. Because trauma survivors may have a tendency to dependency traits, it is important to empower them in their own lives. Setting boundaries gives them a framework within which to work, and this creates structure, safety and independence. It is also important to consider a 'self-care contract' before treatment begins (Table 14.2).

When dealing with *disclosures* the occupational therapist needs to be calm and unconditionally accepting. The occupational therapist's reaction to a disclosure can enhance or destroy the therapeutic relationship. The therapeutic relationship also needs to be built on mutual trust, which may lead to the occupational therapist sharing some personal experiences

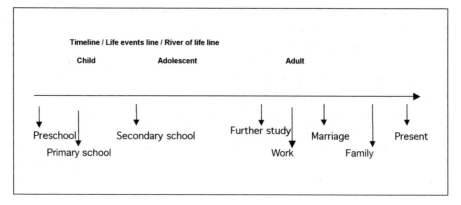

Figure 14.3 Timeline/Life events line/River of life line.

related to the disclosure. The occupational therapist's self-disclosure can be productive, counter-productive or irrelevant. Self-disclosure should be done for modelling, validating the individual's reality and moving past an impasse. Self-disclosures should be brief, 'judicious' and authentic. A thoughtful 'here-and-now' response from the occupational therapist in order to clarify the interactions that are taking place is often preferable and more appropriate.

Clinical reasoning skills are used continually when assessing and treating trauma survivors. The acknowledgement of tacit reasoning must not be underestimated and will often be cited in reflective journals. Reflective journals can enhance an occupational therapist's insight into transference and counter-transference when dealing with trauma survivors. Reflective journals can also elicit an understanding of the development of compassion fatigue.

Assessment

Adequate time needs to be allowed for the initial interview with the trauma survivor, to enable the individual to build up trust with the occupational therapist so that *safety* and *containment* can be obtained. The 'time line', sometimes referred to as Narrative Therapy (Polkinghorne, 1991), is an effective means of obtaining knowledge about an individual's life history and trauma, and contextualizes the trauma event/s (Figure 14.3). Table 14.1 shows a list of headings for a confidential report on the individual, covering all the information obtained and observed.

In a *group setting* the warm-up activities need to be such that the group members feel universality and safety from positive and negative past experiences. This can be facilitated by *circle-sociometry* (group stands in a circle and a member of the group steps forward with a comment about their life experiences – 'I am an orphan', or 'I like to dance' – and if other members of the group are or feel the same they too step forward. Thus connections and observations can be made within the group). Another

Table 14.1 Occupational therapy confidential report example

Occupational therapy confidential report

Client name:	
Age:	
Date of assessment:	
Presenting problem:	
Referred by:	
Medical Aid Fund (if applicable):	
Medical Aid Number:	
Background history:	
Medical history:	
Developmental milestones:	
Traumatic incident:	Initial Repeated
Reaction:	Values:
Habits:	
Physical reaction:	
Stress management:	
Psychosomatic:	
Risky behaviour:	
Psychological reaction:	Cognition: Memory, Concepts, Perception, Volition, Emotive

Social reaction:	Behaviour:
	Support system:
	    Family, Friends,
	    Community

Spiritual reaction:	
Cultural issues:	
Non-disclosure issues:	
Ego strengths identified:	Personal: Interpersonal: Transpersonal / Spiritual:
Plan of action:	
Recommendations:	
Report compiled by:	

method is through the use of *spectograms*, where an imaginary line is created across the floor with a positive and a negative point at each end. Specific criteria are called out and the group members must position themselves on the line according to how they feel about the criteria, e.g. how comfortable are you with touch? *Dyad or triad* warm-ups can also be used. (A useful warm-up tool is to use pictures of animals, birds or insects for the group members to select and to discuss with a partner why they related to that particular picture.) The 'time line' may be completed within the group setting but it is necessary for each group member to work on their own, and the occupational therapist needs to discuss the time line individually as well. This is thus only feasible with a group of three to four individuals.

The time line exercise, which is best used on an individual basis, depicts positive and negative events in an individual's life and enables these events to be put into the context of the individual's life. Dates of incidents need to be recorded, and any links between incidents can be added. Positive experiences may be put above the line, and negative experiences below the line. It is important that the individual completes this diagram themselves. The individual needs to be encouraged to add to the events as the therapeutic relationship develops and when safety and trust is built to enable disclosures. Often, depicting their experiences graphically and overtly making links between incidents within their life context, enables the individual to see themes within their lives, thus improving insight.

During the assessment it is essential to ascertain whether the individual has been a victim or a perpetrator or both. This is very important if the individual is placed within a group, as it will influence the group dynamics. The occupational therapist's ethical, moral and personal emotional attitude towards perpetrators is an important consideration if he/she intends working with this population. The occupational therapist needs to monitor his/her transparency. It is imperative to see the perpetrator in a holistic paradigm, and to analyse why and from where the need for power or control comes, in the individual's background. Perpetrators inevitably have low self-esteem and a poor self-concept, with underlying aggression and a need to be recognized. Action methods in a group setting can effectively enable these individuals to gain insight into their behaviour and its effect on others, and thus promote personal growth and interpersonal learning and relationships when their appropriate ego strengths are acknowledged.

A teenage perpetrator of sodomy – and he was a victim of sodomy himself – depicted his strength in an art therapy session as a penis. When this was acknowledged, he was able to depict other strengths, one being that he actually had a good heart. After six months of occupational therapy his self-esteem had improved markedly and he was more appropriately spontaneous and accepted by his peers.

With an individual client an impact assessment is done to ascertain how the trauma has affected their functioning in all spheres. The use of pre-trauma and post-trauma activity profiles (pie chart) gives information about the individual's actual performance in all the occupational performance areas. Stress boxes can also be used to see how the individual views the trauma and their response to it. This shows their level of mastery with regard to their control and choice over the trauma and what it has done to them. Informal observations within the initial interview give an enormous amount of information. Using clinical skills and clinical judgement regarding the way the interview is conducted can enhance the amount of information obtained. It is also important to ask to interview significant others to gain valuable collateral information.

It is also helpful to use a 'self-care contract' with the trauma survivor before starting therapy to ensure that the trauma survivor uses their available support systems appropriately.

Table 14.2 'Self-Care Contract' example

Self-Care Contract

I,_____, understand that Action Methods sessions may bring up deep feelings and possibly cause me to seek out negative behaviours. I agree to use my support systems wisely to meet my needs appropriately at this time. Should I find myself wanting to engage or actually engaging in self-harming/self-defeating behaviours and thoughts, I agree to take the following actions:

1. _____

2. _____

3. _____

4. _____

I will inform the team about any self-harming thoughts and behaviours I have considered or inflicted on myself during the course of the sessions. I will seek out team members both in the moment and/or as soon as the next session reconvenes.

I further agree not to come to the sessions under the influence of alcohol or drugs and to abstain from their use, or that of other mood-altering substances, for the duration of the sessions. Should I be found to be under the influence at any time during the sessions, I understand that:

My participation will cease immediately at that point.

A team member will contact my therapist and/or other support person(s) to ensure my safety.

Signature: _____ Date: _____

Person to contact in case of emergency: _____

Relationship: _____

Phone number: _____

Treatment – Action methods, theories of activation and occupational therapy theory

Group treatment

Action methods are the group treatment modality of choice as they allow the trauma survivor to access or process trauma material which is not accessed normally in traditional talk therapy (due to Broca's area shutting down during the traumatic incident/event) (Hudgins, 2002). The Therapeutic Spiral Model™ is an example of such a modality that is very effective. If this method is used, in-depth knowledge of the model is necessary and can be found in Hudgins (2002). The conceptual use of strengths and strength building throughout the treatment is essential to promote self-affirmation. The concept of the observing ego is effective in putting the situation in perspective in the here and now, and viewing the self with more clarity. As a result the observing ego often becomes the agent of change, facilitating insight. The facilitation of Yalom's (1985) curative factors within the groups is the foundation and cornerstone of successful group therapy with trauma survivors. It is imperative for the group therapist to facilitate universality and instil hope, cohesion and existential factors to get the desired outcomes with trauma survivors.

Individual treatment

Action methods are also the treatment of choice in individual therapy, together with stress management, teaching coping skills, communication skills and the improvement of self-esteem. The development and concretization of strengths allows the trauma survivor to cope and move on to carry on with their lives. It is also a way of reframing their experiences and changing the perspective of themselves and the situation. Aspects of the Therapeutic Spiral Model can be used in individual treatment, especially the concept of the personal, interpersonal and transpersonal strengths.

Care for the caregiver, or counteracting compassion fatigue

There is a soul weariness that comes with caring and from daily doing business with the handiwork of fear. Sometimes it lives at the edges of one's life, brushing against hope and barely making its presence known. At other times, it comes crashing in, overtaking one with its vivid images of another's terror with its profound demands for attention; nightmares, strange fears and generalized hopelessness (Hudnall Stamm, 1999, p. xix).

Occupational therapists are professionals who have the concept that they can 'handle anything' and tend to work hard in difficult circumstances. The occupational therapist sees and deals with disability, adversity, terminal illness and death, various types of trauma and its effects and the functional problems of individuals within their context of life, together with communities that are plagued by poverty and abuse. The time has come to address the mental health needs of occupational therapists, to keep them resilient and resourceful to carry out the work needed. The tiredness and lack of intrinsic motivation for work used to be called 'burnout', but now secondary traumatization is considered. Compassion stress and compassion fatigue are concepts that have been researched by Figley (1995). Risk factors for secondary traumatization are exposure to the traumatic stories or images, the empathetic sensitivity to their suffering and any unresolved emotional issues that relate to the suffering seen. Occupational therapists need to acknowledge that they are at a high risk of compassion fatigue and that self-nurturing structures need to be put into place to counteract compassion fatigue.

Compassion fatigue is the *state of tension or exhaustion due to working with people in pain*. The facets that contribute to compassion fatigue are what trauma has been experienced in the past and at present (primary trauma) how traumatized the people are that receive help (secondary trauma) and how favourable the working environment is, including how sufficient the resources are to deal with the demands (chronic stress) (Figley, 1995).

The process by which compassion fatigue develops is illustrated in Figure 14.4. Occupational therapists working with trauma survivors may develop compassion stress. This may be disguised and not acknowledged. This compassion stress may develop into secondary traumatic stress and with prolonged exposure to the work with trauma survivors, together with the triggering of own traumatic recollections, compassion fatigue can devel-

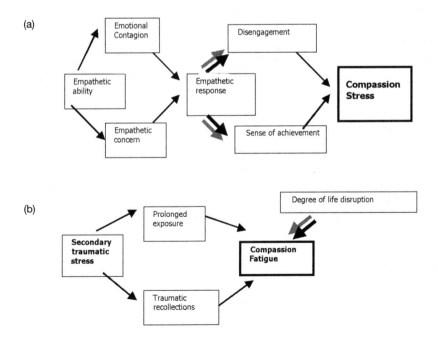

Figure 14.4 (a) A model of compassion stress (b) A model of compassion fatigue.

© 1995 From *Compassion Fatigue. Coping with secondary traumatic stress disorder in those who treat the traumatized* by CR Figley. Reproduced by permission of Routledge/Taylor & Francis Books.

op. This is when an experience or incident disrupts the life of the occupational therapist, which 'tips the balance' of the empathetic attunement. The occupational therapist needs to stop this progression by 'walking the walk', not just 'talking the talk' when it comes to care of self. Occupational therapists are excellent in their treatment of others, but often do not apply their treatment to themselves. They need to make a conscious effort to be constructive, become involved in activities and take time out for self-care as they cannot effectively care for others if they are not resourced themselves. The concepts within the Therapeutic Spiral Model™ pertaining to self-affirmation through personal, interpersonal and transpersonal strengths can be used effectively by the occupational therapist for self-care.

Child abuse

Child abuse or child maltreatment is on the increase throughout the world. It was only in 1960 when Harry C. Kemp and his colleagues coined the term 'battered child syndrome', and began to document such cases, that health professionals began to come out with abuse cases. It was not that abuse did not happen in the past, but that health professionals simply could not bring themselves to believe that such evil took place. As the gradual uncovering of the prevalence of abuse came to the fore, health professionals were forced to look at the causes and the effects of abuse and how to deal effectively with it. Abuse can manifest itself in a variety of ways, such as physical abuse, emotional abuse, neglect, sexual abuse and structural abuse (e.g. legislation that does not protect the vulnerability of children, children in jail). Defining abuse is difficult as there is no consensus on an acceptable definition of child abuse. Crous defines abuse as the continued and deliberate prejudice of children through direct or indirect abuse or the withholding of care (Crous in de Witt and Booysen, 1995). According to the National Institute of Child Health and Human Development, abuse is:

> behaviour toward another person which is: a) outside the norms of conduct *and* b) entails a substantial risk of causing physical or emotional harm. The behaviour included will consist of actions and omissions, ones that are intentional and ones that are unintentional. They will have severe, mild or no immediate adverse consequences (Wenar and Kerig, 2000, p. 304).

Types of abuse

(Western Cape Education Department, 2000)

Physical abuse

Physical abuse is any act or threatened act of violence in which the individual's life, health or safety is threatened or compromised. It can include but is not limited to hitting, burning, violent shaking, kicking and beating.

Profile of physical abusers/perpetrators

The profile of physical abusers/perpetrators is that they often complain that the child is difficult to control, they have little or no knowledge of child development while making unrealistic demands on the child (e.g. expecting toilet control at an early age). They are often secretive about how the child sustained injuries, lying or giving contradictory stories about how the child was injured. They often delay seeking medical attention, and when they do they seem relatively unconcerned about the child's welfare.

Behaviour of a physically abused child

They cannot explain their injuries or remember how the injuries occurred, therefore they give inconsistent explanations. They are wary and afraid of adults, cringe or withdraw if they are touched, are extremely aggressive or withdrawn, attention-seekers and are often overly compliant in trying to please others. They show an avoidant attachment style (Wenar and Kerig, 2000).

Physical indicators of child abuse

The child has injuries that cannot be explained and are inconsistent with the explanation. They have different injuries at different times and at various stages of healing. Injuries are inconsistent with the child's level of development (e.g. babies with head injuries, burn marks, pre-school children with fractures, bruises and burns). They also wear inappropriate clothing to cover up the injuries.

Emotional abuse

Emotional abuse is a pattern of degrading or humiliating the child and can include insulting, ridiculing or name-calling the child, repeatedly threatening to cause harm or emotional harm to the child, breaking down the child's self-esteem and ignoring their developmental needs.

Profile of emotional abusers/perpetrators

The child is seen as the scapegoat and is often blamed for the perpetrator's own problems and disappointments. They express negative feelings about the child, to the child and others. They reject the child by withholding love from the child. They continually try to frighten the child by using bribes and isolating the child in order to prevent them from having contact with others. Emotional abusers often misuse substances and have underlying psychological problems (e.g. depression and anxiety). (This is the same profile as the neglectful caregiver.)

Behaviour of an emotionally abused child

These children are often aggressive and act out in order to seek attention and gain control. Sometimes they can be hyperactive or extremely over-compliant (e.g., being too neat, too clean, too well mannered).

Physical indicators of an emotionally abused child

Enuresis and/or encopresis for which there is no medical cause. Frequent psychosomatic complaints are common (e.g. headaches, nausea and stomach-aches). The child's growth and development are slow in comparison to other children of the same age.

Neglect

Neglect is any act or omission by the parent or the caregiver which results in impaired physical and/or psychological functioning of the child. It can include withholding love, medical care, opportunities to play and social-ize, keeping the child away from school and other places where they will be in contact with others.

Behaviour of a neglected child

These children are listless and lethargic, making very few demands, show-ing no interest in their environment, and showing little or no reaction to strangers' attempts to engage them. These children will beg or steal food, claiming that nobody is at home to look after them. School attendance is irregular. They have inappropriate clothing and hygiene, are always dirty and hungry. Neither their physical nor medical needs receive attention. The child shows an avoidant attachment style (Wenar and Kerig, 2000).

Physical indicators of a neglected child

These are the 'failure to thrive' children. They are pale and emaciated, have very little body fat in relation to their build (low body mass index). They have a 'parchment feel' to their skin as a result of dehydration, and constantly complain of vomiting and/or diarrhoea. Their developmental milestones are not reached within normal limits.

Sexual abuse

This is defined as any unlawful physical act of a sexual nature which is per-petrated against a child and can include an adult or any person significantly older than the child interacting with the child in a sexual manner. Sexual abuse can be divided into contact and non-contact behav-iour. Contact behaviour involves sexual intercourse, kissing the child in a lingering and intimate manner, fondling the child's breasts, inner thighs, buttocks and genital area, or asking the child to touch the perpetrator's genitals, or oral genital contact. Non-contact behaviour includes the exposure of genitals to the child, or directing the child's attention to the perpetrator's genitals, masturbation by the adult in front of the child or involving the child in the making of pornographic material.

Profile of sexual abusers/perpetrators

They are extremely protective and jealous of the child and discourage the child from unsupervised contact with their peer group and with other adults. They accuse the child of being provocative. They often indicate that there are marital or relationship problems in their lives and they misuse alcohol and/or drugs.

Behaviour of a sexually abused child

Inappropriate sexual play with toys, self and others, such as replication of explicit acts and/or inappropriate sexual drawing or descriptions of sex. They show age-inappropriate knowledge of sex, promiscuity and/or prostitution and unwillingness to participate in previously enjoyed activities. There is a sudden drop in school performance due to lack of concentration and intrusive thought about the abuse. They show poor interpersonal relationships with peers and authority, withdrawal and aggressive behaviour, crying without provocation, depression and attempted suicides.

Psychological indicators of a sexually abused child

The child thinks that they are responsible for the abuse and they feel different from other children. They feel dirty or like 'damaged goods', with a feeling that they have been permanently dirtied and that sex is the only value they have to offer other people. They are angry, suffer from depression and anxiety, feel guilty and confused and can be destructive. They can also steal and lie. They are prone to enuresis, encopresis and nightmares. There are changes in appetite and sleeping patterns and they are often absent from school. They often have a lack of respect for boundaries and find it difficult to trust.

Physical indicators of a sexually abused child

These children may show pain or unusual itching in the genital or anal area with torn or bloodstained underwear. Pregnancy, sexually transmitted diseases and urinary tract infections are common. These children often have difficulty sitting and walking due to their injuries and often have throat irritations as a result of forced oral sex.

Occupational therapy intervention

As occupational therapists work so closely with children, it is our duty, both morally, ethically and lawfully, to *break the silence* surrounding abuse by reporting the abuse and helping children overcome the effects of abuse. Silence and secrecy so often go hand in hand with abuse. Child abuse is something that often happens between an adult and a child when they are alone, which further allows the perpetrator to abuse, intimidate and isolate the child. This leads to further secrecy and helplessness. This has profound indications for the therapeutic relationship, which needs to be *open, transparent and supportive*. Therapists need to ensure active and open communication with the child, with an inherent respect for the child, and not adopt the 'adult knows all' stance. The use of a soft toy as an observing ego in the therapy room will allow the child and therapist to have a 'third person's opinion' within the play experience. A squeaky monkey or parrot can play this role.

A moderately mentally handicapped child was displaying acting out behaviour in the occupational therapy playroom. She was an angry lion in a cage. This led to discussions with the multidisciplinary team and it was later found out that her father was physically abusing her. She was overtly tactile defensive during assessment and she had imaginary toy dogs that accompanied her to the occupational therapy sessions. She used the imaginary dogs to talk to as her defence mechanism and to have an aspect she could control in her life.

Always use language that the child understands, and *talk to the child on their own eye level*. Never use punitive punishment. Follow the child's lead, (a true child-centred approach), especially with regard to physical distance and touch. The occupational therapist needs to *model safe touch*.

A five-year-old child kept insisting that she touch the therapist's breasts. It needed to be conveyed to her in a caring non-judgemental way that this was inappropriate, but safe touch like a hug was acceptable. Thus at the end of every session a hug was allowed.

Often if the parent or close family member is the perpetrator, the child will still feel loyal to their family, and still love the person who has abused them. This may lead to a disorganized attachment style. Any attempt by the therapist to degrade the perpetrator can irrevocably damage the therapeutic relationship. The occupational therapist needs to convey a non-judgemental accepting attitude of the child and his/her situation.

A 12-year-old who was sexually and emotionally abused by her father kept running away from foster care to her father's place of work to try and find him. The occupational therapy sessions entailed the child finding her definition of abuse and working through exercises from Johnson et al., 1995. Self-worth was integral in the therapy and when she was ready she was moved into a life skills group. An important aspect of interpersonal relationships was taught, in that we may not love what our loved ones do, but we can still love them. This child was later adopted successfully and is now functioning well.

Occupational therapists working with abused children need to trust themselves and their instinct (tacit knowledge). They always need to show the child that they are also affected by their pain and trauma. When the occupational therapist is no longer emotionally affected by their work, it is a sign of compassion fatigue.

Never make a promise to a child that you cannot keep, as abused children are often betrayed by adults and this will further impede the therapeutic relationship and the child's ability to trust in the future. Honesty and integrity are of utmost importance when working with these children. Children like to work with people not superheroes.

The child needs to know that they are in a safe place and will be treated with respect and dignity. It needs to be affirmed that they are believed and that the abuse is not their fault. The occupational therapist must never talk about the child to the caregiver in front of the child unless it is a positive statement, and confidentiality needs to be respected.

> When a teacher brought the child to the therapy playroom she inadvertently explained in front of the child to the occupational therapist that the child was dirty (clothes). The child misinterpreted this as her 'self being dirty' as a result of her sexual abuse. This resulted in the occupational therapy intervention regressing.

Goals and aims of treatment

Improvement of *self-esteem and self-image* is a priority. This leads to improvement of body image. The child needs to be helped to experience positive adult interaction which is not abusive and will thus help the child to trust other people appropriately. Emotions need to be acknowledged and accepted, and the appropriate emotional response needs to be encouraged. These children need to be taught communication skills and how to have their needs and feeling met appropriately.

Problems regarding their socialization affect their functioning in all spheres of life. These children need to be taught acceptable and appropriate coping mechanisms, and anger management.

> As a warm-up in a group setting each child was given a tub of playdough. The playdough was stretched over the empty tub to form a concave pie cover. Vinegar and bicarbonate of soda were added into the tub, under the pie cover, which caused small explosions. This was to illustrate the consequences of not dealing effectively with our anger. This led to the discussion about dealing with our anger appropriately. Note that this activity is messy so should be done outside.

The play activities need to consider the emotional level of the child's developmental age and not the false emotional maturity that the child portrays.

An eight-year-old had not only taken on the role of sexual partner to her father, but also mothered the four younger step-siblings. In occupational therapy child play activities were used as the main treatment modality in order to allow her to play and experience normal age-appropriate activities. These were mud play, finger painting, doll corner play and swing-ball.

Case study

Karin (12 years old) currently lives with her paternal aunt and uncle, who have legal guardianship over her. She was removed from her biological parents' care a year ago, as her mother was an alcoholic and her father was a multiple substance abuser. Her biological father had sexually molested her on an ongoing basis when she was between the ages of 9 and 11. When the family was involved in a motor vehicle accident due to drunken driving, causing Karin's prolonged hospital stay and multiple surgeries to her leg, she came to the attention of medical professionals and was placed in foster care with her aunt and uncle.

On presentation Karin was showing classic signs of post-traumatic stress. She was unable to sleep at night and experiencing nightmares related to the motor vehicle accident and her sexual abuse. She had intrusive flashbacks during the school day, often just hearing the bang from the motor vehicle accident or the bang of the front door when her parents would return home drunk. She showed signs of hyper-arousal. She was unable to concentrate on her schoolwork and was at risk for failing Grade 5. She had isolated herself from her friends and was not participating in netball, which she had previously enjoyed. Her appetite had increased and she often craved starchy food. She mistrusted most adults and had difficulties relating to her peers and those in authority.

She constantly expressed the wish for life to be 'like it was when I was eight'. She also showed signs of regression, reverting to baby-talk and sometimes enuresis. Karin initially found it very difficult to engage in occupational therapy and form a trusting relationship with the occupational therapist. She showed resistance and would try to keep sessions superficial. Therapy focused on dealing systematically with Karin's traumas – the abuse, the accident and being removed from home.

Initially Karin was seen on an individual basis and later in groups. As Karin's trust in people increased, so did her participation in occupational therapy. Individual sessions focused on Karin's trust issues, her feelings of helplessness about not being able to control the abuse or the accident, forming a positive self-image, acknowledging emotions, venting aggression, experiencing positive peer and adult interaction, and learning how to communicate her needs and feelings. Group therapy focused on self-esteem, social skills and trust-building, as well as task-centred activity groups allowing Karin to express her creativity and thus feel that she could contribute positively.

As time progressed, Karin was able to participate in more age-appropriate activities. At the final therapy session, where Karin was given the freedom to choose the termination activity, she chose to play a board game with the therapist, finger paint and play balloon volleyball with the occupational therapist. Her final words, on parting were: 'It's going to be different now, because I can play again.' That showed the tacit knowledge that occupational therapy had been effective.

Conclusion

Working as an occupational therapist in the field of trauma and abuse is exciting, challenging and never without reward. It is a field within occupational therapy that in the past has received very little attention, yet it is an ever-growing one. Trauma and abuse affect the very core of the emotional and functional being of the individual. Occupational therapists, by the fact that we treat our clients holistically and functionally, are integral members of the multidisciplinary team that treats trauma and abuse survivors. It is an area in which we can truly contribute to the quality of life of the individual, and 'look, learn and listen' qualities need to be incorporated into the therapy. With confidence, experience and expertise occupational therapists can take their rightful place in the treatment of trauma survivors to empower them and make a contribution to Restorative Justice.

Questions

1. What are the different phases of trauma and how do these impact on the occupational therapy services offered to the trauma survivor?
2. What does a trauma survivor need? How does occupational therapy fulfil these needs in the programme?
3. Describe the neurological impact of trauma.
4. Critically compare the different models related to trauma.
5. 'Not all trauma survivors will go on to develop post-traumatic stress disorder.' Discuss this statement in detail.
6. Describe in detail the occupational therapy intervention related to trauma.
7. Describe how abuse can impact on a child's functioning, and link this with the attachment theory. (Attachment theory is covered in chapter 12.)
8. Discuss the occupational therapy aims that would be appropriate for a sexually abused ten-year-old child.
9. What personal qualities does an occupational therapist need to have in order to work in the field of trauma and abuse?
10. How can compassion fatigue impact on our work as occupational therapists?

Chapter 15
A 'bottom-up' approach: the factors influencing a child's emotional, motor and perceptual development for optimal learning

CANDACE LEE BYLSMA

This chapter aims to provide some practical guidelines on how to identify, assess and manage the wide variety of children who present with perceptual, motor and emotional difficulties. The intention is to create an understanding of the possible underlying causes of the presenting problems as well as including occupational therapy treatment ideas. Knowledge of self and the continuous utilization of clinical reasoning are of vital importance and will be emphasized throughout. Because the occupational therapist hopes to foster an understanding of how a child's behaviour frequently provides clues as to the emotional tone of the child, it is vitally important to take this into account during treatment. The chapter will highlight a variety of models and treatment approaches with which occupational therapists should familiarize themselves. Children should never be viewed in isolation, so the author will emphasize the importance of working within the occupational therapy framework of holism and the importance of working within a multidisciplinary team.

Possible diagnoses of children who present with perceptual, motor and emotional difficulties

Mental disorders (DSM-IV-TR™ (American Psychiatric Association, 2000))

Refer to the Diagnostic and Statistical Manual IV (American Psychiatric Association, 1994) for information about 'Disorders Usually First Diagnosed in Infancy, Childhood, or Adolescence'.

Medical conditions

• Cerebral palsy
• Sensory integration dysfunction – Praxic dysfunction: bilateral integration and sequencing, somatodyspraxia; Sensory modulation disorders:
sensory defensiveness, gravitational insecurity, aversive responses to
movement, under-responsiveness (Bundy et al., 2002)

The special challenges of working with children

Working with children is fun, but challenging on many levels for an occupational therapist. In order to develop from a personal and professional
perspective, apply clinical reasoning effectively and get the most out of the
treatment sessions with the child being treated, it is vital to keep the following points in mind. These can be considered to be handling principles:

• It is important for an occupational therapist to know herself very well.
One's own issues, however difficult, should not impact on the occupational therapy sessions. Children are intuitive and can sense when you
are otherwise preoccupied.
• The occupational therapist should be sensitive and use her intuition
when faced with each new child. This will sometimes require that the
occupational therapist regulates or moderates things within herself
that the child may not tolerate well, such as loudness of voice, amount
of imposed touch, perfume due to olfactory sensitivity, etc.
• The occupational therapist should employ a process of reflection,
which will facilitate the best possible treatment process for each individual client and promote self-development. This forms part of the
clinical reasoning process (Creek, 1998).
• Occupational therapy sessions with children should above all be fun.
Use of your (and their) imagination and creativity is of vital importance.
Furthermore, it is very important to be well aware of the normal development of a child (physical, perceptual, cognitive, personality and
social) (Atkinson et al., 1990; Hopkins and Smith, 1988) as well as how
a child plays at each stage of development. Never forget the importance
of play for a child. Play is the child's primary occupation in childhood –
it promotes development of gross and fine motor skills, self-confidence,
expression of emotions, learning of social rules and problem-solving
ability (Oser, 1997; O'Brien et al., 2000). It is not only important to look
at play traditionally – as a functional outcome or predictor of the developmental level of the child – but also to really consider the impact of
pretend play and quality of playfulness on cognitive development. This
has been shown to impact on the development of pre-academic skills of
the child (Stagnitti et al., 2000). Bundy (in Stagnitti et al., 2000) identified three intrinsic qualities of playfulness: those of intrinsic motivation,

internal locus of control and suspension of reality. Having a good understanding and actively promoting playfulness in your occupational therapy sessions will give you invaluable insight about at what level to set your therapy, for optimal achievement and success on the part of the child as well as the therapist.

- Children have a great deal of energy and occupational therapy sessions are physically, emotionally and cognitively intense, as children require your undivided attention and energy. Ensure that you are sufficiently rested, emotionally balanced and can give of yourself without hindrance.
- Reading of signals, such as the non-verbal cues of the child, is very important, as many of the children we deal with 'act out' rather than verbally express their emotions, frustrations and what they would like to do. These signals also give us clues as to how a child is processing the incoming sensory information from the environment and how it is impacting on their arousal levels, thus influencing their ability to learn optimally. (Mercer and Snell in Williams and Shellenberger, 1996). It is important to remember this in every treatment session, because children are dynamic individuals with many internal and external factors impacting on their lives, and their (emotional, arousal) state will change from session to session and even within sessions.
- Accept responsibility if you have graded an activity inappropriately and the child is not able to succeed and derive pleasure from it. The child may even start to exhibit poor behaviours or start to lose interest. Everyone makes mistakes, so just say something like: 'I'm sorry. I made a mistake – this is a really difficult activity to ask you to do.'
- Do not bombard the child with lots of talking. Children generally do not respond to questions well (e.g. How was school today? How are you feeling?, How was that?) – they tend to give typical responses such as 'fine', 'OK' or other monosyllabic answers. A child psychologist taught the author to rather use short simple statements on what you observe. For example, 'You look tired – must have been a hard day at school'; 'By that big smile on your face it looks as if you are feeling happy today'; 'It looks like you are feeling dizzy and didn't really enjoy that activity'. This is a far more effective way to communicate with children, as it makes them feel understood and opens up the channels for unthreatening communication.
- Flexibility and allowing choices is vital in order to engage a child. This promotes internal motivation and ensures interest in the task at hand, making the session meaningful for the child (Williams and Shellenberger, 1996). This does not mean that you hand over control to the child – you are still in control of the environment and therapy process. This promotes feelings of security and facilitates trust between the child and therapist.
- Sincerity is of vital importance, as a child knows intuitively when we really mean what we have said, or whether or not we are not being truthful – honest feedback in simple language is often best.

- The therapist must always be consistent in her approach and set appropriate boundaries in order for a child to feel safe and contained. This fosters trust and reinforces that the child–therapist relationship is unconditional. This will provide safe, pleasurable and satisfying experiences where the child will benefit optimally (Williams and Shellenberger, 1996).
- The therapist should also be aware of her limitations on a professional basis and if not adequately equipped to deal with certain situations, know when to refer on to an appropriate colleague.

The occupational therapy process

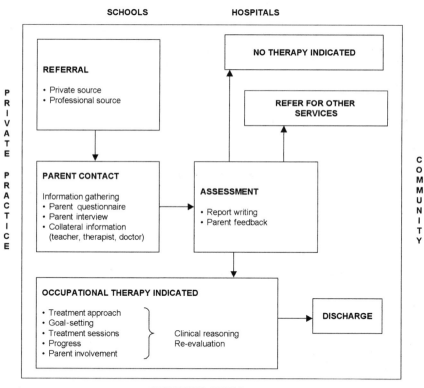

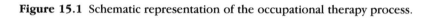

Figure 15.1 Schematic representation of the occupational therapy process.

Referral

This can be from a private source (i.e. other parents – word of mouth), or from a professional source (i.e. medical professionals). Referrals can be in a written format or telephonic.

Information gathering

Assessment scores, although valuable, are not enough to make a differential diagnosis. The context/environment from where a child comes is very important in order to give meaning to the assessment and subsequent treatment of the child (Parham in Bundy et al., 2002). A child has many environments where they fulfil different roles. It is important for the occupational therapist to ascertain how they are coping within these environments, as it will help the therapist to compile a realistic picture of the child and facilitate the goal-setting process and aims of treatment. It is also important to contact (with parental permission) other relevant professionals in the child's life, in order to facilitate a multidisciplinary approach. Furthermore, there may be medical precautions which need to be taken into consideration during your treatment sessions.

Information gathering can be approached in a variety of ways:

- Questionnaires to be completed by the parents/caregivers (see Table 15.1).
- Face-to-face interviews with the parents/caregivers
- Telephonic interviews/discussions – usually with relevant others in the child's life.

Table 15.1 Parent questionnaire

PARENT QUESTIONNAIRE
The following questions are posed to help compile a more complete picture of your child in his/her infancy, early childhood and at present. All information will be treated as confidential.
General particulars
Reason for referral and appropriate reports
Parent description of child – Likes/dislikes, etc.
1) Prenatal history
2) Delivery
3) Birth
4) Post-natal history
5) Developmental history and observable behaviours
6) Medical history
7) Family history
8) Schooling

9) Sensory history
 	
   – Tactile system
   – Gustatory-olfactory system
   – Visual system
   – Proprioceptive system
   – Vestibular system
   – Motor skills

Thank you for your cooperation

If the child is old enough, it is useful to obtain information regarding their perspective on their difficulties and what they would like to achieve. If occupational therapy is indicated later on, this promotes responsibility and commitment to their occupational therapy process and facilitates the goal-setting process (Missiuna and Pollock, 2000).

Assessment

An assessment helps the occupational therapist to ascertain exactly where the child is experiencing difficulties. The assessment results, with additional information gathered, is interpreted and combined into a meaningful whole, which facilitates the treatment approach (Edwards in Wilson, 1998). There are numerous assessments available and it is vital for the occupational therapist to ensure that she is adequately trained to administer the assessment and is able to make the relevant clinical observations within the parameters of the test. Furthermore the therapist should critically evaluate whether or not that particular test will provide useful information to complete the 'whole picture' about the child's functionality in all aspects of daily living, and assist in the treatment planning process (Hayes in Wilson, 1998).

Table 15.2 Appropriate assessments for infants, preschoolers and school-going children

Assessment	Area of function	Age group	Method
Infant/Toddler Symptom Checklist (DeGangi et al., 1995)	Predisposition to developing sensory integration disorder, attention deficit disorder, emotional and behavioural difficulties and learning difficulties	7 months to 30 months	Screening checklist
Sensory Integration Observation Guide (Schaaf et al., 1995)	Information from parents regarding sensory functioning: • tactile-kinesthetic • vestibular proprioceptive • adaptive motor • regulatory	0 years to 3 years	Rating scale
Sensory Profile (Dunn, 1999)	Sensory processing • auditory • visual • vestibular • touch • multi-sensory • oral Modulation Behaviour and emotional responses	3 years to 10 years	Rating scale

Table 15.2 contd.

Assessment	Area of function	Age group	Method
Test of Sensory Function in Infants – TSFI (DeGangi and Greenspan, 1989)	Sensory processing: • Tactile deep pressure • Visual-tactile • Adaptive motor responses • Ocular motor control • Vestibular	4 months to 18 months	Screening rating scale
Bayley Scales Infant Development, Infant Behaviour Record – IBR (Bayley, 1995)	Interpersonal and affective domains, motivational variables and child's interest in sensory experiences	0 years to 4 years	Rating scale
DeGangi-Berk Test of Sensory Integration (Berk and DeGangi, 1983)	Sensory-motor functioning: • postural control • bilateral integration • reflex integration	3 years to 5 years	Screening rating scale
The Screening Test for Evaluating Preschoolers – FirstSTEP (Miller, 1993)	Identifies preschoolers at risk for developmental delays: • cognitive • communication • motor • social/emotional • adaptive behaviour	2 years 9 months to 6 years 2 months	Checklist and rating scale
Strive Towards Achieving Results Together Integrated programme – START (Solarsh et al., 1990)	Developmental screening: • activities of daily living • gross motor • fine motor • receptive and expressive language	0 months to 36 months	Develop-mental screening checklist and graded activity programme
OTA Watertown – Clinical Observation of Sensory Integration (Infant & Pre-school) (Ayres, 1982, revisited OTA staff 2000)	Behaviours related to: • sensory modulation • sensory discrimination • adaptive responses	Infants–preschoolers	Observations and comments
Functional Emotional Assessment Scale – FEAS (DeGangi and Greenspan, in press; Greenspan, 1992)	Parent/child play interaction looking at six levels of emotional development: • regulation and interest in the world • attachment • intentional two-way communication • complex sense of self • emotional ideas • emotional thinking	7 months – 4 years	Videotaped play Observation

Table 15.2 contd.

Assessment	Area of function	Age group	Method
Clinical observations (Adapted by Ayres, 1986)	Neurological functions, eye and hand usage, postural responses, and other neuromuscular conditions related to learning and behaviour	Preschoolers: 3 years to 5 years Older children: 5 years to 8 years	Observation
Sensorimotor History Questionnaire for Preschoolers (DeGangi and Balzer-Martin, 1999)	Performance in: • self-regulation • sensory processing of touch • sensory processing of movement • emotional maturity • motor maturity	3 years to 5 years	Screening rating scale
Miller Assessment for Preschoolers – MAP (Miller, 1988)	School-related difficulties: • cognitive • language • perceptual • motor	2 years 9 months to 5 years 8 months	Screening battery of tests
Southern California Sensory Integration Test – SCSIT (Ayres, 1972)	Detect the nature of sensory integrative dysfunction: • visual • tactile • kinesthetic • perceptual-motor	4 years 0 months to 8 years 11 months Visual perception tests: 10 years 11 months	Diagnostic battery of tests
Sensory Integration and Praxis Test – SIPT (Ayres, 1989)	Diagnose sensory integrative dysfunction, particularly praxis by evaluating: Sensory and neurological processes related to behaviour, learning, language and praxis	4 years 0 months to 8 years 11 months	Diagnostic battery of tests
Southern California Postrotary Nystagmus Test – SCPRNT (Ayres, 1975)	Nervous system processing of vestibular information	5 years to 9 years	Incorporated into SCSIT and SIPT
Movement Assessment Battery for Children – Movement ABC (Henderson and Sugden, 1992)	To assesses developmental coordination disorders – underlying components contributing, both quantitative and qualitative information	4 years to 12 years	Three parts: Classroom screening Assessment battery Intervention strategies

Table 15.2 contd.

Assessment	Area of function	Age group	Method
Bruininks-Oseretsky Test of Motor Proficiency– BOTMP (Bruininks, 1978)	Assessment of motor skills • gross motor • fine motor	4 years 6 months to 14 years 6 months	Screening tool – short version Battery of tests – full version
Goodenough-Harris Drawing Test – DAP (Goodenough and Harris, 1963)	Assesses body image and quality of drawing	3 years to 15 years	Child draws a picture of a man, woman and him/herself
Detroit Test of Learning Aptitude – Primary – DTLA-P (Hammill and Bryant, 1986)	Assesses: • verbal ability • non-verbal ability • conceptual development • structural development • short-term memory • long-term memory • manual dexterity • oral or pointing processes	3 years to 9 years	Battery of tests
Developmental Test of Visual-Motor Integration – VMI (Beery, 1997)	Assesses the child's ability to visually perceive two-dimensional symbols and to reproduce them manually	2 years to 19 years	Three parts: • VMI • motor coordination • visual perception
Developmental Test of Visual Perception 2 – DTPV-2 (Hammill et al., 1993)	Visual perceptual skills: • spatial relations • position in space • form constancy • figure-ground	4 years to 10 years	Battery of tests
Test of Visual-Perceptual Skills (non-motor) – TVPS (Gardner, 1996)	Visual perceptual skills: • visual discrimination • visual memory • visual spatial relations • visual form constancy • visual sequential memory • visual figure ground • visual closure	4 years to 12 years 11 months	Battery of tests
Motor Free Visual Perception Test – MVPT (Colarusso and Hammill, 1972)	Visual perception abilities: • spatial relations • visual and figure-ground discrimination • visual closure • visual memory	5 years to 8 years	Battery of tests

Table 15.2 contd.

Assessment	Area of function	Age group	Method
Coopersmith Self-Esteem Inventories (Coopersmith, 1981)	Measures of self-concept using positive and negative statements	8 years to 15 years	School form: self-evaluative checklist
Piers-Harris Children's Self-Concept Scale (Piers and Harris, 1984)	Measure of self-concept	9 years to 18 years	Self-report checklist

Remember that many of the standardized assessments require practice to ensure that they can be competently administered, and some require formalized training and certification.

When assessing a child always remember the following (Edwards in Wilson, 1998):

- Organize the environment in advance.
- Ensure that there will be no disruptions.
- Accept and respond appropriately to the child's anxiety in a new and unfamiliar environment, under testing conditions.
- Appropriate boundaries need to be in place for children who present with difficult behaviours.
- Accept that at times the child's parent will need to remain in the testing area.
- Read the child's signals appropriately and stop the assessment if you feel that their results will be negatively impacted. Set up an alternative time for the completion of the assessment. This ensures that the test results are reflective of the child's ability.
- When the assessment is complete, always ensure that you place the test items correctly and neatly in the test kit.

Report writing

A written report is the most common means of recording and interpreting the data in a meaningful manner to make available to the child's parents, teachers and other medical professionals (Edwards in Wilson, 1998).

The occupational therapist should develop report-writing skills in order to present the information in a clear, organized, concise and easy to understand manner. Please remember the following when writing a report:

- Whom are you writing the report for – a parent, teacher or medical professional? This will determine the style of writing.
- Occupational therapists are trained in functionality – always link your assessment scores and observed behaviours within the assessment to

how they currently impact, or may impact in the future, on the child's *functional* skills.

- Always include the child's strengths as well as the child's areas of difficulties. This creates a more balanced, holistic view of the child and does not highlight the 'negative' aspects only.
- Make sure that your report is professional in appearance – typed on a letterhead, well laid out with easy-to-read headings, adequate spacing, signed by you as the professional, etc.
- If occupational therapy is indicated, include the goals of therapy, the approach necessary for the child's areas of difficulty and an indication of how long therapy is expected to continue.
- If occupational therapy is not indicated, or additional therapy is indicated, make the appropriate referrals.

Parent feedback

This is a vital part of the OT process. This is the forum where the results of the assessment are reported to the parents and an *understanding* develops about the nature of the child's areas of difficulty, and how they are impacting on their functioning in all aspects. This may also be the first time the parents have come into contact with an occupational therapist, and they will have many questions about the nature of occupational therapy and how it will help their child. When reporting back to the parents it is important to remember the following:

- Have your written assessment report ready, as well as any reports for significant others they may have requested.
- Try to ensure that both parents attend the feedback (if possible). This promotes a unified understanding of the nature of their child's difficulties.
- Allow sufficient time, free from distractions in a private setting, for the feedback to take place.
- Respect their privacy and ensure confidentiality.
- Explain clearly the occupational therapy process and the nature of the assessments administered. Often visual cues are useful, e.g. diagrams, flowcharts, etc. This facilitates a general understanding before you delve into the nature of the child's difficulties. This then allows the parents (and occupational therapist) the opportunity to relate the specific difficulties their child is experiencing to the framework you have already provided. Understanding provides a solid foundation to acceptance by the family, and teamwork between the occupational therapist and the child's family.
- Always start by highlighting the child's areas of strength and then explain that the tests administered are designed to identify problem areas, in order to promote a problem-solving approach to address these difficulties. This creates a more balanced picture and allows for a non-threatening atmosphere to develop. Areas of difficulty can then be discussed.

- Do not judge the parents and their reactions to what you are reporting. Be open and sensitive to their fears. Be prepared for a sometimes very emotional feedback session, e.g. crying, anger, denial, resistance. Above all, listen and allow time for questions.
- At the conclusion of the feedback session (if the parents are ready), discuss suitable times of treatment (if indicated). A contract of terms and conditions of occupational therapy is usually also discussed and a hard copy signed. This promotes parent responsibility and acceptance of the occupational therapy process.

When occupational therapy is indicated

Firstly, it is important to look at the presenting problems and decide on the most effective approach to treatment with each individual child. No two children are the same and therefore your approach with each child will differ. Sometimes your approach with the same child will differ from time to time, depending on the external and internal influences at the time.

What approaches are available for use?

There are numerous models and approaches available to the occupational therapist. It is important to work within a model or use a specific approach as it provides a structure, helps the occupational therapist to formulate aims and facilitates effective treatment using sound principles. Clinical reasoning, too, is influenced by this, as it promotes continuous evaluation of conscious and unconscious knowledge (both objective and subjective) about one's client (Smith Roley et al., 2001). It is beneficial to brush up on your knowledge of some of the commonly used models and approaches shown in Table 15.3 (Hagedorn, 1992).

Table 15.3 Models and approaches

Models	Approaches
Model of Human Occupation (Gary Kielhofner)	Sensory integrative approach
	Neuro-developmental approach
Adaptation through Occupation (Kathlyn Reed)	Sensorimotor approach
	Perceptual motor approach
	Experience-based learning
Adaptive Skills (Anne Cronin Mosey)	Child-centred floor approach
Developmental Model	
Problem Solving Model	
Creative Ability Model (Vona du Toit)	

Often more than one or two models and approaches to treatment are used in any given treatment session.

Goal-setting

According to Bundy in Bundy et al. (2002) goal-setting is a vital part of the planning process, before treatment can begin. It allows the therapist to think clearly and logically, creating an effective working plan of action (Rogers and Masagatani in Bundy et al., 2002) and facilitates collaboration with the child (Missiuna and Pollock, 2000), parents and significant others. Once the goals are set, objectives on how to reach those goals can be drawn up.

Treatment sessions

Intervention can occur on a one-to-one individual basis, two children at a time (either with one or two therapists or a helper) or within a group setting of up to eight children where there is one therapist (or assistant) for every two children (Wilson, 1998). It is important to consider carefully the needs of the child, as well as your experience and what you as the occupational therapist feel you are able to manage best, before deciding on which kind of treatment setting to use. Space, assistants and variety of equipment are further considerations. If two or more children will be working together it is important to match type of difficulties, age and physical build (size) for optimal benefit. Individual treatment sessions usually last for one hour per week, but if the child's endurance is low or they are very young, two sessions a week of half an hour at a time is optimal. Group sessions can be up to one and a half hours in duration, once a week.

Progress

This is an important part of the treatment process. Usually progress notes are made after each treatment session, which allows the occupational therapist to apply clinical reasoning to ensure that she is on track. Verbal or written progress reports are given to the parents and significant others once a term or once every six months as it allows the occupational therapist, parents and significant others to re-evaluate how the child has progressed in terms of the original goals set. This also facilitates parent involvement and carry-over into the home and other environments in the child's life.

Parent involvement

In order for therapy to be successful, the child's parents need to understand and be involved in the occupational therapy process. Carry-over into the home (and school) is vital. For this to occur, regular contact with the parents is important. Sometimes this requires parental involvement in the child's occupational therapy sessions, or observation of their sessions, discussions after treatment sessions, telephonic discussions, etc. The occupational therapist should not bombard the parents with 'homework' tasks, but rather foster an understanding of the general principles used in treatment, and appropriate handling techniques. Provide alternatives/ adjustments to tasks/games which the parent engages in with their child on a daily basis anyway, e.g. adjustments in positioning when playing ball games, creative ways to do school-related tasks, e.g. with shaving cream, sand, tactile letters, and reinforce how important it is to incorporate movement, etc. Remember – the parent should remain the parent, and should not be an 'occupational therapist'! Also remember that the relationship between the parent and child is usually strained when the child has emotional/behavioural problems, and that homework should not exacerbate this relationship. Copious pencil-and-paper activities are of no benefit to anyone!

Discharge

The occupational therapy process with children is a special one, for both the child and the occupational therapist. When the child has achieved all the occupational therapy goals and is proficient in all functional activities necessary, therapy will need to be terminated. This requires sensitivity and preparation (for the child) on the part of the therapist. Usually a period of a few sessions (up to four) is required to prepare the child adequately and promote closure. Do not underestimate the need for this. A discharge summary report is usually compiled for the parents and verbal feedback is given.

When occupational therapy is not indicated

At this stage the therapist will feed back to the parents as described in the previous section, but will explain that occupational therapy is not indicated. Referral to an appropriate source will be made if necessary; or indications will be given that the child needs no intervention and is functioning appropriately in all spheres, or would benefit from a home programme rather than weekly occupational therapy sessions. If this is the case, a home programme will be discussed with the parents and follow-up visits/contact to ensure appropriate implementation will be made.

Interrelation of emotional, motor and perceptual difficulties

The author has chosen to use the following real-life case study to assist in the understanding of emotional, motor and perceptual difficulties, and how they are all interrelated. This is supported by the literature, which states that 'Domains of children's development – physical, social, emotional, and cognitive – are closely related. Development in one domain influences and is influenced by development in other domains' (Sroufe et al., 1992; Kostelnik et al., 1993 in NAEYC, 1997). This is depicted in Figure 15.2.

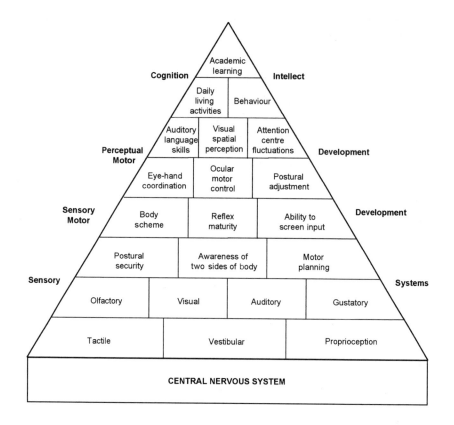

Figure 15.2 Schematic representation of academic learning (Taylor and Trott, 1991 in Williams and Shellenberger, 1996).

Case study

Background information

Monty is a little boy 3 years and 8 months old. He was born at full term, but his mother had to undergo an emergency caesarean section due to placental insufficiency. He weighed 2.35 kg at birth and settled into good feeding and sleeping patterns once at home. Monty reached his developmental milestones of sitting, crawling and walking within normal limits. He is able to dress and feed himself independently, however, these activities are still usually done by an adult. Monty is described as a generally happy little boy, who over-reacts to situations by having temper tantrums, when he lashes out both verbally and physically. He prefers more sedentary play (reading, puzzles, play-dough, painting, etc.), preferably in the company of others (preferably an adult). Monty was recently diagnosed as having asthma, for which he needs two medicated pumps. He has had a tonsillectomy due to recurrent tonsillitis, sinusitis and chest infections. Monty wears glasses as he is exceptionally far-sighted (diagnosed one month ago).

Monty has an older brother Justin (10), who has been adopted by Monty's father and has been diagnosed with attention deficit disorder, hyperactive type (ADHD), and takes Ritalin. Justin has emotional difficulties and attends play therapy on a weekly basis. Furthermore he requires remedial therapy as he is struggling with his schoolwork. (Monty's mother was involved in a physically and emotionally abusive relationship before meeting and marrying Monty's father.) Monty's father is away during the week for business and returns only on weekends. Due to long work hours he is exhausted and sleeps or watches television a great deal when at home. This is a contributor to marital stress. He and his wife have very different parenting styles, which is a source of contention. Boundaries in the family are not optimal, and the children are privy to information that they are not yet able to cope with. Monty's mother is devoted and would do anything for her children. Monty has a loving relationship with all members of the family [looks up to his brother] and is very attached to his mother. The age gap between him and his brother is sometimes apparent, although Justin can be very tolerant a great deal of the time.

Reasons for referral

Monty was referred to occupational therapy by a neuro-developmental paediatrician following the concerns voiced by his teacher. His teacher is concerned about Monty's confidence, his concentration in a group setting, the quality of his gross and fine motor skills, visual perception and that he had not yet established hand dominance. His independence is not yet optimal and he requires a great deal of involvement and encouragement from an adult to engage in an activity and follow it through to completion. Furthermore, the teacher reported that socially he tends to settle disputes with his peers aggressively, which makes inclusion difficult. Monty prefers to play with one child at a time and his play is parallel in nature; often he would rather be an observer than a participant. His teacher has also reported that he avoids rough-and-tumble play, or play that incorporates movement of any kind.

Assessment results

Monty was assessed using the Millers Assessment for Preschoolers, the DeGangi-Berk Test of Sensory Integration, Developmental Test of Visual Perception and the Clinical Observation for Preschoolers. The assessment was administered over two sessions as Monty tired and became uncooperative. He presented as a shy, withdrawn little boy who was not able to separate from his mother [she was present throughout testing]. He did not make good eye contact and was quite anxious in the assessment setting, speaking only when spoken to. He later relaxed somewhat, but frequently responded that the games were 'too hard' or said, 'I can't'. Monty was found to have difficulties with vestibular-proprioceptive processing and had severe gravitational insecurity. His postural control and bilateral integration were poor, which affected the quality of both his gross and fine motor coordination. Primitive reflexes were elicited, which further influenced his movement patterns. Furthermore, hand dominance was unestablished and his eye–hand coordination poor. Perceptually, visual motor integration, visual sequential memory and spatial perception were below expectation. Other perceptual concepts were adequate. Monty was not able to draw a recognizable person, indicative of a diminished body concept. His motor planning ability was within the low normal range and requires further observation. It was observed that he was sensitive to imposed touch during the assessment [supported by the history]. He battled to remain focused on the activities presented and required a great deal of encouragement. Increased distractibility was noticed when there were other people in the occupational therapy room, making task involvement and completion very difficult. Monty was very restless and fidgety when seated at the desk, exhibiting gross postural adjustments.

Behaviour during initial therapy sessions

Monty exhibited fight, flight and fright responses in occupational therapy sessions. He remained unable to separate from his mother for the first three to four months of occupational therapy. He always brought toys from his home into occupational therapy sessions [it was subsequently discovered that he always carried something from home with him wherever he went]. He was anxious and frequently responded with 'I can't' or 'this is too hard'. He found it difficult to follow instructions and could not make choices. Once engaged in an activity, he looked for constant reassurance from the occupational therapist. He tended to give up easily, made poor eye contact and was observed to be easily distracted by visual and auditory stimuli from the environment. He found it difficult to sit still for prolonged periods of time or persevere appropriately with tasks, becoming easily frustrated. He was not able to regulate his emotional responses, which at times resulted in behaviours such as crying, obstinence and withdrawal. In occupational therapy, when his needs were not met quickly or he experienced frustration due to challenges within an activity, Monty sometimes responded in a verbally aggressive way by shouting at the therapist, saying ugly things, or non-verbally by kicking/throwing the equipment. [Aggressive outbursts continued at home and school.] Monty did not seem to take notice of the environment and ask typical questions such as 'why?', as other children his age might do. Due to his severe gravitational insecurity, Monty was extremely fearful of all movement where his feet were off the ground. He even displayed the autonomic nervous system signs of palm sweating, blue ring around the mouth, rigid posture, etc., when on unstable surfaces. Some tactile activities (sticky, wet, lumpy) posed a challenge for him, resulting in avoidance behaviours or emotional outbursts. Furthermore his endurance was poor due to his lowered muscle tone making gross motor activities even more challenging. He tried continually to avoid fine motor and perceptual tasks, often daydreaming or actively resisting when the therapist tried to engage him in these tasks.

Things to consider when dealing with the emotions of a child

What is an emotion? According to Atkinson et al. (1990), intense emotions have many components:

- Physiological reactions triggered by the autonomic nervous system (ANS). This may influence behaviours (i.e. reaction to the emotion) and induce a flight-fight-fright response.
- Cognitive appraisal of the emotion. This plays an important role in the intensity of the emotion.
- Facial expression, which is indicative of the underlying emotion and acts as a communicator to others of that emotion.
- Reaction to the emotion. This is a complex interplay between all of the above components.

It is important to remember that all children have emotions. Emotional expression is a 'window' into the child's internal experiences (Dodge and Gerber in DeGangi, 2000, p.120). They therefore give us an insight into a child's self-regulation ability, as well as his/her perception of self and others. Emotional regulation is vital for the acquisition of adaptive behavioural responses. As a paediatric occupational therapist, regardless of the child's area of presenting difficulty, one may be faced with 'difficult behaviours' (emotional expression), which may be indicative of underlying emotional difficulties. Understanding of the 'whole' picture (i.e. all contributing internal and external factors), and appropriate reading of the child's signals will enable the occupational therapist to respond appropriately in her/his occupational therapy sessions.

It is extremely important to consider in detail the emotional difficulties a child might be experiencing. Many of the children we treat for motor and perceptual problems face problems in this regard. According to Dwivedi (1993) *high states of emotional arousal can impair cognitive processes.* For example, think of how someone's performance can be affected when they are nervous/anxious about doing a practical examination: autonomic nervous system (ANS) symptoms – heart is beating fast, palms are sweaty, mouth is dry, a slightly dizzy, lightheaded or nauseous feeling may prevail. Remembering this may help to give one insight and much needed understanding when one is faced with a child who is displaying 'difficult' behaviour. Children's behaviour is often magnified as they have fewer coping mechanisms than we have as adults.

An understanding of the underlying neurological components involved in emotional control, and how the limbic system is involved in the organization and regulation of incoming sensory information from the environment, is therefore beneficial (Gilman and Newman, 1992; Isaacson in Bundy et al., 2002). This is important to remember when the occupational therapist is reading the child's signals – the child may have the skill, but is not able to participate due to a highly emotional state. Based on work by Ayres and the development of the sensory integration theory, Dunn (1999) developed a new conceptual model, which links children's behaviours to underlying interaction between neurological thresholds. This is defined as 'the amount of stimuli required for a neuron or neuron system to respond' (Dunn, 1999, p. 7). Neurological thresholds can therefore be high (lots of stimuli needed) or low (little stimuli needed). This provides occupational therapists with insight into how a child is processing information from the environment and therefore aids with our treatment intervention to optimize this processing for better behavioural and emotional outcomes. For the occupational therapist it is therefore *vital* to have an understanding of how the sensory systems influence behaviours and emotions. This will help the occupational therapist to employ clinical reasoning to understand accurately all the possible underlying reasons for a child's behaviour or subsequent emotional responses and therefore not just label the child as spoilt, naughty, obstreperous, etc., and react to the behaviour in an unproductive manner.

It is important to remember that you will be employing the following ideas and handling principles into your occupational therapy sessions. Remember, however, that for carry-over to occur you must share and promote an understanding of what works for Monty in all these areas with significant others in his life, such as his parents and teacher. Consistent approaches in other environments than occupational therapy sessions will improve Monty's ability to regulate his emotions and perform more optimally in tasks, using more adaptive behaviours. It will also alleviate some of the caregivers' frustrations and anxieties about how to cope with the emotional demands he makes.

What factors could be influencing Monty's emotional development and impact on his behaviour?

Monty is a very complex little boy with much observable behaviour, which could indicate the following underlying emotions to the understanding and observant occupational therapist:

- Anxiety
- Low self-esteem
- Short attention span
- Poor frustration tolerance

Let us look at each one and discuss what behaviours may cue us in, and how to deal with this in occupational therapy sessions.

Anxiety

Monty displays many of the typical characteristics of an anxious child:

- He suffers from severe separation anxiety from his mother (evident at school for the first three or four months as well).
- He insists on bringing toys from home to occupational therapy sessions (and wherever else he goes). If he has left something behind by accident he experiences severe emotional overload (crying, hitting out, etc.) and will resist coming into occupational therapy.
- Monty requires a great deal of encouragement and involvement from the occupational therapist (or other adult) to engage and persist in an activity, looking for constant reassurance that he is 'doing it right'.
- He exhibits decreased self-confidence as he often expresses that things are 'too hard' or says 'I can't'.
- He makes poor eye contact, seems to withdraw (i.e. 'phases out'/dissociates/daydreams) and talks only when spoken to.
- Monty finds it difficult to make choices and prefers the occupational therapist to make decisions about the activities in therapy.

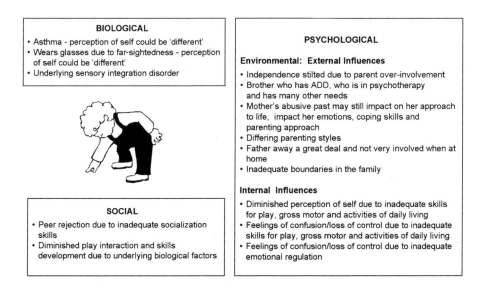

BIOLOGICAL
- Asthma - perception of self could be 'different'
- Wears glasses due to far-sightedness - perception of self could be 'different'
- Underlying sensory integration disorder

SOCIAL
- Peer rejection due to inadequate socialization skills
- Diminished play interaction and skills development due to underlying biological factors

PSYCHOLOGICAL

Environmental: External Influences
- Independence stilted due to parent over-involvement
- Brother who has ADD, who is in psychotherapy and has many other needs
- Mother's abusive past may still impact on her approach to life, impact her emotions, coping skills and parenting approach
- Differing parenting styles
- Father away a great deal and not very involved when at home
- Inadequate boundaries in the family

Internal Influences
- Diminished perception of self due to inadequate skills for play, gross motor and activities of daily living
- Feelings of confusion/loss of control due to inadequate skills for play, gross motor and activities of daily living
- Feelings of confusion/loss of control due to inadequate emotional regulation

Figure 15.3 Biological, psychological and social factors influencing emotions and subsequent behaviours.

- He does not cope well with change or new situations, often over-reacting emotionally.
- He has a short concentration span and is easily distracted by visual and auditory input. This sometimes presents as restlessness and he quickly loses interest in the task at hand.
- Monty has a poor frustration tolerance, which often results in aggressive or emotional outbursts.
- He does not actively notice and explore the environment or ask questions, but merely looks and waits for the occupational therapist to make choices and then responds.
- Monty is afraid of the occupational therapy equipment, particularly that equipment which moves or is unstable. He actively avoids tactile tasks and other activities he perceives to be too difficult.

The literature supports evidence that anxiety is linked to the arousal level of an individual. A person's arousal level is determined by how he/she responds to incoming sensory information from the environment. This is termed sensory modulation. The person can be either under-aroused, have optimal arousal for engagement in activities, which promotes adaptive responses and facilitates learning; or the person can be over-aroused. Kimball stated that 'overarousal led to behavioural disorganisation, anxiety, and potentially negative responses' (Kimball in Bundy et al., 2002, p. 113). The therapist must therefore be aware that anxiety, 'over the top' emotional responses and poor behaviours may be a result of the underlying sensory processing (i.e. poor sensory modulation) occurring within the child. This will ensure correct handling of the situation and structuring of treatment sessions. Anxiety can also result from stress, which is a behavioural response to the environment. There is a relationship between stress and sensory modulation.

Stress responses rely on past experience, e.g. the child may feel stressed when faced with a particular activity in which he/she has previously struggled with, and experienced a sense of failure (Zigmond et al. in Bundy et al., 2002).

What the occupational therapist can do to decrease Monty's anxiety levels in occupational therapy sessions

Handling principles

Understand that Monty has identified underlying sensory modulation difficulties in his tactile (tactile defensiveness), auditory, visual and vestibular (gravitational insecurity) systems, which make it difficult for him to tolerate a great deal of incoming information from these systems. This will explain a great many of his behaviours in terms of his resistance to engage in various tactile activities, the ANS indicators of stress when placed on unstable surfaces, and his resistance therefore to engage in movement activities. It sheds light on why Monty is easily distracted and has a short attention span. This also explains why he prefers to engage in more sedentary activities, avoiding rough-and-tumble play; appears to 'over-react' in certain circumstances and why it is difficult for him to regulate and control his emotional responses. This is seen clearly when he lashes out aggressively in a group dispute situation – his emotions may over-whelm him and he responds in a typical 'fight' manner. It also sheds light on why Monty might find change difficult, as he finds it difficult to adjust on a sensory level to the new environment, especially if he is unsure of what it may hold and how he might feel. When the occupational therapist understands the extent of the involvement of underlying sensory pro-cessing ability in behaviours and emotional regulation, it facilitates the treatment process and appropriate handling of the child.

Find out about Monty's stressors, in order to be forewarned of possi-ble anxiety, which may occur when he is faced with a task in occupational therapy sessions.

Never force Monty to participate in an activity that invokes anxiety. *Try* to encourage or entice him, but stop when it is clear that he is not able to do this. Respect his feelings – they are very real!

An indirect approach is often beneficial with a child like Monty who experiences anxiety. Invitation to play by engaging in the activity and then waiting for him to join in and respond can sometimes work well.

Providing too many choices and too much free time can also be anxiety-provoking as Monty does not know what is expected of him. Limit these choices (usually between two activities), but do not remove choice entirely.

Activity and environmental requirements

Activities should promote success and feelings of achievement – they should therefore fall within Monty's capabilities. Do not grade too quick-ly and make sure that challenges are not going to be too large.

Activities should not make too many demands on too many areas. They should be short and not very complex. This can be graded appropriately as Monty's anxiety lessens, and his competency improves.

Activities should be both excitatory (invigorating) and inhibitory (calm-ing) in nature, to ensure that his nervous system reaches optimal arousal level for adaptive responses to occur, which promotes learning and feel-ings of self-efficacy. *Read* his cues and respond appropriately. This requires continuous evaluation.

Sometimes developing a routine within treatment sessions is beneficial as Monty knows what to expect – i.e. always start with sensory activities, then gross motor, perhaps more sensory and then perceptual and fine motor tasks. Sometimes he developed his own routine and needed to start with the same activity every session in order to cope with the demands later on in the session. This changed periodically. Predictability reduces anxiety – do not take this away from him as it is counter-productive!

Try to keep the environment (treatment areas) looking the same each time. Warn him if it is a mess on a particular day and if any large changes have been made, e.g. equipment been re-covered, moved around, etc. This will lessen his anxiety as he will know what to expect.

Ensure that there is a chair/space provided for Monty's mother to remain and watch occupational therapy, for as long as is required. This too can be graded over time, until he is able to attend an entire treatment session without her. This is ultimately beneficial as it impacts on a child's self-confidence and promotes independence.

Low self-esteem

Monty displays many of the typical characteristics looked for when evaluating self-esteem in children:

- He verbally expresses that tasks are 'too hard' or he is often heard to say 'I can't'.
- He avoids participating in activities that he perceives to be 'too hard' – in therapy, at home and at school.
- Monty can become stubborn and obstinate, openly refusing to cooperate, sometimes experiencing emotional overload by becoming aggressive or tearful.
- He avoids making eye contact, lowering his eyes when spoken to.
- He doesn't persevere with a task, becoming frustrated and giving up quickly when making even the smallest mistake.
- Doesn't like to make choices, wanting the therapist to choose saying things like 'I don't know' or 'you choose'.
- Monty's teacher reports that he lacks confidence.

It is important to realize that not all children who have difficulties in one or more areas of occupation spheres, necessarily have a low self-esteem, or a diminished self-concept (King et al. and Magill-Evans and Restall in Willoughby et al., 1996). It is important, therefore, to use recognized assessment procedures, to ascertain whether or not 'improving self-esteem' is a legitimate treatment goal. Furthermore, Willoughby et al. (1996) caution occupational therapists to critically evaluate whether or not they are actually wanting to increase a child's self-esteem (overall value and feeling of worthiness, i.e. overall evaluation of self). They differentiate between global self-esteem, self-concept (beliefs, ideas and attitudes about self, i.e. description of self) and self-efficacy (estimation of skill level in various activities, linked to motivation to participate or not to participate). There are many models of self-esteem development – it would be beneficial to familiarize oneself with those such as Harter (1983) or Coopersmith (1981). Piers-Harris Children's Self-Concept Scale (Piers and Harris, 1984) and Self- Perception Profile for Children (Harter, 1985) could be used by occupational therapists in an objective manner to evaluate global self-esteem (Willoughby et al., 1996). Always bear in mind the developmental stage of the child, when evaluating self-esteem. Occupational therapists are also reminded to listen to their clients' [children's] perceptions about what they like or don't like about themselves, not only the parents' or teacher's observations, or the results from psychometric assessments.

What the occupational therapist can do to promote Monty's self-esteem in the occupational therapy sessions

Handling principles

- Do not criticize Monty's efforts.
- Do not force him to participate by cajoling, negative statements or comparisons with others.
- Emphasize that he is doing the activity for himself and not 'for me' [the occupational therapist].

Activity and environmental requirements

Monty presents with severe gravitational insecurity and is sensitive to a variety of tactile inputs. Make sure therefore that you grade your activities appropriately and do not challenge him too much. At first, choose activities that Monty enjoys and does successfully. As his sensory processing improves, so too can the diversity and challenges on a sensory level within your treatment sessions. Always watch and respect his signals in terms of overload! Never force him to participate when it is clear that he is not able to do so.

Activities should be short and easily achievable, as he tends to give up quite quickly, exhibiting a low frustration tolerance. As this improves, so you can gradually increase the time and effort demands.

Creative activities with attractive end-products that can be taken home and shown to others are ideal, as this will help Monty receive positive affirmations. Encourage self-evaluation of tasks by reading his non-verbal cues, e.g. 'by the smile on your face it looks like you are proud with the way your picture looks'.

Monty is easily distractible by visual and auditory input. This will therefore impact on his ability to perform optimally in a task and affect his achievement. The occupational therapist must therefore ensure that the environment is free from unnecessary distraction.

Treating individually is always beneficial at first, until he shows improved competence and confidence.

Allow Monty some free exploration time in order to show the therapist (and others) what he is capable of doing. Encourage him to make choices of activities (if he can't choose without help, give him a choice between two) as this promotes confidence because he will feel as if he is in control of the situation. Furthermore, this promotes internal motivation and active participation.

Short attention span

Monty displays many of the typical characteristics looked for when evaluating the attention span of a child:

- He is restless and fidgety when seated at a desk – more so than might be expected for a child of his age.
- He finds it difficult to engage in a task requiring the sustained attention of a child his age. He tends to flit from one activity to another. Sometimes he appears aimless.
- Monty is very easily distracted by external visual and auditory stimuli, and is also subject to internal distraction by his own thoughts – often he will tell the occupational therapist about something totally unrelated to the task at hand.
- He needs instructions repeated many times and tends to struggle to follow through with them.
- Monty needs a great deal of external motivation to become involved in, and to complete, activities.

Diminished sensory modulation ability has an influence over the child's nervous system (internal environment), impacting on attention as well as on many other areas, which in turn results in maladaptive behavioural patterns (external environment) and can therefore affect the learning process (Bundy et al., 2002).

What the occupational therapist can do to facilitate improvement in Monty's attention span

Handling principles

- Facilitating an optimal arousal level for Monty will help with his attention span. This requires an in-depth understanding of, and training in, sensory integration.
- Try to gain his attention by gaining eye contact and then giving short, simple instructions. This is difficult at times as his sensory systems play a role in his avoidance of eye contact. Firm touch before giving an instruction also helps to gain attention. Again, be sensitive to his tactile defensiveness and accept that sometimes this will only serve to overload him further. Read his signals to see what will be more effective at any given time.
- It is often beneficial to acknowledge Monty's efforts to try to concentrate by giving him a tangible reward. This might be in the form of a star/sticker/stamp or allowing him to do an activity of his choice.
- Encourage and redirect his attention back to the task in a non-threatening manner. Employ reflective statements which will help him to feel understood, yet promote understanding of his difficulty (e.g. 'It looks to me like you are finding it hard to concentrate. Maybe the noise outside is bothering you').

Activity and environmental requirements

Always ensure that the activity is fun and motivating for Monty. If possible encourage him to choose the activities, as this ensures intrinsic motivation.

Initially the activities should be short and not complex. This will ensure that an activity is within his concentration span and therefore ensure completion and success. Appropriate grading of activities can then proceed as he becomes more able to attend for longer periods.

Try to ensure that the environment is free from unnecessary distraction. For Monty, try to minimize visual and auditory input in particular. This would be best achieved in an uncluttered, smaller treatment environment. Initially individual treatment sessions are vital and later, as he is able to tolerate more incoming stimuli, parallel sessions with another child and therapist would be an option. Later in therapy, cooperative sessions with another child would be beneficial. Be careful not to grade this too quickly.

Poor frustration tolerance

Monty presents with many of the typical characteristics observed in children who have poor frustration tolerance:

- He gives up easily when he experiences difficulty within an activity.
- He sometimes reacts in an aggressive way (verbal and non-verbal) when experiencing challenge/failure; or when he can't have his needs satisfied immediately.
- Monty sometimes overloads emotionally (crying, withdraws or becomes obstinate) when experiencing delayed gratification and/or challenges within an activity.

Frustration is defined as 'discontented through inability to achieve one's desires' (Concise Oxford Dictionary, 1975). According to Freud, there are two theories regarding frustration and its relation to behaviours, particularly aggressive behaviour. For our purposes, the social-learning theory, which views aggressive behaviour as a learned response, may be beneficial to facilitate an understanding of some of the behaviours which we observe in our treatment sessions. It says that cognition and vicarious learning plays a role in behavioural responses. This theory states that when a person becomes frustrated, the person will experience an unpleasant emotion, which then leads to a behavioural response. This response is determined by what the person has been exposed to, and how they have learned to cope with difficult emotions. Bandura (in Atkinson et al., 1990) explains that the chosen behaviour is usually what relieved the frustration most effectively in the past. He explains that aggressive behaviour is therefore only one of the many other behaviours the person may employ, such as seeking help, withdrawal or trying harder, etc.

What the occupational therapist can do to promote improved frustration tolerance in occupational therapy sessions

Handling principles:

- Do not allow yourself to react to the behaviour when Monty has an outburst – rather use his behaviour to cue you into the underlying emotion that is causing the outburst. This will allow you to remain calm and help him gain insight into why he is behaving in such a way. (It also facilitates your clinical reasoning and ensures you are reading the childs signal's appropriately.) Remember to use reflective statements, which are non-threatening and non-judgemental.
- By reading his signals and understanding the underlying neurological components (sensory impact), which influence emotion and behaviour, you will often be able to anticipate his reactions and be able to stop them before they occur.
- Ensure the safety of Monty, yourself and anyone else in the treatment room. If he is unable to gain control over his emotions and they continue to escalate (which often happened), remove him from the therapy room. Take him into a small, quiet, contained environment, which contains sensory inputs to contain and calm a child, e.g. spandex hammocks, soft music, big beanbags and blankets, other sensory inputs such as vibration; or use specific calming techniques such as the Willbarger Brushing and Joint Compression (Willbarger in Bundy et al., 2002). Make sure that you are sufficiently qualified to use and administer this kind of input.

Activity and environmental requirements

- Ensure that the activity requirements are not too high – Monty initially needs to achieve success.
- The duration of activities is important for him as he has a short attention span and he finds it difficult to wait for a delayed outcome. Initially, short one-step activities with quickly achieved end products are necessary. Thereafter, as his attention and frustration tolerance improves, more steps can be added, making the activity longer and more complex.
- Ensure that the environment is safe from unnecessary hazards.

Now that we have a better understanding of Monty's emotional difficulties and we have a better idea of what some of the underlying causes are and how to deal with them, it is important to address his motor and perceptual difficulties.

Motor development

Learning is multi-sensory process, which according to Ayres (1981) involves the organization of sensation for use, by giving them [the sensations] meaning. This process is known as sensory integration. The first seven years of life are known as the sensory-motor developmental years, as the brain is primarily interested in receiving and responding to incoming sensations by moving the body in relation to those incoming sensations. Children do not develop abstract thought or reasoning until they are about 7 or 8 years of age and this sensory-motor stage of development lays the 'concrete knowledge' about self and the child's environment, which forms the foundations for later 'intellectual, social and personal development' (Piaget in Ayres, 1981, p. 24). It is believed that if the sensory-motor processes are well organized and integrated, later learning will be easier. Children naturally seek out information from the environment, and if it is a fun, satisfying experience, will continue to do so, thus facilitating their own ability to integrate incoming sensations in an orderly manner. Sometimes this process is interrupted, which will influence the child's development in numerous ways, impacting on his/her ability to perform optimally in the necessary occupational performance spheres. When this occurs, a child is referred to occupational therapy.

What factors could be influencing Monty's motor development?

The occupational therapist must consider the **underlying reasons** for the presenting problems. A bottom-up approach is therefore used. Appropriate activities can then be incorporated into therapy sessions. It is important to realize this, as the occupational therapist wants to improve the child's underlying components necessary for skill development, and not teach the child how to do specific tasks, i.e. development of splinter skills.

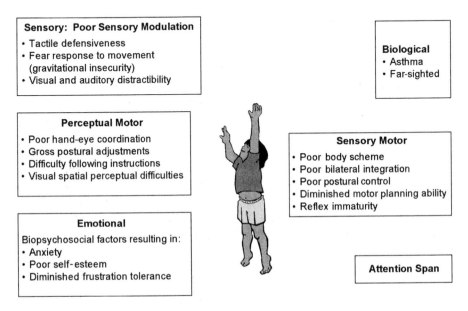

Sensory: Poor Sensory Modulation
- Tactile defensiveness
- Fear response to movement (gravitational insecurity)
- Visual and auditory distractibility

Biological
- Asthma
- Far-sighted

Perceptual Motor
- Poor hand-eye coordination
- Gross postural adjustments
- Difficulty following instructions
- Visual spatial perceptual difficulties

Sensory Motor
- Poor body scheme
- Poor bilateral integration
- Poor postural control
- Diminished motor planning ability
- Reflex immaturity

Emotional
Biopsychosocial factors resulting in:
- Anxiety
- Poor self-esteem
- Diminished frustration tolerance

Attention Span

Figure 15.4 Factors influencing motor development.

Facilitate the child's understanding (in simple language) of why you are doing certain activities and what area they are working on, e.g. 'this game makes your tummy muscles strong, so you won't get so tired when you are sitting at the table doing work'. This incorporated cognitive approach works particularly well with older children and allows them to feel a sense of control, facilitating motivation.

If treatment for Monty's motor development is to be effective, the therapist will have to address his sensory modulation difficulties and facilitate his emotional development.

In occupational therapy, each area will need to be addressed using age-appropriate activities and relevant occupational therapy treatment principles to foster the development of his sensory-motor and perceptual motor components.

Children consolidate what they learn through practice, so allow for this in your therapy sessions and grade appropriately to promote further development for more complex skills.

Perceptual development

Traditionally perceptual development, particularly the development of visual perceptual skills, was often considered by occupational therapists (and other disciplines) as an indicator of academic learning potential. If a visual perceptual difficulty was identified, copious pencil-and-paper exercises were given to the child, or many other table-top activities such as puzzles were done. This promoted the development of isolated skills. It did not, however, encompass the general development of visual skills, which are needed for complex activities such as reading. It is important for the inexperienced therapist to realize that using this method alone to treat visual perceptual deficits is outdated. Based on the work by Jean Ayres and the development of sensory integration, therapists now employ a bottom-up approach to visual perceptual development. The integration of incoming sensory information from the environment and sensory-motor development is a foundation for the development of visual perceptual skills (Ayres, 1981) (see Figure 15.4). Once these underlying areas have been treated and the child is able to sufficiently organize incoming sensory information (i.e. visual sensory processing has been addressed) it may then be appropriate to incorporate desk-top, puzzle-type activities and pencil-and-paper activities to further promote visual perception. If the child's problems in this area persist, referral to a specialized optometrist to develop the eye muscles may be beneficial. This bottom-up approach facilitates academic learning.

What factors could be influencing Monty's perceptual development?

- Once again the occupational therapist must take into consideration the underlying reasons for Monty's presenting problems. This will allow

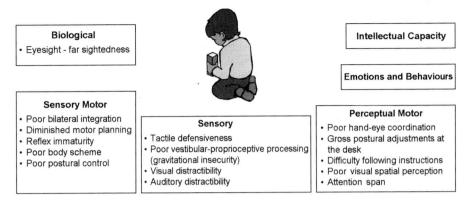

Figure 15.5 Factors influencing perceptual development.

her to choose appropriate activities to stimulate and develop general visual sensory processing.
- Always use a kinesthetic approach first, i.e. incorporate whole body movements, use touch and various tactile modalities, auditory input such as tapping, clapping, rhyming and visual feedback such as mirrors, etc.
- Next move on to three-dimensional (3D) activities, i.e. gross motor activities, games.
- Lastly incorporate two-dimensional (2D) activities, i.e. classic pencil-and-paper activities.

    Remember some factors, such as Monty's eyesight (he is far-sighted) and intellectual capability may have a 'top-down' effect on his abilities in this sphere. This may restrict his development in this area, and the development of his underlying areas of difficulty will have to be understood within these parameters. At this stage his intellectual capacity is not known, but it is something to consider in the future should this turn out to be an area of difficulty. Also, his far-sightedness is now being remediated by wearing glasses, however for a crucial period (first three years of his life), when a great deal of development was occurring in the underlying areas, this was not known and would have impacted on his visual sensory processing.
- Also remember that at any given stage Monty's sensory modulation difficulty can impact on his arousal level, emotional regulation and subsequent behavioural outcomes. This can have a top-down effect and will influence his ability in this regard. If the therapist is aware of this, she will read his signals appropriately and his performance will be attributed to his arousal level and not his actual capability!

Conclusion

The author has emphasized and created an understanding of the underlying components, which influence the emotional, motor and perceptual development in a child, and how they are interrelated. It can be seen that the child forms part of a complex system and a multidisciplinary and holistic approach is therefore vital to occupational therapy outcomes. The trend today is towards early identification and intervention, which allows optimal timing for intervention to occur, in order to circumvent some of the difficulties the child may face in later life.

Questions

1. What must the occupational therapist employ at all times when working with children to ensure optimal outcomes of treatment sessions? Discuss this process briefly to show your understanding.
2. How does this impact on the occupational therapist's handling of the child within treatment sessions?
3. What do we hope to gather from assessing a child? What do you need to remember when entering this assessment process?
4. What is the single most important thing to convey to the parents, and why?
5. Why work within a model, framework or use a specific approach when treating children?
6. Catherine, a little girl of five, enters your assessment room clinging to her mother. She avoids all eye contact with you and makes no spontaneous conversation. Her eyes appear to be constantly brimming with tears and she looks to her mother for constant reassurance. She appears 'immobilized' and distracted. You start a formalized assessment, but you can see that she is struggling.

   a) Do you continue with the assessment?
   b) If not, what would you do?
   c) Looking at her behaviours, what underlying emotions could you assume were present?

7. Storm, an eight-year-old boy, arrives at your occupational therapy rooms. He is shouting at his mother as they enter and he slams the door shut behind him, kicking the plant at the door as he passes. His eyes are sunken, his cheeks are red and his brows are knitted together. His mother raises her eyes and leaves hastily, without a backward glance. All your efforts to engage him in an activity are thwarted and he starts to become abusive and aggressive.

   a) What underlying factors could be influencing his behaviour?
   b) How would you deal with these difficult behaviours in order to engage him in your therapy session?

8. Why should you incorporate choices into your occupational therapy sessions, and when can they be counterproductive?
9. If a child were to be referred for visual perceptual difficulties, poor pencil grip or inattention in class, would you merely assess these areas of deficit? What else would you incorporate into your assessment and why? Explain this process to show your understanding of a 'bottom-up' approach.

Chapter 16
Sensory integration in mental retardation and pervasive developmental disorders

ANNAMARIE VAN JAARSVELD

The role of sensory integration in the functioning of an adult or child can no longer be ignored. Between the late 1960s and the 1980s, A.J. Ayres did groundbreaking work in researching, defining, describing and developing the theory and practice of sensory integration. Initially Ayres focused her research on sensory integration as a dysfunction, especially in children with learning and behaviour problems, and on the role of motor control and visual perception on learning. Her research also included other sensory systems, namely the vestibular, proprioceptive and tactile systems and the impact that these systems had on a child's ability to learn. Standardized tests were developed to measure these sensory systems. She also developed clinical observations that evaluate neuromotor maturation, including observations of muscle tone, primitive postural reflexes, postural control, eye movements, balance and gravitational security. Through these standardized tests and observations Ayres was able to identify dysfunctions in the sensory processing of the vestibular, proprioceptive, tactile and visual systems that interfere with motor functioning, cognition, language, behaviour and emotional wellbeing (Ayres, 1983).

Today there is no doubt about the importance of sensory integration in normal, everyday function. If an individual does not have normal integration of the different senses he/she will experience difficulties in making adaptive responses to the challenges presented not only by the individual's own body but also those in the environment. This does not only have an effect on activity performance but also on the individual's occupations and in the long run on health. Bundy et al. (2002) and Smith Roley et al. (2001) state in no uncertain terms that sensory integration is the foundation for occupation.

It is a fact that pathology can interfere with the process of integrating sensory information. If sensory information cannot be integrated or is integrated in a dysfunctional way, it will contribute to the way the individual makes sense of their world and this could often be disorganizing, as seen in children with mental retardation and even more so in children with pervasive developmental disorders (PDD). It is a known fact and stated in literature (Ayres, 1979; Kaplan and Sadock, 1998; Murray-Slutsky and Paris, 2000) that children diagnosed with both the above-mentioned conditions experience difficulty with making adaptive responses. The ability to make adaptive responses relies heavily on sensory integration (see spiral process of self-actualization) (Fisher et al., 1991).

Occupational therapists in South Africa who wish to use sensory integration in treatment will be introduced to the techniques at an undergraduate level, but require specialized postgraduate training to become expert at the techniques.

Sensory integration as a model

Kielhofner (1997, p. 197) states: 'sensory integration is clearly the most researched conceptual model of practice'. It not only has a very well-described theoretical basis but also thoroughly developed assessment and intervention procedures. This model is underpinned by neuroscience, and because of the rapid growth of neuroscience the model and the strong research efforts surrounding it have undergone a great deal of change. This is likely to continue to be the case.

Understanding the organization and functioning of the brain is central to this model. The theory of sensory integration is based on several assumptions:

1. Neural plasticity: The brain has the ability to change or to modify.
2. Developmental sequence: Sensory integrative capacities take place in a developmental sequence and this sequence unfolds as a result of the interaction between brain maturation and accumulating sensory experiences.
3. Integrated brain function: One part of the brain is dependent on other parts of the brain for effective function.
4. Brain organization and adaptive behaviour: The fact that the brain is an organized system allows for adaptive behaviour (which involves processing of sensory information), and adaptive behaviour impacts brain organization (see section on spiral process of sensory integration, below).
5. Inner drive: Individuals have an inner drive to participate in sensory-motor activities that supports the sensory integrative process (see section on spiral process, below).

The need for integrated sensations

Ayres (1983) has described sensations as food that nourishes the brain. Sensory integration theory states that the tactile/proprioceptive and vestibular/proprioceptive systems are in continual interaction with the visual and auditory systems to provide multimodal sensory information that is needed to make meaningful motor responses (Smith Roley et al., 2001). If the environment, or pathology, causes deprivation of sensory nourishment or integration thereof, it will leave the individual deficient in the integrated sensations which will lead to dysfunctional participation in activities of daily living.

Spiral process of sensory integration

A model of the spiral process of sensory integration that emphasized self-actualization was proposed by Fisher and Murray (Fisher et al., 1991). This model proposes that 'inner drive provides the impetus to become involved in meaningful activities that are the source of sensation' (Bundy et al., 2002, p.14). The participation in meaningful activity is central in this model. An activity, according to Fisher and Bundy, is meaningful when the individual is in control and able to make sense of the experience. Sensory intake is one of the first steps in the process of sensory integration. Integrated sensations are critical in making adaptive responses. Adaptive responses are the ability of the individual to process sensations, organize and integrate them to form a meaningful outcome (Ayres, 1979).

When sensations are integrated it gives rise to the planning of an adaptive response/interaction that is appropriate to the initial demand that was made from the environment. Once the adaptive response is planned, the response (behaviours that can be observed, evaluated and changed) takes place. Adaptive responses then give rise to outcome feedback. Outcome feedback arises from the body and informs the individual about how it felt to make an adaptive response; in other words, whether it was successful or not. Bundy et al. (2002, p. 14) sum it up by saying, 'planning an adaptive interaction means knowing "what to do" and organizing "how to do it"'.

Every time a successful adaptive response is made, a neuronal model of an action is developed and is stored in the brain. It can now be used to plan new and more complex responses.

Within this model the core assumption of occupational therapy is also reflected, namely that humans have an occupational nature and adaptive responses are the basis of occupational behaviour. Within this core assumption two other core assumptions of occupational science are also reflected, first that 'humans have an innate need to participate in occupation and that is intrinsically motivating and secondly that humans develop meaning, satisfaction, confidence, self-control and a sense of mastery from participating in occupation' (Bundy et al., 2002, p. 14). Planning, organizing and executing adaptive responses includes both sensation and volitional components. Successful adaptive responses lead the individual to experience a sense of mastery and belief in their own abilities. This in turn enables the individual to become self-directed and more involved in participation in meaningful occupation. It is thus hypothesized by Fisher and Murray 'that the spiralling process of self-actualisation, sensory integration, and adaptive interactions leads to organised and effective occupational behaviour (e.g. self-care, self-management, play, academic performance)' (Bundy et al., 2002, p.16).

Sensory integration and the developing child

A child learns through play. Play is the main occupation of a child. During play children will seek opportunities to take in tactile, vestibular and proprioceptive stimulation (Smith Roley et al., 2001). The multisensory nature of play provides the child with necessary building blocks that contribute to development. Play is thus a critical component in development.

Normal children have an innate drive to take part in play activities that provide their own optimal sensory environment. Children who, because of pathology, do not use play activities optimally are deprived for various reasons (e.g. lack of inner drive, poor sensory integration) of 'balanced sensory nourishment'. This in turn can lead to developmental obstructions, which can vary in nature and intensity. If a child cannot play in a meaningful and purposeful way, it will affect the child's self-actualization process and in the end the child's occupations.

Dysfunctions in sensory integration

Dysfunctions are described mainly according to Bundy et al. (2002) unless otherwise indicated.

Sensory modulation disorders

Sensory modulation abilities within the framework of sensory integration are described as

> the capacity to regulate and organize the degree, intensity and nature of responses to sensory input in a graded and adaptive manner. This allows the individual to achieve and maintain an optimal range of performance to challenges in daily life (Smith Roley et al., 2001, p. 57).

Sensory modulation dysfunction (SMD) can be defined as a problem in regulating and organizing the degree, intensity and nature of responses to sensory input in a graded manner. SMD decreases the individual's ability to achieve and maintain an optimal range of performances, as well as the ability of the individual to adapt to challenges in daily life.

Children with SMD demonstrate hyper-responsivity, hypo-responsivity, or lability in response to sensory stimuli. These problems with responsivity directly influence their level of arousal, which is detrimental to the readiness of a child in becoming involved in any activity. They can also display unusual patterns of sensory seeking or avoiding. Emotions that children with SMD have to deal with include anxiety, lability, fear, aggression, depression and hostility. Attention problems are common with these children due to hyperactivity or hypo-activity. Functional performance is also restricted, e.g. they have problems with activities such as dressing, eating, bathing and socializing. Their play activities are also negatively influenced (Smith Roley et al., 2001). It is clear that children with SMD are not only restricted in terms of sensations, but also in terms of attention, emotions and activities of daily living.

SMD can manifest in several different ways and four types of modulation disorders are included in sensory integration theory:

1. Sensory defensiveness (including tactile defensiveness)

This type of defensiveness is often linked to poor limbic or reticular processing as a fight-or-flight reaction that is elicited by sensation that others would consider non-noxious.

Sensory defensiveness is usually a dysfunction in the anterolateral system, which is responsible for the mediation of pain, crude touch, light touch and temperature. Most of the fibres of the anterolateral system terminate in the reticular formation (responsible for arousal, emotional tone and autonomic regulation). Projections are sent from there to the thalamus (integrating centre that coordinates information and relays it to the cortex) and the limbic system (sets the tone for emotional and motivational aspects of behaviour and attention). This system is thus associated with many aspects of touch, arousal, emotional tone, attention and autonomic regulation. It is important to note that defensiveness can occur in all sensory systems and that sensory defensiveness is an over-reponse to sensory stimulation.

Emotions that these children exhibit include anxiety, fear and aggression. In particular they have problems with attention in terms of hyperactivity, distractibility, impulsiveness and hostility. They will avoid activities that will expose them to the sensation to which they are defensive.

2. Gravitational insecurity

Here the reaction is also out of proportion to the stimulus, which could vary from just being out of the upright position, fear of certain movements, or having one's feet off the ground. This insecurity is associated with poor otolithic processing.

Their emotions are also very much involved in that they can become extremely fearful when they have to take part in activities that require gravitational security. If they are fearful and anxious it will also influence their attention and the way they will partake in an activity.

3. Aversive response to movement

Rather than otolithic processing, aversive responses are thought to reflect poor processing of semicircular canal-mediated information. Aversive response to movement that most individuals would consider non-noxious is a characteristic of this disorder. Movement elicits autonomic nervous system reactions.

Because of the fact that unfamiliar movements elicit an autonomic nervous system reaction, these children tend to be fearful and can become aggressive when they are exposed to movements that are unfamiliar to them or make them feel uncomfortable. They tend to be very uncertain of themselves.

4. Under-responsiveness

Each of the already mentioned SMD involves an over-reaction to sensations but there are some individuals who are under-responsive to sensation. It seems as if they do not notice sensation or their response is far less than expected. A delayed reaction to sensation may also be implicated within this disorder. Under-responsiveness to sensation can occur in all sensory systems.

These children can appear to be lethargic and are slow to warm up. It seems as if the world is passing by without them noticing (as if they are living in their own world). Their attention levels are also implicated in that it is not easy to get their attention and a lot of input is needed to keep their attention.

It is important to note that children may demonstrate a fluctuating defensive response within a particular system.

Practic dysfunctions

Praxis, according to sensory integration theory, refers to the ability to plan new movements. There are two different types of practic dysfunctions: bilateral integration and sequencing (BIS) dyspraxia and somatodyspraxia. BIS deficits are associated with vestibular and proprioceptive processing, whilst somatodyspraxia is associated with tactile, vestibular and proprioceptive processing.

Dyspractic children are clumsy, may need more help than their peers, their speech development can be delayed, they will use additional visual or other cognitive clues to be successful in the execution of an activity and they experience problems with getting themselves organized.

Postural deficits

It is assumed that posture is the outward manifestation of vestibular and proprioceptive processing and although a postural deficit on its own is not a practic disorder, it reflects the basis for deficits in BIS and sometimes for somatodyspraxia. Relevant postural indicators to include in assessment and observation are:

- extensor muscle tone (observed in a standing position)
- prone extension
- proximal stability

- ability to move neck into flexion against gravity (part of supine flexion)
- equilibrium
- post-rotary nystagmus reactions (often part of this group of indicators, in which case the cluster may be called 'postural ocular').

Children with postural deficits will have problems with postural control and stability. They will have problems with maintaining postures (e.g. they will lean on their arms whilst working at a table, curl their legs and feet around chair legs, or assume a 'lying' position in a chair). They need assistance from their environment to help them with postural demands.

Deficits in tactile discrimination

Tactile discrimination deficits are assumed to be an outward manifestation of tactile processing and thought to be a basis for somatodyspraxia.

These children usually have problems with body scheme, gross and fine motor skills, oral control and motor planning. They may appear clumsy in performing motor skills, be accident-prone, mouth objects or drool, and depend on using their vision for successful completion of tasks. Behaviour can vary from controlling and demanding to showing no interest (in a shut-down mode in the sense that their nervous systems can not handle any more sensory input). Emotions that they have to deal with include frustration, aggression or in the latter case, apathy. Cognitive problems such as perceptual and academic problems can also be a direct result of this disorder.

Somatodyspraxia

Individuals with somatodyspraxia have difficulty with the whole spectrum of gross motor tasks. That means that they have difficulty with both feedback (from their own body and the environment after the action was completed, e.g. was it successful/unsuccessful) and feedforward-dependent motor actions (before the action is carried out they need information from their nervous system on the 'how' of the actions; for example in an action like catching a ball, the individual needs to get his/her limbs to a particular place in time to act). Any activity that depends on sound somato-sensory feedback will provide problems for them (e.g. identifying shapes by touch, without seeing them). Fine motor tasks are often also involved.

This type of dyspraxia is more severe than BIS dyspraxia. For a diagnosis of somatodyspraxia to be made the individual must have deficits in somatosensory processing.

Deficits in bilateral integration and sequencing

Individuals with BIS dyspraxia experience difficulties in using the two sides of the body in a coordinated manner and also have difficulties with the sequencing of motor actions, and specifically anticipatory projected movements which are very much feedforward dependent. As already mentioned the vestibular and proprioceptive systems are the basis for adequate BIS actions and as can be expected, the visual system also plays an important role in guiding of movements.

Except for the fact that these children also experience the same problems as the somatodyspractic children (excluding the somato-sensory problems) they can also experience problems in using the two sides of their bodies in a coordinated way, crossing their midline and establishing a skilled dominant side. They will avoid any unfamiliar activities and thus have a limited range of activities in which they partake. They also suffer emotionally and, because of their inability to experience success, they usually have a very low self-esteem and their motivation is low.

Postural-ocular movement disorder

A postural-ocular disorder is described in the literature as the behavioural manifestation of a vestibular-proprioceptive processing disorder and is hypothesized to be the basis for the BIS disorder (Fisher et al., 1991). Poor processing of vestibular-proprioceptive input is believed to hamper the development of posture and ocular control.

These children will experience problems with posture-related demands, e.g. righting and equilibrium reactions, flexion and extension postures, postural stability, and lateral flexion and rotation. In terms of ocular control they will experience problems with activities, e.g. where they have to follow an object with their eyes, visually fixate and dissociate eye from head movements. Their form and space perception, as well as eye–hand coordination, will be poor.

Mental retardation

The Diagnostic and Statistical Manual of Mental Disorders (DSM-IV-TR™ (2000)) defines mental retardation as 'significantly sub-average general intellectual functioning with an onset before the age of 18' (Kaplan and Sadock, 1998, p. 1137). Although intellectual functioning is sub-average it is also accompanied by impaired adaptive skills and possible physical disabilities.

Adaptive skills for daily functioning are those daily living skills needed to live, work and play in the community. Included are self-care, home-living, social skills, leisure, health and safety, self-direction, functional academics (reading, writing, basic maths) and community use and work (see www.thearc.org/faqs/mrqa.html for more details). Thus it is very important for the mentally retarded child that the family accept the child as he/she is, and to encourage the development of adaptive skills. The family needs to overcome the stigma of mental retardation, and create an environment conducive to the child's maximal development in daily functioning. The family members need to be supported to overcome the denial, guilt, shame or ambivalence towards the child relating to the stigma of mental retardation. Support groups for the parents in the community can be formed for this purpose.

The tenth revision of International Classification of Diseases and Related Health Problems (ICD-10) views mental retardation as a condition of 'arrested or incomplete development of the mind characterised by impaired developmental skills that contribute to the overall level of intelligence' (Kaplan and Sadock, 1998, p. 1137). It is also stated that adaptive behaviour is almost always impaired.

Both the above-mentioned classifications allow for categories that specify the extent of the impairments. Different terms are also used for this condition, such as 'intellectual disability', 'mental handicap', and 'mentally challenged'.

Developmental characteristics vary depending on the degree of mental retardation. In profound cases some motor development is present and they may respond minimally to limited training in self-help, during school age (6–20 years old). In severe cases they can talk or learn to communicate, be trained in elementary health habits and profit from systematic habit training. In moderate cases they can profit from training in social and occupational skills but are unlikely to progress beyond second grade academically. In mild cases they can learn academic skills up to approximately sixth grade by their late teens and can be guided towards social conformity (US Department of Health, Education and Welfare, 1989).

Other features that were identified by surveys according to Kaplan and Sadock (1998) include a greater frequency of several clinical features than in the normal population. They include hyperactivity, low frustration tolerance, aggression, affective instability, repetitive, stereotypic motor behaviours and various self-injurious behaviours. In terms of psychosocial factors a negative self-image and poor self-esteem are common features of mildly and moderately mentally retarded people. They are well aware of being different and experience repeated failure and disappointment in not meeting expectations.

Taking the above into account it is clear that the mentally retarded person should be exposed to a setting which includes a comprehensive programme that addresses adaptive skills training, social skills training, and vocational training (Kaplan and Sadock, 1998). Their sensory integration enables them to make sense of the world around them from a physical and psychological perspective, so normalizing their adaptive responses encourages development. They have a right to quality of life!

Pervasive developmental disorders

Recent literature describes pervasive developmental disorders (PDD) as a Spectrum Disorder (Murray-Slutsky and Paris, 2000; Smith Roley et al.,

2001), because of its varying degree of symptoms. According to the DSM-IV-TR™ (American Psychiatric Association, 2000), PDD disorders 'include a group of psychiatric conditions in which there is an impairment in reciprocal social skills, language development, and a range of behavioural repertoire' (Kaplan and Sadock 1998, p. 1179).

The ICD-10 states 'these disorders are characterised by qualitative abnormalities in reciprocal social interactions and in patterns of communications, and by restricted stereotyped, repetitive repertoire of interests and activities' (Kaplan and Sadock 1998, p. 1179). It is important to mention that a high percentage of these spectrum disorder children are also mentally retarded, although mental retardation is not required for the diagnosis.

Disorders that are included in the PDD spectrum of disorders include Autism, Rett's Disorder, Childhood Disintegrative Disorder (Heller's Syndrome), Asperger's Syndrome, Schizophrenia and Pervasive Developmental Disorder not otherwise specified (Kaplan and Sadock, 1998). Murray-Slutsky and Paris (2000) also include within this spectrum other disorders with autistic-like symptoms. They are Fragile-X Syndrome (Martin-Bell Syndrome), Landau-Kleffner Syndrome, Mobius Syndrome, Sotos Syndrome (Cerebral Gigantism), Tourette Syndrome and Williams Syndrome. What is significant in children with a PDD spectrum disorder is their marked lack of ability to make adaptive responses.

The role of sensory integration in the above pathologies

The fact that literature and practical experience both support the observation that children with mental retardation and PDD spectrum disorders have difficulties in making adaptive responses justifies the use of a sensory integration model in the intervention of these children.

Adaptive responses can be on various levels, which include motor and behavioural responses. Adaptive responses in terms of sensory integration therapy will be mainly motor responses but when therapy is successful it will impact on behavioural responses as well. A child who can make sense of his sensory world will be able to cope better with the demands of the environment, and a child who can cope with the demands of his environment has a better chance of being adaptable, balanced and well functioning.

Sensory integration and mental retardation

Although there are conflicting opinions in the literature on the use of sensory integration with children with mental retardation, the author is of the opinion that if you are a trained sensory integration occupational therapist and you withhold sensory integration treatment from them, you are doing them an injustice. There are more than enough functional problems to indicate that most of these children experience sensory integration dysfunctions. Clinical reasoning further supports the use of sensory integration as a model of practice. Mentally retarded children do not have the cognitive abilities to use their environment and the objects in their environment to their full potential. Their motor and dispositional abilities are also affected by the fact that they are mentally retarded and that will further limit their participation and effective use of their environment. A child's development is dependent on many important experiences and one of these experiences is sensory, especially touch and movement. If a child is deprived of these because of cognitive, motor and dispositional restrictions, then there is no reason why they could not be provided to them through a therapeutic environment.

Sensory integration and the PDD spectrum

Ayres and Tickle (1980) described sensory dysfunctions accompanying autistic disorders in terms of both sensory-seeking and sensory-avoiding behaviour, e.g. in terms of movement autistic children would often involve themselves in rocking or rhythmic motions (considered to be calming or organizing) or twirling and swinging motions (considered to be alerting and activating). Ayres also stated that the objective of sensory integration therapy for the autistic child is to improve sensory processing to enhance registration and modulation of sensations so that the child will be able to form simple adaptive responses as a means of helping the child to learn and organize their behaviour.

According to Smith Roley et al. (2001, p. 366) recent research done by Kemper and Bauman on autistic children has 'found consistent abnormalities in the number and size of cells within the limbic systems, particularly in the amygdala and hypocampus'. Aspects of emotions and behaviour are controlled by the amygdala whilst the hippocampus plays an important role in learning and memory. Autopsy studies on individuals with autistic disorder by the same researchers have demonstrated cerebellum abnormalities. It is postulated by them that cerebellar abnormalities have an effect on the modulation of emotions, mental imagery, anticipatory planning, aspects of attention as well as aspects of language processing. Damage to the posterior inferior region of the cerebellum was also demonstrated in these studies and this has implications for the function of the vestibular system, as there are direct connections between this part of the brain and the vestibular system. The inhibitory role of the cerebellum on brainstem structures is specifically implicated.

In a study on sensory modulation done by Miller, Reisman, McIntosh and Simon (Smith Roley et al., 2001) on children with different diagnoses, it was found that children with Autistic and Fragile-X Syndromes had impaired sensation. Although the characteristics of the impairments did vary between the two groups there was no doubt that their modulation of sensation was impaired.

In a study done by Parham et al. (2000) on high-functioning autistic children, it was found that they tested significantly low on all tests for praxis, as well as poor tactile, vestibular and proprioceptive sensory processing compared to children in the normative developmental range.

From the above-mentioned studies it is clear that there are sufficient indications of sensory integration disorders within these children. They have dysfunctions that are part of the neural substrates for sensory perception, attachment of meaning, drive, and initiation of purposeful action and are likely to demonstrate diminished inner drive for purposeful interaction, limited ideation, and impaired planning and participation in a new or novel activity (Smith Roley et al., 2001). These authors also state that the intervention process should start by establishing a means for engaging the child in activity, in which meaningful sensory experiences is orchestrated.

Children with mental retardation and PDD are, because of their pathology, restricted in functioning. Although sensory integration disorders may only be a small part of the full picture, these children also have the right to make sense of their world to the best of their abilities, and providing them with sensory integration therapy will help them do so.

Assessment

Formal sensory integration assessment of children with mental retardation and PDD is limited, depending on the severity of the condition. The occupational therapist often has to rely on a sensory history, sensory checklists (of which there are several available) and collateral information. Probably the most important form of assessment of these children is observations. Because the children have limited resources they will provide themselves with the sensory stimulation that is organizing for them (although often in an unacceptable way), or they will avoid sensory stimulation that disorganizes them. Thus, analysing these children's sensory processing, their sensory registration and their planning abilities will give a wealth of information on the status of their sensory integration. If all the above-mentioned information is plotted onto a sensory integration worksheet it will not only be possible to make a diagnosis of the type of sensory integration dysfunction of a specific child but it will also help to direct treatment.

Each child will be evaluated individually and a treatment programme will then be planned to address the child's underlying problems. Constant reassessment and modification of the programme, based on the child's response, is essential.

Intervention

For the purposes of this chapter it is appropriate to discuss a few distinct problems of children with mental retardation and PDD that could be addressed through the use of sensory integration. The discussion of the intervention cannot take place without the acknowledgement of the work done by Murray-Slutsky, Paris and Smith Roley.

Sensory modulation dysfunction (SMD)

Intervention will depend on the type of SMD that the child is experiencing and the state of the child's arousal levels. The ultimate state is that of calm-alert, but we often see that these children are either under-aroused or over-aroused, or are fluctuating between these two levels. For planning intervention the occupational therapist also needs to know whether the child is experiencing problems with arousal/attention, sensory registration or orientation and in which sensory system is the problem (problems could be in one or more of the sensory systems). With the autistic child you will also need to know whether problems occur in a specific environment or at a certain time of day.

With all these questions answered intervention can be planned.

Over-aroused children

Such children are overexcited, anxious and hyperactive and may also be defensive to certain forms of sensory stimulation. Because of this state of over-arousal their nervous systems are not able to filter out important from the non-important sensory stimulation, and information processing is poor. They appear to be out of control and in constant non-functional motion. The aim is to get them from this over-aroused state into a calm-alert state and therefore inhibitory techniques should be used. Activities that include deep-touch and proprioception as well as resistance are the best to use. Activities should be slow, repetitive, rhythmic and provide neutral warmth.

Examples of such activities are: leopard crawling on a carpeted floor, wheelbarrow walking and making a 'hot-dog' by rolling the child in a blanket and applying deep pressure.

Over-aroused children need to organize themselves again and often they benefit from having a small enclosed area (e.g. play tent) where stimuli are decreased and they have control over them. They often enjoy having soft, heavy objects like blankets and cushions available in this enclosed space. They should have the freedom to go in there and stay there as long as is needed to organize their nervous system.

Over-aroused children may also go into a state of shutdown and the occupational therapist must be very aware of this state because it seems as if they are under-aroused but their nervous system is just not able to cope with any more sensory input. If the occupational therapist reads this state incorrectly she will start using arousal techniques and this will be the last thing the child needs. In doing so she will only disorganize the child further. She needs to also use inhibitory techniques to get the child into a calm-alert state again.

The therapeutic environment should be well organized and stimulus-free as far as possible. Lighting should be low and noise levels must be as low as possible. The occupational therapist can use herself in a therapeutic way by talking in a soft, monotonous voice, and she should behave in a calm and peaceful way.

Under-aroused children

These children have difficulty with either the registration or processing of sensory information and they need to be brought into the calm-alert state. They will benefit from activities that arouse the nervous system. Fast, repetitive movements that have a stronger impact on the nervous system are effective. Linear vestibular movements combined with deep touch and proprioception help to arouse the nervous system. Movements that are irregular, jerky and fast can also have an arousing effect but should be used with care because these movements could also be disorganizing.

Examples of activities:

- scooterboard activities
- linear swinging in a hammock
- bouncing on a therapy ball
- jumping on a trampoline.

When exposing under-aroused children to activities they should be carefully observed for their reactions. Facial expression is always one of the best indicators of whether a sensory experience is having the desired effect – look for increased responsiveness and processing of sensory information.

The therapeutic environment should be bright and colourful. The occupational therapist can also use herself in a therapeutic way by talking in a louder voice, being energetic and making use of gestures and animation; in other words, there should be 'energy' in the environment as well.

Children who fluctuate between arousal states or who have defensive disorders

These children are often difficult to identify and to treat. Intervention strategies should therefore be selected very carefully. One fact that must always be remembered is that these children's nervous systems are unstable and will be very sensitive to sensory input. Within minutes they can fluctuate between over-arousal and under-arousal. To get these children into a calm-alert state the occupational therapist needs to know their defensive behaviours and exactly how they respond to certain types of stimulation. These children are usually highly emotional and their high anxiety levels should also be addressed. Activities that are threatening to them or cause them to fluctuate between arousal levels should be avoided.

Examples of activities:

1. Children who have difficulty with integrating/processing tactile sensations:
   - Use deep pressure activities first, e.g. firm stroking.
   - Do resistive activities that provide deep proprioceptive input e.g. tug-of-war.
2. Children who are gravitationally insecure:
   - Use deep pressure activities as well as deep proprioceptive input.

- When lifting the child off the ground, keep his body close to your body while providing deep touch input.
- During activity, verbalize what is going to happen so that the child can mentally prepare himself.

Always remember that what is calming and organizing for these children at one moment can be disorganizing the next moment, so the occupational therapist must be prepared to adapt or modify activities, the environment and the way that she uses herself in therapy. It is important to use clinical reasoning skills continually with these children.

Tactile discrimination disorders

Because the dorsal column medial lemniscal system (DCMLS) is mainly responsible for tactile discrimination the occupational therapist must work through this system, providing enhanced sensory input. Stimulation of the tactile, vibratory, touch pressure and proprioceptive receptors should be included in activities to result in improved discriminatory skills. Vestibular activities must be mainly linear as this is the type of vestibular stimulation that is processed by the DCMLS.

Examples of activities:

- Swinging in a hammock: Child in prone position in the hammock and while the child is swinging in a linear plane, he/she can be asked to throw heavy bean bags at a target, depending on the child's ability.
- Jumping on a trampoline (child must have the necessary postural control).
- Crawling through a tunnel made of stretchable material to provide deep touch and heavy proprioceptive input. The child can also be asked to push a therapy ball through the tunnel.
- Scooterboard activities, where either a rope or hula-hoop is used onto which the child must hold on and sustain a flexed posture.

Although the DCMLS is involved in the processing of tactile and vestibular input, it is also involved with selective attention, orientation and anticipation, the programming and execution of movement sequences, skilled manual dexterity and the manipulation of objects in space (Fisher et al., 1991).

Problems with body scheme, gross and fine motor control as well as oral motor control will also be addressed through sensory integration therapy depending on the occurrence and severity of the problems.

Practic dysfunctions

Praxis requires the ability to: 1) Conceptualize a plan. Sensory registration and the ability of the child to get into a calm-alert state of arousal plays an important role here. 2) Plan, sequence and organize the sensory information. This requires sensory integration in terms of planning and sequencing, body scheme, development of normal neuronal models (memories of movements), feedback and feedforward. 3) Carry out the sequence. Here active participation is needed to make the necessary adaptive response.

Intervention will start with the conceptualization of a plan (1). Intervention will be focused on sensory registration and getting the child into a calm-alert state.

Once this has been achieved, intervention will focus on the planning and sequencing of the activity (2). The vestibular and proprioceptive systems play an important role in terms of providing information on the body's movement through space, muscle tone, balance, coordination of the two sides of the body and the timing and sequencing of movements. Proprioceptive processing is especially involved in the programming and planning of projected action sequences (feedforward). It also provides the necessary information regarding the body and its movement through space which affects the rate and timing of movements.

Intervention will also depend on the cause of the dysfunction. If the dyspraxia is due to poor tactile discrimination, then activities that provide tactile-proprioceptive input and facilitate an adaptive response will be used. If the dyspraxia is caused by a bilateral integration and sequencing disorder, the focus of intervention will be on activities that provide vestibular and proprioceptive input and require an adaptive response. It is hypothesized by Fisher et al. (1991) that the basis of a bilateral integration and sequencing disorder is a vestibular-proprioceptive processing disorder.

The third part of intervention is where the sequencing part of an activity has to be carried out (3). Once a child is able to conceptualize the plan and organize the information of an activity/task, the execution of the task will follow. In sequenced task execution it is important first to provide the child with the foundation skills needed to execute a task (as discussed in 1 and 2), because once they understand their body scheme and how it relates to the outside world, their sense of self will improve and their 'library' of neuronal models from which they can draw to carry out the functional part of an activity/task will also expand. Functional tasks must include play, school and personal care activities. Some sequential tasks need to be taught (e.g. tying shoelaces, bicycle riding and writing). The success of sensory integration therapy will be indicated by the ability of the child to generalize the skills taught, to carrying out other tasks that demand the use of similar movements. If a child can only carry out the task learnt and is not able to generalize skills, then the child has been taught splinter skills and sensory integration has not taken place.

Somatodyspraxia, because of its multisensory integration basis (tactile in terms of discrimination and vestibular-proprioceptive in terms of planning), is the most severe form of dyspraxia. It also impacts on every aspect of a child's functioning.

Classified under practic disorders there is also a visuodyspraxia which is thought to be the end result of a somatodyspraxia. These children have poor form and space perception, their visual motor skills are poor and visual construction (e.g. dot-to-dot designs) is also poor. In terms of intervention, the somatodyspraxia will first be addressed and then the visuodyspraxia.

Sensory seeking and self-stimulation behaviours

Stereotypic, disruptive and self-stimulatory behaviours can be typical under the PDD spectrum children but can also be seen in children with mental retardation (especially institutionalized children – see 'Effects of institutionalization'). Typical behaviour of children who are sensory seeking or self-stimulatory includes head banging, shaking of extremities, finger or ear flicking, scratching, biting (self or others), mouthing or chewing, grinding of teeth, rubbing of hands, rocking, spinning, scratching, humming (or any other form of vocalization), smelling and sniffing of objects.

There are many reasons why a child will engage in these types of behaviours but one of the reasons is that the child has a sensory integrative dysfunction; thus the cause of the behaviour could vary, e.g.:

- It could be that the sensation derived from the behaviour provides the child with enhanced sensory input.
- It may be a way for a child to communicate with his environment, in terms of attention received, obtained or avoided.
- It could provide the child with a method to indicate his needs in terms of sensory input (touch, vestibular, proprioceptive, auditory, visual, olfactory or smell).
- It could be due to an already identified sensory integrative disorder, e.g. somatosensory or tactile discrimination disorder.

The role of the occupational therapist will be to use clinical reasoning to analyse these behaviours by first identifying the reason for the behaviour as mentioned above. The behaviour also needs to be analysed to identify which sensory systems are involved, e.g. where movement is involved like rocking, spinning and running the child is providing himself with vestibular input. The type of vestibular input should also be identified (linear, rotatory, angular or vibratory). A child that hangs upside down or positions himself with his head in an inverted position needs intense vestibular input. Where behaviours such as jumping, crashing, hitting, pinching and teeth grinding and chewing are involved, the child is providing himself with proprioceptive stimulation (some of the mentioned behaviours also have an element of vestibular stimulation). The type of proprioceptive input should also be identified, e.g. proprioceptive or deep proprioceptive. Where behaviours such as scratching, biting, masturbating and head banging are involved the child is providing himself with touch and proprioceptive input. The type of touch stimulation should also be identified (light touch or deep touch). Where the child engages in activities such as finger or hand flicking, spinning himself with open eyes, there is definitely an element of visual stimulation involved. Behaviours which involve smelling and sniffing provide olfactory stimulation and behaviours involving sounds provide auditory stimulation.

All of these types of stimulation in which the child engages are usually dysfunctional and disruptive, therefore the occupational therapist will, depending on the sensory reason for the behaviour, plan intervention. The main goal of intervention in these types of behaviours is to diminish the behaviour by providing the child with a 'sensory diet' that will provide the stimulation that his nervous system needs. It is also done in such a way that the child is actively participating (requiring adaptive responses) and is functional and not dysfunctional.

Self-injurious behaviour

Although self-injurious behaviour is also a form of self-stimulation as described above it is more severe and disruptive. Varney-Blackburn (1985) has described a treatment protocol for the treatment of self-injurious behaviour in children with mental retardation and autistic behaviour. Varney-Blackburn (in Crouch and Alers, 1997) describes a treatment session as follows: Start with a tactile rubdown (unless the child is tactile defensive), which has a primal, pervasive, preparatory influence, lasting for up to 30 minutes. This has an alerting effect on the nervous system and allows for maximum response to further sensory input. Various textured articles (e.g. sponges, cotton wool, loofahs, brushes, hand cream and body lotions) are applied according to sensory modulation principles. In the past it was thought that tactile stimulation should be applied in the direction of the hair growth and not across the midline, but Wilbarger and Wilbarger (1991) have found this not to be a limiting factor. The development of eye contact and auditory stimulation is encouraged and naming the body parts where the stimulation is applied also encourages body concept.

Excitatory stimulation as well as a vibrator will then be applied to the areas that the child self-injures. A vibrator should always be used with great caution, particularly in the facial area. Vibration provides a potent form of touch-pressure and proprioception. When ice is applied it should be done fast and with light strokes (slow icing has an inhibitory influence).

The child could also be placed in a snowbox (large box filled with shell-sized polystyrene pieces) at any time during the session as this provides a great deal of tactile input and warmth. There are definite precautionary measures that should be taken note of. A child who has problems with bladder and sphincter control should wear a nappy as the warmth and comfort provided by the snowbox tend to relax the bladder and sphincter muscles. The child could be asked to find objects hidden in the snowbox (adaptive response is then required).

Vestibular equipment can be used either to calm or alert a child depending on the need (see modulation disorders). Varney-Blackburn emphasizes that random vestibular stimulation has a disorganizing effect. Careful observation is necessary throughout the session to make sure that the input has an organizing effect and if necessary, adaptations need to be made.

It is also recommended that vestibular stimulation should be used to enhance language and communication. The use of singing is also recommended, especially action songs that describe what is taking place, movements and body parts. Language is processed in the left hemisphere and music in the right hemisphere, so for the child who has language difficulties music can be used to enhance communication.

Treatment sessions for reducing of self-injurious behaviour usually last for approximately three-quarters of an hour and should be continued for a few months (research by Varney-Blackburn (1985) showed that most children show a positive response after two to four months) and then the child could be included in a maintenance programme twice or three times a week. Some children respond very quickly and others take longer before improvement in self-injurious behaviour is seen.

Drooling

Drooling is often present in the profoundly mentally retarded child and by exposing the child to an oral stimulation programme combined with a sensory integration programme the drooling can be greatly reduced or eliminated (Varney-Blackburn in Crouch and Alers, 1997).

The oral stimulation programme should be applied as follows: The occupational therapist sits with the child on her lap, facing away from her. If possible the child can be looking into a mirror. A block of ice wrapped in a cloth is used to apply stimulation around the mouth area. Movements should be light and fast. This is repeated five times, the mouth area is then dried and the application repeated. Next a vibrator (an electric toothbrush wrapped in a cloth is very effective) is used to provide stimulation to the facial prominences (chin, cheek bone and jaw bone). A vibrator should once again be used with caution. After this a few drops of lemon juice/essence is dropped onto the child's tongue (an eye dropper can be used). The production of saliva is stimulated and the child can now use the tone that has been built up in the previous steps to swallow the saliva. Flavoured lip balm can be applied to the child's lips to enhance the awareness of the mouth area. It is also suggested that textured finger food be given to the child to eat.

The oral stimulation activity ideas presented by Oetter et al. (1995) may also be incorporated into this programme. For maximum results the child should be exposed to a full sensory integration treatment programme.

Hyperactivity

Hyperactivity is often seen in mentally retarded children as well as in the

PDD spectrum child. The reticular formation in the brain plays an important role in organizing and promoting alertness (Ayres, 1983) and helps to keep activity levels within the normal range. Hyperactivity caused by poor sensory registration/processing or poor inhibition of the reticular formation can be treated successfully with sensory integration therapy and could be seen and approached as a sensory modulation disorder (SMD).

Seizures

Seizures may be overt and easy to observe or they can be masked as momentary inattentiveness, change in muscle tone with no obvious reason, fluttering of eyes, drooling or sudden change in behaviour. If a child does have seizures the occupational therapist must be extra cautious during therapy but there is no reason why children with seizures could not be exposed to sensory integration therapy.

It is true that vestibular stimulation can elicit a seizure but it depends where in the brain the lesion is that causes the seizure, as it could be situated in any one of many different areas of the brain. Therefore it cannot be assumed that vestibular, or any other type of sensory stimulation will aggravate the epilepsy (Varney-Blackburn in Crouch and Alers, 1997). The occupational therapist using sensory integration treatment should just be extremely cautious. If any signs are observed that may suggest that the treatment has an aggravating effect on the seizure the treatment should be terminated immediately, the intervention used must be analysed and the necessary adaptation should be made to the programme. Children with registration, attention and arousal difficulties are at especially high risk for seizures because they have medical-neurological problems (Murray-Slutsky and Paris, 2000).

Institutionalization

Although institutionalization is not a factor within the child, it is a factor within the environment that can cause sensory deprivation and aggravate already existing sensory integration dysfunctions. A high percentage of the children with mental retardation and PDD spectrum disorders are found in institutions and this should be taken into account when intervention is planned, especially in terms of the sensory world the child is exposed to within an institution. Within this deprived sensory world he has to still develop despite of his already existing pathology.

Cermak in Smith Roley et al. (2001) state that although recent research on the effects of institutionalization indicates that not all children in institutions show problems in sensory integration, these children are at significant risk. Extensive research has been done on the effects of institutionalization on the development of a child. The importance of sensory experiences (especially touch and movement) in development is well described in the literature. Children living in an institution are not only deprived of sensory experiences but are also exposed to infrequencies of interaction (also on a sensory level) by caregivers.

In research done by Gale Haradon (in Smith Roley et al., 2001) it was found that institutionalized children experienced many sensory processing and sensory modulation disorders. Intervention studies discussed by Cermak (Smith Roley et al., 2001) indicate that the effects of deprivation and institutionalization can be reduced but therapy must be multifaceted and interdisciplinary. The provision of sensory integration treatment should definitely be one of the strategies for minimizing the effects of institutionalization on the development of children.

General sensory integration treatment principles

- First and most important, always remember that if sensory registration does not take place in a meaningful way, neuronal models or memory are not formed and therefore learning will not occur. So always work for meaningful sensory registration.
- To facilitate sensory integration make use of enhanced sensory activities that will provide the necessary input in those sensory systems that need integration in a specific child and in accordance to the goals set in the treatment plan for the child.
- Principles to remember when using vestibular activities: Angular movement provides stimulation to the semicircular canal and facilitates phasic, fleeting postural reactions whilst linear movements (up and down and forward and backwards) provide stimulation to the utricle hair cells and facilitate tonic postural extension and increased muscle tone which is needed in maintaining an anti-gravity extensor posture.
- Whilst linear vestibular movements facilitate postural extension, only heavy work can promote postural flexion. First work for total flexion through phasic fleeting movements and then grade to activities that promote tonic sustained flexion.
- Always work for an adaptive response which is challenging and motivating, because functional outcomes create integration (if sensory stimulation is provided without active participation and adapted responses from the child no integration will take place!).
- Talk in short concrete sentences, as listening places an extra demand on the sensory systems and both the mentally retarded and PDD spectrum child have language difficulties as well.
- Routine and structure provide a lot of security to both the mentally retarded child and the PDD child, both of whom have problems in handling change.
- Decrease anxiety as far as possible by allowing your treatment session to flow, keeping activities familiar (challenges within the activity could vary), and help them to anticipate change.

- Detailed reports should be kept on the child's responses to treatment and progress. Feedback on the child's progress should be given regularly to other members of the team.
- The production of adapted responses indicates progress and the grading of the programme should be guided by the adapted responses of the child.

Precautions

- Never leave a child unattended in a sensory integration area, as the apparatus used without supervision and guidance could cause serious injuries.
- Doctors, other staff members, parents and caregivers should always be informed that a child is exposed to sensory integration treatment. Doctors should also be consulted about any condition that might be aggravated by especially vestibular stimulation (e.g. epilepsy and ventricular shunts). Feedback received from them plays a valuable part not only in the adaptation of the programme but also in its success. Effective sensory integration treatment will lead to more functional behaviour and skills.
- Equipment must be kept in a good condition and mattresses should always be placed under suspension apparatus to reduce the chance of injury. Polystyrene chips should be changed regularly as they disintegrate easily and there is a risk that small pieces might be swallowed or get stuck in body cavities.
- Activities should never be forced onto a child. A golden rule is that if a child does not enjoy, his nervous system is not integrating and thus no learning is taking place.
- As many of these children are not able to communicate effectively it is of the utmost importance to observe them very closely and, according to Varney-Blackburn (in Crouch and Alers, 1997), this observation should be continued by caregivers for at least two hours after treatment. Any signs of distress, which indicate autonomic nervous system reactions, should be reported and treated accordingly. Signs of stress include the following: paleness, sweating, tachycardia, nausea or vomiting, extreme fear and/or agitation, constant yawning, over-excitement, constant crying, falling asleep or losing consciousness. Depending on the symptoms the necessary intervention should be made by either exposing the child to inhibitory or excitatory activities. If a child loses consciousness because of over-inhibition of the brainstem, give excitatory stimulation such as light touch applied to the soles of the feet and face or ice applied to the face. It must always be remembered that these children's nervous systems can be much more sensitive to sensory stimulation and adverse reactions can easily occur!

Use of groups in sensory integration treatment

When practising as an occupational therapist in developing countries one is faced with realities that do not always allow for individual sensory integration treatment but do allow for a lot of creativity and challenge. Factors such as cost, patient numbers, manpower and facilities often force the occupational therapist to make use of groups in treating children with sensory integration dysfunction. Although not the ideal, it is better treating children in groups than excluding children from treatment that could help them to be more functional. The following are a few guidelines that could be used when treating children in sensory integration groups:

- Include children with similar dysfunction in the same group.
- Include children who could benefit from the same types of stimulation activities in the same group.
- Include children with similar arousal levels in the same group (under-aroused children together and over-aroused children together because the nature of the stimulation will differ vastly between the two groups).
- Group children also according to their level of creative participation (see Chapter 1). The adaptive responses made by children who function on the different levels of creative ability will vary because of their differences in action, volition, handling of tools and materials, relating to people, and task concept. The planning of activities in terms of the adaptive responses required will be much easier when the children in the group function on the same level of creative ability.
- Support staff are essential when working in groups. If the staff have received additional training in sensory integration they could really be of great value and could help to make the group session that much more effective. The more capable hands available in group treatment the better the chance to address individual needs within the group.
- If available, a video of a group session could help the therapist to plan intervention more effectively because by viewing the tape the therapist could look at individual needs and make the necessary adaptations to the programme.

Conclusion

The use of sensory integration as a model within the population of mentally retarded children and PDD spectrum children is essential, and cannot be carried out in isolation (Varney-Blackburn in Crouch and Alers, 1997). This is not only in terms of controlled stimulation and a stimulating environment but also in terms of multidisciplinary teamwork. Sensory integration treatment should always be done under the leadership of a trained sensory integration occupational therapist and progress should not only be measured by the child's sensory integrative abilities but also by the child's functioning in all spheres of life.

Questions

1. Describe the role that sensory integration plays in normal functioning using the spiral process of sensory integration as a departure point.
2. Describe how the mentally retarded child/PDD spectrum child could be affected by a sensory integration dysfunction.
3. Describe in your own words what you understand under the following sensory integration dysfunctions:

   a) Sensory modulation disorders
   b) Practic dysfunctions.

4. Which symptoms that are typical of mentally retarded children and PDD spectrum children can be related to sensory integration dysfunctions?
5. Why do children engage in sensory seeking and self-stimulation behaviours?
6. Describe how you could use sensory integration treatment in children with:

   a) Self-injurious behaviour
   b) Drooling.

7. What effects could institutionalization have on the sensory integration abilities of a child?
8. Name the precautions that should always be taken when using sensory integration treatment with children who are mentally retarded or PDD spectrum.

Chapter 17
Specific occupational therapy intervention with adolescents

LOUISE FOUCHÉ

Adolescent psychiatry has long been neglected in many parts of the world. Adolescents are usually treated with children or with adult clients, frequently resulting in inefficient treatment. Adolescents' development plays a large role and their specific needs, behaviours and problems must be kept in mind continuously if treatment is to be therapeutic and effective.

Overview of the adolescent

Adolescence is the time between childhood and adulthood and the term adolescence, from the Latin word *adolescere*, means 'to grow up' or 'to grow to adulthood' (Louw, 1990). The phase of adolescence extends from 12 to 18 years for girls and 13 to 20 years for boys (Louw, 1990).

Adolescence is a time characterized by unique development. Some believe it to be a tumultuous time (Hurlock in Mpe, 2001), while others are of the opinion that it is not as turbulent as it was previously thought to be, and that the majority of adolescents negotiate their way through this life phase successfully (Louw 1990; Wiener 1991; Szabo, 1996). How easily the adolescent makes the transition depends on various factors, for example speed and length of transition, discontinuity in training, ambiguous status, degree of realism and motivation, environmental aids or obstructions and on adult expectations within the culture. However it occurs, adolescence remains a time of transition in which individuals develop from a child into an adult, after which they will be recognized by society as mature adults with all the accompanying responsibilities.

Adolescence is divided into three periods, namely Early (ages 11 to 14 years), Middle (ages 14 to 17 years) and Late (ages 17 to 20). These divisions are arbitrary, as growth and development occur along a continuum that varies from person to person (Kaplan et al., 1998).

Trends in adolescent psychiatry

Due to limited resources including human resources, few private psychiatric clinics and state psychiatric units can afford to address the specific needs of adolescents. Serrett (in Wilson, 1996) suggests that the trend in psychiatry is less concerned with self-expression and personal growth and more concerned with activities related to occupational competency. Space and facilities are becoming more limited and all options involving costs are scrutinized. The result is that adolescents are usually either accommodated in adults' or childrens' wards. In both cases their unique needs are not being addressed optimally. The emphasis on placing clients back into the community as fast as possible also plays a role.

The emergence of psychopathology during adolescence that continues into adulthood is recognized (Rutter in Szabo, 1996) and therefore the appropriate treatment regime is crucial in attempting to prevent chronicity and consequent disability (Szabo, 1996). This emphasizes the importance of adolescent psychiatry. Szabo (1996) noted that the diagnostic trend in adolescent psychiatry, within a South African context, has changed. Adolescents admitted are, psychiatrically, more ill. There has been a decrease in adjustment disorders diagnosed, but an increase in anxiety, mood and psychotic disorders.

In the psychiatric field in occupational therapy it has also been found that less emphasis is placed on adolescent psychiatry within the occupational therapy curriculum. This is cause for concern and the question may be asked, 'Why are adolescents viewed as less important?' although literature is clearly emphasizing the need for specialized care (Wiener, 1991; Szabo, 1996).

Assessments

According to Vance and Pumariega (2001) there is a change occurring in the assessment of children and adolescents in psychology. The shift is being made from standard assessment batteries consisting of projective instruments to computer-based, focal and behavioural assessments. Structural psychiatric interviews, neuro-psychological test batteries and new cognitive batteries are also being used. The reasons for the shift are: to determine a clearer baseline against which the effect of treatment can be measured; to accommodate a greater variety of settings; to provide almost immediate results; to be used cross-culturally; and to help choose appropriate treatment modalities (Vance and Pumariega, 2001).

Lougher (in Creek, 2002) is of the opinion that occupational therapists do not use standardized tests routinely but appear to use a more descriptive approach. The occupational therapist should investigate the advantages of each assessment and decide what would work best within the clinical setting.

Assessments should include all the performance components, performance areas and the client's social skills and interpersonal relationships. The different assessment methods that may be used include interviews, collateral information, observations in structured and unstructured situations, participation in craft and functional activities such as ADL and formal and informal tests.

Interview

Depending on the role divisions within a multidisciplinary team, different members may perform the first interview. Since interviewing is a generic skill, it does not matter who conducts the interview. It is, however, important that all necessary information is obtained and a rapport is established with the client. The interview should, if possible, include the mother, father and the client. Even if the parents are divorced both should be present. Later in the interview the parents can be requested to leave so that more personal questions can be asked. The therapist should observe the client's relationship with both parents and their relationship with each other first hand.

The occupational therapist starts with open-ended questions (Morrison and Anders, 1999) and follows up with milestones and general background history. The occupational therapist should remember to ask questions regarding the client's performance areas. The client's school progress and recent functioning at school is important. A decline in schoolwork is a positive indicator of emotional problems in children and adolescents. Asking about the disciplining of the child is also valuable. The first part of the interview should end by asking the parents if there is any additional information that they think is necessary for the therapist to know that was not raised in the interview.

After the parents have been asked to leave, the interview will continue with the client. It is important to reassure the client of confidentiality, explaining that the information will be shared with all the team members to ensure optimal treatment but that his parents will not be informed unless he gives permission. If you do this, it is more likely that the personal information concerning sexual development, relationship with peers and use of substances will yield truthful answers. The way the questions are posed and the occupational therapist's non-verbal communication is vitally important when the sensitive questions are asked. The therapist should ask, 'Have you experimented with drugs?' instead of 'You haven't used drugs before, have you?' The therapist gains insight when asking the client two or three fantasy questions, e.g. 'If you could wish for three things what would they be?' or 'If you were left on an island who would you like to have with you?' (Scott and Katz, 1988; Morrison and Anders, 1999). Other meaningful questions are 'What would your best friend say if I asked him about you?' Questions about suicidal ideation and attempts are vital.

The occupational therapist can ask the client to make a collage of him/herself and then ask for an explanation. The therapist should assess the client's mood. The interview could also include assessment questions concerning other performance components e.g. 100 – 7 concentration test or recalling seven numbers to assess immediate memory (Kaplan et al., 1998).

The occupational therapist should ascertain what performance areas are the most problematic for the client and what they would like to change. Questions such as, 'What do you do after school?' or 'What do you do with your friends?' are helpful (Morrison and Anders, 1999).

Irrespective of the questions asked the occupational therapist must remember that she is interviewing an adolescent who sometimes approaches interviews with suspicion, hostility and indifference (Hoge, 1999). It is therefore important that time is spent building a rapport. The occupational therapist must be non-judgemental, empathetic, warm and trustworthy. Adolescents are particularly sensitive to adults who come across as 'fake' and therefore the therapist must be congruent and monitor transparency. Initial resistance, vulgar language or testing behaviour should not shock the occupational therapist as adolescents use these to test the therapist. However, the therapist is advised not to try to be a peer by using slang and vulgar language in return. The interviewer should find a middle ground between being excessively formal and inappropriately familiar (Morrison and Anders, 1999). According to Morrison and Anders (1999), it is important to project the occupational therapist's genuine fondness for the adolescent, during the interview.

Collateral information

Select appropriate people for each individual case. The nursing staff who observe the client continuously in the ward provide valuable information. An aunt or uncle in the family may provide information from another perspective. The current and/or previous schoolteachers, friends, siblings, previous therapists, medical doctor, holiday job employer, etc., are possible sources of information. However, it is essential that the occupational therapist receives permission from the client and his parents (as he is still a minor), in writing, before gathering collateral information.

Activities

The client's participation in known and unknown activities will yield a wealth of information to the occupational therapist. The functional activities are essential in assessing adolescents. Craft activities also help the occupational therapist in assessing performance components and performance areas. A variety of different methods should be used to assess adolescents, as they become bored easily. This, however, indicates the importance of assessing adolescents' psychological endurance. Their cognitive abilities should be assessed to ascertain what cognitive development has been achieved. The therapist will then know what cognitive abilities she needs to stimulate during the treatment and which are reliable. The adolescent's mood must always be assessed. However it should be remembered that adolescents' moods tend to be short-lived and labile. Repeated mood assessments over time are therefore more accurate (Morrison and Anders, 1999).

The occupational therapist frequently makes use of a collage as an assessment activity since it is an easy, affordable and effective method of assessing numerous different abilities and skills. The adolescent is provided with paper/cardboard and asked to make a collage of whatever he likes. These instructions are unstructured and the activity is therefore projective. The selection of pictures as well as how and where they are placed are noted. It is important that the occupational therapist does not make any interpretations but rather asks the client 'Explain why you selected this picture', and 'What does this picture symbolize for you?'

The occupational therapist can assess the following by means of the collage: thought processes, concentration, decision making, memory, introspection, insight, motivation/drive, psychomotor activity and affect. Depending on the pictures selected the occupational therapist will also be able to determine self-esteem, mood, peer and/or parental relationships. The themes of the collage can give the occupational therapist an indication of issues that are uppermost in the client's mind. Another advantage of making a collage is that it is non-threatening to adolescents and they can express themselves freely and creatively. The collage can also be used to assess numerous prevocational skills, especially work competency which includes planning, neatness, accuracy, ability to evaluate own work, ability to recognize mistakes, perseverance, etc.

The occupational therapist could make use of additional activities, e.g. craft activities such as making cards, leatherwork, etc., to assess the remaining performance components, so that all aspects are covered; namely disposition, cognition and emotional components. If there is any indication of possible problems from the interview, history or observation, additional sensory-motor and neurological components should also be assessed.

Functional activities

All areas of functioning should be assessed.

Leisure time

The same leisure time assessments used for adults can be used for the adolescent population. If adolescents do not have any constructive leisure time the exact reason should be examined. Adolescents tend to be passive and lazy and the occupational therapist should not view their lack of leisure time as an indication of pathology. Adolescents often listen to music while lying on their beds. This is viewed as 'passive' leisure time and is still considered constructive leisure time, since it is age-appropriate.

The therapist could ask herself the following questions to ascertain possible reasons for poor use of leisure time. Is the adolescent unsure of what he enjoys? Is it part of finding his identity? Does he have no energy for it (as in mood disorders)? Does he have a financial problem with continuing the hobby? These are some possible reasons for poor leisure time functioning.

One would expect the client to spend most of his free time with his peers, as this is the norm for the developmental phase. If this is not the case, the reason behind this should be investigated. The therapist should ascertain whether the leisure time with friends could be viewed as constructive or destructive. The occupational therapist may find that the client hangs around with friends who abuse substances or vandalize property in their free time, indicating a clear problem of destructive leisure time.

Work

When assessing the performance area of work the therapist should focus on assessing prevocational skills especially work endurance, work habits (which include personal and social presentation and work competency) and work motivation. Life skills such as time management, planning of work, etc., may also be assessed. These areas are prerequisites to vocational skills that are essential for the client to secure full-time employment.

School

Occupational therapists often neglect the area of school in the adolescent client's assessments. If a schoolteacher is part of the multidisciplinary team, he could be asked to assess the client's level of school functioning by doing maths or language and comprehension tests on the required academic level. However it still remains important that the occupational therapist liaises with the teacher and does not take it for granted that teaching staff are assessing these aspects. The occupational therapist may need to suggest methods of adaptation for clients' problems and should contact the school (with the parents' permission) to ascertain problems experienced there. Modapts (modular arrangement for predetermined time standards) could also be used to assess the client's reading and writing speed.

Activities of daily living (ADL)

According to Occupational Therapy Practice Framework there are two types of activities of daily living, namely personal and instrumental ADL.

The therapist should thoroughly assess the client's personal ADL.

According to du Toit (1991) adolescents should be able to complete most of the *personal activities of daily living*. These include bathing, showering, dressing, eating, feeding, mobility, personal device care, personal hygiene and grooming, sexual activity, sleep/rest and toilet hygiene.

There are some areas which the adolescent is not expected to have mastered yet, including personal device care, i.e. contraceptives and sexual devices, sexual activity, and personal hygiene and grooming, i.e. applying and removing cosmetics, shaving and management of supplies, e.g. knowing when to buy cosmetics.

The area of sexual activity is a sensitive one that therapists should approach without being judgemental and with understanding and tact. The therapist may ask if the adolescent is experiencing any problems in this area that he/she would like to address in treatment. Although the adolescent may initially say there are no problems, the topic will have been acknowledged and the channels of communication opened. At a later stage the adolescent may be more comfortable with the therapist and then voice his problems. The therapist must remember not to enforce her values on the client and be cognisant of her counter-transference issues regarding sexual behaviour.

The more complex ADL, otherwise known as *Instrumental ADL* (Occupational Therapy Practice Framework, 2002), are those orientated towards interacting with the environment and include caring for others, care of pets, child rearing, communication device use, community mobility, financial management, health management and maintenance, home establishment and management, meal preparation and clean-up, safety procedures and emergency responses and shopping. The occupational therapist should not expect the adolescent to perform these instrumental ADL tasks independently under normal circumstances but may wish to incorporate them during prevention programmes in the community or at schools in order to enhance development. However, in the case of young teen mothers who have chosen to take care of their children or where AIDS orphans are taking care of their siblings, these ADL tasks will have to be assessed to determine where the client needs assistance or methods of compensation. It may even be necessary for the therapist to teach the adolescent some of these tasks.

Social skills

Social skills and forming interpersonal relationships are vital aspects of being functional. In essence social skills are necessary to function in all the above performance areas. If the client has a problem with his social skills, it will have a detrimental effect on his ability to form peer relationships, which is needed to form mature relationships later in life.

Standardized tests

The occupational therapist must ensure that the standardized tests used during assessments are suitable for the client's culture as well as age group. Assessment results of tests standardized for adults cannot be generalized to the adolescent population group. Similarly, tests standardized for children cannot be used for adolescents. For example the Developmental Test of Visual-Motor Integration (Beery, 1997) is reliable for adolescents only up to the ceiling age of 15 years (Neistadt and Crepeau, 1998).

Numerous informal questionnaires are available on the internet. However, when using any self-reporting questionnaire, the occupational therapist should ensure that the client has the necessary insight and introspection to be able to answer the questions; otherwise the answer will be invalid and unreliable.

Tests such as the Canadian Occupational Performance Measure (Law et al., 1998), Hospital Depression and Anxiety Scale (Milne, 1992), Inventory of Interpersonal Problems (Milne, 1992) and Coping Responses Inventory (Milne, 1992) are tests that occupational therapists may administer to adolescents.

The clients may also be referred to a counselling psychologist for additional tests, e.g. personality, aptitude and study skills.

Groups

Groups are highly recommended as a method of assessing adolescents, as peer relationships are essential to their development. The occupational therapist should note if the adolescent replies to others only when spoken to and if he has a problem initiating a conversation. The adolescent may prefer making contact with others on a one-to-one basis and feel intimidated in a group. The adolescent may also have better skills conversing with adults than with his own peer group. His ability to make contact with members of the same and the opposite sex should be distinguished.

The adolescent's non-verbal communication should be observed to assess if it is congruent with his verbal skills. Often misunderstandings and conflict can arise between the client and his parents when his verbal and non-verbal skills are incongruent. The ability to reciprocate in a relationship can also be observed within a group setting. The occupational therapist should assess if the adolescent is able to look beyond himself and focus on others by giving support, listening to them, taking turns and being able to give and receive in a relationship. When observed within a group setting, the client's ability to be assertive (and not aggressive or passive) will reflect his abilities more realistically. All the observations should be placed in a developmental perspective before deciding whether it is a problem that needs to be addressed in treatment.

Observations

During the above assessments the occupational therapist should observe both content (i.e. what is he actually saying) and process (for example, What does he avoid? When is he animated? What has been left unsaid?) Additional observations can be made when the client is in an unstructured situation, e.g. eating lunch, playing outside in free time or during sport. These observations may bring new insights. It is especially useful when assessing clients suffering from anxiety disorders as their anxiety can influence test results.

Treatment can only be scientific and effective when it is based on accurate assessment results. The therapist should view all the information and select the priority areas to treat. The therapist must be able to understand the client in his context and select the treatment goals that will be most beneficial. The occupational therapist should therefore ensure that a thorough assessment is completed before treating the client.

Treatment

The selection of a treatment approach, treating performance areas and selecting activities is important in the adolescent treatment programme.

Treatment approaches

Developmental approach

Since profound development occurs within the adolescent phase, it is essential for all therapists to counsel, assess and treat adolescents against a developmental framework. In order to use the developmental approach the occupational therapist must have knowledge of the development that occurs during adolescence and the effect it has on them. During adolescence development takes place within all areas: namely physical, cognitive, emotional and social. An overview of the main developments in each area will be discussed. Thought needs to be given to the developments within the context of a preventative, habilitative, remedial, rehabilitative and maintenance treatment programme.

When incorporating the developmental theories in treatment, it is important to refer not only to the adolescent phase, but also to the development that precedes it. If the adolescent has not mastered the tasks from the previous developmental phase, he will not be able to accomplish the tasks of the current phase. The occupational therapist will then have to treat the preceding life tasks before stimulating those of the adolescent phase.

Occupational therapists who are interested in working specifically with adolescents are advised to study the development of adolescents more comprehensively as well as the developmental theories of Erickson, Kohlberg and Havinghurst's life tasks of the adolescent phase (Meyer et al., 1988; Louw, 1990; Neistadt, 1998) as these will not be covered in this chapter.

1. Physical development
During adolescence, the body starts to change and grow. The changes that occur include an increase in body size, increase in the growth rate (due to growth hormones) and development of secondary sexual characteristics

(due to oestrogen and testosterone) as well as an increase in sexual libido and reaching sexual maturity (Louw, 1990).

Often adolescents in their mid-teens look lanky and awkward, because different parts of the body grow in different phases and at different rates. They are often passive and 'lazy' because so much energy is being used for these biological changes. The hormones can also cause acne problems, which cause them to be self-conscious. Adolescents have to readjust to their body image as the body keeps changing, and they have to learn to deal with sexual maturation.

2. Cognitive development

An expansion in the style of thought occurs that broadens awareness, imagination, judgement and insight during adolescence. Abstract thoughts start to develop during this phase, which is also known as the stage of formal operations, according to Piaget's theory (Wiener, 1991). The following cognitive abilities are now possible:

* starting to speculate
* looking at different possibilities/options and not just at the immediate facts
* able to formulate, test and evaluate their own hypotheses
* able to combine more variables and find solutions therefore they become more skilled at solving complex problems
* developing plans that have been thought through
* evaluating their own thoughts
* becoming introspective and can evaluate themselves
* starting to challenge everything and reject old boundaries and ideas
* becoming more open and creative thinkers (Louw, 1990).

Adolescents start to develop their own value systems due to the development of their thought processes. They become more critical of their parents' behaviour and values. They question and test all limits, boundaries and convictions. This is necessary to enable them to become clear on their own thoughts and feelings about various subjects. They may become rebellious as well, as they can formulate hypotheses and respond to parental demands with possible alternatives (Dusek, 1987). They begin to believe themselves invulnerable and may settle on a world cause to fight for. Adolescents are now capable of conceptualizing their own as well as others' thoughts. They do, however, find it difficult to separate their thoughts from the thoughts of others. Since they are absorbed with thoughts about themselves, they feel others should be too (Dusek, 1987).

3. Emotional development

Hormonal changes that occur during adolescence cause emotional lability in the early teenage years. The adolescent has to deal with all the physical changes that occur as well as adapt to new roles and behaviours expected from their environment. The cognitive changes (e.g. introspection and egocentrism) cause them to be more aware of their own concerns and feelings and may intensify their emotions.

Emotional development can cause the adolescent to experience the following:

* antagonism
* boredom
* emotional lability where they find it difficult to control their emotions
* uncertainty about their own feelings and thoughts
* fear of making fools of themselves
* lack of self-confidence
* strong need for independence.

4. Social development

Social development is one of the most important developmental areas in adolescents. Adolescents who do not develop socially are at risk of being unable to form mature interpersonal relationships later in life. Due to the adolescent's cognitive skills and ability to understand others, they can now share on a more intimate level in relationships.

The peer group becomes extremely important for adolescents. It acts as a mini-society in which the adolescent can experiment with social behaviour and relationships because it is viewed as a safe environment. Adolescents now become more interested in the opposite sex, where previously they were only interested in friends of the same sex.

Their friendships change in that they view friendships as more intimate, loyal and faithful. As these become more crucial, they compete less with each other and share more equally (Montemayor et al., 1990). They wear the same clothes as their peer group and use the same language. This creates a sense of belonging and unity. Their peer group helps them to develop their identity in terms of who they are and what is important to them. The majority of adolescents receive sex education from their peer group (Louw, 1991).

If the peer group does not meet with the approval of the adolescent's parents, conflict may arise. The conflict will then be exacerbated by the adolescent's need for independence and their need to form their own value system.

It is important when treating adolescents that the life tasks and all areas of development are kept in mind and continuously integrated within the treatment programmes. Adolescents have their own unique interests and needs that should be addressed during their treatment programmes. All subsequent approaches will also be described, keeping the developmental approach in mind.

Humanistic approach

The humanistic approach is an excellent approach to use in developing a therapeutic relationship with the adolescent. By making use of reflection, being warm and congruent, a rapport will be established with greater ease, without the therapist being authoritarian or trying to be the client's friend.

The belief that the client has his own answers within him and that the therapist merely facilitates a therapeutic process ensures that the adolescent takes responsibility for his choices and ultimately for his own life. This empowers the adolescent who may feel disempowered within his/her family or social situation. Additionally giving the adolescent control (by providing him with choices) leads him to take more responsibility which stimulates one of his life tasks. It will also help him in forming his identity (What do I like? or What is more important to me now?). During treatment the occupational therapist should not come across as authoritarian. The adolescent may be asked, 'Here are the objectives we have identified together as problem areas, which aspects would you like to focus on?' or 'I have selected three activities to address your poor time management skills; which would make the most sense to you?'

Another humanistic characteristic is to develop a positive self-concept. Fortunately an adolescent client is still developing his self-concept which means that therapeutic interventions can play a great role in the development of his self-concept. This in turn contributes to autonomy and the realization that he does not have to be a captive of his past.

The humanistic therapists exploit the potential of creative activities (Finlay, 1997). The occupational therapist can therefore make use of different creative activities during treatment to encourage creative and spontaneous expressions, thereby enabling the client to reach his potential and improve his self-esteem (Finlay, 1997).

The humanistic approach is, however, not suitable for clients with mental retardation or concrete thoughts. Clients should have developed sufficient cognitive abilities to understand the concept of responsibility and must be in the process of developing their own identity. Intellectual insight is also a prerequisite for selecting the humanistic approach for adolescent clients.

Psychoanalytical approach

The same principles and techniques for adult clients apply to the treatment of adolescents. However, the client should have some abstract thoughts and intellectual abilities in order to gain insight when projective techniques are used. Maximum effectiveness can be obtained by presenting projective techniques within a group of adolescents. As adolescents are in tune with each other and know how other adolescents think, they can be surprisingly accurate with their observations and questions posed to each other about, for example, pictures drawn, clay models made and selection of symbols during psychodrama. Occupational therapists should ensure that they have the necessary training before selecting a psychoanalytical approach.

Interactive approach

Because the development of peer relationships as well as heterosexual relationships occurs during adolescence and because so much value is placed on peer relationships, the interactive approach is an important one. During a group session adolescents are exposed to a simulated 'peer group' and can learn, experiment and practise their social skills within the 'safe' and therapeutic group context. Specific feedback concerning the client's maladaptive behaviour can be facilitated from the group members. This technique is especially powerful for adolescents when facilitated in the here-and-now as they are more likely to listen to feedback coming from a peer than from a therapist or parent. Additionally, skills learnt during the group therapy are transferred to society once they are discharged (Yalom, 1995).

When facilitating the curative factors (Yalom, 1995) for an adolescent group, the therapist should focus on the following:

• *Cohesion*: Cohesion is essential in adolescent groups. Often adolescents who have emotional problems withdraw from their friends and therefore do not have a peer group to which they belong. It is important that an adolescent feels that he belongs to the group, so that he can start to experiment with social skills and take more interpersonal risks. The therapist therefore needs to facilitate cohesion in order to address these needs and facilitate effective group therapy. Additionally, adolescents who are members of a group with strong cohesion disclose feelings and experiences on a deeper level. In a sense the therapy group becomes a substitute for the peer group. Therapy groups should therefore include members of the same age group and of both sexes.
• *Imparting of information*: The adolescent's peer group is of more value to him than parents or therapists. Adolescents believe that other adolescents are going through the same experiences as they are and will therefore pay more attention to advice or solutions offered by group members.
• *Existential factors*: Facilitating existential factors can be curative as adolescents have a strong external locus of control. Sometimes the cohesion may become so strong that the group members start to take responsibility for other members' problems. The therapist should avoid this by letting the group members realize that each individual is responsible for his own choices.

Cognitive approach

The adolescent's cognitive development must have reached a stage where he is able to reason abstractly. As different complex thoughts are developing during the adolescent phase, this approach may be implemented successfully. However care should be taken not to allow the adolescent to intellectualize. This may happen because adolescents' cognitive abilities develop faster than their emotional abilities.

Since the adolescent feels invincible, the danger exists that they are unrealistic about their abilities and their problem solving may not always be realistic for their circumstances. The therapist can then make use of the other cognitive abilities that are developing, e.g. being able to see different variables that influence a problem, in order to facilitate more realistic problem solving.

As an adolescent becomes more introspective, the client can begin to identify his own irrational thoughts or negative thoughts. The process of challenging negative thoughts and trying to replace them with more rational or positive thoughts is possible during adolescence. The added advantage is that the sooner the client learns to identify the existence of irrational/negative thoughts, the easier it will become to identify them as he grows older.

Cognitive-behavioural approach

Giles and Allen state that

> this framework is the best suited to occupational therapy due to its focus on functional problem-solving which in turn helps the client to identify and practise alternative behaviour to problem situations' (Giles and Allen in Henderson, 1998).

It can be applied successfully for life skills or pre-vocational skills training. Before the client is taught a specific technique, tips, compensation methods, etc., he should understand the importance of it in his life, how to utilize it and how the process works. It should then be followed up by repetition, practising the skill and receiving coaching in order for the client to master the skill. Social modelling (Bandura in Meyer et al., 1988) may also be used especially during role-plays to train clients' social skills.

Neuro-physiological approach

Adolescents are normally passive and have little energy; therefore by stimulating the vestibular system their activity levels increase. This approach can help in providing them with feedback about their new body image, and also helps to develop their self-concept (which is part of identity). Adolescent psychiatric clients often have aggression bottled up inside and the aggression can be channelled by means of sport or physical activities that help them to dissipate some of these emotions.

Aerobic exercises have been found to elevate adolescents' mood (Brollier et al., 1994), indicating the effectiveness of a neuro-physiological approach for adolescents with mood disorders.

Behavioural approach

A purely behavioural approach can be used to focus on changing a specific maladaptive behaviour e.g. self-mutilating behaviour or in eating disorder clients to increase their body weight. However the approach may come across as being authoritarian where the adolescent is given minimal control or choices, which in turn can increase feelings of antagonism. This will cause the therapeutic relationship to suffer. When selecting the behavioural approach it is suggested that an additional occupational therapist monitors and enforces the behavioural programme so as not to interfere with the rapport that has been established.

Human occupational approach

The Model of Human Occupation (Kielhofner, 1995) views the client from a perspective unique to occupational therapy. The model is applied in the same way as with adult clients where the three subsystems – namely, volition, habituation and performance systems – are assessed for problems which are then treated. There are, however, some differences which should be kept in mind when working with adolescents.

- Volition subsystem: The adolescent has a need for independence and develops his own value system. He begins to consider choosing an occupation since he becomes more future-orientated, has a sense of pride in his work responsibilities, has a sense of enjoyment in leisure and develops a concept of productive and leisure activities. Due to the increase in his maturity, interests, expression of self-identity and peer group pressures, he may develop new leisure time interests (Sholle-Martin, 1987).
- Habituation: As described in the life crisis of Erickson, the adolescent experiments with different roles. The most dominant roles of adolescents are those of scholar, friend and part-time worker (Sholle-Martin, 1987). Adolescents should be encouraged to have a part-time job or do voluntary work as they can then develop budgeting skills, be exposed to a work environment, explore job skills, improve their own budgeting and develop a sense of pride in their accomplishments. The client will start to learn to balance work and leisure. The adolescent should be given more responsibilities in managing his own time, routines and work habits, thereby stimulating him to develop more specific routines and habits.
- Performance subsystem: Refer to section on treatment approaches, and literature detailing the development that occurs during adolescence.

Treatment of performance areas

The occupational therapist should select the most appropriate approach and activities, within a developmental approach, in order to achieve the objectives identified. The treatment programme will depend on the individual client and the setting and resources available and therefore it is difficult to provide more specific guidelines for treatment.

The aspects that will be addressed for an adolescent's leisure time will depend on the exact nature of the problem identified. For problems in social functioning the client should be referred for family therapy or the occupational therapist could address social skills training within group therapy. The occupational therapist should advise teaching staff on how to adapt to the client's scholastic problems, e.g. when severe reading speed problems occur oral exams or helping the client with time management or planning of his school work could be suggested. The ADL problems may be addressed within didactic or discussion groups or even in individual sessions. Some hospitals/clinics/schools have pre-vocational programmes which address different skills needed in the work area. The occupational therapist can make use of creative ways to address the pre-vocational skills; for example, make use of the ward newspaper, which the clients have to compile. The activity could attempt, among other things, to facilitate an increase in self-expression and social interaction; improve time management; identify own interests and values, etc. (Nelson and Condrin, 1987).

Activities

Numerous activities may be selected depending on the objective and approach being used. Activities selected for treatment need not be elaborate, complex or expensive. Adolescents tend to intellectualize, therefore activities focusing only on cognitive abilities will reinforce the intellectualization. The occupational therapist should incorporate more emotional aspects by asking clients for examples of their own life or by reflecting on their emotions. The occupational therapist should try to be creative and ensure an element of experiential learning and fun as adolescents learn best through experience. Many games can be adapted to suit the occupational therapist's objectives.

Active games and movement diminish anxiety and decrease the adolescents' passive nature. Research shows that adolescents tend to talk more about their feelings after a motor activity (MacLennan and Dies, 1992). Activities that include food and music are also effective.

- Self-concept puzzle: Draw a puzzle on paper. The occupational therapist may facilitate the improvement of his self-concept by designating specific puzzle pieces to represent various aspects of a self-concept, for example, relationships, life dreams, interests, personality, etc. Other pieces could answer the following questions: 'How do others experience me?' or 'What do I know about myself that no one else knows?', etc.
- Projective exercises: Represent each member of their family using a symbol and draw them close to or far from themselves to symbolize how close the relationship is. Or draw their life as a journey that they are undertaking.
- Expressive exercises: Express what they are feeling towards themselves or express how they are feeling now. A wide variety of media can be used, for example, white chalk on black paper, finger paints, clay, drama, texture collages, etc.

- Sport activities: Many sport activities may be selected e.g. volleyball, adapted 'survivor' game, obstacle course, broom hockey, balloon volleyball, etc.
- Music: Adolescents usually identify strongly with music and it can therefore be used expressively, for quiz games or for social interaction.
- Cooking and baking activities may be used for specific performance components or ADL objectives.
- Discussion group: Numerous topics may be discussed, e.g. career interests, relationships with the opposite sex, sexually transmitted diseases and contraceptives.
- Newspaper reviews where the adolescents are provided with an opportunity to voice their opinions and feelings on current events.
- Board games
- Value clarification groups
- Poetry
- Role-playing
- More activities can be found in the following books *Talk with teens* (Peterson, 1995), *Activities for adolescent in therapy* (Dennison, 1998) and *Activity manual for adolescents* (Karp et al., 1998).

Some specialized techniques that could be applied in the treatment of adolescents include theraplay, psychodrama and sensory integration. Occupational therapists should ensure that they have the necessary training before applying these techniques.

Culture

It is interesting to note that the majority of the developmental tasks are universal irrespective of culture (Louw, 1990). However, what does differ from culture to culture is the age at which children are viewed as being mature and therefore ready to take on adult responsibilities.

One of the differences is that in rural communities there seems to be a lower prevalence of adjustment disorders or conduct disorders (Chiland and Young, 1992). Another difference is, for example, the method of committing suicide. The method of suicide is linked to the availability and accessibility of different methods. The methods used to commit suicide among young black South Africans were railway-related suicides and the use of the following self-poisoning or over-dosages: rat poison, over-the-counter medication, paraffin and cockroach poison; depending on availability, firearms were also used.

Acculturation is a process by which a culture changes due to systematic and continuous influence of other culture(s). It is a reality for South African people, as more people are moving to the cities and becoming westernized. A prominent problem among the youth is that they find it difficult to form an identity. In a sense they feel that they cannot identify with one specific culture group. Some follow Western traditions when attending school or tertiary education while returning to their traditional rituals over weekends or on returning home. They are therefore faced with a more complex task of forming their identity. It has, however, been found that as soon as trauma or tragedy strikes, a person is inclined to return to the rituals and beliefs of his childhood.

The occupational therapist must therefore assess clients individually to ascertain whether they have a problem in this regard and to find out how they view mental illness and what life philosophy they are developing, in order to understand the client better. With this understanding, more holistic and individualized treatment programmes can be implemented. If a client's beliefs concerning the cause of his illness are not addressed in treatment, or if the 'why' is never resolved, then the client will remain uneasy and stressed, which has a negative effect on his wellbeing and progress (Heggenhougen and Shore, 1986).

It should be kept in mind that the majority of South African clients (between 60 and 80 per cent) see both a psychiatrist and their traditional healer (Pretorius, 1995). The occupational therapist should therefore not disregard the client's and his family's beliefs and values but rather acknowledge them and try to allow both therapies to work complementarily to each other, rather than exclusively.

Prevention programmes

There are many interventions that enhance the positive health and adjustment of children and adolescents or reducing the subsequent rate of problems, or both types of outcomes (Durlak, 1997). The increasing trend of treating clients within their community indicates a greater need for prevention programmes that will enhance the resilience of adolescent clients. Providing counselling services when problems arise ensures that problems are addressed immediately and may prevent the development of a mental disorder. Monasterio (2002) identified the following protective factors for youth:

- individual characteristics ('better' cognitive skills, strong communicators, sense of humour, positive self-concept and greater conscientiousness)
- parenting patterns (authoritative – not authoritarian – parenting style, clear parental and child role definitions, parental warmth and involvement with the adolescent)
- connectedness (sense of belonging, caring relationships with other adults and meaningful role in the broader social context)
- available opportunities (supportive adults at crucial junctures and opportunities to develop skills).

The above aspects can be addressed by means of preventative programmes within the communities.

Multidisciplinary team

The occupational therapist should always work within a multidisciplinary team and the domain and function of the occupational therapist does not differ when working in adolescent psychiatry. There are, however, some pitfalls that need to be mentioned.

Adolescents are often self-disclosing in a group in which they feel comfortable. The occupational therapist should make it clear to the group beforehand that she needs to give feedback to the team members and she is obliged to inform the team of anything that is relevant to the client's treatment. This will give the responsibility to the client to decide how much he wants to disclose within the group. Being open and honest with the client and providing feedback to the team can prevent manipulative behaviour on the part of clients who may try to play team members off against each other. The client will also not feel that the occupational therapist has broken any confidentiality agreements.

In some cases the team members will select a specific approach and handling principles to use, e.g. the behavioural approach. It is then imperative that the occupational therapist adheres to it, to ensure consistent and therefore efficient treatment.

Conclusion

Adolescent psychiatry is a specialized field and the most important aspects of treating these exciting and challenging clients have been highlighted. This chapter is, however, by no means comprehensive. Any occupational therapist wishing to work in the adolescent psychiatry field is encouraged to read more on the subject.

Adolescent psychiatry is gaining recognition in the psychiatric field. It is, however, unclear why this is not the trend in occupational therapy. Research to determine possible reasons is strongly recommended in order to rectify the problem as a matter of urgency. Further it is recommended that the effect of the different conventional treatment methods be investigated to ascertain how effective they are with an adolescent population group.

Working as an occupational therapist in the adolescent psychiatric field poses many challenges and offers numerous opportunities. It can bring enormous job satisfaction and is to be recommended.

Questions

1. Explain the importance of treating adolescents separately from children and adults.
2. Explain how the assessment of an adolescent differs from that of an adult.
3. Explain the cognitive development that takes place during adolescence and discuss how an occupational therapist should incorporate this knowledge in her treatment.

4. Explain the importance of adolescents' social development and the effect it has on them.

5. An adolescent is referred to occupational therapy with the following problems:

   - poor concentration
   - irritability
   - very passive
   - rebellious
   - withdraws from his peer group
   - drop in school marks.

Discuss the treatment of the client by setting realistic objectives and by selecting appropriate treatment approaches and activities.

PART FOUR
ADULTS

Chapter 18
Post-traumatic brain injury

SYLVIA BIRKHEAD

Few illnesses, injuries or diseases result in the devastating and overwhelming damage which accompanies brain injury. The acute rehabilitation and medical care address primarily the physical aspects of the injury, and involve the whole hospital medical team. Survivors, family members and professionals are painfully aware that the most disabling consequences of brain injury are usually cognitive and behavioural deficits, and these are usually only fully apparent once the head-injured person has been discharged home from hospital. The individual who sustains a brain injury is no longer the same person: he or she may behave differently, think differently and in fact be a different person than before the injury. The differences may be large or small, but they are differences nonetheless. And when one member of a family changes, the entire family changes (Falconer, 1998).

The pattern of recovery after neurological damage is usually one of rapid gains soon after injury, and much slower gains, and even pauses, in recovery thereafter (Gronwall et al., 1999). The trend amongst the medical fraternity is to tell families of head-injured people that maximum recovery occurs in the first 6–18 months and thereafter any improvement is minimal or a bonus. With the development of activity centres and support groups for head-injured people who have completed rehabilitation, i.e. who are 18+ months post-injury, it is becoming apparent that there is no limit to the extent to which individuals who have sustained head injuries can be rehabilitated. Focus needs to be on achieving maximum rehabilitation. Rehabilitation can be lifelong. Until recently, this was not the case – once the physical problems had been addressed, it was, more often than not, left to the family members to deal with the more long-term residual cognitive and behavioural problems.

This chapter will deal with management of the post-traumatic brain-injured person with specific reference to cognitive and behavioural aspects. The information is occupational therapy-specific but is also relevant to the whole rehabilitation team as well as for families and carers of head-injured people. Although each individual who sustains a head injury is unique and therefore will need individual attention, the deficits which result and the most appropriate rehabilitation goals for head-injured people have a commonality and can be applied generally.

Client group profile

Gutman (in Pedretti and Early, 2001) states that 80 per cent of individuals who sustain head injuries are males between the ages of 18 and 30, and that alcohol use is a leading contributor to traumatic brain injury (TBI). Figures quoted by the then director of the Headway Support Group in Johannesburg in 1997, were that 80,000 head injuries occurred per year in South Africa, the majority caused by motor vehicle accidents. The injuries are therefore mostly 'closed' head injuries caused by acceleration, which leads to multiple areas of the brain being damaged. In the United Kingdom approximately 150,000 people sustain minor head injuries a year, while 10,000 people suffer moderate head, and 11,600 suffer severe head injury (www.headway.org.uk). Traffic accidents account for between 40 and 50 per cent of these injuries.

It is known that the effects of traumatic brain injury depend on which area of the brain is damaged. This chapter will primarily consider injury to the brain behind the forehead (the frontal lobe), because damage to this part of the brain results in changes in behaviour and loss of self-restraint and insight. The widespread tearing of nerve fibres to specific areas of the brain results in all working areas of the brain being affected to some extent, hence the multitude of other problems, such as physical aspects. Cognitive and behavioural problems more commonly prevent successful reintegration and return to employment of the brain-injured person.

Rehabilitation

No two cases of head injury are alike, so no fixed treatment programme can be implemented. Rehabilitation should focus on facilitating behaviours that are expressed in non-treatment or naturalistic settings. Diller (in Christensen and Uzzell, 1994) describes new treatment modalities as being:

- advances in group methods, where groups range from basic skills, e.g. organizing schedules, to stress reduction or self-regulation
- use of coaches, who facilitate obtaining and holding down a job, assist clients and families with cognitive and personal problems in the home, adjust to community re-entry and to teach family members to distinguish deficits from behaviours that may ordinarily be viewed as non-cooperation, stubborn, anger or emotional disturbance
- newer methods in vocational rehabilitation and applications of computers as assistive technologies.

General management approaches and philosophy

Howard and Bleiberg (1997) wrote a Manual of Behavioural Management Strategies for TBI adults in which they listed the most commonly found intellectual (cognitive) and emotional (behavioural) problems. Specific management strategies are discussed for each of the identified problems but 12 generalized management philosophies or approaches are prescribed. These are as follows:

1. *Interdisciplinary management of the client is a must!*

Team members such as the therapists, caregivers, employers, families and doctors must work together to provide management consistency, which in turn provides stability to the head-injured person.

2. *Treat the client as an adult*

Give the client as much control, respect and responsibility as their behaviour will allow, even if they behave in a child-like manner.

3. *Rehabilitation from brain injury is a learning process*

The rehabilitation process is much more a learning process than a medical process, where the outcome is to facilitate behaviour change in the head-injured client.

4. *Be patient*

The client has an impaired capacity for learning new things, so change occurs slowly. The client often needs time to consolidate new skills and repetition and practice are paramount.

5. *Try not to overstimulate the client*

Clients can become overwhelmed and confused if presented with too much stimulatory input. They can often process only one thing at a time, so although they need ongoing stimulation in order to recover, this must be done gradually.

6. *Be consistent in managing behaviour*

Provide the client with stability by having everyone involved on the team (including the family members) manage the client in the same manner. This will help the client understand the impact of his behaviour on others.

7. *Clients often become worse during the course of treatment*

As clients improve cognitively, they often then become more insightful and deteriorate emotionally as they realize the implications of the head injury on their lives. This reaction needs to be dealt with in therapy so it does not become a block to further progress.

8. *Model calm and controlled behaviour for the client*

Calm demeanour on the part of the occupational therapist will help reduce the client's fear and anxiety.

9. *Expect the unexpected – variability is the rule*

Brain-injured clients exhibit fluctuations in mood, behaviour, concentration and functional ability from minute to minute in some cases. Try to help the client remain as stable as possible in daily activities.

10. *Brain-injured clients are more sensitive to stress*

The performance of brain-injured people is altered easily by minor stressors. They often have to put in a lot of extra effort to achieve what they used to be able to do without thinking, and any disruption, even to a minor task, can make them ineffective. Stick to routines and provide structure and guidance, as well as providing opportunity for them to rest, or lessen the difficulty of demands to reduce stressors.

11. *Treat the family as well as the client*

The family members need information, guidance and counselling in order to learn to love the 'new' person and mourn the loss of the former person. They also need to provide information to the rehabilitation team as to how the client was before the accident and be involved in the management so they know how to continue the rehabilitation process at home with minimal supervision and input from the medical team.

12. *Redirect the client*

When the client is being aggressive or displaying negative behaviours, it is often most effective to simply redirect their attention to another topic, rather than trying to confront them.

Frames of reference

From the learning frame of reference, behavioural and cognitive aspects might be used to address social skills training and memory management in the brain-injured person. A compensatory or rehabilitative frame of reference could also be used. Personality and behavioural changes are best dealt with using behaviour modification, i.e. to extinguish unwanted behaviour or shape existing behaviour into a more socially acceptable pattern (McWilliams in Turner et al., 1997). Behaviour modification programmes may be necessary to address behaviours that are hindering rehabilitation efforts.

A remedial or adaptive approach is needed to address the cognitive aspects that are affected by traumatic brain injury. Behavioural learning methods are most effective to develop awareness of appropriate social goals, develop skills in social behaviours and facilitate successful social interactions. Family counselling may also be necessary to resolve negative feelings and to help relatives cope with the reality of the client's abilities. One needs to look at the client's ability to be reintroduced into the community and also to encourage independence in leisure skills (Scott and Dow in Trombly, 1995).

Selection of recreational activities requires that the individual's specific cognitive and behavioural problems be taken into account. Some head-injured people go on to further academic skills and others recover sufficiently to be employed, whether in sheltered, coached or open labour employment. Rehabilitation services such as job coaching need to be considered to ensure ongoing improvement of the injured person's overall functional ability.

Intellectual or cognitive problems

The cognitive impairments that are considered are those that become evident in hospital after coming out of coma, but which persist once the brain-injured person has been discharged home. These include:

- impaired alertness and delayed processing of information
- attention and concentration deficits
- problems with memory and learning
- perceptual and language difficulties
- impaired initiation and termination of activities
- poor ability to transfer or learn new skills
- difficulties with abstract thinking, planning, judgement, insight, problem solving and other executive (higher-level cognitive) functions.

Behavioural, emotional or psychosocial problems

The problems in these areas of function that affect most brain-injured people and that need to be addressed in order to rebuild occupational and social roles, are:

- lack of drive, motivation or initiative
- decreased frustration tolerance leading to increased irritability, anger and aggression
- loss of social roles leading to isolation, inability to form or maintain relationships, feelings of dependence and lack of personal control. The brain-injured client as well as the family will experience the stages of loss as described by Kübler-Ross (1973), i.e. denial, bargaining, anger, depression and acceptance or resignation
- affective changes include increased lability, depression, anxiety or emotional blunting

- disorientation and diminished ability to comprehend social situations or non-verbal cues
- social inappropriateness, disinhibition and impulsiveness
- self-centredness and egocentrism.

Aspects to consider during therapy

Individuals who have sustained head injuries have the ability to recover old skills and learn new skills. They can be taught to modify their behaviour and lead satisfying and productive lives, as long as they are provided with the appropriate learning strategies and environments. The whole rehabilitation team can play a part in the treatment of the brain-injured person's cognitive and social skills. The TBI person's assets as well as weaknesses need to be assessed and this should preferably be done in the home setting where it is easier to see how the family and the client deal with behavioural and cognitive problems. Rehabilitation must consider the 'complete' person at all times and therapies cannot be carried out in isolation. As therapists, we need to understand the person behind the brain that was injured and so need to discover hidden strengths and weaknesses, in order to restore that person to a more functional life.

Occupational therapists and families of brain-injured people generally tend to overestimate or underestimate the cognitive and behavioural abilities and limitations, and fail to understand the practical implications of the deficits.

The plasticity of the brain is a concept still to be explored and researched but the present thinking is that there are many as yet untapped tools for rehabilitation of the brain-injured person. There is a suggested hierarchy that needs to be considered when embarking on a rehabilitation programme for TBI clients. The therapist needs to focus on the 'executive functions', e.g. attention and concentration, distractibility, initiation, planning and sequencing, which need to develop before addressing the more specific skills such as memory, learning and perception. Attention and concentration need to be addressed before the brain-injured person can be expected to improve memory. Behaviour does still need to be controlled to some extent during the cognitive and physical rehabilitation phase, but not as a structured behaviour management programme at this stage. This means that occupational therapists must try to give accurate and realistic feedback to the client on their behaviour and its consequences, so that they learn what is acceptable, and don't become more isolated because of driving others away with unacceptable behaviour. This realistic feedback needs to be given in a tactful but overt manner to facilitate understanding and insight.

Behaviour management can be introduced once the injured person has better concentration and the ability to remember. The occupational therapist must balance the focus on behaviours that the brain-injured person needs to stop with those that need to be encouraged, i.e. behavioural goals must not all just be negative and related to behaviours that have to be stopped, but include the behaviours that are positive and acceptable. Reward the small steps achieved in reaching appropriate behaviour and give immediate feedback.

Inability to initiate may be due to poor planning or organization or the injured person may say 'it just never occurred to me'. Once the injured person's behaviour is under control in the home setting, then community or recreational activities can be introduced, preferably with a stepping stone such as a 'TBI support group' or 'activity centre', before attempting to mainstream in the community.

The client needs to practise skills learnt in occupational therapy, in all different situations, as often as possible in order to make new behaviours habitual. Occupational therapists should be aware that the client needs time to consolidate new information and there may be periods where there is very slow progress. Learning occurs slowly after head injury and requires a great deal of practice before the injured person can retain and retrieve the new information reliably. Include activities in the programme that the client knew how to do before the injury, i.e. activities where re-learning not new learning is required to carry them out. Also include activities that the client performs well and enjoys doing so that they remain motivated. Although repetition and consistency are key words in addressing cognitive problems, remember that the brain-injured person will benefit most from compensatory methods for improving their ability to remember things. Use both auditory and visual presentation to ensure maximal opportunity for comprehension. Activities should be selected which rely as much as possible on the most intact functional areas.

One of the hallmarks of head injury is fluctuating performance, and this could be due to environmental variables, the brain-injured individual's variables such as fatigue, and interpersonal variables such as the mood of the person working with the brain-injured person.

The environment needs to be structured to maximize remaining abilities and provide the injured person with opportunities to re-acquire skills. The person with TBI will improve more effectively if working to a daily schedule, which must initially allow for the decreased speed of performance. Those activities which are essential for daily function (personal management tasks such as bathing or eating) should be used mostly in the initial stages of the client's homecoming. However, almost any task can be used for cognitive retraining from dressing in the morning to playing scrabble or going shopping.

The client will need a tight structure as it helps to reduce the demands placed upon him or her to function independently on a cognitive and creative level, and also helps to reduce the demands placed upon the family and caregiver.

Support groups

As stated earlier in this chapter, the cognitive and behavioural aspects of function in the TBI client are factors that need to be continually addressed, long after the client has been discharged from hospital. Often individual therapy is discontinued after the 6–18-month medical and physical rehabilitation period, and the best method of ensuring ongoing professional input is for the client to attend a head injury support group. Gutman (in Pedretti and Early, 2001) has outlined the specific benefits of group treatment for TBI clients by saying it enables the individual to meet others experiencing the same life concerns (thus decreasing feelings of isolation), offers exposure to peer reactions to behaviours (particularly helpful if the individual is exhibiting socially inappropriate behaviours), and facilitates problem solving by providing the opportunity to speak to others who have dealt successfully with the same or similar problems.

Support groups in the form of activity or day care centres can incorporate the holistic principles of occupational therapy which include working with each client as a whole and focusing on improving or maintaining all aspects of function, i.e. physical, cognitive, psychological, social and spiritual, by providing support and opportunity to be involved in a variety of activities which are relevant to each individual. A support group provides an environment where traumatically brain-injured people and their families can feel accepted, comfortable and secure; can become competent and confident to the best of their abilities. Such a group can also create challenges and opportunities to help enable the members to achieve these goals. A support group provides a place of 'belonging' for head-injured people, where they can take part in meaningful activities and socialize with others. In this environment they are able to relearn old skills and learn new skills, which will better enable them to reach their maximum potential and return to as normal a life as possible.

Activities that could be used in an occupational therapist-coordinated activity centre for TBI clients

Perhaps a reminder of the basic principle of the occupational therapy process will clarify why an activity centre works so effectively with head-injured clients.

Through the use of selected activities or tasks, the occupational therapist promotes, restores and maintains the client's ability to perform their activities of daily living and roles, so essential to a productive, participative and satisfying life, in spite of their disability. All aspects of function are important, i.e. work, self-care and leisure activities, and each individual is looked at as a whole. The client is not just a passive recipient of a treatment procedure though, but rather is actively engaged in his own therapeutic programme. Activity means to be meaningfully active physically and/or mentally and/or socially. If the correct activity is chosen, it can influence the mind and body, the senses, emotions and movement as well as motivation and behaviour. Purposeful (i.e. meaningful to the client) activity is the agent for change and the very core of occupational therapy, so no activity should just be randomly selected.

A balanced programme should include seven types of activity (Cornish 1975):

1. Physical, e.g. group exercises/walking/ball games and other sports
2. Mental, e.g. discussions/quizzes/word and board games
3. Individual, e.g. crafts/jigsaws/letter writing/computer games
4. Small group, e.g. indoor games such as cards/specific tasks such as nail-care
5. Social, e.g. parties/sing-alongs/picnics/outings
6. Service to others, e.g. saving stamps for charity/fund raising activities
7. Cultural, e.g. book groups/music groups/crafts.

Conclusion

The effects of traumatic brain injury are many and they have a devastating effect on the overall function of any individual because they can impact on physical, cognitive, emotional and social aspects of function. The medical and physical impairments are usually dealt with by the rehabilitation team in the hospital and as outpatients, for a maximum of about 18 months. Thereafter it is left largely to the family to deal with the lifelong behavioural and cognitive deficits resulting from TBI. This chapter has highlighted the rehabilitation techniques that can be used by the family and professionals in addressing the cognitive and behavioural effects of head injury specifically. Behaviour management is considered extremely effective and the other suggested handling principles have been recommended by psychologists and occupational therapists specifically, as seen by the references used in formulation of this chapter. The chapter concludes with suggested activities to be used in a support group setting.

Future research that would be particularly beneficial to occupational therapists and the occupational therapy profession would be to measure the effectiveness of such a structured activity programme in preparing TBI clients for return to society either in a functional role in the home situation or in some form of employment – be it sheltered or open labour – having dealt with the behavioural and cognitive impairments caused by the head injury.

Questions

1. List the areas of deficit after TBI and say which are the two areas that were most neglected by the rehabilitation team until recently.

2. List the 12 generalized management philosophies or approaches used when addressing cognitively and behaviourally impaired TBI adults.
3. Seven major deficits in each of the cognitive and behavioural problem areas have been identified. Name three from each problem area and say how you think this problem could affect the TBI person's ability to carry out daily function.
4. Why is it important to structure the environment for a TBI person?
5. Describe why learning of new skills is difficult for the TBI adult.
6. What are the benefits of a support group?
7. Give at least one example of an activity that could be used specifically for treatment of TBI adults, in each of the seven activity types prescribed for a balanced activity programme.

Chapter 19
Occupational therapy with anxiety and somatoform disorders

MADELEINE DUNCAN

Gaining control

Anxious people often feel out of control; as if some impending disaster is about to erupt upon their lives leaving them vulnerable and abandoned. Worries and bodily ailments preoccupy their thinking, making it difficult for them to participate optimally in life. Occupational therapists work alongside anxious people to support their efforts at recovery by guiding their participation in valued occupations, tasks and roles. Occupation is placed at the centre of helping them regain control when it feels as if they are 'losing it'.

The aim of this chapter is to provide a 'how to think' framework for clinical reasoning about the occupational consequences of debilitating anxiety. It suggests occupational therapy action with individuals, groups and populations. Triggers for critical thinking and reflective practice are suggested to guide problem solving and solution generation in collaboration with persons who are troubled by anxiety and somatoform disorders or who are at risk of developing these conditions.

Anxiety and somatoform disorders: a medical perspective

Stress is an external pressure that is brought to bear upon the individual (Keable, 1989). Anxiety is a normal human response to stress. A healthy measure of anxiety is essential for survival because it serves as an emotional protective system; almost like armour around the psyche that helps the person adapt to and cope with the stresses of daily living. Anxiety and somatization become disabling when they occur in the absence of an appreciable degree, or kind, of threat or danger or medical condition. Either is considered to be a disorder when it causes subjective distress, impedes functioning and results in excessive physiological arousal as well as cognitive, emotional and behavioural disturbances.

The DSM-IV-TR™ (American Psychiatric Association, 2000) describes the signs, symptoms and diagnostic criteria for the anxiety and somatoform disorders. To establish a common frame of reference, the following summary lists the most salient features of this group of neurotic disorders.

Anxiety and somatoform disorders in a nutshell

What: anxiety is a subjective feeling of heightened tension and diffuse uneasiness. It sometimes involves a reportable internal experience of intense dread and foreboding unrelated to an external threat, which differentiates it from fear. Somatoform symptoms such as pain, gastrointestinal, sexual and pseudo-neurological complaints occur in the absence of diagnosable medical illness; they are presumed to be psychologically based and outside the person's conscious control.

Why: anxiety and somatization are viewed as interactive processes between psychological, biological and environmental factors. Somatoform symptoms may mask anxiety or depression.

- Biological factors point to genetic transmission with concordance of 30 per cent for panic disorders in monozygotic twins. Certain substances stimulate anxiety, such as sodium lactate and caffeine.
- Cognitive, learning and behavioural theories suggest that anxiety and somatization may be attributable to a learnt response contributing to a highly strung personality style.
- Psychodynamic theory links anxiety to unresolved, unconscious psychological conflict that originates in the ego as it tries to moderate intense challenges from the id and superego. The ego resorts to a range of defence mechanisms to contain anxiety, such as somatization.
- Humanistic, existential and socio-cultural theories attribute anxiety to loss of a sense of self; concerns about the meaningfulness of life; and the need for self-actualization.
- Culture-bound explanations may attribute mental and emotional distress to ancestral communication, curses or omens.

When: anxiety and somatization may be precipitated by chronic and acute stress, emotionally charged environments and by coping strategies becoming overtaxed or defence mechanisms becoming ineffective. Cultural timing suggests that the distress occurs at a particular transitional life phase or as an ancestral call to pursue a particular course of action.

Who: Type A personality traits may be prone to anxiety whereas cluster-B personality disorders (histrionic) may somatize. Unassertive persons as well as those with low self-esteem or learned helplessness and maladaptive behavioural patterns are also vulnerable.

Where: in situations of societal, transpersonal, interpersonal and intrapersonal upheaval.

How: presentation of illness behaviour according to diagnostic categories for example panic disorder with or without agoraphobia, social phobia, phobic disorders, obsessive-compulsive disorders, post-traumatic stress disorder, acute stress disorders and generalized anxiety disorder. Somatoform disorders are classified into five specific types: somatization disorder, conversion disorder, pain disorder hypochondriasis and body dysmorphic disorder (Bothwell, 1998; American Psychiatric Association, 2002).

Disabling anxiety and somatic complaints: an occupational perspective

Psychiatric signs and symptoms tell a particular story about the person's internal turmoil, coping skills and residual capacities. A personal history and an occupational narrative provide clues about three possible factors exacerbating the anxiety or somatic complaint:

1. precipitating (what triggered the episode or illness process? what was the 'last straw' event or series of life incidents? what occupational crisis overwhelmed the person's coping capacity?)
2. perpetuating (what 'feeds' the anxiety or physical complaint, i.e. what keeps it going? which occupational dysfunction or risks prevent the person(s) from breaking the cycle of anxiety or somatization?) and
3. predisposing (what made the person vulnerable in the first place? which occupational risks or consequences inclined the person/group towards an anxiety or somatic illness?).

The focus of occupational therapy is usually to assist the distressed person to:

- understand the biopsychosocial and occupational factors that predispose
- alleviate, where possible, any biopsychosocial or occupational factors that precipitate, and
- minimize, where possible, those biopsychosocial or occupational factors that perpetuate the presence of anxiety or somatization.

While interested in and informed about the signs, symptoms, causative factors and functional consequences of anxiety and somatoform disorders, the occupational therapist is most interested in another set of data. This is information that, according to Hasselkus (2002), tells the client's 'phenomenological story about occupation' (p. 68). She suggests that 'occupation is a powerful source of meaning in our lives, meaning arises from occupation and occupation arises from meaning' (Hasselkus, 2002, p. 14). Being able to 'do' in daily life and finding fulfilment in such doing is the essence of wellbeing and lifelong development (Wilcock, 1998b). Living with disabling anxiety or (perceived) persistent somatic complaints changes the person's ability to perform and enjoy those tasks, activities, occupations and roles that bring meaning and purpose to life (Christiansen and Baum, 1997).

It follows that, if mental ill-health leads to the loss or disruption of familiar occupations and therefore meaning and purpose in life, the primary role of occupational therapy should be to address the occupational implications of anxiety and somatoform disorders. The main goal is, therefore, to help the client re-author a more hopeful story through perspective transformation about the self as occupational being.

Uncovering needs

Change is possible, according to occupational therapy philosophy, by facilitating the innate capacity and drive of humans to be creatively occupied (Wilcock, 1998a, b; Yerxa, 1998; Christiansen and Townsend, 2004). This capacity becomes stunted or obscured by the disabling effects of anxiety and somatization or by the contexts in which people live, work and play. The occupational therapist, taking both an occupational (Christiansen and Townsend, 2004) and a biopsychosocial (Stein and Cutler, 2002) approach to uncovering needs, uses a range of formal and informal assessment methods based on the principles of collaboration, empowerment and client-centred practice. The focus of assessment may be an individual, a group or a community or the context/environment within which people are occupationally engaged.

Uncovering needs: Principles

Collaborative inquiry; empowerment; client-centred information gathering

Methods

1. Observation: attending to and interpreting the meaning and purpose of verbal and non-verbal behaviour in structured and unstructured settings. The identification of co-morbid psychiatric conditions in patients with somatic complaints requires astute observation.
2. Measurement: use of standardized tools to provide objective data against which to measure extent of problem; determine priority domains of concern, outcomes of intervention and provide feedback on progress. For example:

   a) Battery of Anxiety Questionnaires (Powell and Enright, 1991)
   b) Occupational Self-Assessment (Baron, Kielhofner et al., 2002)

3. Evaluation: use of multi-axial taxonomies to diagnose disorder or ascertain level of functioning. For example:

   a) DSM-IV-TR™ multi-axial evaluation (American Psychiatric Association, 2002)

b) International Classification of Functioning (World Health Organization, 2001a)

4. Interview: semi-structured information gathering. For example:

   a) Canadian Occupational Performance Measure (Law, Baptiste et al., 1998)
   b) Occupational Performance History Interview (Kielhofner, Mallinson et al., 1998)

5. Narrative: occupational storytelling and story-making. For example:

   Stories of 'doing', 'being' and 'becoming ' through preferred occupational choices across the life span (Clark, Ennevor et al., 1996; Wilcock, 1998a)

6. Consultation: gathering and sharing collateral information from and with significant others (for example family, partner, employer, teacher); team members and role players such as community and inter-sectoral representatives. For example:

   Surveys and community forums: participatory inquiry and action methods to determine scope of need and expectations within a group/community (Kniepmann, 1997).

The occupational implications of disabling anxiety

Table 19.1 offers a framework for uncovering needs; determining the focus of action and ensuring a comprehensive, holistic and occupation-based approach to practice. It presents an integrated, holistic profile of the occupational human whose life has been disrupted by the onset or chronic presence of disabling anxiety or whose mental health is vulnerable because of occupational risk factors. It suggests six domains of interest that warrant attention during occupational therapy including a phenomenological interpretation of the illness experience. The reader is invited, where possible, to adjust the interpretation of Table 19.1 according to the cultural diversity and indigenous health practices of a particular client, group or community.

The occupational implications of disabling anxiety and psychogenic somatic complaints may be understood by using:

- biopsychosocial and occupational performance taxonomies (Christiansen and Baum, 1997);
- an occupational perspective of health (Wilcock, 1998b);
- the International Classification of Functioning (ICF); (World Health Organization, 2001), and the
- Diagnostic and Statistical Manual DSM-IV-TR™ (American Psychiatric Association 2000).

Table 19.1 The occupational implications of disabling anxiety and stress

Occupational risks (Wilcock, 1998) axis 4: DSM IV-TR (APA, 2002)	Experiencing anxiety (Patel, 2003)	Performance component impairments ICF (WHO, 2001) axes 1,2,3: DSM IV-TR (APA, 2002)	Occupational performance limitations ICF (WHO, 2001) 5: DSM IV-TR, (APA, 2002) Christiansen and Baum (1997) axis	Participation restrictions Bronfenbrenner (1977); ICF (WHO, 2002)	Occupational consequences (Wilcock 1998b) pp 137–151
LIFE EVENTS e.g. • occupational deprivation during childhood, e.g. limited play opportunities, poor role modelling of adaptive occupational performance • enduring trauma leading to learned helplessness or poor sense of agency in occupational behaviour NATURAL ENVIRONMENT e.g. • pollutants decreasing resilience of body and mind TEMPORAL ENVIRONMENT e.g. • lack of financial/practical means to do occupations of choice • few or too many	'I'm lethargic' 'I'm always tired and nauseous' 'The constant headaches get me down' 'I'm losing it, feeling out of control; like I'm going crazy' 'Something dreadful is going to happen; I can't stop expecting disaster any moment' 'My vision is blurred; things change size' 'My heart beats very fast and I feel like	COGNITIVE e.g. • poor concentration • indecisive problem solving • distorted, irrational ideas • obsessions, e.g. guilt, doubt • catastrophic thinking • self-critical thoughts • low self-esteem DISPOSITIONAL, e.g. • excessive drive, i.e. restlessness	SELF-MAINTENANCE e.g. • excessive sweating causing body odour • chapped hands with eczematoid appearance from excessive washing • gum lesions from excessive teeth cleaning • unkempt appearance from hair pulling TEMPORALITY e.g. • disorganized habit patterns and routines result in untidy living/working space • poor time management, e.g.	MICRO-SYSTEM • preoccupation with self and illness experience leads to avoidance behaviour, e.g. unable to participate in activities that promote independence and autonomy such as driving, shopping, visiting friends MESOSYSTEM • strained participation in relationships with significant others, e.g. • fear of people	OCCUPATIONAL IMBALANCE • restricted engagement in occupations that meet unique physical, social, mental or rest needs • insufficient time for a range of chosen and obligatory occupations, e.g. worker role overload means neglecting other roles • occupational forms appear irrelevant to survival; is more concerned with symptoms OCCUPATIONAL DEPRIVATION • illness behaviour keeps person from

Table 19.1 contd.

Occupational risks (Wilcock, 1998) axis 4: DSM IV-TR (APA, 2002)	Experiencing anxiety (Patel, 2003)	Performance component impairments ICF (WHO, 2001) axes 1,2,3: DSM IV-TR (APA, 2002)	Occupational performance limitations ICF (WHO, 2001) 5: DSM IV-TR, (APA, 2002) Christiansen and Baum (1997) axis	Participation restrictions Bronfenbrenner (1977); ICF (WHO, 2002)	Occupational consequences (Wilcock 1998b) pp 137–151
choices leading to occupational boredom or overload SOCIO-CULTURAL ENVIRONMENT e.g. • cultural values, e.g. gender roles and indigenous practices regulate or restrict occupational choice • decline of nuclear family and social networks leading to role overload; anti-occupations such as crime-related activities • changing patterns of work e.g. migrant labour, unemployment stress or executive burnout	fainting; sometimes I do' 'A suffocating and choking feeling in my throat...like I could die' 'It's like ants crawling over my hands, like pins and needles' 'Worry, worry, worry...that's all I do; in fact it stops me doing anything else' 'I go hysterical; I panic just thinking of... (phobia)' 'It's like a movie in my mind; I experience flashes	• demotivation • increase in activity levels • secondary AFFECTIVE, e.g. • irritability and tension • mood swings • aggression • depression 'burnout' BEHAVIOURAL e.g. • excessive substance abuse • difficulty sleeping • accident-prone • loss of libido • altered eating patterns • social withdrawal	compulsive cleaning therefore neglects other tasks • reduced PRODUCTIVITY e.g. • over-conscientious and perfectionism leads to work overload and their lifestyle • work habits decline as worry or phobias increase • unable to meet deadlines/commitments i.e. compulsions waste time LEISURE/PLAY/ CREATIVITY AND SPIRITUALITY • reduced pleasure and self efficacy in	reinforced by overprotectiveness of parent/partner gain, e.g. manipulation to keep relationships intact • family adjust around illness behaviour of client leading to resentment or co-dependency EXOSYSTEM • patterns of avoidance leading to withdrawal from formal and informal social structures, e.g.	acquiring, using or enjoying life opportunities occupational engagement leads to sensory deprivation or repetitive compulsions lead to sensory overload that in turn exacerbates anxiety symptoms OCCUPATIONAL ALIENATION • illness behaviour separates and estranges anxious person from the mainstream of society; becomes disconnected from the networks of community

Table 19.1 contd.

Occupational risks (Wilcock, 1998) axis 4: DSM IV-TR (APA, 2002)	Experiencing anxiety (Patel, 2003)	Performance component impairments ICF (WHO, 2001) axes 1,2,3: DSM IV-TR (APA, 2002)	Occupational performance limitations ICF (WHO, 2001) 5: DSM IV-TR, (APA, 2002) Christiansen and Baum (1997) axis	Participation restrictions Bronfenbrenner (1977); ICF (WHO, 2002)	Occupational consequences (Wilcock 1998b) pp 137–151)
	of it over and over' 'I'm on edge; hyper-alert; irritable; ready to blow up' 'I check and recheck, over and over; checking takes over my life' 'Everyone notices my nose; it's hideous'	PHYSICAL, e.g. • high blood pressure • migraine • stomach ulcers • asthma • cancer • skin rashes • diarrhoea/ spastic colon	previously valued hobbies, interests and 're-creation' activities • boredom or frenetic participation with little appreciation of restfulness	refuses social invitations; restricts lifestyle to cope with or focus on symptoms MACROSYSTEM • restricted participation in community/civil society, i.e. neglects civic duties	

A range of taxonomies and classification systems such as those used here are indicated because of the diverse contexts within which occupational therapy services are available to the public. This applies particularly in a developing context where the primary healthcare approach is used to interpret needs and identify critical action. The implications of pathological anxiety do not proceed in a linear direction from risks to consequences because each person's (group or community) vulnerability or illness narrative is unique and multifaceted. There are, in other words, no categorical distinctions between the implications presented in each domain in Table 19.1; only an attempt to make use of existing taxonomies to promote understanding, guide assessment and direct action.

Purposes and processes

The purpose of occupational therapy is to collaborate with clients in understanding and managing the occupational implications of their anxiety or somatization. Making sense and responding appropriately involves a four-stage cyclical process of reflection and action (Schön, 1983):

1. naming (identifying critical occupational and developmental needs)
2. framing (identifying principles and guidelines for action)
3. acting (implementing occupational therapy through reflection-in-action)
4. evaluating (ensuring relevance through reflection-on-action).

During this cycle, the occupational therapist makes use of a range of clinical reasoning skills and capacity development methods. In collaboration with the client (group or community), a plan of action is devised to meet the following purposes through occupation:

- promote mental health, wellbeing and quality of life
- prevent the onset of anxiety-related illnesses and disorders
- remediate performance component impairments or
- rehabilitate occupational performance dysfunctions stemming from disabling anxiety or psychogenic somatic complaints
- develop capacity for self-determination, full inclusion, participation and equalization of opportunities for persons with chronic anxiety or somatoform disorders.

The focus of comprehensive (prevention, promotion, therapeutic/curative, rehabilitation) occupational therapy may however be directed at different facets and stages of risk or recovery as depicted in Figure 19.1.

Occupational therapists, working in therapeutic programmes, help clients move beyond 'symptom pre-occupation' to 'symptom control and prevention' by acquiring self-helping habit patterns through health promoting occupations. These patterns of living promote functional adaptation to the challenges of life by organizing time and effort around valued occupations within chosen roles.

Prevention, promotion and psychosocial rehabilitation programmes aim to support the equalization of opportunities; social integration and self-determination of mental health consumers. In developing contexts occupation-based projects may become the means for poverty alleviation and capacity development, as well as inclusion of people living with disabling anxiety or other mental health concerns.

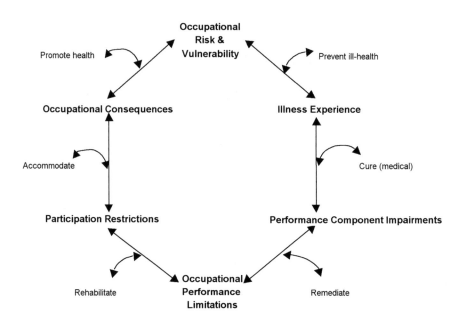

Figure 19.1 The integrated, comprehensive occupational therapy cycle.

Determining and sequencing priorities

The decision to assess or address the mental health, occupational or developmental needs inherent in any domain in Figure 19.1 will be informed by:

- whether an individual, group or population focus is indicated
- degree of vulnerability and risk
- stage of illness or recovery
- level of healthcare service or sector where action will occur
- context of service delivery
- type of occupational therapy programme indicated
- available resources and support.

A curative approach may, for example, be indicated for a patient with obsessive compulsive disorder who is admitted to an acute care facility at a tertiary-level state hospital. The aim of admission will be to contain the intensity of distress experienced by the individual and their significant others. Remedial, therapeutic action will be taken to address performance component impairments, for example cognitive restructuring for obsessions; sensory modulation or medication for restlessness; and therapeutic activities that channel compulsions. Interactive reasoning and teamwork will inform the most appropriate handling to shift the patient's sense of personal causation and agency.

As the person's internal turmoil subsides, attention may shift to addressing productivity limitations and participation restrictions. Psychosocial rehabilitation strategies such as supported employment and reasonable accommodation in the workplace may be indicated. By linking the client with consumer support and empowerment groups, action is taken to prevent relapse, promote wellbeing and create a feeling of solidarity against the oppression of the illness and social attitudes. The best timing for the client to join with others who share a common appreciation of the lived experience of anxiety and somatoform disorders will depend on stage of recovery, accessibility and availability of such support systems.

The occupational therapist who works for a local authority or with a primary healthcare team may direct his or her efforts not only at individuals, but also at groups and populations. Preventive and promotive occupation-based programmes within a particular community or geographical area may address occupational risk factors (for example, poverty and violence) that contribute to the development or exacerbation of anxiety and somatoform disorders. Smith (2003), for example, states that:

> patients presenting with somatoform symptoms are seen in a variety of medical settings and are a source of frustration because of their incessant visits and resistance to reassurance. Despite their relatively small numbers they are liable to consume a disproportionately large share of the available resources because of excessive consultations, special investigations and treatment. This imposes an important responsibility on doctors, particularly at primary care levels, to identify and manage these patients timeously (p. 156).

Preventative strategies such as support groups, income-generating projects or skills training workshops become useful forums for managing 'revolving door' clients (i.e. those who repeatedly enter and exit the health services). Psycho-education and occupational development offer containment to people who may otherwise seek medical support from an overtaxed health system. Skills training such as coping with anxiety and stress, awareness-raising about occupational deprivation, alienation and imbalance and education about the benefits of occupation for mental health and wellbeing may be conveyed (Wilcock, 1998b).

The mental health of families may, for example, be enhanced by introducing indigenous play (culture-bound or heritage games) sessions as part of occupational enrichment projects at health promoting schools. Play becomes the means by which youth may be coached in stress, conflict, and anxiety-management skills and learn about themselves as occupational beings. Community members (who may be mental health consumers themselves) develop resilience through training as lay stress counsellors or conflict mediators. Job creation projects become the vehicle for prevention and mental health promotion. The emphasis is, in other words, not on life skills training but on developing life skills through occupational empowerment (Duncan 2004). Health and quality of life are promoted and vulnerability contained through enriching and enabling the occupational repertoire of individuals and communities.

Action: grounded in theory and policy

The most appropriate plan of action is one that is based on an understanding of the occupational implications of disabling anxiety or psychogenic somatic complaints; an occupational perspective of health (Wilcock, 1998b) and an occupational development approach to therapy (adapted from Townsend, 1999, 2000). This is a plan that recognizes and taps into the benefits of both the social and medical models of disability (World Health Organization, 2001a) at appropriate stages in the helping process whilst remaining grounded in occupational therapy practice models such as:

- Person-Environment-Occupational Performance Model (Christiansen and Baum, 1997)
- Ecology of Human Performance Model (Dunn et al., 1994)
- Model of Human Occupation (Kielhofner, 1995)
- Person-Environment-Occupation Model (Law et al., 1996)
- Occupational Adaptation Model (Schkade and Schultz, 1992).

(for a helpful summary of these models refer to Christiansen and Baum, 1997, pp. 86–100).

Working within the context of a developing country also requires that therapists be grounded in community development and transformation models such as:

- Human Scale Development (Max-Neef, 1991)
- Education: the Practice of Freedom (Freire, 1974)
- Transformation through Occupation: a prototype (Duncan and Watson, 2004).

These models are particularly helpful for framing group- or population-based comprehensive mental health programmes.

Grounding in the therapeutic principles of the following biopsycho-social theories of anxiety and psychogenic medical complaints is also indicated, especially when addressing performance component impairments in individual clients:

- Physiological explanations: for example, Selye's (1976) seminal theory of stress.
- Behavioural and cognitive theories: for example, Beck and Emery (1985) and Astin (1997).
- Psychodynamic theories: for example seminal theories such as Freud's 1936 work on defence mechanisms and group analytic theorists such as Brown and Zinkin (1994) who describe the dynamics of socio-cultural influences on individual and group behaviour.
- Integrative models: for example, seminal work such as Holmes and Rahe (1967) sociological life stress theory.

A word of caution is appropriate here. All of the above theories are heavily influenced by a Western world view and are mostly inappropriate for explaining and addressing the origins of anxiety according to indigenous African world views. Occupational therapists working cross-culturally should therefore familiarize themselves with indigenous explanations of anxiety or persistent somatic complaints such as the role of ancestors and curses (Swartz, 1998).

Another useful source of information to frame any plan of action, especially programme development at all levels of the national health service, is a range of relevant policies affecting services for persons with mental health concerns such as:

- Psychosocial Rehabilitation Policy documents (World Health Organization, 1996; Department of Health, 2003).
- Ottawa Charter for Health Promotion (World Health Organization, 1986).

Becoming familiar with international and national mental health policies helps the occupational therapist to situate practice within the public health domain or within alternative, appropriate sectors.

Clinical reasoning: making sense of the client's health journey

According to Mattingly (1991) clinical reasoning in occupational therapy 'is a largely tacit, highly imaginistic and deeply phenomenological mode of thinking. It involves more than the ability to offer explicit reasons for clinical actions because it is based on tacit understanding and habitual knowledge gained through experience' (p. 979).

Types of clinical reasoning (Neistadt, 1998)

Procedural reasoning: the process of defining the client's (group/community) occupational performance, performance component and performance context needs or problems, selecting appropriate theoretical principles and developing guidelines for action.

Narrative reasoning: process of uncovering the client's (group/community) occupational story as told through preferred activities, habits and roles including the story of living with anxiety or a persistent somatic complaint. It may also become the client (group/community) and therapist's story of building a more hopeful future through shared problem solving and solution generating.

Interactive reasoning: understanding what happens and informs the interpersonal relationship between client (group/ community) and significant others, including the therapist.

Conditional reasoning: the process of understanding how, why, where, when and with whom to revise the action moment to moment within the change facilitation process. It involves 'thinking-on-your-feet' and 'reflecting-in-action'.

Pragmatic reasoning: consideration of the practical and logistical factors that impact on the outcome of action such as financial and social resources or infra structures in the action context and beyond, i.e. consideration of micro, meso and macro systems

Ethical reasoning: awareness of the moral, ethical and/or human rights and responsibilities that inform the helping relationship; professionalism and accountability to the client, public, self and employer.

Different types of clinical reasoning (Neistadt, 1998) may be used simultaneously or sequentially in tacit ways to address the problems of living that arise as a result of disabling anxiety or somatization. The various forms of clinical reasoning are applied here in somewhat linear and reductionistic ways so as to capture the essence of occupational therapy practice with anxiety and somatoform disorders. Refer to chapter 3 for more detailed information.

The examples under each domain in Table 19.1 may serve as helpful triggers for clinical reasoning and are described in greater detail below.

Domain one: occupational risks

According to Wilcock (1998b) occupational risk factors leading to vulnerability and ill-health include occupational alienation, deprivation and imbalance; lack of opportunity to develop potential, overcrowding, loneliness, ecological breakdown, substance abuse and a range of other socio-political precipitants. Stress and the onset of anxiety may be linked to life events and environmental factors that are occupationally compromising such as limited play opportunities resulting, for example, in the child not acquiring basic self-assertion skills or a sense of personal agency. Poor role modelling of adaptive occupational functioning or enduring stress and trauma may predispose the individual to adopt a fearful attitude and avoidance behaviour towards occupational challenges. Natural, temporal and socio-cultural environments also precipitate or perpetuate occupational dysfunction. The onset of anxiety and agitated depression may, for example, be linked to pressured jobs, boredom or enduring poverty.

Environments either press for over- or under-use of capacities. Wilcock (1998b) suggests that:

> if capacities are overused, people feel fatigue, stress and burnout, which can lead to increased susceptibility to accidents or illness. If capacities are under-used, they will atrophy, cause disturbance to equilibrium, and produce a decline in health. The balanced exercise of personal capacities to enable maintenance and development of the organism is perhaps the most primary and least appreciated function of human occupation (p. 118).

It follows then that occupational therapists have a contribution to make in the prevention of anxiety disorders and the promotion of mental health by addressing the occupational contexts within which people live, learn, work, play and worship (Wilcock and Townsend, 2000; Duncan and Watson, 2004).

Domain two: experiencing and living with anxiety

Anxiety is disabling because it immobilizes coping strategies. As Leslie Dallion explains:

> Anxiety? For me ... sometimes just going into a store and going to the check-out lane can be hard ... sometimes I have severe anxiety because I am worried about what they are thinking about me ... I also don't drive because of fear of accidentally getting into a wreck or hitting someone (I am 25 and not being able to drive is very limiting because I can't come and go as I like). I also have fears about someone breaking into my home, killers, it's an endless list of fears and it does alter one's life.
>
> > (www.livingwithanxiety.com; livingwithanxiety@groups.msn.com; www.panicportal.com. Accessed 12/9/03).

Occupational therapists are, in some ways, much like 'brokers' for living. By seeking to understand the person's phenomenological experience of anxiety, they are able to recommend a range of self-help resources and support networks. The purpose of such resources and networks is to:

- build a sense of solidarity in facing the challenges of living with an anxiety disorder
- share information and develop alternative coping strategies
- contribute to research and policy
- advocate for the rights of people with psychiatric disabilities (National Council on Disability, 2000; http://www.psych.org/psych/htdocs/public_info/bill_rights.html).

There is a growing mental health consumer lobby as well as information about the resources and support services available in South Africa such as the:

- Obsessive Compulsive Disorder Association of South Africa
- Mental Health Information Centre of South Africa
- Depression and Anxiety Support Group. These resources can be accessed at: www.sun.ac.za/local/academic/med/menhealt/index.htm

Particular attention needs to be paid to the ethical dimensions of practice. A few critical ethical issues that may arise in working with this group of psychiatric disorders are addressed in the box entitled 'Triggers for ethical reasoning'.

Triggers for ethical reasoning

Non-maleficence: be aware of your own anxiety and potential for being over-conscientious or punitive. Being too helpful will encourage passivity and dependence. Some people with somatoform disorders are exceptionally taxing and may evoke punitive (unconscious) responses from the therapist, such as deliberately over-treating a trivial condition.

Veracity: do not suggest that the person is dishonest; avoid any hint of criticism and never confront the person with an interpretation of his/her unconscious motivations without the necessary support. Beware of perverse benefits such as exploiting the patient's pathological illness behaviour (e.g. hypochondriasis or pain disorder) for financial gain.

Beneficence: take precautions pertaining to the side effects of medication, for example hypertension and drowsiness. Acquire an updated, basic knowledge of anxiolytics to feed back observations to the doctor or nursing staff.

Justice: where possible ensure equitable access to comprehensive occupational therapy and advocate for occupational justice (Wilcock and Townsend, 2000).

Human rights and responsibilities: promote the rights of mental health consumers to appropriate, affordable and accessible healthcare including occupational therapy and educate consumers about responsible health behaviours such as occupational balance.

Domain three: anxiety-related performance component impairments

The International Classification of Functioning (World Health Organization, 2001) provides a detailed description of current thinking about impairment. It suggests that impairments are significant deviation or loss in body function or structure (including psychological problems).

Anxiety causes a range of cognitive, dispositional, affective, behavioural and physical performance component impairments that restrict effective and efficient occupational performance.

Conditional reasoning in action

Handling a panic attack

A panic attack usually occurs suddenly and unexpectedly. It is an intense feeling of apprehension and impending doom, and is accompanied by a wide range of physical sensations such as dizziness, palpitations, nausea, paraesthesia of hands, feet and mouth, and chest constrictions. The person feels compelled to scream, run or hide and may be convinced that the symptoms are due to a serious medical condition such as heart disease or impending madness.

If a panic episode occurs during occupational therapy, the occupational therapist should:

- calmly tell the person that they are able to exercise control by slowing down their breathing. Provide systematic instructions that encourage smooth, slow, regular and fairly shallow breathing
- provide clear, rational suggestions that counteract the sense of desperation and urge to flee. Focus the person's attention on the surroundings rather than on negative thoughts and sensations
- encourage the person to recall relaxation principles and to slow down, especially breathing, in a similar manner
- cup hands over mouth so that no air from outside enters the lungs for a few minutes until the carbon dioxide calms the breathing down
- use firm handling to overcome lost initiative: clearly state what will happen next. Encourage the person to stay rather than avoid the situation
- review the incident with the person, allay fears and devise practical ways to cope with future episodes
- report the incident to the health team if indicated.

Handling a hysterical seizure

Some people may have both genuine and hysterical seizures, so distinguishing between the two can be quite difficult. Some features of a hysterical seizure are:

- it usually occurs in front of an audience and in relation to some emotional upset or to draw attention
- the person seldom gets hurt when falling; does not lose consciousness and there is no associated post-ictal confusion, drowsiness or amnesia as would be the case in an epileptic seizure
- movements are exaggerated and bizarre and do not conform to the typical tonic-clonic sequence of an epileptic seizure

- autonomic manifestations such as frothing at the mouth, cyanosis, incontinence and tongue biting are absent
- the hysterical episode may end gradually and is often decreased by inattention
- follow team recommendations for handling to ensure a uniform approach
- reassure other people in the vicinity that the situation is under control.

Occupational therapists, working within the medical model, focus on remediating impairments such as poor concentration, low self-esteem, free-floating anxiety and psychomotor agitation. Substantial use is made of procedural and conditional clinical reasoning to ensure suitability of fit between presenting complaints and remedial action. Short-term treatment aims in tertiary (specialist) psychiatric services are usually formulated to address performance component dysfunction of acutely ill persons. Attention is paid to the selection and structured presentation of activities and techniques that will afford therapeutic gains in a range of debilitating symptoms such as obsessions, compulsions, phobias, panic attacks and conversions.

Principles supporting therapeutic action are drawn from behavioural, cognitive behavioural, psychodynamic, existentialist and humanistic theories and occupational therapy models. The occupational therapist acts, amongst other roles, as teacher, model, motivator and facilitator. Use is made of a range of therapeutic and psycho-educational change modalities such as:

- anxiety and stress management training (Keable, 1989)
- relaxation therapy (Kennerly, 1995)
- task and socio-emotional groups
- social skills training including assertiveness and conflict resolution
- systematic desensitization i.e. gradual exposure to anxiety provoking situations (Powell and Enright, 1991)
- role-play and a range of behaviour modification methods such as modelling, role reversal, doubling and role rehearsal in simulated problem situations. Feedback, repetition and homework assignments are used to facilitate transfer of learning to everyday life
- psycho-education: videos, handouts and lectures about diagnosis and medication and information about support groups.

Triggers for procedural reasoning (acute settings)

Rationale: The distressed person may view activity participation as irrelevant to his/her immediate needs and problems. The usefulness of activities as a way of achieving better self-awareness and understanding of emotional difficulties can be clarified through education about occupation, joint recovery planning, goal-setting and regular evaluation of progress.

Planning: Starts after needs assessment and requires a clear understanding of precipitating, predisposing and perpetuating occupational, social and health factors as well as appreciation of occupational resources and enablers.

Presentation:

- demonstration and explanation in a matter-of-fact, logical manner. Focus attention on one component at a time and avoid urgent, hasty presentations and rapid changes during activities. This will increase tension and precipitate a negative response such as 'I'll never cope'
- repeating instructions as anxiety interferes with the ability to concentrate
- modelling a relaxed, problem-orientated, rational approach to hitches such as spilt paint or incorrectly followed directions that arise during activity participation. Review stress related sensory data, feelings and tensions that arise and discuss possible self-help solutions
- coach the anxious or somatizing person to 'listen' to his/her self-talk and to take charge over incapacitating responses through mindfulness principles
- encourage in vivo relaxation, i.e. relaxation response in action.

Criteria for selection of activities:

- activities that direct attention away from the self and rumination about symptoms. Provide opportunities to do things for, and with, others
- activities that foster communication and evoke a positive response from others. Examples are restoring broken toys for a children's home or making a gift for a relative
- activities that allow the anxious person to practise anxiety and stress management methods in action. For example, identify a series of activities, graded from least to most threatening, around a phobic situation or object. Select and implement these activities in consultation with the primary psychotherapist and the client. For example, the hospitalized agoraphobic who was housebound prior to admission may progress from a simple activity such as a manicure or a facial with the occupational therapist to a baking session with one other person to eventual participation in a group outing to a place of interest to transfer of training in personal life space
- select activities that will not be affected by physical symptoms such as sweaty, trembling hands or blurred vision
- activities that allow for constructive use of restlessness, i.e. aimless,

agitated behaviour, can be sublimated into goal-directed activity. Avoid fine coordination and dexterity (e.g. wood carving) and start instead with gross to medium range movement. For example, a brisk walk, swingball and table tennis may involve one-to-one contact with the occupational therapist who can, during the game, educate the anxious person about the value of exercise in the reduction of anxiety

- concrete activities that stimulate logical thought will promote decision making, improve self-esteem and reduce self-negating thought, for example, making (and flying) a kite or making (and driving) a wire car for and with a child
- activities that provide opportunities to experience, identify and express a wide range of emotions, e.g. sublimation of anger into physical actions (chopping, sawing, hammering)
- activities that allow the anxious person to discover the meaning of their symptoms. The assisted uncovering of conflicts and defence mechanisms should go hand in hand with opportunities to acquire and practise alternative, adaptive responses to anxiety-provoking life situations. For example, where depression is a feature, the resolution of guilt and anger may be indicated. Evocative media such as art, music and drama within a socio-emotional group context is helpful. Close cooperation with team members, and particularly the individual psychotherapist, is strongly advised
- activities that accommodate cultural mores and support indigenous healing practices.

Recent resurgence of occupation as the core purpose of occupational therapy, as well as the adoption of the primary healthcare approach, have challenged the profession to move beyond the biopsychosocial model and its emphasis on individual functioning. Attention is turning to critical-emancipatory (liberation through education, i.e. the individual is empowered through collective action) and hermeneutic (interpreting the socio-cultural contexts of living) models. These models position the individual in a system, group or community and situate the potential for personal transformation within socio-cultural processes.

Occupational therapists are, in other words, creating opportunities for the transformation of the occupational human (in illness and health) within a network of social systems rather than focusing primarily on the remediation of performance component impairments. Individuals living with disabling anxiety are supported in seeking meaning and purpose as occupational humans first and foremost. Life skills training and performance component remediation are seen to occur through occupational development (see below).

Domain four: occupational performance limitations

The chronic persistence of performance component impairments can have a disabling effect on the anxious person's ability to meet role demands. Free-floating anxiety, anticipation of imminent calamity, restrictions imposed by agoraphobia and time-consuming compulsions limit or restrict productivity and the constructive use of innate creative resources and time. For example, anxious people are seldom inclined towards hobbies, creative or sport interests because all available emotional energy is spent trying to keep anxiety under control. They may over-indulge in watching television or reading, abuse substances or eat excessively in an attempt to control or alleviate tension. People living in poverty do not have the luxury of 'over-indulgence' when they are very anxious; for them survival is an additional enduring stress that erodes their ability to adapt to role demands.

The detrimental side effects of insular, sedentary activities (for example, obesity and substance abuse) need to be considered. Excessive sweating, loose bowel movements, increased salivation, poor diet and lack of exercise all contribute to neglected self-care, compromised work habits and deteriorating role performance. Time spent on avoidance behaviour or compulsive rituals may, for example, lead to reduced productivity.

Hygiene and grooming may be problematic for some individuals, in particular those with secondary depression, hygiene-related phobias (for example, fear of germs) and time-consuming compulsions. Being overly preoccupied with one compulsion such as hand washing may cause the anxious person to neglect their appearance and general hygiene. Tense people also seldom rest well and complain of sleep disturbances. Chronic fatigue reduces productivity and leads to irritability and interpersonal tensions, as well as general lethargy. A range of valid and reliable occupational performance assessments is available (Law et al., 2001), making outcomes-based practice easier for the occupational therapist.

Attention may be paid to self-identified occupational performance areas of concern through structured participation in or education about:

1. Leisure/play pursuits: Reawakening an interest in a neglected hobby, introduction to alternative, economically viable, creative or sporting activities; education on the value of constructive leisure pursuits and awareness raising about available, affordable and accessible community facilities.
2. Self-maintenance:
   a) Exercise and rest: Exercise is a reliable means of symptom control, especially when anxiety is associated with repressed anger. Physical fitness strengthens the immune system and increases the endorphins that act as natural tranquillizers. Sport, aerobics, yoga and physical training, walking and drumming are some alternatives to add variety to an exercise regime (Keable, 1989). Collaboration with a physiotherapist is recommended.

b) Sleep: Self-management skills to deal with events that lead to poor sleep may be needed. An information leaflet covering topics such as sleep requirements for different age groups, stimulus control before bedtime, coping with difficulties in getting to sleep or waking during the night and sleep goals can be made available. In cases where withdrawal from medication is attempted, the person may experience severe symptoms such as perceptual distortions, panic attacks and insomnia (Powell and Enright, 1991).

c) Diet: Over- or under-eating may be associated with tension relief and secondary problems such as malnutrition or obesity. Basic information on the use of diet to control tension can be shared and referral to self-help organizations such as Weight Watchers and Alcoholics Anonymous may be indicated.

3. Spirituality and recreation: Spirituality, cultural and religious activities may offer respite from intrusive anxiety. Encourage meditation, contemplation and spiritual guidance as important dimensions of occupational balance.

4. Productivity: Anxiety erodes productivity. Time management and motivation decline, as does the energy to sustain effective and efficient work habits. Temporal disorganization exacerbates a sense of 'being out of control' and output standards drop, putting the anxious person's job at risk or reducing their capacity to maintain order in their working environment. This is especially important in countries where unemployment is high and there are few state benefits for the unemployed. The number of jobs in South Africa declined from 5.2 million to 4.8 million in 1999. Maintaining mental health and productivity is therefore essential for survival, especially if the anxious person has to be motivated enough to find alternative ways of generating income as a result of unemployment. Attention to skills development for goal-directed productivity, worker rights and income-generation strategies will go a long way towards alleviating anxiety, especially if the individual uses somatic defences to cope with work-related stress.

Domain five: participation restrictions

The International Classification of Functioning, Disability and Health (WHO, 2001) defines participation restrictions as

> problems an individual may experience in involvement in life situations or the "lived experience" of people in the actual context in which they live and conduct their lives. The context here refers to all aspects of the physical, social and attitudinal world (p. 122).

People with chronic anxiety or somatoform disorders may, for example, be restricted from participating in major life areas such as education, employment and community activities because of un-accommodating services and negative attitudes of other people.

Triggers for pragmatic reasoning

The illness behaviour associated with anxiety and somatoform disorders can be regulated internally by the individual and where needed, accommodated externally by the contexts within which they live, work, enjoy recreation and play. For example:

- pacing: setting realistic time frames and goals to compensate for time spent ruminating about illness complaint or for reduced attention span
- positioning: structure the environment to accommodate compulsive rituals or social phobia by, for example, enabling the individual to come and go (within reason) as the needs of anxiety dictate, and to participate at a level with which they feel safe and in control
- press: sufficient pressure to participate with graded support. The development of agoraphobia is, for example, exacerbated by avoidance and a restricted activity schedule. The less the agoraphobic does, the more time he/she has available to think about the first panic attack. Occupational press breaks the rumination/avoidance cycle
- habituation: anxious people get flustered easily, and while they may appear busy, they seldom experience the sense of achievement that comes from doing a job well. Developing effective habits for responding to routine demands in a timely and orderly manner can reduce day-to-day irritations and feeling out of control. Timetabling can be introduced with particular emphasis on those activities that the individual feels able to handle. Every time the person avoids doing something, it becomes harder the next time it has to be done, e.g. someone with body dysmorphic disorder who avoids mirrors and therefore does not groom. Adapting activity participation within a structured timetable and enabling graded exposure/desensitization can counteract the loss of confidence due to such avoidance
- contingency: set up contingency plans to deal with productivity decline and participation restrictions, e.g. panic attacks, conversion symptoms and compulsions may occur at work. Fear of being ridiculed, the stigma of psychiatric intervention and the loss of self-confidence may indicate the need for gradual reintegration into the worker role with support from the therapist and employer.

Reasonable accommodation and equalization of opportunities may be indicated based on the promotion of human rights of persons with mental disorders, for example:

- extra time for writing examinations in a suitable space, e.g. no distractions, close to a toilet or a room where person can pace up and down if needed
- supported employment, e.g. negotiated job adjustments to accommodate fluctuations in productivity

- access to generic medication if medical costs are too high
- counselling for significant others in the household or awareness raising workshops in the workplace to facilitate shifts in stigmatizing
  attitudes
- occupational justice, i.e. ensuring the right to health promoting occupations and occupational opportunities is exercised (Wilcock and
  Townsend, 2000).

Occupational therapists can make a significant contribution towards creating optimal environments because they are trained to enhance social
support systems in collaboration with disabled persons (McColl, 1997).

Domain six: occupational consequences

Note: domain six is closely linked to domain one, indicating the circularity and integration between the domains in Table 19.1.

Chronic anxiety is a risk in itself because it isolates, alienates and deprives
the individual (group or community) of qualitative engagement with life
opportunities. The long-term consequences of disabling anxiety may
therefore be occupational imbalance, deprivation and alienation (Wilcock,
1998b). A client-centred approach enables both the client and the occupational therapist to discover ways in which purposeful 'doing' may enhance
a sense of agentic 'being' that counteracts the powerlessness so often associated with anxiety. Occupation is presented, in consultations with the
client, as the primary method or means by which mental health may be
promoted. Meaningful and purposeful occupational engagement in a
range of valued roles and a personally satisfying occupational repertoire is
envisaged as the end point or outcome of wellbeing.

This may, however, be too optimistic given the contexts of pervasive
poverty and social disorganization in which many clients live. These contexts precipitate the onset or exacerbate the incidence of stress and
prevalence of anxiety and somatization disorders. It becomes crucial
under these circumstances that the client-centred approach be revisited
to include a community development perspective. The individuals as well
as the community become the 'client'. The occupational therapist adopts
an empowerment and development (as opposed to a therapeutic)
approach to mental health promotion and engages the capacity of individuals and groups to be self-determining by endorsing adult education
principles and empowerment through education (Freire, 1974). Both
client and therapist are able to make informed decisions about the way
forward in occupational therapy once a shared understanding of the
occupational implications of pathological anxiety and prolonged stress is
achieved and critical domains of action identified. To do this, the occupational therapist enlarges the client's (group and community) liberty and
responsibility by using participatory inquiry principles and action-reflec-
tion methods.

Client-centered practice revisited

Change may be facilitated through the client seeking assistance from a health professional in managing some aspect of his or her life; in this instance, the occupational disruption that ensues from pervasive and overwhelming anxiety or somatization. The core principle of client-centred practice (Christiansen and Baum, 1997) is the belief that the client, as primary agent of change, knows what he or she needs from therapy and that his or her interests, opinions and goals should therefore prevail during comprehensive occupational therapy processes. The occupational therapist may base his or her interactive reasoning on the following guidelines for handling persons with disabling anxiety or somatic complaints.

Triggers for interactive reasoning

Reassurance

Reassurance is one of the most helpful methods of allaying anxiety. Reassurance is however unlikely to shift concerns about somatic complaints in somatoform disorders and should be used in combination with firm limit setting. Reassurance can be offered by:

- validating the person/group's fears, physical and emotional distress and indicating that improvement is possible
- expressing an appreciation of the imposition of unwanted thoughts and acts on occupational performance
- pointing out positive, realistic attributes to counteract negative self-assessment
- acknowledging that symptoms are distressing but not dangerous, for example 'choking is a sign of anxiety and cannot hurt you' or 'the urge to check is a way of bringing your anxiety under control'
- engaging with the suppressed need for attention and affirmation. For example, people with conversion disorder may display 'La Belle Indifférence' towards their physical symptoms, i.e. they appear unperturbed by their physical condition. Offer reassurance by focusing on progress rather than physical complaints.

Encouragement

Encouragement helps the person/group build up feelings of personal security, ability and self-acceptance. It supports attempts towards adaptive, independent actions by focusing on strengths and resources. Encouragement is offered by:

- promoting realistic self-evaluation of performance, highlighting assets and personal responsibility for the outcome of actions and attitudes
- acknowledging attempts to get in touch with feelings as opposed to using maladaptive defence mechanisms

- providing opportunities to share and express emotions such as anger, guilt or sadness
- helping the person/group to be precise when describing feelings, behaviours and precipitating events. This prevents over-generalization; for example, people avoid a variety of situations on the basis of one anxiety-related incident that they have blown out of all proportion in their minds
- being practical about dramatic ideas by using cognitive restructuring principles, e.g. a hypochondriac or panic-stricken person who is convinced s/he is dying
- using persuasion and expressing faith in the person/group's ability to succeed. Helping them realize that facing, rather than avoiding, problem situations is the only sure way to improve; that mistakes are part of learning and that adaptive functioning is possible in spite of apparently incapacitating symptoms
- evoking a 'here and now' awareness of feelings during activity participation and helping people to deal with feelings and thoughts in-vivo, for example, using a suitable relaxation response; mindfulness strategies or changing negative self-statements into positive ones during occupational performance
- encouraging first-person statements ('I' rather than 'one') as these increase self-awareness and train the person to identify their own stress responses in body, behaviour and thoughts. By identifying discrepancies between actual events and internal experiences, the person can be shown that his/her assumptions may be distorted and need to be challenged.

Acceptance

Acceptance means allowing the person/group to be autonomous. It creates a sense of security in the helping relationship that frees individuals/group to take risks in facing up to problem situations. Acceptance is conveyed by:

- keeping any hint of criticism, frustration or resentment at bay. These emotions are likely to occur in response to the unreasonable demands of somatoform disorders for attention, frequency and extent of treatment
- setting realistic demands in terms of current and past abilities and offering justifiable recognition for responsible participation and commitment to occupational engagement
- accommodating idiosyncrasies such as rituals, tics and conversion symptoms.

Analytic attitude

Psychogenic pain or anxiety is essentially ego-dystonic, i.e. the person is distressed by the invasion of the symptoms (whether imagined or actual) as 'unfamiliar'. They use a range of defence mechanisms to cope with the unwanted/unpleasant affect. The analytic attitude enables the therapist to:

- offer the person/group some understanding of their defences
- remain aware of the possibility of counter-transference and take steps to work with transferences
- resolve the tension between empathy and apathy, under- and over-involvement and feeling 'drained' by the demanding behaviour of the patient/group.

Support and confrontation

Support and confrontation are both essential to promote change. Support without confrontation is insipid, and confrontation without support is destructive. Support and confrontation can be offered by:

- being available, within reasonable limits, to listen and counsel. It is particularly important to clarify limits of what therapy may offer and to set fixed appointment times especially with somatizing individuals
- investigating realistic courses of action, problem solving and decision making; sensitive use of reflection and interpretation
- modelling alternative, adaptive ways of being assertive
- giving honest, sensitive feedback or encouraging similar feedback within a supportive climate from group members as to the effect of behaviour on others. Encourage realistic self-appraisal in the light of such feedback
- evoking a 'here and now' awareness that clarifies feelings, motives, needs and response patterns and enables 'try-out' of newly acquired behaviour.

Integrated, comprehensive practice

Figure 19.2 depicts an integrated approach to occupational therapy practice. It juxtaposes domains of concern arising from anxiety and somatoform disorders with occupational interventions and solutions. Here the praxis between occupational enablers and strengths and occupational development forms the crux of occupational therapy.

Figure 19.2 is also a tool for educating clients about themselves as occupational beings and for promoting an occupational perspective of health. The anxious person is coached, with reference to the diagram, towards an appreciation of him/herself as the primary agent of change. By helping the client to externalize anxiety (i.e. it is a problem that can be proactively managed) and to internalize an occupational identity, their capacity for self-regulation is enhanced.

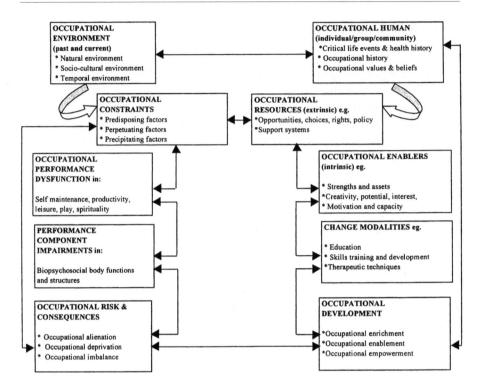

Figure 19.2 Occupational dimensions of integrated occupational therapy practice (Adapted from Wilcock A (1998b), Townsend E (1999)).

Descriptors: the occupational dimensions of integrated comprehensive practice

Occupational risk (adapted from Wilcock, 1998b):

Systemic and contextual factors that render the individual, group or community vulnerable or at risk of developing health disorders or conditions. (Risks and consequences are mutually inclusive, i.e. two sides of the same coin. Refer to circularity between domains in Table 19.1)

Occupational consequences (adapted from Wilcock, 1998b):

The outcome or results of long-term exposure to occupational risks, enduring adversity, vulnerability, 'disease' or disabling health concerns.

- *Imbalance*: Disruption of balance or equilibrium within and between intrinsic and extrinsic physical, mental and social capacities.
- *Alienation*: Estrangement or diversion from innate, natural creativity leading to separation from self, others, activities and products.
- *Deprivation*: Being restricted, kept or hindered from acquiring, using or enjoying innate capacities, interests and skills

Occupational constraints

Critical precipitating, perpetuating and predisposing problems and/or needs arising from occupational risks and/or consequences; occupational performance dysfunction and performance component impairments.

Occupational resources and enablers

Favourable extrinsic (contextual) and intrinsic (personal) factors that promote the attainment of positive outcomes or enhance the change process.

Change modalities

A range of specialized methods, techniques and strategies (such as relaxation therapy, life skills training, psycho-education, group work, art/music/movement therapy, meditation, psychodrama and alternative therapies e.g. Reiki, aromatherapy) aimed at promoting occupational performance.

Occupational development (adapted from Townsend 1999, 2000):

A core focus of the change and development process may be:

- *Occupational enrichment*: Expanding access, opportunity, scope, choice and balance of occupations
- *Occupational empowerment*: Promoting human potential, creative participation and productivity by addressing the balance of power, rights and responsibilities of the individual, group or community
- *Occupational enablement*: Facilitating competencies for creative participation in occupational opportunities.

This perspective on occupational therapy practice views occupation as more than the means by which health gains can be made; it also becomes the end. The anxious person is guided towards an understanding of him/herself as an occupational being whose identity, purpose and meaning are inextricably linked to 'doing'. The individual is empowered to view anxiety as an external (as opposed to an internal, medicalized) problem within his control through valued occupation. Non-prescriptive exploration of the occupational self across the life span enhances the client's appreciation of:

- his idiosyncratic occupational preferences
- occupational balance for sustained mental health and wellbeing
- activity analysis in making health promoting occupational choices
- socio-cultural influences (for example, gender and culture) in regulating occupational choice, access and participation.

The challenge for the occupational therapist is to think divergently about populations, communities and groups and convergently about individuals.

Different forms of thinking about practice will be required depending on whether service is direct (hands on with individuals or groups) or indirect (programme development/project management, consultation, policy implementation, etc.). The following box contains some examples of how Figure 19.2 may be used as a tool for critical thinking.

Critical thinking for integrated, comprehensive practice

- *Occupational environment*: what obstacles or facilitators currently exist in the micro (personal), meso (community) and macro (societal) environments in which this individual, group or community live, work and play? Which historical life events impact on the current and future adaptive capacity of the individual, group or community?
- *Occupational human*: what does the longitudinal occupational profile of the individual, group or community reveal about values, beliefs, interests and capacities? What do current occupational choices and time use patterns suggest about the health and development needs of the individual, group or community?
- *Occupational constraints*: which factors predispose, perpetuate or precipitate occupational risk in the individual, group or community? Which risks deserve priority attention and why?
- *Occupational performance dysfunction*: what self-maintenance, productivity, leisure or recreation (rest, creativity, spirituality) needs have been uncovered in the process of collaboration with this individual, group or community?
- *Performance component impairment*: which biopsychosocial performance components are amenable to remediation and what strategies are indicated for achieving change?
- *Occupational risks and consequences*: what evidence exists for the impact of imbalance, deprivation, alienation or injustice on human potential
- *Occupational dysfunction and maladaptation*: what adaptations (behavioural or temporal) have been made by the individual, group or community to cope with internal and external stress? How effective or ineffective are these coping strategies?
- *Occupational resources and enablers*: what assets, strengths, skills, capacities and potential are available (either within the person or the environment) that can be mobilized to promote health and wellbeing?
- *Change modalities*: what techniques, methods, models or strategies (e.g. use of self, group dynamics, social power) are best suited to enable participation, enhance potential and empower capacity?
- *Occupational development*: In which ways can occupation be used to achieve the goals and objectives of comprehensive (promotion, prevention, therapeutic, rehabilitation) healthcare? How may the ability of the individual, group or community to exercise their rights, responsibilities and self-determination be promoted?

Narrative reasoning: making sense of the occupational story

Listening deeply, respectfully and appreciatively to a client's narrative in order to extrapolate the occupational (as opposed to pathological) essence requires practice. All the types of clinical reasoning are applicable throughout the occupational therapy process but narrative reasoning may be the most challenging as it requires appreciation of ethnographic nuances. For example, there may be substantial differences between clinician and client in terms of age, culture, language, socio-economic and educational status as well as life experience. The following stories pose trigger questions for the application of narrative reasoning as well as integration of the perspectives described in the chapter.

Stories to elicit narrative reasoning

Story 1

A young man in his late twenties is admitted to a mental hospital with a conversion disorder involving paralysis of the right arm. His premorbid personality is described as extroverted with healthy interpersonal relationships and a wide range of interests. He is a committed member of a religious group that requires an oath of silence for extended periods of time. He converted to this religious order two years ago and has distanced himself from his traditional ethnic customs. His hysterical paralysis was quite advanced before it was noticed by members of the religious community where he lives. His left arm (non-dominant) has developed a mild contracture.

Questions

- What might the occupational disjunction be for this young man between his occupational history and preferences and the current occupational demands of the context within which he lives and practices his faith?
- What meaning might his paralysed right arm hold for him as the means by which he may re-engage with valued occupations?
- What might social anthropology and theology contribute to understanding this man's occupational needs?

Story 2

A middle-aged female is admitted to a private mental health clinic with severe claustrophobia and hypomanic behaviour. The police have brought her in because she was found running naked down a main street of the town. She has on a number of occasions during the past few months driven aimlessly for hundreds of miles in a panic-stricken attempt to get away from what she calls 'prison'. Investigations by the social worker reveal that this woman is virtually housebound by a severely disabled husband. He had a bilateral amputation eight months ago then suffered a stroke that has left him uncommunicative and he is too heavy to transfer easily. He did not receive rehabilitation, was sent home with a cumbersome, non-folding wheelchair and is unable to cope independently with self-care activities. The couple live on a farm and are isolated from social and support systems.

Questions

- In which ways might this woman's illness behaviour be a maladaptive response to occupational deprivation, alienation or imbalance?
- What is the interface between her mental health and her husband's health story and what might a more hopeful future story for them entail?

Story 3

Thandi, a 25-year-old Xhosa-speaking woman, presents with (apparently) bizarre choreoform movements of her face and hands including rolling eyes, protruding tongue and wringing gesticulations. She witnessed the gruesome murder of her uncle, with whom she had a close relationship, three months ago. She now ruminates about ways in which she could have prevented his death. She feels compelled to perform these movements to appease the ancestors whom she says spoke to her through the cow that was slaughtered at his funeral.

Thandi works as a cleaner in a clothing factory and lives with five other people in a small shack in an informal settlement that is renowned for crime, violence and poverty.

Questions

- Which occupational domains, in order of importance, will you address? Why and how?
- Which occupational risks rendered Thandi vulnerable and what might the occupational consequences be if she does not receive mental health intervention?
- What are the ethical and moral implications of pathologizing Thandi's behaviour when it may in fact be culture-bound? How might mental distress/illness and culturally appropriate behaviour be differentiated?

Story 4 (group)

Moira is a young housewife who has joined a support group for people with anxiety disorders being offered by a local mental health clinic. The group (approximately 6–8 people) meets once a week for one and a half hours. Shortly after the birth of her first child Moira felt compelled to wash the baby's nappies repeatedly and to hang them on the line in perfect symmetry with 90-degree corners. She is obsessed with the hygiene of the nappies. She is spending so much time performing these compulsions that both her child and general domestic responsibilities are being neglected. She seldom leaves the home and has difficulty bonding with her child. Prior to becoming a mother, she held a pressured job as a design consultant for a women's magazine.

John, another member of the group, is a 27-year-old accountant who recently got engaged. He is very comfortable in a small, close circle of friends but his worst fear is going to a party with his fiancée; even worse, the thought of the wedding ceremony sends him into panic. He has struggled with social anxiety disorder for a number of years anticipating that he will embarrass or humiliate himself whenever he has to talk in public.

Peter, also a member of the group, is a 57-year-old electrician who is recovering from a third laparotomy (investigative abdominal surgery) for chronic pain. He was referred for psychiatric assessment by the surgeon and physician as neither could find any medical cause for his pain. Peter has shared with the group that his wife is dominating, highly competent in her job and makes him feel redundant. They have no children, live in a small flat and seldom socialize.

Questions

- If the group were to listen to Moira, John and Peter's stories with the aim of getting to know them as occupational beings, what questions might other members of the group ask them?
- In which ways do Moira, John and Peter's occupational choices, interests and needs differ and which occupational development strategies will best suit each of them?

Story 5 (population)

South Africa is a very violent society. Law enforcement officers are particularly at risk of developing post-traumatic stress disorder. The incidence of suicide, substance abuse and domestic violence amongst this population is increasing, as are admissions to mental health clinics for a range of anxiety and depressive disorders. Police officers work long hours and seldom access counselling services, although they are available, and many apply for extended leave of absence due to work stress. One proactive police commander of a metropolitan district has launched a mental health promotion and prevention service for law enforcement officers (and their families) under his command.

Questions

- In which ways might violent (anti-)occupations in society become re-enacted by these officers in their personal lives as occupational humans?
- What information, using the comprehensive occupational therapy cycle, might emerge about the occupational needs of this population?
- In which ways might occupational justice be an issue in this scenario?

Conclusion

Recent developments in occupational therapy suggest a recommitment to occupation as the cornerstone of health and the foundation for the art and science of living (Wilcock, 1998b; Townsend, 1999; Whiteford et al., 2000; Christiansen and Townsend, 2004). According to Hasselkus (2002) this emphasis on the 'embeddedness of occupation in the lifespan human development may be the most powerful dimension of the relationship between occupation and well-being ... more powerful than occupation as therapy for recovery or improvement after disability ...' (p. 66). Some perspectives on how these developments may be operationalized in occupational therapy with people at risk of developing, or who are living with, disabling anxiety or somatization have been presented. Triggers for clinical reasoning have also been provided in the belief that competent practice is based on reflection and critical thinking about the impact of disabling anxiety on the occupational human.

Chapter 20
Three approaches and processes in occupational therapy with mood disorders

MADELEINE DUNCAN

This chapter suggests three complementary approaches and occupational therapy processes that may be followed in working with adults who have mood disorders. The *positivist* approach focuses on biopsychosocial interpretations and management of the mental illness or psychiatric disorder. It uses medically orientated processes to address mental health problems. The *narrative* approach is concerned with understanding the meaning individuals attribute to their life and illness experiences. It uses hermeneutic (interpretative) processes to explore meanings and turnings of an individual or group story. The *developmental action* approach is aimed at promoting collective action against the socio-cultural oppression that marginalizes people with psychiatric disabilities. It uses participatory action processes to promote the inclusion of, and equal opportunities for persons living with mental health concerns. Two case studies of people with mood disorders are used to illustrate the application of the three approaches and processes.

An overview of mood disorders

By 2020, depressive disorders are expected to be the second biggest cause of disease burden worldwide (Patel and Kleinman, 2003). This category of psychiatric illness is therefore of critical importance to mental health practitioners and communities that need to collaborate in stemming the tide of disease burden. 'Mood' refers to the internal emotional state of an individual and 'affect' to the external expression of emotional content. Mood disorders have a disturbance in mood as the predominant feature and may be divided into two broad categories, namely the *depressive* and the *bipolar* disorders.

Depressive disorders

Depression has been called the common cold of mental health problems.

The term can apply to a transient mood, a sustained change in affect, a symptom, a syndrome or a psychiatric disorder (Checkly, 1998). People with a depressive mood disorder report an ineffable and all-pervading depth of despair and hopelessness far beyond normal experience. Physical, social and personal role functioning is also greatly impaired (Checkly, 1998). Depressive disorders may present and be managed in five ways:

- *Adaptation disorder with depressed mood.* This is usually a reactive depression occurring in response to a stressful life event which the person fails to handle with their available coping skills. Intervention aims to support the person in coming to terms with the precipitating problem or to change their perception of the trigger events so that they can adapt to the challenges facing them. Psycho-education and life skills training such as management of stress and depression, guidance on how to lead a balanced lifestyle and support in conflict resolution will usually promote a rapid return to pre-morbid functioning.
- *Dysthymia.* This is a low-grade, neurotic depression situated in the personality of the individual who tends to find it difficult to cope with relatively minor life events. Intervention is aimed at personality maturation and the development of emotional and functional resilience through psychotherapeutic methods such as transactional analysis, cognitive behavioural therapy and assertiveness training. Occupational coaching may strengthen the individual's capacity for productive participation in significant life roles.
- *Major depression.* This is a serious mood disturbance with significant performance component impairments (for example, insomnia, anhedonia, loss of libido) and occupational performance dysfunction (for example, decreased productivity at work, inability to socialize and restricted participation in valued activities). Intervention is aimed at regulating neurotransmitter receptor dysfunction through antidepressant medication and at reducing the person's vulnerability to stress through insight-orientated psychotherapy and occupational adaptation.
- *Major depression with melancholia.* This is a very deep depression requiring hospitalization and carefully monitored pharmacological intervention. If the person does not respond to medication and a supportive psychotherapeutic environment, electroconvulsive therapy may be indicated, especially if the person is a serious suicide risk. Occupational therapy may, in the early stages of admission, focus on sensory integrative activation followed, in the later stages, by the same methods that apply to a major depression.
- *Major depression with psychosis.* This condition is very serious and the person usually requires protracted hospitalization. A dopamine blocker is usually prescribed together with an antidepressant and/or electroconvulsive therapy. Occupational therapy will be particularly concerned with the reintegration of the individual into his or her life roles after discharge with the aim of preventing relapse through reasonable accommodation and psychosocial rehabilitation. Optimal

participation in a range of meaningful occupations with appropriate support will facilitate wellbeing.

Signs, symptoms and functional consequences of depression

Table 20.1 Signs, symptoms and functional consequences of depression

Mild/moderate depression	Functional consequences	Severe depression
Indecisiveness Self-criticism Poor attention and concentration Worrying Questions the meaning of life	Insufficient drive and self-loathing may result in poor self-care, an unkempt appearance and a disorganized, untidy or dirty environment at home and at work	Vigorous self-denunciation Delusions of guilt or nihilism Excessive rumination about some imagined or actual wrong-doing
Sadness and pessimism Somatization e.g. headaches Irritability Low self-esteem Loss of spontaneity Inability to have fun Withdrawn	Secondary gain may be to adopt the 'sick role'. Avoidance behaviour leads to unproductivity which in turn reinforces low self-esteem, setting up a vicious cycle of occupational deprivation and imbalance	Deep sense of despair or rage Extreme feelings of unworthiness, hopelessness and helplessness
Chronic fatigue Apathy, loss of energy Insomnia Loss of interest in life tasks Weight loss or gain Loss of libido	Person avoids role-related responsibilities leading to strained interpersonal relationships at home, work and at play	Excessive agitation or psychomotor retardation Suicide risk Marked weight loss Severe sleep problems
Uncharacteristic behaviour such as temper outbursts and accident proneness	Masked depression may present as occupational imbalance or a self-destructive lifestyle for example: • 'workaholic' behaviour; person spends much time on the job without being effective or efficient • impulsivity in the use of substances/gambling/ sexual acting out	Psychotic behaviour such as bizarre motor tics; catatonic posturing or foetal positioning with loss of contact with reality

Bipolar disorder

People with a bipolar disorder experience both depressive and manic episodes. Swinging from one affective state to the other will vary from person to person and depends on how stabilized the person is on medication. The manic episode is characterized by 'an abnormal and persistently elevated, expansive or irritable mood at least once a week' (DSM IV-TM (American Psychiatric Association, 2000, p. 357)).

Mania is an extreme state of excitation and the person is clearly psychotic. In the early stages of mania (called hypomania), however, family and friends might experience the person as being 'quite fun' and the mood is definitely infectious! A person's sense of well-being and increased productivity may lead them to ignore more severe aspects of the illness, such as irritability, argumentativeness, insomnia and poor judgement. They may engage in sexual and other high-risk behaviors without appropriate appreciation of the consequences (Kaplan and Sadock, 2000).

Hypomanic symptoms can profoundly affect the person's social life, family life and employment if the illness is not medically managed. Kay Redfield Jamison, a psychiatrist who has experienced manic-depression at first hand confesses that 'I am too frightened that I will again become morbidly depressed or virulently manic – either of which would, in turn, rip apart every aspect of my life, relationships and work that I find most meaningful – to seriously consider any change in my medical treatment' (Jamison, 1997, p. 212).

Psychopharmacology is of utmost importance for functional integrity but the medication may produce severe side effects. People with a bipolar disorder therefore have a high relapse rate, i.e. 50 per cent in the first five months and 80 to 90 per cent within the first year and a half, because of a lack of compliance with medication. This is a clear indication to the occupational therapist that psycho-education must be a priority in treatment, for both the client and the family. As with depression, holistic treatment should also include exercise, support groups, vocational guidance, counselling, leisure enhancement, psycho-education, stress management and the creative arts. Relaxation therapy can be carried out only as the hypomania subsides. It is not indicated, nor is it successful, in the early stage of the illness because of the increased psychomotor activity.

Signs, symptoms and functional consequences of hypomania

Table 20.2 Signs, symptoms and functional consequences of hypomania

Hypomania	Functional consequences
Elevated mood, euphoria and irritability. An increase in sexual activity and lack of inhibition.	May be too agitated to care about taking a bath or washing hair
Racing and pressurized thoughts, flight of ideas, tangential or extreme circumstantial thinking. Jokes and punning are common and may have rude or vulgar connotations.	Grooming is overdone: for example, makeup is thickly applied
	Quantity of productivity is high but of poor quality
Hyperactivity, restlessness, distractibility and psychomotor agitation.	Starts projects impulsively with little foresight about feasibility or outcomes
Ideas of grandeur, unrealistic expectations, religiosity and the indiscriminate spending of large sums of money (if available).	Expansive interpersonal relationships without regard for others' wishes to communicate
	Occupational overload and imbalance
Loss of sleep that can occur for as long as three days.	

The positivist approach: biopsychosocial process

The term 'biopsychosocial' originated from the third Diagnostic and Statistical Manual of Mental Disorders III (DSM III) (American Psychiatric Association, 1994, p. xvii). This was the first nomenclature to introduce a multiaxial system for classifying mental disorders based on a biopsychosocial understanding of etiology.

> 'Biopsychosocial' approach implies that an etiology of a disease has biological, psychological, and sociological determinants such as genetic, developmental and environmental factors. In treatment biopsychosocial implies a holistic multimodal treatment approach encompassing medication, psychological counselling, exercise, nutrition, stress management and cultural considerations (Stein and Cutler, 2002, p. 616).

The biopsychosocial approach is helpful in defining, categorizing and assessing clinically significant behaviours and in offering the health team a common language for directing therapeutic and rehabilitative measures. The interpretation of psychological, social and occupational (as in work) 'functioning' on Axis V: Global Assessment of Functioning (GAF) Scale of the DSM-IV (American Psychiatric Association, 1994, p. 32) is strongly linked to the presence or absence of symptoms. It therefore medicalizes the concept of 'functioning' and reinforces a reductionistic approach to intervention, i.e. it focuses on the remediation of performance component impairment such as hypomania, depression, anxiety and low self-esteem and uses these as indicators of optimal psychological, social and occupational (work) functioning.

'Functioning' from an occupational therapy perspective is much broader than the absence of symptoms. Optimal functioning is linked to wellbeing, quality of life and the person's self-efficacy and mastery in choosing, organizing and performing those occupations he or she finds useful and meaningful in various living environments. Occupational therapists are concerned with enabling the person to live life fully by also addressing issues such as inclusion, reasonable accommodation and equal opportunities in the contexts where they live, work and play.

The biopsychosocial approach in occupational therapy is most useful in acute clinical settings where medically orientated processes and actions apply (Stein and Cutler, 2002). Techniques such as social skills and assertiveness training and evocative techniques may be used to promote insight and to equip individuals with basic self-regulation strategies. Activities, for example crafts, baking or sport sessions, may be used to 'improve functioning' in self-care, productivity and the constructive use of leisure time. Alternative healing therapies that offer clients self-help through art, drama, exercise and spirituality also promote the attainment of performance component health.

Table 20.3 Three approaches and processes in a nutshell

Positive approach	Developmental approach	Narrative approach
Biopsychosocial occupational therapy process (Stein and Cutler, 2002, p. 189)	**Participatory-action occupational therapy process**	**Hermeneutic occupational therapy process (Adapted from Schön, 1983 and White, 1995)**
1 Initial interview mental state examination commences	Invitation to participants to act as co-investigators of 'limit situations' and opportunities	Naming the problem or critical issue: • externalized descriptions of problems or issues i.e. objectifying and naming the core issue(s); • mapping the history of the externalized problem or developmental need, i.e. defining how the problem/ issue influences the person and how the person influences the problem/issue
2 Assessment (diagnostic category, problem identification	Exploration 'real-talk' (sharing of lives) i.e. participants uncover what they collectively experience as marginalizing and what brings hope and liberty.	Framing the action • co-authorship through power-sharing dialogue • joint process of creating an alternative hopeful story
3 Establish goals: long-term (LTG): functional performance short-term (STG): performance components	Identify patterns seek commonalities and differences; identify critical actions for change; negotiate roles and responsibilities.	Acting • intentional 'doing' to find unique occupational outcomes • continuous detection of clues to confidence in 'doing', 'being' and 'becoming'. • actively assembling an alternative story using externalized knowledges of capacity and hope to defy the problems' persuasion and oppression or theoretical issue's impact
4 Implement treatment: operationalize STG	Supply information add new knowledge, generate ideas, educate for transformation, draw on analytic ability of participants	Evaluating • creating an appreciative audience to cheer the client on • documenting evidence to serve as a permanent record of progress e.g. using reflecting teams, letters
5 Reassess/evaluate	Enable experiential learning practise skills in action, develop a learning/doing culture	Cyclical exploration, interpretation of text and discovery of meaning
6 Readjust treatment	Revision in hindsight	
7 Closure/follow-up to ensure symptoms stay in remission	Iterative participation and action	

Developmental approach: participatory-action process

The South African national rehabilitation policy is based on the principles of community development, primary healthcare and the social integration of disabled persons. Psychosocial rehabilitation (PSR) is a strategy that:

> facilitates opportunities for individuals with impairments, activity or participation restrictions due to mental health concerns, to reach their optimal level of independent functioning in the community. It implies both improving individuals' competencies and introducing environmental changes in order to create a life of the best quality possible for people who have experienced a mental disorder, or who have an impairment of their mental capacity which produces a certain level of disability (World Health Organization, 1996, p. 2).

PSR is a strategy within community-based rehabilitation (CBR). Both are philosophies to service delivery and are not services in themselves. In other words, CBR and PSR do not refer to 'what' is done but 'how' things are done (Department of Health, 2000, p. 6).

The objective of psychosocial rehabilitation is to instill hope and to create opportunities for people with mental health concerns to be successful and satisfied in their environments of choice with the least amount of professional intervention. An emancipatory perspective places the power in the hands of consumers who, through collective action, develop the capacity to direct their own healing and development. This is achieved at a macro level by building strategic intersectoral partnerships; challenging public opinions and attitudes; monitoring legislation; promoting quality assurance of mental health services and conducting research. At an individual level it may be achieved by addressing personal needs and promoting competencies in four PSR life areas: housing, working, socializing and learning. PSR technologies may include awareness-raising, symptom control, case management, psycho-education, life skills training, vocational enablement and income generation, social support and advocacy.

PSR: mobilizing community action

Occupational therapists are advocates for occupation. Their distinctive contribution to PSR is being agents for, and with, people who have mental health concerns, to move themselves collectively towards optimal participation in valued life roles and occupations of choice. This orientation is based on a belief in the capacity of human beings to help each other grow and develop, irrespective of the extent of need and disability. Occupational therapists are specialists in identifying and mediating the effects of occupational disruption, restriction and dysfunction on the mental health of individuals, groups and communities (Wilcock, 1998a). They do this through collaborating with consumers and multi-sectoral service organizations in setting up appropriate, affordable and accessible occupation-based resources and support systems based on community development and primary healthcare principles such as capacity building, local accountability and fostering partnerships.

Community development helps people transform existing environments that they find oppressive of their human needs into ones that meet their human needs. The participatory-action approach enables collective reflection and action upon the world. Through this consumers gain a sense of 'we-feeling' that propels them to change their circumstances. They participate actively in planning, delivering and evaluating PSR services for themselves and by themselves with minimal assistance from healthcare professionals. For example, income-generating projects such as breadmaking, recycling and gardening become the hub for peer support, psycho-education and life skills development (Duncan, 2004).

The occupational narrative approach: hermeneutic process

Narrative refers to the spoken or written account of connected life events in order of happening or in order of significance. Stories provide the structure of life and, if externalized or objectified through conversation or writing, provide the means by which to understand how the self is constituted (Polkinghorne, 1991). Many dominant stories or narratives are generated in the wider social discourses in which we live and the language (for example, metaphors and idioms) we use to describe our lives. Discourse refers to the taken-for-granted assumptions that lie beneath the surface of many conversations in a particular social context; for example statements about what is considered normal or conventional (White, 1991). Hermeneutic action explores and interprets these tacit meanings and helps people discover areas of competence, ability and agency that lie hidden within their personal narrative.

Instead of locating the illness problem in the person (as the biopsychosocial approach does), the narrative approach begins to locate problems and solutions in the cultural landscape of the person's story. This enables the construction of a hopeful storyline (which isn't always possible when a symptomatic or medicalized approach to therapy is followed) by exploring the meaning that persons attribute to their experience of a particular set of problems or events and how these meanings shape their lives.

Re-authoring an occupational identity.

Michael White (1991; 1995) introduced the notion of 're-authoring' to the narrative lexicon. He describes it as 'the process of facilitating the generation of and/or resurrection of alternative stories by being curious about preferred outcomes' (White, 1991, p. 29). As people separate from the dominant or 'totalizing' stories that constitute their lives (for example, the total invasion of depression into the fabric of thinking, acting and feeling or the control of hypomania over productivity and role performance), it becomes possible for them to orient themselves to aspects of their experience that contradict these knowledges.

Occupational narrative (storytelling and story-making) (Clark et al., 1996; Mattingly, 1998) seeks to externalize the meanings attributed to and purposes of significant tasks, activities, roles and occupations as these constitute the person's identity. By externalizing conversation about depression or hypomania (that is, situating it outside the person as a socially constructed phenomenon), its oppression over occupational engagement and performance may be challenged. The person comes to view themselves as an occupational being with control over the problems of living with a mood disorder by harnessing occupation as a means of personal power.

According to White (1991):

> as persons become engaged in these externalising conversations, their private stories cease to speak to them of their identity and of the truth of their relationships – these private stories are no longer transfixing of persons' lives. Persons experience a separation from, and alienation in relation to these stories. In the space established by this separation, persons a free to explore alternative and preferred knowledges of who they might be; alternative and preferred knowledges into which they might enter their lives (p. 29).

Occupational landscaping

Bruner (1986, in White, 1991, p. 28) points out that stories are composed of dual landscapes, i.e. 'a landscape of action and a landscape of consciousness'. The landscape of action provides a thematic unfolding of chronological events; in other words, happenings are linked in a particular sequence according to a particular plot through past, present and future. Occupational storytelling and story-making focus on the landscape of action in favoured occupations throughout the lifespan.

The term 'occupational being' refers to a person who is actively engaged in 'doing'; in being productive and in action, experiences a sense of self-worth and self-efficacy (Clark et al., 1996).

The landscape of consciousness contains the interpretations that the teller and the reader/listener make of the characters and events in the story. This landscape unfolds through reflection, speculation, realization and conclusions about the intentions, motives, characteristics, beliefs, preferences, etc. of the characters in the story. By acting as a life coach, the occupational therapist guides the client towards envisaging a hopeful future by asking questions that evoke an optimistic sense of self as occupational being (see Table 20.5, pp. 470–3).

Application of the three approaches and processes

The three approaches and processes described above are applied to two case studies with the aim of clarifying some key principles and procedures of occupational therapy with mood disorders.

Case study one: Andiswa's story

Andiswa, a 48-year-old Xhosa woman, was brought by the police to the female admission ward of a psychiatric hospital. She was found running naked in the street outside her home shouting that she was Ms. South Africa. Andiswa is well known to staff on the ward as she has had numerous admissions over the years because she is non-compliant with medication. She had her first hypomanic episode at the age of 28 and has been admitted to hospital approximately every two years since then, usually in a manic phase followed by a depressive episode.

Andiswa describes her life as uneventful until the birth of her third child. She recalls not being able to get out of bed, leaving the house in a mess and not caring what happened to her children. Her husband started beating her and when this did not work, he took her to a traditional healer. She took the medicine he gave her and slowly started feeling better. About a year later she remembers waking up one morning feeling very happy so she went out to find work. The next thing she remembers was waking up in hospital believing that she had been bewitched. Since then she has been in and out of hospital many times.

Andiswa and her husband live in a two-roomed brick and corrugated iron dwelling in an informal settlement. Their three adult children live close by but are unable to assist financially because they are all, like Andiswa, unemployed. When she is well she takes whatever casual cleaning jobs she can get to supplement her disability grant. There is a communal water tap and toilet in the street outside the shack. They have an electrical box but cannot always afford the pre-payment cards. There is no space for a garden, a lot of litter is lying around and in winter, when it rains, flooding occurs. Andiswa does most of her shopping at the spaza shops (home-based trading stores) in the neighbourhood. She uses a taxi to get where she needs to go as they are easily available. Andiswa is a member of the Women's League of a political party and of the local Methodist church. Her husband, a long distance truck driver, is often away from home. He beats her when he is drunk and he has had numerous extramarital affairs.

Table 20.4 depicts the use of the biopsychosocial process with Andiswa during an acute admission for bipolar disorder (manic episode).

Table 20.4 Andiswa – the positivist approach and biopsychosocial process

DSM IV-R Multi-Axial Evaluation DSM-IV (American Psychiatric Association 1994, p. 26)	Presentation of Hypomania (on admission) (Kaplan and Sadock, 2000)	Intervention		
		BIO (Example)	PSYCHO (Acute and subacute phase)	SOCIAL (adapted from World Health Organization, 1994)
Axis 1: (Clinical disorder) Bipolar 1 Disorder (most recent episode manic)	Flight of ideas Talkative Distractable Low frustration tolerance Psychomotor agitation Inflated self-esteem Irritable and argumentative Intrusive, impulsive and demanding Social irresponsibility (sexually disinhibited)	Haloperidol – antipsychotic 10 mg 2/day Side effects: akathisia, muscle stiffness and motor retardation, drowsiness Diazepam – anxiolytic 5 mg 2/day as needed No side effects reported Lithium carbonate – mood stabilizer: 1000 mg at night Side effects: tremors, nausea, thirst, diarrhoea, indigestion	**Handling of hypomania:** • unconditional acceptance with clear boundaries, structure and support • provide feedback on what is difficult about her behaviour and encourage her to take responsibility for controlling it herself • monitor and intervene if her behaviour affects other patients adversely	Commence PSR case management as soon as possible by focusing on: **1. Symptom control** referral to primary healthcare clinic close to Andiswa's home with recommended dosage of medication **2. Psycho-education** inform Andiswa and husband about bipolar disorder and importance of compliance **3. Social support** accessing wellness self-help/support groups close to home; marital counselling **4. Awareness raising** enable Andiswa to educate Women's League and church about her illness and needs; inform her about services for abused women.
Axis 2: (Personality disorder) Deferred dependent traits	When she is well she tends to be retiring, passive and subordinate	If tuberculosis or HIV is confirmed, the appropriate medication will be prescribed and referral to relevant support organizations will be made	**Choose tasks and activities that:** • are age, culture and gender appropriate; have purpose and hold meaning for her. • promote attention, logical thought, concrete judgement and post-ponement of gratification.	

Table 20.4 contd.

DSM IV-R Multi-Axial Evaluation DSM-IV (American Psychiatric Association 1994, p. 26)	Presentation of Hypomania (on admission) (Kaplan and Sadock, 2000)	Intervention		
		BIO (Example)	PSYCHO (Acute and subacute phase)	SOCIAL (adapted from World Health Organization, 1996)
Axis 3: (General medical conditions) ? tuberculosis, ? HIV (for investigation)	Eczema/ skin rash; unexplained weight loss, coughing, persistent low-grade temperature	**Education about medicine:** • Explain bipolar disorder and how medicine helps • Involve family to monitor and encourage use of pills • Explain and minimize side effects by regulating dose (liaise with doctor/nurse) • Stick to simple dosage schedules e.g. once a day • Stress regular check-ups and not stopping pills without consulting doctor	• direct restlessness into constructive outcomes • promote intellectual and emotional (at later stage of recovery) insight **Structure the treatment environment to:** • support or precipitate change in functioning such as interpersonal skills and work habits • Protect against exploitation • Prevent exhaustion (e.g, sexual/financial)	**5. Economic empowerment** link Andiswa with income-generation project run by mental health consumers such as bread baking and container mulch gardening **6. Life skills coaching** mental health promotion strategies, e.g. stress reduction; conflict resolution; budgeting **7. Advocacy** enhancing awareness of consumer rights and responsibilities.
Axis 4: (psychosocial environmental problems) problems with primary support system, economic problems	Marital discord Inadequate finances Neglected personal hygiene, over-dressed Gets by on very little sleep Disregards the rights and boundaries of others; Strained relationships Disorganized work habits, i.e. excessive quantity but poor quality of output; low endurance and unable to postpone gratification			
Axis 5: (Global Assessment of Functioning) Score: current 40 pre-morbid 65				

Case study two: Ronald's story

Ronald, a 31-year-old male with tetraplegia, was admitted to the psychiatric ward of a state hospital with a provisional diagnosis of adjustment disorder with depression. He was referred by his general medical practitioner who felt that Ronald would, in addition to anti-depressant medication, respond positively to psychotherapy and assertiveness training.

Ronald had recently moved from living with his family to a group home for severely physically disabled persons. He had no movement in his lower limbs but had sufficient movement in his right upper limb to direct his motorized wheelchair. Diagnosed with Hodgkin's Disease when he was four years old, he started losing his balance and sensation at 16 and became increasingly disabled after developing Syringea Myelia two years previously. He had partial bodily sensation; a syringo pleural shunt to relieve pressure on the spinal cord and experienced tiresome spasms. He received physiotherapy when indicated.

Ronald had a loving family and many supportive friends who enjoyed his good sense of humour. He completed a diploma in library information services and worked briefly as a liaison officer for an alarm company before his function decreased too much for him to continue working. The company could not afford to make adaptations to the workstations that he required. He lived with his parents until a place became available in the group home – a move he requested in order to broaden his social contact.

He always had what he called a 'rotten' self-esteem but began to strongly dislike himself soon after moving to the group home. He lost faith in his abilities to do anything and felt 'useless', 'good for nothing' and 'worthless'. His despair was made worse by insomnia, loss of appetite and an increasing resentment at the invasion of his privacy because of his dependence on a care attendant to meet his physical needs. He started ruminating about suicide, became agitated and lost interest in friends and family.

Table 20.5 Ronald's story

Ronald's story	Occupational narrative approach
Ronald: 'I was rock bottom when I went to hospital. Let's face it, who wouldn't be unhappy with a story like mine? I still struggle with depression and times of despair but knowing what it is and how to manage it helps a lot. The anti-depressant medication made a huge difference. I started feeling better after ten days. The mental health team helped me understand the vicious cycle of helplessness into which I had lapsed: loss of control left me feeling hopeless and therefore helpless which in turn made me passive and feeling more out of control. My negative thinking also went	**The aim of occupational narrative (story-telling and story-making) is to:** • determine the assumptions and meanings that lie beneath the texture of everyday life activities • enable the client to interpret their actions, choices and values in a range of occupations across the lifespan • help the person discover areas of competence, ability and agency in the face of occupational dysfunction • promote the development of a more satisfying and appealing story line aligned personal occupational preferences.

Table 20.5 contd.

Ronald's story	Occupational narrative approach
in circles: hating myself led to a negative view of the world and to a hopeless appraisal of the future. Life just didn't seem worth living anymore'. **OT:** 'Whilst gathering information at the start of our contact, Ronald showed me a one-page copy of his life story that he and his care attendant had compiled. It was a detailed account of his medical history rather than of his identity as an occupational being. This alerted me to the option of writing an occupational narrative with him. Storytelling and story-making would enable him to direct and lead the process from beginning to end thereby promoting his sense of agency and motivation to try something new. By remembering all the occupations that define his interests, innate abilities and skills over the years, his negative self-appraisal would possibly shift. He would come to appreciate that his life has been rich in productive activities and could potentially remain rich and rewarding albeit in a different form. An alternative occupational story may unfold as Ronald gains an appreciation of the link between doing, being well and becoming fully himself.' **Ronald:** 'I gained a lot from talking to the psychologist about my feelings and from group discussions. Life skills sessions were also helpful but the turning point in my mood really started when I came to appreciate myself as an agent in accessing occupational opportunities. I had given up hope but felt encouraged by Sacha's (OT) narrative approach to uncovering my practical needs. In the past people tended to concentrate on what was physically wrong with me and only ever asked about my health- or disability-related problems. She suggested that I become her partner in identifying what I was able to do as opposed to unable to do. I had become so preoccupied with my loss that I was unable to appreciate that I was still me in spite of being disabled.' **OT:** 'I decided that it would be easiest to write the occupational memories down on a large sheet of cardboard so that we developed a mind map or pictorial representation of those occupations that defined Ronald as an occupational being from childhood to the present. He chose to divide his life into two stages; childhood/ adolescence and early twenties to the present. We rated each memory on a scale of 1–10 in terms of the value, meaning and	**The core assumptions of the narrative approach (adapted from Epstein and White 1991) include:** • humans live their lives according to stories (*Once upon a time when I was able-bodied I ...*) • the stories we live by are not produced in a vacuum (*... I then ended up in a group home with other disabled people, kind of shoved to one side by society...*) • social discourses lie embedded within stories (for example, the taken-for-granted assumptions that lie beneath conversations in a social context about what is considered 'normal' for example being disabled or mentally ill is assumed to mean 'abnormal') • people align themselves with a range of contradictory and alternative social discourses (for example, social constructions of gender, power, race, ethnicity, sexual orientation etc. introduce a range of discourses) • dominant cultural discourses impose severe limitations on people seeking to create change in their lives (*it's hard to break through the stigma of disability; people seem to think that because you are in wheelchair you are also intellectually impaired and don't give you a chance*) • deconstructing dominant cultural discourses raises new possibilities for living (*understanding how cultural assumptions about privilege and power operate made me see my disability in a new light*) • there is always some dimension of the lived experience that does not get encapsulated in a story (*some dimensions of the disability experience are intensely spiritual and personal; beyond words or definition*) **The storytelling and story-making process (adapted from Clark, Ennevor and Richardson, 1996) consists of:** *1. building a communal horizon of understanding* • negotiate co-authorship • power-sharing dialogue • respectful relationship • curiosity, optimism and tentativeness • vigilance about dogma and cultural stereotypes • pre-eminence of person's knowledge • inclusion of the ordinary so that therapist suspends self and experiences the world of the client as closely as possible

Table 20.5 contd.

Ronald's story	Occupational narrative approach
enjoyment. The recalling of memories was initially difficult for Ronald but once he got the essence of occupation, the rest flooded back. As he responded to the medication, his affect became more animated whilst recalling favoured occupations. At times memories returned in order of occurrence and at other times he jumped all over the place as some occupations reminded him of others at a different time of his life. I kept in touch with the psychologist he was seeing to ensure that the occupational narrative process did not impede his psychotherapy.' **Ronald:** 'Sacha was a really good listener. She was very involved with my stories, asking questions that got me thinking about who I became when I was actively engaged in meaningful occupations. At the end of each session she helped me identify the underlying themes and gave me some reflective homework assignments. At least I had something purposeful to occupy my thinking when I struggled with insomnia! It became clear to me that I was a group-orientated person who enjoys socialising, spending time outdoors and that animals inspire me. I had her in stitches with my stories of cowboys and crooks; a game I played with a gang of boys. Sacha then introduced the idea of occupational story-making and building a future story line. She suggested that I start thinking of viable ideas to give expression to who I was as an occupational being in spite of being severely disabled.' **OT:** 'Ronald started proposing ideas linked to the themes that emerged from his storytelling sessions. The first addition to his life was linked to his love for animals. He enjoyed watching the birds outside his window and came up with the idea to install a birdfeeder. Purely by coincidence I had one I no longer used and offered it to him. This in fact led to our first outing into the world of activity. We went to buy birdseed and while visiting the pet shop, investigated another idea Ronald had of getting some fish for his room because the upkeep would be minimal and he longed to share his room with another living thing. He led the entire shopping expedition and was decidedly proud of his initiative. As with all his ideas, he initially sees them as impossibilities and doesn't have the faith or belief in himself to attempt any. My support enabled him to break the negative rumination and inactivity cycle. I also made regular use of curiosity,	*2. Occupational storytelling* • probing the history of the client in his or her world of activity as an occupational being across the lifespan • elicit stories in time and by value • story analysis and synthesis: finding common threads, themes and a central plot *3. Occupational story-making* • constructing a meaningful future based on an appreciation and vision of the self enacting valued occupational plot(s) • coaching: making links between wellbeing and 'doing', assembling an alternative/ modified activity repertoire • enabling participation: adapting strategies • creating place: harnessing environmental opportunities for engagement *4. Affirmation* • appreciative audience • documenting achievement, e.g. letters, reflecting teams (see example of letter below) White (1991) suggests a range of questions that enable the landscapes of action and consciousness to be externalized, scrutinized and reconstituted. A few examples of questions, for the purposes of an occupational narrative, have been adapted from White: • What can you tell me about your history that would help me understand you as a 'doing' individual? • What have you witnessed in your life up to now that could give you some hint about what inspires your activity choices? • I would like to get a better grasp of how and why you do certain occupations. What did you notice yourself doing, or thinking, as a younger person, that could have provided some clue that your particular interests in this occupation was on the horizon? • What do these discoveries tell you about what you need and want from the activities that you participate in? • Let's reflect for a moment on your occupational history. What new conclusions might you reach about your tastes; about what is appealing to you; about what suits you as a person? • If I had been a spectator to your life when you were a younger person, what do you think I might have witnessed you doing then that might help me understand what your occupational needs are now?

Table 20.5 contd.

Ronald's story	Occupational narrative approach
i.e. I enabled him to re-author his occupational sense of self by posing questions that challenged the hegemony of depression.'	• Exactly what activity choices would you be committing yourself to if you were to more fully embrace this knowledge of yourself as an occupational being?
Ronald: 'Once I got the hang of linking my activities to my essence as an occupational being, I came up with the idea of doing volunteer work at an old age home. My first visit was rewarding because I was able to give to others. It certainly snapped me out of my preoccupation with my limitations. By this stage I had been discharged and was seeing the OT as an outpatient. We cooked up the idea of fundraising through selling tickets for organisations at a busy mall close to the group home. I could get all the talking I so enjoy while doing something really worthwhile for society. My first attempt was enriching; a morale-boosting experience that I have repeated many times. In fact, I now have a reason to get up in the mornings and have started to write a book about my life living with a disability.'	• What conclusions might those persons who know you reach about your intentions to build a stronger occupational foundation for a balanced life? • If you could attribute a name to the depression what would it be? In which ways have you taken steps to ring fence the influence of (name of depression, for example, 'terminator') on your participation in mothering (sport, holding down a job, self care, etc.)?
OT: 'It was important to do a contextual assessment to identify, with Ronald, those opportunities available in his immediate environment and within easy access to the group home that could be harnessed to enrich his life. We discovered that four of the residents owned voice-activated computers and immediately started thinking of ways in which Ronald could work towards acquiring one. The anticipation of e-mail contact and making new friends on the Web motivated him to save enough to buy one, which he eventually did. I terminated therapy after three months and bumped into Ronald a year later at an amusement park. He had arranged for a friend to take him on a roller coaster ride …. he said he was choosing to live fully.'	**AFFIRMATION:** letter to Ronald (an example) Dear Ron, What a wonderful anti-depression event our outing to the pet shop proved to be. I was privileged to witness you taking a stand against the oppression of depression through seeking out an occupation that would bring purpose and meaning to the time you spend in your room. You spoke excitedly about the inspiration you gain from watching birds and about the potential of expanding this occupation to include a fish bowl and birdfeeder. How may you continue to use your understanding of occupational enrichment to resist the invasion of depression? What may participation in alternative occupations enable you to become?
Ronald: 'During my last session with Sacha we reflected on the unfolding narrative of my life and the power that lay in my own hands to construct a more hopeful future. I realized how many of my occupations involve friends, family and other people, all of whom accept me and choose to spend time with me. I know that my medical prognosis is poor and that depression is a realistic response to loss. I also know that doing something with and for someone else is, for me, the best anti-depressant I can take when the future seems bleak. Sacha wrote me a number of letters after every occupational breakthrough. I often refer to these when the going gets tough'.	You sounded particularly motivated to try out a visit to the old age home and to volunteer to sell tickets at the mall. I can see a good fit between the innate properties of these two activities and your occupational essence. You thrive on connecting with and serving other people. What conclusions can you reach about other occupations that match your interests and abilities? How may
OT: 'On reflection, I came to appreciate the need for occupation in Ronald's life and how the lack of it was negatively influencing his wellbeing. I was able to grasp the bigger picture of enabling participation and of occupational enrichment instead of becoming too focussed on his performance component dysfunction. We did find solutions for some of his functional difficulties such as an assistive device to facilitate independent eating. His assertiveness skills and self-	

Table 20.5 contd.

Ronald's story	Occupational narrative approach
esteem developed through occupational engagement and was reinforced by psychotherapy and maintained by anti-depressant medication. Once he owned and acted on the story-making process he began to see potential for change.'	your proactive stand against depression and occupational deprivation enable members of the group home to join you in opposing the marginalization of disabled persons? Wishing you lots of fun discovering new dimensions of your occupational self! Cheers for now, S

Capturing change: outcomes-based practice

In this clinical setting use was made of the International Classification of Functioning and Health (ICF) (World Health Organization, 2001) as an outcome measure of Ronald's progress in selected domains of functioning, activity and participation in his lived environment. The ICF is a health and health-related classification that incorporates The Standard Rules on the Equalization of Opportunities for Persons with Disabilities (World Health Organization, 1994). It does not classify people, but describes the situation of each person within an array of health or health-related domains. The ICF is a

> 'conceptual framework for information that is applicable to personal health care, including prevention, health promotion, and the improvement of participation by removing or mitigating societal hindrances and encouraging the provision of social supports and facilitators' (World Health Organization, 2001, p. 7).

It offers psychosocial occupational therapists access to a common, universal language for mapping functioning and psychiatric disability of individuals and populations. Users are strongly recommended to obtain training in the use of the classification through WHO and its network of collaborators.

In a clinical setting the ICF:

- may be used as a uniform reporting framework from the person's entry point into the service system through to their reintegration into society
- allows the involvement of the person in the definition of outcomes
- may be used to describe the situation of the person within an array of health and health-related domains
- enables the occupational therapist to complement and expand the global assessment of functioning on Axis 5 of the Diagnostic and Statistical Manual (American Psychiatric Association, 2000)
- is a useful research and statistical tool to measure outcomes, quality of life and environmental factors.

The ICF has two parts, each with two components:

Part 1: Functioning and Disability (classifies body functions, structures and activities and participation). This part captures information on impairments as well as activity limitations and participation restrictions.

Part 2: Contextual Factors (classifies environmental factors and personal factors). This part captures information on the physical, social and attitudinal environment in which people live and conduct their lives. Each component in the two parts can be expressed in both negative and positive terms and consists of various domains and categories that are the units of classification. These may be coded and qualified, i.e. by adding qualifiers to the allocated code, and the extent or magnitude of the functioning (performance and capacity). Disability may be described as well as the facilitators or barriers impacting on social integration and participation.

Interpreting meaning: ICF and occupational therapy

The ICF does not classify personal factors such as the particular background of the individual, gender, race, lifestyle, habits, values, interests, education, past and current life experiences, overall behaviour and character style, individual psychological and a range of other idiosyncratic features. It is therefore not holistic and client centred in the way that occupational therapists define these concepts as therapeutic stances. The ICF does not, for example, take into account the richness of purpose and meaning that people derive from functioning in the world, from occupational engagement and social participation. The ICF definition of functioning is, in other words, not aligned with occupational therapy philosophy or theory about humans as meaning-making beings through functioning, participating and occupational engagement.

Activity for the occupational therapist is more than the ability to perform a skill or a function; it is a communication process whereby thoughts and feelings are expressed non-verbally and the means whereby human growth and development occur. Occupational therapy theorists agree that 'through action on and interaction with the environment, humans grow and develop those skills and abilities that enable them to be competent members of society and to gain a sense of self and social worth' (Miller and Walker, 1993, p. 267). Through interaction with objects and people in their environment, humans respond to an innate need to be meaningfully and purposefully engaged in the process of exploring and mastering their environment.

Through action-orientated experiences, humans test skills, clarify relationships; integrate and develop sensory, motor, cognitive and psychological functions; become socialised to cultural norms and roles and gain competence as social beings (Miller and Walker, 1993, pp. 266–267).

Occupational therapists believe that 'doing is becoming' and that activity is directed by the 'being' or essence of the individual (Wilcock, 1998b). The occupational nature of humans is, in other words, the core business of the profession and the occupational therapist who uses the ICF as a tool for outcomes-based practice needs to bear this orientation in mind. Despite the discrepancies in interpretation of core constructs, it nevertheless offers a useful means for communicating across disciplines and for demonstrating the outcome of intervention with reference to funders and quality assurance mechanisms.

ICF coding: an example

It is useful to identify a set of generic domains for coding (there are four levels, each more complex and detailed than the previous) for a particular occupational therapy service. In the mental health setting, adult clients may present with any of the psychiatric disorders classified in the Diagnostic and Statistical Manual IV-TR (American Psychiatric Association, 2002). Sets of cross-diagnostic critical indicators were therefore selected in each of the components (body function and structure, activities, participation and environmental factors) to provide a baseline (i.e., only first level coding) health information system for the occupational therapy service in the psychiatric unit.

The ICF components are denoted by prefixes (*b, s, d, e*) in each code followed by a dot and a qualifier (for example scale of severity) from 1–4:

- *b* for body functions. For example b7302.1 describes body (*b*) impairment of power of muscles of one side of the body (*7302*). A MILD (5–24%) impairment would be recorded as *.1* (b7302.1). A point two (*.2*) would mean MODERATE impairment (25–49%), *.3* = SEVERE impairment (50–95%) and *.4* = COMPLETE impairment (96–100%).
- *s* for body structures. Similar qualifiers are used after the dot as for body function impairments. A set of three qualifiers may follow the dot in which the first digit describes the extent, the second the nature and the third the location of the body structure impairment. For example *s110.181* describes the structure of the brain with mild impairment (*.1*), not specified (*8*), on the right side (*1*).
- *d* for activities and participation. For example d710.12 describes basic interpersonal interactions with mild (*.1*) performance difficulty and moderate (*2*) capacity.
- *e* for environmental factors. For example *e310. +03* describes the support and quality of relationships of the immediate family (*310*) as no barrier (*0*) with substantial (*+3*) facilitation.

Each client is assessed on a predetermined set of outcomes-based practice indicators on admission and at discharge and the data are processed at regular intervals to describe service outcomes.

Table 20.6 The ICF codes used as outcome measures: an example

Component	Client	Folder No.	Domain	Codes and Qualifiers (Entry Date)	Codes and Qualifiers (Exit Date)	Outcomes
Body function and structure	R.S	XYZ	Global psychosocial functions	*b122.3* (severe impairment)	*b122.1* (mild impairment)	*.2* improvement in function
Activity and participation			Community and social life (recreation and leisure)	*d920.41* (complete difficulty)	*d920.2* (moderate difficulty)	*.2* improvement in functioning
Environment			Attitudes (individual attitudes of personal care providers/ assistants)	*e440.2* (moderate barrier)	*e440 + 2* (moderate facilitator)	*.4* improvement in external world that has an impact on Ronald's functioning

Conclusion

Mood disorders are on the increase and deserve serious attention in comprehensive healthcare services. This chapter has highlighted three alternative and complementary approaches to occupational therapy with mood disorders. Examples of how the approaches may be applied in acute settings, in community-based rehabilitation and in people's homes have been suggested. The use of the ICF as an outcome measure for all three approaches has been explained using one case study as reference. Flexible approaches are indicated in the South African context due to the vast disparity that still exists between resources in established mental healthcare facilities and grassroots clinics. A balance between the social and medical models of practice is also advisable to accommodate the needs of clients from acute admission through to community reintegration.

Acknowledgements

Appreciation is extended to Ingrid Magner, occupational therapist and lecturer at the University of the Western Cape, for sharing Andiswa's story. Sacha Percy did the innovative occupational narrative work with Ronald (pseudonym) during her final fieldwork placement as an undergraduate occupational therapy student at the University of Cape Town during 2001.

Details of the stories and context have been modified to convey principles of practice rather than factual accuracy.

Questions

1) List advantages and disadvantages of an occupational vs performance component focus in occupational therapy with mood disorders.

2) What, in your opinion, may be an appropriate description of Ronald and Andiswa's occupational status at the time of their admission to hospital (e.g. occupational deprivation, alienation, imbalance)?

3) What are the occupational justice issues that you may consider raising with the management of the group home where Ronald is residing or with policy makers in the health district where Andiswa resides?

4) What do you envisage as a reasonable outcome for Ronald and Andiswa after OT?

Chapter 21
Understanding and treating people with personality disorders in occupational therapy

ANN NOTT

> It is worse to be sick in soul than in body, for those afflicted in body only suffer, but those afflicted in soul both suffer and do ill. (Polish proverb)

Personality refers to the characteristics and behaviour that make up an individual's adjustment to life and includes major traits, interests, values, self-concept, abilities, drives and emotional patterns.

Personality traits are the enduring, subjective patterns of perceiving and relating to oneself and one's environment in a wide range of social and personal contexts. These behaviour patterns should be relatively stable, predictable and consistent. When one's personality traits become inflexible, maladaptive and rigidly pervasive, and deviate from cultural standards, it can be said that a personality disorder exists (DSM-IV-TR™, (Gillis, 1986; Profis, 1992; American Psychiatric Association, 2000).

Personality disorders have an onset in adolescence or early adult life and continue through most of life. As behavioural patterns interfere with function, causing significant impairment in social and occupational spheres, occupational therapy is an integral part of treatment assisting the individual to be more functional in daily life.

The personality disorder group is seen in 10–20 per cent of the general population (Gillis, 1986; Robertson et al., 2001).

The person with a personality disorder is clinically less impaired than those with other disorders of mental health but functionally more disabled. Superficially they may present as stable, have relatively good jobs, are intelligent and seem to cope with life. On closer examination, deeply ingrained maladaptive behavioural patterns are operational with no feelings of anxiety about their present behaviour. This is compounded by symptoms that are alloplastic (blame is put on others) and egosyntonic (their behaviour is right). That is, someone with a personality disorder is much more likely to refuse psychiatric help, point out the therapist's problems, and persist in fixed behavioural patterns perpetuating problems for which they seek assistance and causing scepticism from colleagues in other disciplines on the competence of psychiatric treatment (Robertson et al., 2001; Sadock and Sadock, 2003).

People with personality disorders are associated with poor treatment outcomes as they are very time-consuming due to their locus of control being external. People with personality disorders typically lack insight, have motivational problems, are resistant to change, are anxious or agitated with behaviour that is manipulative and overtly or covertly self-defeating.

The occupational therapist requires a good understanding of this condition because, behind a façade of seemingly coping and competent behaviour, is a person who may have all or a combination of the following problems:

- Struggles to cope with stressful situations.
- Is lonely and isolated.
- Has fluctuating labile mood.
- Has poor self-concept with low self-esteem.
- Is unable to cope with responsibility, decision making.
- Feels inadequate.
- Has reduced social skills (especially assertiveness skills).
- Struggles to form mature relationships.

As will be seen, this group of clients exhibit a wide range of impairments and disabilities in performing their roles in society. It is established that their problems may relate to crime, alcohol and drug abuse with elevated levels of separation, divorce and child custody hearings.

Long-term prognosis can be poor with a revolving door syndrome of repeated hospital admissions. Contributing factors are: reduced potential for insight with an inability to self-regulate behaviour, co-morbidity on Axis 1, reduced support systems as relationships are superficial, abusive or turbulent, and impaired occupational functioning with either a fluctuating or chaotic work record, conflicting or awkward work relationships, etc. However, some features such as aggression become less apparent as the person enters middle age (Galder et al., 1996).

Conversely, some individuals have a good prognosis in excellent work histories, supportive networks and willingness for therapy.

This chapter aims to give a broad outline of personality disorders and to clarify issues surrounding them. It will provide different models, treatment approaches and techniques that will enhance the quality of occupational therapy.

Using an eclectic approach in which different theories and models are studied, the occupational therapist becomes equipped with knowledge so that occupational therapy is given from a solid foundation.

What is a personality disorder?

Diagnosis of personality disorders is based either on the DSM-IV-TR™ (American Psychiatric Association, 2000) coding on Axis II or using the ICD-10 Classification. The World Health Organization (1992) classification, ICD-10, makes a basic differentiation between organic personality disorders, enduring personality changes derived from catastrophic experiences, habit and impulse disorders, gender identity and sexual disorders, and personality abnormalities that reflect a residue from some mental illness. It also outlines nine specific personality types (Rutter and Taylor, 2002; World Health Organization, 1992). The DSM-IV-TR™ (American Psychiatric Association, 2000) system specifies 11 types. Features must be seen as separate from the mood and panic disorders found on Axis I. If personality disorders from different clusters occur together, a mixed personality is specified. When there are overriding features such as a depressive, passive-aggressive, sadomasochistic and sadistic personality, the disorder is described as personality disorder not otherwise specified (Sadock and Sadock, 2003). For the purposes of this chapter the focus will be solely on the three clusters as outlined by the DSM-IV-TR™.

The occupational therapist analyses the person's ethnic, cultural and social background to ascertain whether symptomatology is an expression of habits, customs, cultural adaptations and belief, rather than a disorder. Relevant pointers include attitudes to illness, religious beliefs and moral standards (Galder et al., 1996). Certain cultures may enforce submission to authority and contribute to development of a personality disorder (Robertson et al., 2001).

Gender distribution differs among the personality disorders. Predominantly in men, there are the antisocial, schizoid and obsessive-compulsive personality disorders; the avoidant and dependent personality disorders are seen more frequently in women (Robertson et al., 2001). Sexual identity disturbances are clinically observed to suggest homosexuality with the male borderline person and with the woman presenting with antisocial personality disorder features. However, social stereotyping is contraindicated.

In order to treat this disorder effectively, the occupational therapist requires knowledge of the types of personality disorders and their psychodynamics. This will direct choice, selection and focus of treatment.

Cluster A

'Odd' or 'eccentric' behaviour characterizes this cluster with the onset occurring in early adulthood. This group comprises paranoid, schizoid and schizotypal personality disorders (Sadock and Sadock, 2003). They are also termed the 'sensitive and suspicious personalities' (Galder et al., 1996).

A pattern of pervasive distrust and suspiciousness of others is a distinguishing feature of a paranoid personality disorder.

There is an inability to take responsibility for their own feelings and a tendency to interpret others' actions as being deliberately demeaning, threatening and exploitative. A tendency to be pathologically jealous occurs in this group (Profis, 1992). Brief psychotic episodes may occur during times of stress (Robertson et al., 2001).

The schizoid personality has an indifference, detachment and discomfort in social relations. They may pursue their lives with little need for emotional ties and give the impression of being cold and aloof. They are reclusive and pursue solitary tasks (Robertson et al., 2001).

The schizotypal person is strikingly odd, strange and eccentric and displays magical thinking, ideas of reference and derealization. Differentiation of own feelings is a struggle, but sensitivity in detecting the feelings of others is prominent. Thought disorder is absent but communication is disturbed with observed peculiar behaviour and social detachment (Sadock and Sadock, 2003).

Cluster B

This cluster is characterized by 'emotional', 'dramatic' and 'erratic' behaviour, and incorporates the 'extroversion' concept of Carl Jung (1933). Other terms described are the 'dramatic and impulsive' and 'aggressive and antisocial' personalities (Galder et al., 1996).

The histrionic has a high degree of attention-seeking behaviour, with exaggerated thoughts and feelings. Temper tantrums and false accusations (if not the focus of attention) with seductive behaviour are common. Relationships are superficial, inconsiderate, vain and demanding with manipulative threats, e.g. suicide, being displayed. This group seem to mature with age (Sadock and Sadock, 2003).

Narcissistic personalities, due to their heightened self-esteem, consider they have the right to special treatment and are grandiose and self-absorbed, with reduced empathy. They handle criticism poorly by expressing indifference or rage, or by humiliating others. Narcissistic rage is often linked with some crimes. Due to high levels of ambition and selfishness they are exploitative in interpersonal relations. Clinically, they were found difficult to treat as ageing is poorly handled – as a result of beauty and youth being so overvalued (Profis, 1992).

A pervasive pattern of instability in mood, relationships, behaviour and self-image characterizes the borderline personality disorder. Relationships vacillate between idealization and devaluation. Impulsivity is ever-present with inappropriate anger and loss of control as in suicidal threats, self-mutilation or temper tantrums. Identity disturbance relating to sexual orientation or self-image can be present. There are marked shifts in base-line mood from depression to irritability. Chronic feelings of boredom or emptiness are a common symptom.

The antisocial person has an inability to conform to social norms, with a disregard for law and order. As they have a veneer of charm and seduction, only collateral information will reveal truancy, lying, thefts, fights and abuse of others. No remorse is expressed unless they are caught and one should guard against them using the treatment facility as a hideaway from prison.

Cluster C

This group is characterized by anxious and fearful behaviour, and reflects Jung's (1933) introversion concept. Other descriptions would be anxious, moody, prone to worry, low self-esteem and confidence (Galder et al., 1996).

The avoidant person presents as socially inhibited, inadequate and hypersensitive to negative evaluation. Socially they are timid, fearful and uncomfortable. They tend not to have close friends outside their family circle as they avoid rejection and fear of social embarrassment (Profis, 1992; Sadock and Sadock, 2003).

A pattern of dependent, submissive relationships is part of the profile of the client with dependent personality disorder. They are unable to make decisions and allow others to decide for them. Their behaviour is passive and abuse by others is common. They are easily hurt by disapproval and criticism and preoccupied with abandonment.

The obsessive-compulsive personality is perfectionist, inflexible and rigid in their approach to life with excessive control, extreme devotion to work, unreasonably high demands on others and a preoccupation with rules, order and details. Affect is restricted and indecision common. (This differs from obsessive-compulsive disorder in that there is no anxiety base, the obsessions and compulsions are not recurrent and no distress is experienced.) Inherently, there is a rigid personality framework whereby lifelong patterns and standards are imposed on self and others (Profis, 1992; Robertson et al., 2001), and crisis occurs when order is disrupted or change enforced.

Understanding the etiology and development of personality disorders

Personality disorders result from an interaction of genetic with upbringing factors (Galder et al., 1996).

Incorporation of both genetic and constitutional factors in the causation of personality disorders has been well documented (Profis, 1992; Sadock and Sadock, 2003).

One should look at a combination of these four separate theoretical frameworks:

1. Dynamic model – is based on internal organizing psychology resulting from conflict experienced in early life, with emphasis on developmental factors.

2. Trait model – this considers all possible personality types with inter-personal behaviour as the core.
3. Biological model – personality is ascribed to genetic or biological pre-dispositions.
4. Sociological model – regards personality as shaped by social circum-stances; pathology is based on deviance from social norms and harm to society.

Freud believed that fixation at a stage of development led to a certain per-sonality types, e.g. oral fixation contributed towards dependency and an anal fixation led to obsessive-compulsive personality traits (Robertson et al., 2001).

The basic cause appears to be faulty childhood rearing, resulting more from the parents' attitude than their actions. Onset is at an early age and is precipitated by parental neglect, rejection, loss or lack of adequate parental models for identification. The results manifest in late adoles-cence, when behaviour becomes a fixed, pathological way of coping with life (Gillis, 1986). It was noted that dysfunctional parenting in childhood was associated with the dramatic and anxious DSM clusters but not with Cluster A (Rutter and Taylor, 2002).

Genetic factors such as the XYY chromosome appearance, abnormal EEGs and a high threshold for emotional stimulation are the complexed components of the antisocial personality disorder. Clinical experience suggests father to son inheritance of the antisocial person. Biological studies showed shortened rapid eye movement (REM) latency, sleep con-tinuity disturbances, soft neurological signs, abnormal Dexamethasone Suppression Test and an abnormal Thyrotropin Release Hormone test with borderline and antisocial personality disorders. There is an etiologi-cal correlation of borderline personality disorder with childhood sexual abuse (Rutter and Taylor, 2001). Children with borderline intelligence are at risk for personality disorders (Sadock and Sadock, 2003). The most clear-cut finding from family studies is the association of schizophrenia and schizotypal personality in the biological relatives (Robertson et al., 2001; Rutter and Taylor, 2002).

Millon (1984) analysed personality and brought about a renaissance of theory and assessment, whereby he stated that there were very rarely pure personality types, and thus devised eight diagnostic criteria providing a descriptive and comprehensive guide to personality disorders. The occu-pational therapist will gain valuable insight by referencing these (given in Table 21.1) as emotional and cognitive factors recorded which are absent in DSM-IV-TR™, where the emphasis is on behavioural components. From this, the Millon Clinical Multi-axial Inventory was devised to screen peo-ple with these disorders.

Knowledge of background history is essential for comprehending the dynamics and the basis for therapeutic intervention.

Table 21.1 Millon's chart of personality theory and assessment

INTRAPSYCHIC ORGANIZATION	MEAGRE	FRAGILE	UNDEVELOPED	DISJOINTED	SPURIOUS	UNBOUNDED	COMPART- MENTALIZED	DISCORDANT	FRAGMENTED	DIFFUSED	INELASTIC
Internal composition	Indifferent	Avoidant	Immature	Shallow	Contrived	Pernicious	Concealed	Irreconcilable	Chaotic	Incompatible	Unalterable
Self-perception	Complacent	Alienated	Inept	Sociable	Admirable	Competitive	Conscientious	Discontented	Estranged	Uncertain	Inviolable
Unconscious mechanisms	Intellectual-ization	Fantasy	Introjection	Dissociation	Rational	Acting out	Reaction formation	Displacement	Undoing	Regression	Projection
Affective expression	Flat	Anguished	Pacific	Fickle	Insouciant	Hostile	Solemn	Irritable	Distraught or insentient	Labile	Irascible
Cognitive style	Impoverished	Distracted	Naïve	Flighty	Expansive	Personalistic	Constricted	Inconsistent	Autistic	Capricious	Suspicious
Interpersonal conduct	Aloof	Aversive	Submissive	Flirtatious	Exploitive	Antagonistic	Respectful	Ambivalent	Secretive	Paradoxical	Provocative
Behavioural presentation	Lethargic	Guarded	Incompetent	Affected	Arrogant	Fearless	Disciplined	Stubborn	Aberrant	Precipitous	Defensive
Personality	Schizoid	Avoidant	Dependent	Histrionic	Narcissistic	Antisocial	Compressive	Passive-aggressive	Schizotypal	Borderline	Paranoid

According to Galder et al. (1996), assessment to determine personality disorder should be validated by four sources:

1. client's own description of personality
2. client's behaviour during the interview
3. client's account of behaviour in a variety of past circumstances
4. views of relatives and friends.

The occupational therapist has a multi-functional approach and with the use of diverse activities would confirm the diagnosis.

Common defence mechanisms

The occupational therapist needs to understand the defence mechanisms used by the person with a personality disorder, i.e. the unconscious mental processes that the ego uses to resolve conflicts.

Splitting

This is predominant with histrionic and narcissistic personality types and is used, for example, to divide staff members or self into the 'good' and the 'bad'. As a result, the client may play one off against the other.

If regarded as 'good', the occupational therapist can be emotionally seduced and may start colluding, to the detriment of progress and therapeutic intervention.

Denial

This is a defence mechanism commonly found with the introversion cluster of personality disorders (avoidant and dependent). Confrontation is essential for behavioural change and is best achieved within a group context by a fellow member.

Repression

This is common with schizoid and obsessive-compulsive personality disorders. Feelings and needs are repressed and denied.

Projection

This defence mechanism is common in most personality disorders, especially paranoid. The personality disorder clients may try to merge their personal boundaries with those of the therapist and will point out faults, rather than face the pain of confronting their own problems. Awareness of this manipulative mechanism will allow the therapist to differentiate from the over-intrusive client and not get hooked into pathological dynamics.

Introversion

This mechanism is mostly seen with the borderline personality who participates in self-damaging acts which are the end result of an internal struggle against depression, anger and frustration and converted into self-mutilation. The occupational therapist should be aware of the person's internal struggles and allow for externalization of aggression in a constructive way to relieve the pain.

Models of treatment intervention and teamwork

Personality disorders are more likely to frequent Accident and Emergency units and crisis centres, and to call telephone counselling services.

Treatment usually takes place in a psychiatric unit, clinic or outpatient department. The person with a personality disorder usually tends to settle easily within the contained environment of the hospital. Therapy in a rehabilitation facility where the team has a unified treatment approach and frame of reference is recommended. Family involvement and early establishment of supportive networks is essential in successful outcomes. Post-discharge should look at maintaining support and containment through case management, ongoing review, self-help groups and ongoing individual or group therapy.

Behavioural approaches

Because it is difficult to change personality structure and stereotypical behavioural responses to stress, many theorists opt for a behavioural approach to teach appropriate responses to stressful situations. It is a long-term process consisting of operant behaviour (positive feedback for appropriate behaviour and ignoring negative behaviour), which allows the person to experience feelings of wellbeing and success by participating in positive tasks, even if they are not always continually reinforced (classic conditioning). Occupational therapy interventions such as relaxation and assertiveness training are behavioural in essence and by observing appropriate behaviour in all social settings, the avoidant and dependent persons can practise new skills.

Dialectical behaviour therapy

Linehan (1993) found that cognitive behavioural treatment was the best procedure for borderline personality disorders and expanded this theory to create a model called Dialectical Behaviour Therapy (DBT), which includes skills training based on biosocial and psychosocial theories. Dialectics refers to both the fundamental nature of reality as well as persuasive dialogue/relationships and refers to the treatment approach the therapist adopts to effect change.

With personality disorders there is an interrelatedness of stresses and processes and as such skills need to be learnt simultaneously to bring about change. Thus the occupational therapist may need to teach self-regulation skills, e.g. assertiveness, together with skills for positively influencing the environment such as stress management in the workplace.

As reality is not static and requires change in acquiring skills, there is positive validation and a shift in others' opinions. It is a dynamic model of intervention and may benefit other personality disorders.

Cognitive behavioural approaches

Cognitive therapy is used to treat symptoms and abnormal behaviours which persist because of the way the client *thinks* about them and behaviour therapy is used to treat symptoms and behaviour because *of actions* taken to relieve distress. Because *thought and action* often occur together a cognitive behavioural approach is used (Galder et al., 1996). Most cognitive behavioural therapies require specialized training; less complex procedures can be accomplished by a competent occupational therapist such as anxiety management, relaxation, etc. (Scott et al., 1989). Clinical experience has shown that obsessive-compulsive disorders benefit most from this approach. Applications such as assertiveness are useful for avoidant personalities.

The therapeutic community model

The therapeutic community comprises a containing environment in a ward of a hospital/clinic or a rehabilitation centre. The entire psychotherapy unit is involved and a supportive, consistent environment is created to allow for emotional growth and behavioural change. Important aspects to achieve this goal include: effective communication on all levels (covert, overt, verbal and non-verbal); group meetings, for example, climate meetings, goals groups and feelings groups; cooperation in programme planning and specified task roles for the team members.

Within the unit are structural elements to contain the personality disorder client in their state of crisis, so that they are able to mobilize their internal and external resources (Branch, 2003).

These structural elements consist of the following:

- Limit setting – the client is provided with the knowledge of rules and is encouraged to take responsibility for behaviour by signing contracts focused on containing destructive behaviour, e.g. self-harm, substance use and treatment contracts (see Appendices 1a, b and c, pp. 503–4).
- Early decision on discharge date – certain disorders such as dependent and borderline personality disorders display behavioural regression when there is mention of discharge, which takes the form of self-injurious behaviour, anxiety and panic or suicidal attempts. A clear knowledge of the process and length of hospitalization alleviates this and allows for personal and family planning.
- Goal-oriented approach – a collaborative approach in treatment encourages the person to set realistic goals which can focus occupa-

tional therapy, treatment and selection of groups based on specific
needs (Appendix 2, pp. 504).
• Family feedback – family feedback on coping skills and behaviours during hospital leave allows for change to be monitored and treatment
modified (Appendix 3, pp. 505).

Pharmacological interventions

The personality disorder presents on admission in crisis, with polypharma-
ceutical interventions in a desperate attempt to cope. Consolidation of
medication becomes a necessity. Medication is prescribed to deal with specific symptoms such as agitation, anxiety and depression. With 'at risk'
clients with a tendency to dependence, benzodiazepines are restricted to
short-term use. It has been suggested that they are avoided because of
dependency (Robertson et al., 2001). Anti-psychotics are often required for
acute control of impulsivity and damaging behaviour, psychotic episodes
and long-term behaviour management. Minor tranquillizers assist when
there is drug and alcohol withdrawal. If there is a presenting eating disorder, antidepressants are considered (Profis, 1992). Anxiolytics and selective
serotonin re-uptake inhibitors (SSRIs) may help to blunt the symptoms of
the obsessive-compulsive personality disorder (Robertson et al., 2001).

The multidisciplinary team

With people who have personality disorders it is important to focus on
the here and now, and not the 'then' of past traumas, even though support and individual psychotherapy are encouraged to resolve those
issues. The approach is crisis intervention, prioritizing problems and goal-
setting with the multidisciplinary team working cohesively together
towards a common aim (Branch, 2003).

Due to intrapsychic conflicts, the clinical psychologist offers psychotherapy on either an analytic or a supportive level with group therapy
supporting that premise. Psychoanalytic-orientated therapy seems more
effective with borderline, avoidant and dependent personalities.
Psychodynamic therapy offers the client an opportunity to understand
how he/she is received in society and develops accountability within the
client; as such a certain amount of insight is required in order to be able
to benefit from this therapy. Diverse difficulties in all areas of function
indicate occupational therapy providing intensive functional and occupational assessments and treatment.

Among other things, the social worker makes a relevant contribution to
positive family and personal relationships, and will coordinate relationship group, using a family systems approach (Minuchin, 1974) as well as
victims' groups. She may also conduct individual social needs. The nursing manager and the nursing team are ward coordinators and contain the
therapeutic environment by running daily morning groups, climate

meetings, etc. The psychiatrist monitors medication closely, and provides psychotherapy and overall case management.

Occupational therapy

When someone with a personality disorder is admitted to a therapeutic community or other treatment facility, they would benefit from occupational therapy intervention.

Aims of occupational therapy

Occupational therapy intervention aims to:

* stabilize fluctuating mood
* improve self-concept and self-esteem
* improve insight and judgement
* assist in forming mature interpersonal relationships
* teach constructive ways of coping with stress and anxiety
* allow for appropriate expression and ventilation of feelings to bring about conflict resolution
* develop social skills and assertiveness skills
* promote behavioural change.

The occupational therapist should also build on strengths, identify provoking/stress factors, treat abuse of substances and provide help for families (Galder et al., 1996). It is helpful, after identifying behaviour patterns, to understand the value the behaviour gives to the person, what maintains the behaviour and what the consequences for changing the behaviour are. If the spiritual realm is important and gives comfort to the person, then this cannot be excluded but should be supported and encouraged in a healthy way.

General occupational therapy principles for intervention

A useful list of do's and don'ts in treatment provides the therapist with a guide to preventing pitfalls in establishing a therapeutic relationship (Profis, 1992)

The occupational therapist should:

* focus on behaviour and not explanation of behaviour
* establish a stance of collaborative sharing in the problem
* confront and not interpret defence mechanisms
* set limits and provide structure
* allow for participation in groups and helping others
* assist in processing the consequences of intended actions.

The occupational therapist should not:

- listen to repetitious complaints
- insist on a contract
- try to save face if fooled or resort to blame and punitive acts
- try to rescue or encourage dependency
- offer interpretations or insights in early stages of treatment
- lie or present conflicting non-verbal messages
- present self as an emotionless screen.

Specific occupational therapy intervention principles applied to the three clusters

Cluster A

It has been suggested that schizotypal and paranoid personality disorders should be excluded from group therapy (Robertson et al., 2001; Sadock and Sadock, 2003). This can be a generalization as those with more intact ego strengths would benefit from non-threatening, structured task-centred groups. Schizoid personality disorders also benefit from group therapy but need the occupational therapist to protect them from over-intrusive group members. It has been noted that social skills should be introduced gradually (Robertson et al., 2001). Clinical experience has shown that they benefit most and can integrate and resolve conflicts as a passive member. As they are unable to cope with excessive attention, and may become withdrawn and defensive when demands are made on them, the occupational therapist provides support during the early stages of group therapy. Modelling unconditional acceptance of their limitations ensures acceptance by other group members.

- *Paranoid personality:* A relationship of predictability and constancy is important here. The therapist needs to be honest, straightforward and open in answering questions and if accused of a fault offer an apology rather than become defensive (Profis, 1992), as trust is a difficult area. Situations and people's reactions should be interpreted gently so that faulty interpretations can be shifted. 'Delusional' accusations should be dealt with gently, without humiliation.
- *Schizoid personality:* A fairly businesslike, factual, but friendly approach, which presents a stable reality concept, rather than compliments and praise, will create a therapeutic bond. The occupational therapist should guard against pushing for closeness. Structure in group settings is vital as long silences are harmful and the client may need protection from aggressive group members (Profis, 1992).
- *Schizotypal personality:* A supportive therapeutic approach is recommended for treatment (Robertson et al., 2001). The occupational therapist is careful not to ridicule cults or express scepticism about unusual beliefs.

Cluster B

The extroversion group benefit from evocative groups and dialectical behaviour therapy (Linehan, 1993). Transference and counter-transference issues emerge frequently. Conflict is often evident as a 'crisis is always present'. Confrontation is most effective in groups, elicited by fellow group members.

- *Histrionic personality:* Attention-seeking behaviour must be ignored and situations created where attention is received in socially acceptable ways. The occupational therapist should guard against dependency and assist in replacing negative behaviour, e.g. manipulative suicidal threats with positive coping mechanisms, e.g. clarifying and verbalizing real feelings.
- *Narcissistic personality:* A therapeutic, empathic rapport must be established, even if the therapist is disconcerted by the superior, disdainful stance presented. At all times, the occupational therapist encourages empathy, awareness of feelings and others' points of view. Issues relating to transference and counter-transference need to be dealt with effectively (Robertson et al., 2001).
- *Antisocial personality:* Long-term behaviour-orientated inpatient programmes are suggested (Robertson et al., 2001) but prognosis is often poor and success more prevalent with adolescents. Self-help groups are useful but compliance is not always ensured. Firm limits are essential to deal with destructive behaviour. The occupational therapist must be vigilant to overt and covert manipulation and explore alternative behaviour styles.
- *Borderline personality:* A structured, reality-orientated approach is more useful than interpretation (Profis, 1992) and clear, firm limit-setting and boundaries will prevent regression and self-destructive behaviour. Be prepared for impulsivity and unpredictability and aim to react calmly. Watch out for physically harmful tools and provide activities channelling aggression and relieving pain. The consequences of destructive behaviour for the family need to be addressed (Robertson et al., 2001).

Cluster C

The introversion group benefit from the structure and containment found in task-centred groups approaches; but the obsessive-compulsive personality should be exposed to expressive therapies such as art and clay work. Homework should be given so that these people actively practise skills to increase confidence (Robertson et al., 2001).

- *Avoidant personality:* The first step is to develop trust by conveying an accepting attitude. Do not encourage avoidance at any level, for example by putting off decision making or avoiding problem areas so that responsibility for own actions is taken. Approach confrontation with great caution to allow for exploration of appropriate social behaviour and assertiveness, providing knowledge of the negative consequences of avoidance and the reality that no one can predict outcomes.

- *Dependent personality:* At all times, encourage independence in thought, decisions, responsibilities and function. Assertiveness training based on cognitive restructuring and support to test out negative thinking patterns, is imperative. Self-esteem is built up by involvement in concrete, short-term goals and success in attainment. The person and not the therapist must assess own feelings, needs and behaviour, to avoid reinforcing dependency. Dependency and the negative effects this has on others should be exposed during group therapy sessions so that more positive behavioural patterns can emerge.
- *Obsessive-compulsive personality:* The occupational therapist should create a relaxed atmosphere and aim to reduce tension, as it is usually the precursor to compulsive behaviour. Perfectionism can be used constructively in choice of tasks and activities but completion is compulsory. Encourage awareness that alienation from others is caused by compulsivity and facilitate expression of affects, especially anger, tension and anxiety. Promote enjoyment, fun and the positive impact these feelings have on mood, thought and action.

Intervention methods

Individual occupational therapy

The occupational therapist has a unique skill in the functional and work spheres. Analysis of these spheres highlights areas of stress, productivity, relationship problems and coping skills. Assessments focus on life circumstances, relationships, leisure and social pursuits, role expectations, mood and energy levels, habits and time planning.

Clients can also practise on a practical level what they learn from groups and other therapy modalities.

Assessment of job context and content allows for exploration of difficulties and problem solving. An individualized programme focusing on these areas alleviates tension and anxiety in treatment intervention.

Occupational therapists are called upon to be case managers by doing functional work and supportive counselling (Branch, 2003).

Group work

Group therapy brings about behavioural change and develops emotional insight. Because of defence mechanisms, the person accepts and learns more from others in the group than from the therapist and can identify, share information and move towards a process of behavioural change and conflict resolution.

Yalom's (1985) curative factors in group therapy applicable to personality disorders are:

- *Universality.* A shared, common feeling that the person experiences when group members express similar feelings, and conflicts.
- *Imitative behaviour.* This occurs during the working phase of the group, when the individual 'copies' others and adopts new behaviour patterns. This behaviour might not last but it does allow for alternative communication patterns.
- *Interpersonal learning.* The group acts as a social microcosm. Through group interaction, the personality disorder is faced with different situations that stimulate coping skills, problem solving and conflict resolution.
- *Socializing techniques.* Group therapy teaches ways of expressing feelings, needs and conflicts, thereby stimulating social contact and developing interpersonal relationships.
- *Corrective recapitulation of the primary family.* The group represents the primary family and allows for working through family conflicts.
- *Instilling hope.* Despair, frustration and anger are common feelings expressed in group therapy, and members benefit from the feeling of hope that develops within the group.

Selecting groups – a team approach

The multidisciplinary team provides information on the best type of group therapy intervention. Emphasis placed on supportive psychotherapy requires a structured, containing and goal-orientated therapeutic approach. Occupational therapy reinforces this stance by focusing on task-centred groups that work on confidence, self-esteem and coping skills. Explorative socio-emotional groups, e.g. expressive therapies and psychodrama, would be non-productive due to their evocative approach. If psychotherapeutic and psychiatric interventions consist of psychoanalysis, hypnosis, narco-analysis or non-directed psychotherapy, socio-emotional groups will facilitate conflict resolution and insight and provide the team with valuable information. Clinical experience has shown that having psychotherapy after an art therapy group provides material for the psychotherapy, and dynamically enhances therapeutic intervention. Another benefit of working within a close, multidisciplinary team is that maladaptive behavioural patterns and defences such as splitting and acting out are minimized. A consistent ward environment and treatment approach removes tension, increases motivation and maximizes participation.

Socio-emotional group work

1. Expressive groups
Expressive group therapy using art, clay, movement and music is used to release pent-up emotions. Catharsis with abreaction allows for resolution.

Experiencing and exploring feelings and themes such as anger (through art), family structure and support (through clay modelling), self-image and esteem, and future planning, actively provides a healthy outlet for anger and frustration and externalizes stress and anxiety, hence allowing the development of problem solving. For example, in 'Family sculpting', each group member takes a turn to sculpt her family, using the group members as parental or sibling figures, and positioning the 'family' at emotional distances from herself. This allows the person to work out family conflicts, understand relationships and support systems, and so on. It should only be used during the 'working phase' of the group, when trust and cohesion are established.

2. *Self-awareness groups*

These groups are termed 'encounter' or 'evocative' groups. As with most groups, one develops favourite and preferred exercises. This is based on observed successes and the nature of group interaction where trust, cohesion, communication and insight are apparent. Such activities include:

- Coat of arms The patients are asked to create their own coat of arms containing the following information:

Table 21.2 The 'Coat of Arms' layout

My emotional self	My social self
Three things I'd like to change in myself	Three things I'd like to be recognized by
My achievements	Where I want to be in six months' time

- advertisement of myself
- auction of qualities
- trust games, for example Blind Walk (Remocker and Storch, 1982)
- self-esteem declaration.

3. *Dialectical behaviour therapy (DBT)*

The components of DBT are outlined as problem solving, exposure, skills training and contingency management. The person begins to reframe suicidal and dysfunctional behaviours as strengths are utilized and positive emotional expression is validated.

Five problem areas are impacted on:

1. dysregulation and lability of emotions by teaching regulation skills
2. interpersonal dysregulation in relationships that are chaotic or intense by introducing IPR effectiveness skills
3. behavioural dysregulation such as impulsivity and suicidal ideation which are maladaptive problem-solving behaviours as a result of not

tolerating emotional distress and acting out by teaching distress tolerance skills

4. dysregulation of self with feelings of emptiness AND

5. brief non-psychotic cognitive disturbances such as depersonalization by teaching 'mindfulness skills' by consciously experiencing and observing oneself and surrounding events.

All groups require clients to do homework and practise skills and then feed back to the group their progress before new material is handed out. Groups run for 6–8 sessions of one and a half hour's duration. The occupational therapist can contribute to all the four training skill components: core mindfulness skills, interpersonal effectiveness skills, emotional regulation skills and distress tolerance skills.

Task-centred groups

Social skills groups

An important dimension of a treatment programme should address social skills, and the nature of the programme should vary according to needs. The introverted personality disorders (schizoid or dependent) benefit from non-verbal or verbal skills, conversation skills and assertiveness training. Assertiveness training comprises protective techniques (fogging, broken record) and expressive techniques ('I' statements).

In contrast, the extroversion cluster (histrionic and narcissistic) presenting as over-assertive and aggressive benefit more from an insight-orientated approach whereby the modes of communication and behaviour are explained. Anger management and self-regulating behaviour is explored (Linehan, 1993). The short- and long-term consequences of being passive-aggressive, indirect or aggressive in communication are examined.

The following techniques are successful in communications groups:

- *Dyads or a 'carousel'* (Blatner, 1992) are used effectively in early stages of group development, so that discussions are done in pairs rather than the entire group; this works well with Cluster C. Selected conversation topics such as giving or receiving criticism, saying 'no', asking for help, complimenting and apologizing, and expressing anger, are discussed. Exploring childhood messages, such as fear of rejection, ridicule and 'children are seen and not heard' hinder assertive behaviour and need to be expressed. Guilt feelings provide insight into the rationale for stereotyped behaviours.
- *Role-play* is the follow-on technique in which stressful social situations are enacted out using assertive behaviours, such as

    – General situations such as coping with queue jumping, giving compliments, returning defective articles to a store, introducing people, initiating and maintaining a conversation.

 – Personal situations such as expressing affection, asking for help, say-ing 'no', coping with destructive criticism, and negotiating and compromising.

Persons with a personality disorder need to practise appropriate expres-sive verbal skills rather than resorting to defensive communication such as adopting 'you' statements in an accusatory or manipulative manner. The technique of 'I' statements express feelings appropriately, reduces stress in relationships and assists in taking responsibility for own feelings and actions.

Values clarification groups

Values clarification can be used effectively with people who have person-ality disorders, to help reassess life values, resolve conflicts around these values, and look at consequences of present values in developing alterna-tive values; within a process which inter alia promotes behavioural insight. It has been noted that the techniques of values clarification with people with personality disorders were beneficial and initiated change to a more adaptive lifestyle of appropriate coping mechanisms (Roper, 1985).

Values clarification aims at consciously planning one's life to reach ful-filment. Within this planning is the freedom to choose, accept or reject values. Exercises are done in dyads, followed by group discussions and homework tasks when needed.

Examples of tasks are:

• Exercise 1: 'My values' emblem

Table 21.3 My values emblem layout

What has been my greatest achievement?	What has been my greatest failure?
What three things do people admire in me?	What do I need from people?

• Exercise 2: The influence of other people's values on my life. For exam-ple, family, authority, friends and someone I love.
• Exercise 3: Alternatives and consequences. Clients discuss their per-sonal alternatives and consequences. For example: Getting better – happier, better lifestyle versus not getting better – no work, unhappy.

Stress management and relaxation therapy

All persons with personality disorders display symptoms of distress and anxiety. They react in a stereotyped way to a variety of life stressors (Gillis, 1986), particularly in interpersonal relationships, work and everyday pressures. Stress is the precipitating factor in admission; therefore stress management is imperative in teaching coping strategies. Maladaptive stress-inducing coping strategies are alcohol, over-the-counter medication, drugs and excessive eating, and these must be identified. Self-help groups play a part here, and joining them should be organized whilst in hospital to initiate this ongoing support network.

Useful exercises for stress management should look at assessing stress, introducing balance in life such as leisure and sport, and addressing emotional support needs.

To achieve this, the occupational therapist uses handouts, self-assessment exercises, brainstorming, thought restructuring (challenging negative thinking), time planning and goal-setting.

Each session should begin or end with relaxation therapy which includes exposure to a variety of relaxations, such as simple meditative exercises, systematic muscle relaxation, imagery and music. A healthy lifestyle of correct nutrition, exercise, sport and hobbies is considered. Examination of support systems, such as in individuals, church groups or self-help groups e.g. Alcoholics Anonymous, Weight Watchers or eating disorder support groups, is explored.

Other task-centred occupational therapeutic activities

These activities are incorporated into the programme as they provide respite from intense socio-emotional group work and are functional in approach. Because of their content, these groups are goal-orientated, constructive and can be a tool for assessment or treatment. An element of fun, laughter and enjoyment is introduced in the process.

They may include:

- newspaper (cultural-type groups)
- concentration (cognitive exercises)
- educational (medication, mental health)
- life skills (support system network, constructive leisure time)
- work issues (coping with conflict situations, handling a job interview, work preparation).

Recreational activities

The value of recreational activities in an occupational therapy programme is that they allow for externalization of aggression and frustration and have a motivating factor by reducing apathy and negativity. They reintroduce the individual to the value of exercise/sport/hobbies as a release from stress and a positive way of coping with tension. These informal group activities are an important social assessment tool and provide a model for constructive leisure time use. To ensure their success these activities could be chosen on a democratic basis at ward climate meetings.

Some recommended activities include:

- *inter-ward sport and recreation* (volleyball, adapted baseball, tennis, Trivial Pursuit, Pictionary and Scrabble)

- *therapeutic outings* (cinema, picnics, art galleries, museums and theatre)
- *ward barbecues or cooking* (pancakes, fudge)
- *parties* (barn dances and discos)
- *concerts* (talent shows and singalongs)
- *fundraising* (sale of goods, cake sales).

Creative activities

Clinical experience strongly supports a creative occupational therapy programme as an integral part of the treatment. Rather than a rigid approach where activities are chosen for the client, the occupational therapist provides social time in the programme where the atmosphere is informal and relaxed and the setting conducive to exploring activities. In other words, respite from the other intensive therapies is offered.

Individuals with personality disorders are found to be highly creative and artistic, and the structuring of the environment should allow for resuming old or developing new leisure time interests. Music creates a relaxing atmosphere and recreational games and domestic activities can be incorporated here. The individual is encouraged to do these activities post-discharge for a healthier, balanced lifestyle. Aims of treatment include:

- time to practise social and assertive techniques
- taking responsibility and encouraging independent decision making
- improving motivation and initiative
- stress release
- improving self-esteem and confidence.

Outpatient, community and follow-up treatment programmes

Due to the dynamics and structural composition of personality disorders, treatment should consist in the main of group therapy. A full day's programme that includes healthy activities and addresses all issues pertaining to the psychodynamics should be planned and coordinated with all team members. Prior to the completion of treatment the occupational therapist focuses on work integration issues by doing job preparation and job liaison or coaching. On discharge, DBT groups continue to provide support.

With follow-up, the ideal setting for this person is to obtain support by the occupational therapist through home visit and programmes and a work visit. This input would provide the necessary structure and support within the external environment.

It is essential that the person be provided with community resources for self and family by linking up to community centres, sport clubs and self-help groups. This link-up ensures constructive use of time and continued outlets for emotion and stress in socially appropriate ways. Family counselling and psycho-education are imperative for successful reintegration.

The international trend is moving towards case management in which the person is assigned a mental health professional most suited to their needs. That is, a person needing more work and leisure time support would be assigned an occupational therapist whereas if the focus were more pharmacological, the psychiatrist would be the case manager. This approach seems more economically viable and allows for post-discharge monitoring in alleviating the revolving door syndrome.

Case studies to demonstrate occupational therapy intervention

Two cases are presented to illustrate how vital occupational therapy is in changing maladaptive behaviour patterns and responses to stress, improving quality of life and thereby inducing a healthier mental state.

Case study 1 – Cluster B

Background

Jack is an 18-year-old adolescent, with severe behavioural problems. He has antisocial and borderline personality traits. On admission, he was confused and tended to drift in his life with no stable job. He dressed in torn, black clothes and had long, dirty and unkempt hair. At face value he presented as quiet and withdrawn although able to communicate easily with fellow clients and staff. A closer assessment revealed underlying tension, loneliness, isolation, anger and confusion with erratic outbursts and self-mutilation, i.e. slashing his wrists.

Occupational therapy

The occupational therapist aimed at establishing a relationship that was accepting and non-critical so that he could vent his feelings. He found using the medium of art most conducive in expressing ideals, fantasies, conflicts and feelings (especially anger). Free expression of art was allowed. It was suggested that he take the drawings to individual psychotherapy to use as a catalyst to talking and resolving issues. The occupational therapist retained the drawings and prior to discharge looked at this tangible evidence of his progress and process towards recovery. Reviewing the drawings, one could see movement from explosive, angry and destructive art to more contained, structured and focused drawings. The self-mutilating behaviour was simultaneously abating. Jack began to feel more whole and less fragmented, developing a stronger base for emotional growth.

Other interventions included assertiveness training, stress management, pottery and leatherwork. Gradually work-related tasks were introduced. Jack became less egocentric and more involved in the occupational therapy activities by planning recreational and sporting activities.

He was in treatment for three months and prior to discharge the occupational therapist and Jack considered various goals and future plans. He started attending a technical college and began studying graphics.

Follow-up was carried out with regular sessions for counselling and support. No further admissions have been recorded.

Case study 2 – Cluster C

Background

Marie is a slightly overweight, middle-aged woman. She is married with three children. She has a stable job as a senior shop assistant. She had two previous hospital admissions within the space of two years. Marie was admitted with a diagnosis of dysthymic disorder with dependent personality disorder on Axis II.

At work, Marie displayed maladaptive behavioural traits such as acting out, passivity and manipulation. At home, her behaviour interfered with her functioning and disrupted the harmony in the home. She felt unable to express her needs, feelings and desires and was passive-aggressive in communication. Rehabilitation was short-term (due to dependency traits) and structured and focused, using a goal-orientated approach. The medical team worked together to achieve this.

Occupational therapy

The therapeutic approach of the occupational therapist was consistent, calm, matter of fact with persuasive and firm handling when Marie started manipulating, avoiding or being passively aggressive. The programme focused primarily on improving Marie's social skills, especially self-assertion, and teaching stress management.

Role-plays were perceived as most effective as she could practise situations in which she felt threatened or rejected, e.g. refusing unreasonable demands placed on her by her work or family. Initially, she was unable to benefit in the assertiveness training and would back down for fear of rejection or escalating anxiety and guilt. Although the social skills taught Marie alternative ways of dealing with difficult communication situations, she felt insecure and uncomfortable about implementing them. Structural homework with regular feedback to the group encouraged her to do this. Her husband was educated on assertiveness so that Marie would be supported and a new behavioural style adopted at home. Marie benefited from learning the short-term and long-term effects of her passive/indirect behaviour and this greatly improved her insight and motivation. Another dimension of occupational therapy included stress management and goal-setting. As her self-esteem improved, she took up past interests of sewing and tapestry, and regained confidence in the recreational sphere by resuming badminton with her husband. All these activities, which she termed short-term goals, were self-initiated. As Marie showed typical signs of reduced responsibility, lack of confidence and helplessness, this self-initiation in activity showed a definite shift in behaviour. The occupational therapist encouraged her always to acknowledge her feelings and use problem-solving and assertion techniques to empower and motivate her in being successful.

Creative activities were chosen so that when they were executed the end result would gain recognition and praise from others. These included baking, e.g. making cakes for ward tea, Florentine tapestry and découpage. In this way, her strengths were used and expanded upon.

As there was a great deal of underlying aggression and anger, sports such as volleyball and adapted baseball were selected. Goals groups helped her to deal with her aggression constructively by owning negative feelings and working on them constructively.

Marie was discharged after three weeks of occupational therapy, feeling more confident and responsible for her own life. Telephonic contact with her confirmed that she had continued with the goal-setting and felt sociable, less needy on her family and was happier. She reported that the social skills group was the most helpful of all occupational therapy.

Conclusion

Personality disorders comprise a complex field of psychiatry; however the occupational therapist working in this area will be extended on both a professional and an emotional level in a discipline that is exciting, rewarding and challenging. A cohesive, united team makes work much easier and prevents pitfalls as outlined above. It is a gratifying experience when the occupational therapist sees shifts in the client from turmoil and chaos to resolution and peace of mind, with productivity and healthy functioning as a bonus.

Good therapy grows out of healthy self-analysis, with flexibility, knowledge and teamwork being core elements to dynamic and fulfilling occupational therapy. This is an area for the brave-hearted, and well worth it.

Questions

1. List the clusters and types of personality disorders according to DSM-IV-TR™. How does the occupational therapy programme differ for each cluster?
2. What defence mechanisms are prevalent amongst personality disorders? Explain their dynamics.
3. What are counter-transference and transference and how do they impact on therapy?

4. Discuss the curative factors of group therapy with personality disorders.
5. What criteria can be used in choosing occupational therapy intervention for persons with personality disorders?
6. List the three types of behavioural approaches and what the occupational therapist will do in each approach.

Appendix 1 Limit Settings Contracts

Appendix 1a) No Self-Harm Contract

I,   hereby declare that for the duration of my stay in Hospital, I will contract not to harm myself in any way.

This contract is inclusive of any leave that I am granted during my admission.

If at any time I feel that I am unable to control an urge to hurt myself, I will do the following:

- Speak to my therapist or a nurse therapist or any other available professional staff member.

- Use appropriate ways of distracting myself from the harmful urges, i.e.:

  - sit with others;
  - watch TV;
  - go for a walk with someone;
  - find a puzzle, game or other activity to keep me occupied;
  - do some kind of physical exercise;
  - practise some relaxation techniques.

I understand that any self-injurious behaviour is considered as counter-productive to a healing constructive treatment plan.

Consequences of breaking the contract are possible discharge or transfer to a safer environment.

SIGNATURE   DATE

WITNESS   DATE

Appendix 1b) Anger Management Contract

I undertake that, in the event of a situation arising during my stay at Hospital that upsets me to the extent I feel angry and aggressive and at risk of becoming out of control, I give a commitment to take responsibility for my emotions by:

- utilizing a healthy technique to distract myself
- walking away from the situation
- seeking assistance from a staff member.

At all times I will control my anger and will not express it inappropriately.

SIGNED: DATE:

WITNESS:

Appendix 1c) Substance Abuse Contract

Substance abuse is the improper use of drugs or alcohol. It is established, and agreed, that due to your excessive use of _____

a) You have become dependent on this substance.
b) Your functioning has been impaired due to this substance.
c) Your relationship with self and others is impaired.

In order to be effectively treated the following commitment will be expected from you.

1. Personal commitment to attend all ward activities:

   Sport
   Occupational therapy
   Open groups
   Closed groups
   Individual therapy
   Outings

2. Initiating contact with Community Resources, obtaining mentor, and making appointment with said service.
3. No weekend privileges for first 3–4 weeks according to assessment.
4. No outside appointments during the first four weeks other than those stipulated by the unit, e.g. medical appointments.

Any deviation from the above commitment may result in immediate discharge from the Ward.

SIGNED   DATE

WITNESS

COMMUNITY RESOURCES:

Appendix 2: Goals

NAME: DATE:

Welcome to the Psychotherapy Unit. We have found that it is helpful when you are admitted to our unit that you think carefully about what you hope to gain from your stay. This helps both you and the team to understand your problems and needs, and to devise the best treatment plan possible.

Please take time to answer these questions:
1. What are your goals for your stay?
2. What are the areas/topics/issues/problems you need to work on in occupational therapy?
3. How do you feel we (the team) can help you to reach these goals?
4. How will YOU know when you are ready to be discharged? (What will be different for you? How will you feel?)

THANK YOU: Please hand this to your occupational therapist when completed.

Appendix 3 Family/Friend Report Back Form

Weekend date............

DEAR FAMILY MEMBER

To confirm that the treatment (medication and therapy) is effective, we need you to complete the following questionnaire as he/she will be spending time with you over the weekend.

This information will also help us to decide if further treatment is necessary or whether discharge from the Ward is possible.

Please hand the questionnaire to the case manager or send it back in a sealed envelope addressed to the Sister in charge. Thanking you for your cooperation.

FAMILY/FRIEND REPORT BACK FORM:

Please complete the following questions relating to:

1. Did he/she have any SOCIAL CONTACT, if so, did the patient initiate it?
   i.e. went to visit or received visitors. Did patient make acceptable social contact?

2. What was the patient's SLEEP PATTERN (too little or too much) and what do you think was the reason for this? (Morning, afternoon, evening).

3. Was the patient's SELF-CARE satisfactory? i.e. hair care, nail care, eating habits and etiquette, bath and toilet, make-up, etc.

4. Did the patient help with any CHORES? If yes, specify cooking, cleaning, ironing, washing dishes, making beds, etc.

5. Did the patient spend his/her FREE TIME by doing hobbies or any other activity? If yes, specify.

6. Did you observe any STRANGE BEHAVIOUR? i.e. strange thoughts, too active, aggression, side effects of medication.

7. Did patient take MEDICATION as prescribed and did you notice any effects thereof?

8. Do you think the patient is ready for DISCHARGE? Why?

9. Any other comments?

SIGNATURE:_____ RELATION: _____

PRINT NAME:_____ DATE:_____

Thank you

Chapter 22
Activation and psycho-education: major principles in the occupational therapist's approach to schizophrenia

ROSEMARY CROUCH

Schizophrenia is one of the most insidious, slowly progressive and disabling of the mental disorders. It seems to attack by producing severe disability during the potentially most creative and productive years of a person's life (Kaplan and Sadock, 2000). People with schizophrenia are often extraordinarily intelligent and creative young people who become seriously demoralized when they realize the impact that the illness can have on their lives. Schizophrenia involves dysfunction in one or more major areas of functioning, e.g. interpersonal relationships, work, education and self-care (DSM-IV-TR™ (American Psychiatric Association, 2000)) and it is for this reason that occupational therapy plays a vital part in the rehabilitation of people with this illness.

This chapter will discuss the work of major theorists on activation and describe psycho-education. The use of these techniques as part of the occupational therapy intervention for persons with schizophrenia in both hospital-based and community rehabilitation programmes will be described in detail.

The cause of schizophrenia is not yet fully understood, but there are many indications that several factors play a part. These are heredity, disposition or vulnerability, infections, damage to brain tissue and excessive stress.

Dopamine levels are affected and normal brain function is disrupted. However, 'with the advent of the seratonin-dopamine antagonists, many persons with severe illnesses have their symptoms controlled enough to make them candidates for rehabilitation' (Meninger in Kaplan and Sadock, 2000, p. 3193).

The full description and classification of the illness of schizophrenia can be found in:

- The Diagnostic and Statistical Manual of Mental Disorders, DSM-IV-TR™ (American Psychiatric Association, 2000)

- The Comprehensive Textbook of Psychiatry, 7th edition (Kaplan and Sadock, 2000)
- The ICD-10 Classification of Mental Disorders (WHO, 1992).

There are some important features of schizophrenia that should be high-lighted if one is to fully understand the focus of intervention of the occupational therapist. These are as follows:

- Schizophrenia presents primarily as a disorganization of thinking which can result in grossly disorganized behaviour, including inappro-priate sexual behaviour, silliness and argumentativeness, and a deterioration of ADL skills such as unusual dress and a lack of hygiene.
- Symptoms of schizophrenia can be divided into:
  - positive symptoms: delusions, hallucinations, disorganized speech and grossly disorganized or catatonic behaviour.
  - negative symptoms: flattening of affect, a lack of fluency and pro-ductivity of thought and speech (alogia) and avolition (DSM-IV-TR™ (American Psychiatric Association, 2000)).

- Other symptoms of concern to the occupational therapist include:
  - lack of interest in eating (delusions may interfere)
  - abnormalities of psychomotor activity, e.g. pacing and rocking
  - concentration, attention and memory difficulties
  - non-compliance with treatment
  - poor psychosocial functioning
  - depersonalization
  - somatic concerns, e.g. digestive or weight problems
  - derealization
  - anxieties and phobias
  - motor abnormalities such a grimacing and posturing, odd manner-isms, stereotyped behaviour
  - suicide. Ten per cent of people with schizophrenia succeed at sui-cide and 20–40 per cent make an attempt (again it is often related to delusions or hallucinations).

In 1974 Lorna Jean King, occupational therapist, hypothesized that patients with acute schizophrenia show defects in proprioceptive mecha-nisms which result in a lack of sensory integration. Working on the original work by Jean Ayres (1983), King has discussed the vestibular com-ponent of proprioceptive feedback being underactive and under-reactive in the person with schizophrenia, in its role in the sensory integration process. This person may therefore exhibit an apparent gross motor or motor planning problem resulting in lack of perceptual constancy, poor body image and fatigue, which often causes postural patterns.

These handicaps have been noted as resulting in severe emotional stress and they also predispose to hallucinatory phenomena in the person with schizophrenia.

From about 1970 to 1990 sensory integration therapy was conducted with chronic patients with schizophrenia with good results. However, these results were not sufficiently empirically proven and research funding in the USA devoted to sensory integration in psychiatry was diverted from schizophrenia-focused to autism-focused research.

This trend was also influenced by the movement of the chronic schizophrenia patients out of the institutions and into the community. In the community setting, facilities for clients with schizophrenia are far from adequate throughout the world but real attempts are being made to accommodate them in their home context. Primary healthcare clinics are administering chronic medicines from the clinics and to the home base. Clients with schizophrenia are followed up on a regular basis, although some clients do slip through the system. In the developing countries the diagnosis of schizophrenia tends to be more frequently used than bipolar mood disorder when clients exhibit bizarre behaviour. Support groups can be an effective medium to normalize this behaviour within the community context. The occupational therapist working in the community setting needs to coordinate groups for these clients to encourage them to form support groups. The families can be encouraged to acknowledge their strengths and enable them to carry out household duties rather than disregarding them and thus increasing their stigma. The client suffering from schizophrenia needs to be empowered to participate in meaningful, purposeful activity, however modest that activity may be. Sensory stimulation activities (tactile and vestibular stimulation) can be fun and pleasurable, and are thus is a good starting point for these groups.

Occupational therapy theory, purposeful activity and activation

If one looks at the above symptoms of schizophrenia, the various theoretical models of occupational performance come to mind, i.e. Reed and Sanderson (1992), Kielhofner (1992) and Canadian Association of Occupational Therapy (1991). Gardener (in Creek, 2002, p. 230) states that

> within these models cognition is seen as a performance component or skill which contributes, along with many other performance components, to a person's ability to function competently, and to their own satisfaction, in a given occupational area'.

Although some theorists in occupational therapy view dysfunction as a relationship between emotion and action (Christiansen and Baum, 1997), cognitive skills are the primary focus of treatment by occupational therapists with the person with schizophrenia.

Purposeful activity is the cornerstone and the major tool of intervention in occupational therapy. Hagedorn (1997, p. 143) describes activity as 'an integrated sequence of tasks which takes place on a specific occasion, during a finite period, for a particular purpose'.

However, it must be remembered that an individual with the illness of schizophrenia may have an impaired capacity for the performance of purposeful activity if any of the necessary precursors is missing, or if one or more of the additional components is lacking (Creek, 1998). Models such as The Person Environmental Occupational Performance Model (Christiansen and Baum, 1997) identify those factors contributing to self-identity which might be missing, and thereby influences both wellbeing and occupational performance.

Linking to theories on the performance of purposeful activity is the research undertaken by a South African, du Toit, in 1983 (de Witt in Crouch and Alers, 1997). She intimates that creative capacity varies from one individual to another and is influenced by factors such as intelligence, personality structure, mental health, environmental factors and security (see chapter 1). Du Toit describes volition as being central to creative theory and this is pivotal in the illness of schizophrenia. Du Toit describes volition as motivation and action. The motivational component represents the energy source for occupational behaviour and this motivation governs action. We know that one of the central aspects of schizophrenia is loss of volition. This is the link and the critical axis at which change can occur through the occupational therapy process. Creative purposeful activity as a central part of occupational therapy intervention is extremely important in improving and maintaining function in persons with schizophrenia.

Treatment of schizophrenia

Elpers (in Kaplan and Sadock, 2000, p. 3190) states that with schizophrenia 'psychosocial rehabilitation goals can range from complete restoration of function to limited improvement in the patient's ability to handle self care'.

Medication in the form of a new generation of neuroleptics makes it possible today to alleviate the negative symptoms of schizophrenia and in doing so opening the door to rehabilitation for the person with this illness. With the correct approach to the treatment of schizophrenia, many of those afflicted are able to live as normal a life as possible in the community. Treatment can be hospital-based or community-based depending on the severity of the first episode and also on the treatment facilities available. Wherever treatment takes place occupational therapy is a vital part of the holistic approach to rehabilitation.

Elpers (in Kaplan and Sadock, 2000, p. 3193) believes that today all persons with schizophrenia do or will need rehabilitation and focuses essentially on the person's remaining capacities, not the residual symptoms. Rehabilitation must emphasize the person's individuality, their responsibility and sense of self-reliance rather than the residual symptoms, illness and dependency. Liebermann et al. (in Kaplan and Sadock, 2000, p. 3218) state that:

The growing recognition that a large proportion of persons with schizophrenia and mood disorders experience a poor quality of life with long-term disability, persisting symptoms or a relapsing course of illness, has given way to the field of rehabilitation.

'An essential ingredient of rehabilitation is hope' (Elpers in Kaplan and Sadock, 2000, p. 3193) and this hope must be transferred to clients with schizophrenia and their families.

Hospital-based rehabilitation/treatment

People with schizophrenia, if admitted (or committed by certification) to a hospital, are usually in an acute, psychotic state and need to be hospitalized because they are a danger to themselves or others.

Even though most countries are striving to convert to community rehabilitation in psychiatry, there is still a place for the containing, acute and long-term care psychiatric units worldwide, particularly in developing countries. This will remain a reality for a long time yet, until adequate community facilities are available.

Moya Willson (Willson, 1983, p. 140) states that 'Activities are the major therapeutic measures used within occupational therapy. Each activity needs to be selected for its relevance to the functional and personal needs of the patient.' Willson details excellent programmes and activities for long-term treatment of patients with mental disorders such as schizophrenia. She uses physical activities, creative writing, the use of music, remedial drama, recreation, personal activities, and work and constructive activities.

Early intervention and effective treatment of acute episodes of schizophrenia, with the specific alleviation of symptoms, are very important for minimizing long-term disability. Hospitalization undoubtedly has a major role to play in this.

'Hospital treatment characteristically involves a multidisciplinary group of mental health professionals' (Meninger in Kaplan and Sadock, 2000, p. 3212).

Short-term or extended treatment programmes are focused on evaluating strengths, weaknesses, skills and impairments at this early stage. The occupational therapist is the key professional in this process.

During the hospitalization period the rehabilitation needs of patients must be individually assessed within the context of what they wish to do with their lives, and their opportunities to fulfil this. The occupational therapy programme is a programme of activation and psycho-education.

Assessment

All treatment by the occupational therapists is focused by good, thorough assessment. Every patient must be assessed before treatment takes place. As stated by Meninger (in Kaplan and Sadock, 2000, p. 3213) the occupational therapists must 'evaluate strengths, weaknesses, skills and impairment'.

Many good standardized tests are available to the occupational therapist today. Examples of these tests are as follows:

- The Canadian Occupational Performance Measure (COPM, 1998) is an excellent client-centred assessment of function that is frequently used in the psychiatric field.
- Assessment of ADL of Personal Life Skills (PLS): The Milwaukee Evaluation of Daily Living Skills (MEDLS) (Leonardelli in Hemphill, 1982); The scorable self-care evaluation (SCORE), Clarke and Peters, 1994) and the Klein-Bell Activity of Daily Living Scale (Klein and Bell, 1979).
- ADL and some components of performance and cognitive ability: The Bay Area Functional Performance Evaluation (BaFPE) (Bloomer and Williams, 1986).
- Leisure and Activity Configuration (Mosey, 1973); Activity Card Sort (Baum and Edwards, 2001).
- Assessment of Motor and Process Skills (AMPS) (Fischer, 2001).

Once the assessment has been carried out, individual aims of treatment can be formulated for each patient.

Principles of handling the person with an acute episode of schizophrenia

During hospitalization of the patient with schizophrenia, the occupational therapist is often confronted with bizarre, psychotic behaviour. It is important for the occupational therapist to handle the patient in a calm and consistent manner to bring them in touch with reality.

Guidelines of handling are as follows:

- The patient must never be ridiculed or laughed at because of their bizarre ideas, delusions or hallucinations.
- These ideas, delusions and hallucinations must not be condoned or endorsed by the occupational therapist but the patient should be gently reminded of reality. When psychotic thought and perceptions are present, the occupational therapist must not try to 'talk' the patient out of it. The best way to bring the patient back to reality is by engagement in a concrete activity. Their thought pattern is fixed!
- Gently remind the patient of the time of day and date, and orientate them to place.
- Use touch and close proximity with care as this may become part of the delusional thought (except in the sensory integrative activities).
- Handle aggression calmly and try to channel it into activity with wide movements.
- Gently correct unacceptable behaviour. Do not be punitive in approach.

Guidelines for other principles of treatment, according to the patient's level of creative ability, such as requirements and presentation of activities, as well as grading, can be found in chapter 1.

A balanced occupational therapy programme

An effective occupational therapy programme must contain 'elements of practicality, concrete problem-solving for everyday challenges, low-key socialisation and recreation, engagement of attainable tasks, and specific goal orientation' (Libermann et al. in Kaplan and Sadock, 2000, p. 3227). Social skills training, when the psychotic features are diminished, is very important in order to counteract pervasive deficits in social functioning.

A balanced weekly programme should consist of the following:

- Personal care groups/self independence and assistance in the family's daily tasks.
- Psycho-educational groups.
- Creative activity groups which can include cooking and hobby or leisure pursuits. Learning the skill of using leisure time is very important.
- Music and recreation.
- If there is no sensory integration programme, simple exercise groups, walks and sport, such as volleyball, are very important for physical fitness.
- Social skills training such as stress management, and coping and communication skills training. These should preferably take place in groups and should be focused on the reintegration of the patient into the community.
- Individual sessions on subjects such as child management or budgeting, when appropriate.
- Vocational assessment and rehabilitation which should be carried forward into community care.
- Discharge planning.

Psycho-education

The effectiveness of psycho-educational programmes with persons with schizophrenia has been demonstrated by Kissling and Baum (1994). They are the two main developers of what is known as the Prelapse Programme. Kissling and Baum have provided recommendations based on experience in the framework of their Munich study and on the experience of leaders of comparable studies. They have found this type of programme to be very successful not only with the patient but also with the family.

The purpose of implementing this type of programme is to:

- promote insight into the illness of schizophrenia
- encourage compliance with medication and to understand the role of medication in the control of the illness.
- prevent relapse
- educate the families.

The programme consists of eight sessions, which address the following issues:

- What is schizophrenia?
- What are the causes of schizophrenia?
- How can schizophrenia be treated?
- Psychosocial treatment strategies.
- Relapse prevention.
- The role of relatives.

The multidisciplinary team carries out this programme, but in many hospitals it is seen as part of the occupational therapy programme. Subjects such as understanding the medication are best presented by a psychiatrist who is an expert in this field, whilst psychosocial treatment strategies would be best presented by the occupational therapist. Separate groups are best for patients and families. Families often find it difficult to speak out and discuss the problems with the patient present.

Psycho-education is also seen as a very important part of community psychiatry.

Community-based rehabilitation for people with schizophrenia

Today community-based rehabilitation is recommended as the best alternative for the successful treatment of the person with schizophrenia.

> The goal of psychiatric rehabilitation is to teach skills and provide community supports so that the individual with mental disabilities can function in the social, vocational, educational and familial roles with the least amount of supervision from the helping professionals (Liebermann et al. in Kaplan and Sadock, 2000, p. 3218).

Rehabilitation is an essential component of the continuum of services necessary for people served by the public sector (Elpers in Kaplan and Sadock, 2000). A community-based rehabilitation programme is often an extension of the hospital programme, but some clients are able to join a community-based programme shortly after being diagnosed and placed on medication.

Various types of rehabilitation programmes exist in different parts of the world. Day programmes are offered by some hospitals and community centres and in the USA, South Africa and Australia the Life-skills/Fountain House model of community service has proved to be very successful. In South Africa, Canada and other Western countries, occupational therapists in private practice can offer effective community-based programmes for schizophrenia clients of a middle to high socio-economic status.

Elpers (in Kaplan and Sadock, 2000, p. 3193) underlines the fact that for the person with schizophrenia being seen 'to exist in the community without being shunned or appearing bizarre, is essential to rehabilitation'.

Liberman et al. (in Kaplan and Sadock, 2000) also emphasize a biopsychosocial approach to comprehensive care of the person with schizophrenia in the community, by stressing the following aspects of rehabilitation:

- training in social and independent living skills
- family psycho-education
- self-management of medication and awareness of symptoms
- assertive clinical case management by the community health professionals
- supported housing and employment.

What has come to light in community-based rehabilitation is that the client with schizophrenia requires a continuing, supportive and positive relationship with a suitable health professional/religious counsellor/carer. 'This is central to the overall strategy for treating the patient with schizophrenia, no matter how much drug or psychosocial treatment contributes' (Libermann et al. in Kaplan and Sadock, 2000, p. 2865). Often the occupational therapist is in the position to provide this type of community care. The relationship between occupational therapist and client must be firm and trusting, to make it possible to correct the life skills of the client in a positive and frank way without lowering the client's self-esteem and in this way building up confidence.

It is important also to realize that clients require continuous rather than short-term efforts to achieve and maintain improved functioning. Kaplan and Sadock (2000) suggest that it is ideal that patients have the same therapists or caregivers throughout their illness as this brings about continuity of care.

Occupational therapy as part of the community rehabilitation programme

Rehabilitation of the client with schizophrenia in the community is a collaborative, multidisciplinary effort. Control of the client's medication is an important aspect of the holistic approach to rehabilitation, and compliance by the client in this respect must precede efforts at psychosocial rehabilitation. This is a team effort and must be addressed by every person in the rehabilitation team. Often some of the positive symptoms of schizophrenia, such as hallucinations, remain for a long time. It has been found, however, that clients can function quite well despite this and rehabilitation can proceed.

Wherever the rehabilitation takes place, the occupational therapist should focus on the client's strengths and on skills necessary for their survival in the community. These are:

- tolerating others
- dressing in an appropriate manner, self-care and grooming

- polite social interaction and communication/social skills
- time management principles and discipline such as keeping appointments
- the preparation of food, attention to diet, shopping and storing food
- dudgeting and money management
- vocational rehabilitation. Work is an extremely important component of the client's sense of self-worth and their participation in society (Kaplan and Sadock, 2000).

The skill of occupational therapists in the use of group work is of utmost importance, as it is in groups that the person with schizophrenia learns to relate to others in the community. Occupational therapists are involved in both group work and individual treatment in community centres, day centres, early intervention programmes in schools and, in some countries, in private practice, with persons with schizophrenia who are living in the community.

> Without continuous attention to their psychosocial rehabilitation these individuals deteriorate over time and cost the mental health programs great sums of money (Kaplan and Sadock, 2000, p. 3190).

Case study

Mary is a 40-year-old married woman who lives in a suburb of Johannesburg, South Africa. She is a highly intelligent woman with a university degree.

When she was studying at university she met her husband who has to this day faithfully supported her through her illness.

Shortly after they were married Mary began to experience hallucinations and delusions of a paranoid nature. She heard the next door neighbours tapping on the walls of her flat, day and night, and her activities of daily living were drastically reduced. She eventually became so psychotic that she had to be certified. She spent two weeks in the acute ward of a mental hospital where she was treated individually by an occupational therapist.

She was diagnosed as schizophreniform disorder (DSM-IV-TR™ (American Psychiatric Association, 2000)) and was placed on neuroleptic medication. Six months later she was diagnosed with schizophrenia of the paranoid type on the DSM-IV-TR™.

When Mary was discharged from hospital she was referred to a day clinic in the community where she was assessed by the occupational therapist and had aims of treatment drawn up which incorporated activation and psycho-education. She then took part in the occupational therapy programme.

The psychiatrist and occupational therapist interviewed her husband and guidelines for Mary's recovery were discussed. He was alerted to the side effects of medication such as extra-pyramidal effects.

Mary's programme consisted of individual sessions where her day's programme and a balanced lifestyle were discussed, including attending a gymnasium three times a week. She was encouraged to attend to her appearance and to a balanced diet for herself and her husband. The group sessions for social skills training were introduced by the occupational therapist too early in treatment, and Mary was extremely aggressive towards the other group members, as she did not trust them. Instead she was included in the creative activities group, where she began to regain her confidence despite the fact that some of the positive symptoms were still present. She was included in the psycho-education group once a week and after the eight sessions she could talk freely about her illness with selected people. The occupational therapist undertook social skills training with Mary on an individual basis.

Mary's treatment continued in occupational therapy on a part-time basis for a year, and she also began vocational rehabilitation. There has been a slight decline in cognitive ability and in order to keep her stress levels low, a less demanding type of work has been suggested for her.

The occupational therapist and psychiatrist, working together, have carefully watched her progress and assessed her regularly for symptoms. She has not relapsed and has been maintained at a functional level.

Summary and conclusion

This chapter has highlighted both the theoretical and practical implications of the use of everyday, practical activities in the treatment and maintenance of the functioning of the person with schizophrenia. The theories of activation, occupation, sensory integration and holistic care have provided a base for the discussion. Psycho-education has also been introduced as a successful intervention.

Advances in neuroleptic medication, as well the move of the profession of occupational therapy into the field of health sciences and psychosocial care, has provided a much more scientifically based, realistic, holistic, client-centred approach to the treatment of the person with schizophrenia. This chapter includes intervention in the acute phase, the reintegration of the person into the community and, most importantly, the maintenance and survival of the person in the community. The multi-disciplinary approach has been emphasized throughout.

Questions

1. Discuss the importance of activating the person with schizophrenia. Discuss at least two theorists in this regard.
2. 'Schizophrenia is a debilitating illness.' Discuss this statement with reference to the everyday activities of a person with schizophrenia.

3. Hospital-based occupational therapy programmes are often necessary in the acute stage of the illness of schizophrenia. Describe a balanced occupational therapy programme and principles of handling the patient.
4. Community-based programmes are preferred for the person with schizophrenia. Why is this so? Describe briefly the focus of community-based rehabilitation programmes for persons with schizophrenia.
5. What is psycho-education and why is it important?

Chapter 23
The recovering alcoholic and occupational therapy intervention

ROSEMARY CROUCH

Lee Wilcocks has stated that 'Alcoholism is the most treatable, untreated disease!' (Wilcocks, 1992, p. 3). There are a number of factors contributing to this fact, the most important one being the denial that bedevils the person suffering from alcoholism. Wilcocks continues by saying that 'Alcoholics can be helped and the sooner they are helped the greater the chance of recovery' (p. 3).

These statements are a positive way of introducing a way of thinking or an attitude towards the illness/disease of alcoholism, which is often neglected, or considered secondary to other dilemmas such as HIV/AIDS and cancer. Only in sophisticated developed countries is alcoholism considered a priority, yet it is one of the most seriously debilitating conditions which affects not only the individual but the whole community. It occurs in both developed and in many developing countries as well.

Alcohol is the root cause of many motor vehicle and industrial accidents, child and spousal abuse (particularly in the rural areas and crowded urban areas of a country like South Africa), divorce, the destruction of relationships, violence, drowning and numerous other social problems. The illness affects the economy of a country through loss of working hours, in medical costs as a result of the excessive use of alcohol, and contributes greatly to poverty. It is stated in the DSM-IV-TR™ (American Psychiatric Association, 2000) that 'In most cultures alcohol is the most frequently used brain depressant and is a cause of considerable morbidity and mortality' (p. 212). 'Once a pattern of compulsiveness develops, individuals with dependency may devote substantial periods of time to obtaining and consuming alcoholic beverages' (p. 213).

The DSM-IV-TR™ (American Psychiatric Association, 2000) describes both alcohol abuse and alcohol dependence. The definitions are as follows:

- *Substance abuse:* 'The essential feature of substance abuse is a maladaptive pattern of substance use manifested by recurrent and

519

significant adverse consequences related to the repeated use of the substance' (American Psychiatric Association, 2000, p. 198). The possible consequences are described as:

- failure to fulfil major role obligations
- repeated situations which are physically hazardous
- multiple legal problems
- recurrent social and interpersonal problems, e.g. divorce, physical and verbal abuse, rape, child abuse
- repeated absences at work/school and poor work/school performance
- neglect of childcare and household duties
- aggressive behaviour.

• *Substance dependence:*

The essential feature of substance dependence is a cluster of cognitive, behavioural and physiological symptoms indicating that the individual continues use of the substance despite significant substance-related problems. There is a pattern of repeated self-administration that can result in tolerance, withdrawal and compulsive drug-taking behaviour. 'Craving' is a feature of this disorder (American Psychiatric Association, 2000, p. 181).

The criteria for this disorder are described as follows:

• use of alcohol in larger amounts or over a longer period than intended
• a persistent desire to cut down or regulate intake
• often persistent, unsuccessful efforts to decrease or discontinue
• a great deal of time spent obtaining alcohol, using it and recovering from drinking it
• all daily activities revolve around the use of alcohol
• social, occupational and recreational activities are reduced and there is withdrawal from family activities and hobbies
• despite psychological and physical effects, the person continues to use alcohol.

Both alcohol abuse and alcohol dependence are classified as illnesses and will be referred to collectively as 'alcoholism' in this chapter.

Denial is the defence mechanism that is extremely strong in the alcoholic and often prevents the person from seeking treatment before the body and mind are damaged. There are a number of reasons for this, one of which is that alcoholism is still seen as a social disgrace in most cultures, and the stigma prevents the alcoholic from acknowledging the problem. There may also be religious taboos against the use of alcohol.

Other frequently encountered defence mechanisms include intellectualization, selective recall and euphoric recall, repression, projection, rationalization and minimizing. All of these defence mechanisms are used to protect the alcoholic from being attacked and hurt by others. The defences become an integral part of their coping (Wilcocks, 1992).

Alcoholism is a relapsing illness. Relapse is a process, not an event, and is often part of the rehabilitation process, but is understandably unwelcome to family and friends. It is an after-effect, which builds up with following warning signs:

- **H** – Hungry (for alcohol – craving)
- **A** – Angry (forced to lose a good friend called alcohol)
- **L** – Lonely (no friends, only drinking friends)
- **T** – Tired (no energy, which was previously obtained from the high-carbohydrate alcohol).

In South Africa the problem of alcoholism is so overwhelming at all levels of society that even a major effort may only scratch the surface of the problem. Only community-based projects that involve the schools, community and religious leaders, and the perpetrators of the problem such as the 'shebeens' (traditional taverns), bars and off-licences, will have any hope of trying to prevent alcohol abuse.

Treatment is available for the more privileged members of society. Private hospitals, religious organizations and NGOs, as well as the state, provide facilities offering short-term treatment for alcoholics. Unfortunately not all alcoholics can be treated in short-term facilities. Chronic cases of alcoholism are usually catered for in long-term treatment centres, which in South Africa are provided by the state. The mental hospitals house a frightening number of people who are permanently disabled by alcohol, with conditions such as alcohol amnestic disorder.

The emphasis today is on short-term treatment, and the client is encouraged to resume contact with society as soon after the 'dry-out'/detoxification period as possible. Detoxification is considered a medical emergency and should take place only under close medical or nursing supervision. Detoxification is, however, only the start of the treatment of the alcoholic. Developing insight into the condition, skills training, lifestyle change, treatment of underlying conditions such as depression, psychotherapy where necessary, and ongoing support, are the essential ingredients for the next phase of recovery.

This is where the occupational therapist comes into the team approach to rehabilitation.

The occupational therapist may encounter the alcoholic client in various treatment settings, for example in the orthopaedic or general medical unit or the psychiatric unit. Here the client's alcoholic illness may be complicated by other conditions such as multiple fractures from a motor vehicle accident, heart complaints, diabetes, anxiety or depression. The occupational therapist is trained to treat the client in totality and should always take serious note of the alcoholic pathology, as this may be a focus for intervention.

Most importantly the alcoholic is encountered by the occupational therapist at grassroots level where no facilities are available. The versatility of the training of occupational therapists worldwide makes them ideal for taking part in the intervention within the client's own environment, taking into consideration all the performance areas of their life, i.e. the performance area, the performance components and the performance contexts (American Occupational Therapy Association, 1994). These areas are well defined in Chacksfield and Lancaster (in Creek, 2002, p. 519).

Occupational therapy and the rehabilitation of the alcoholic

The occupational therapist has a vital role to play in helping the recovering alcoholic take part in a sober lifestyle again.

Various theories of occupational therapy provide a sound basis for this intervention.

Wilcock (1998a) describes three factors that cause a breakdown of health, and it can be seen that these factors are very applicable to the alcoholic:

1. Occupational imbalance, which is a lack of balance between work, rest and play. This causes a loss of harmony between internal bodily systems and between the person and the environment. The alcoholic develops difficulties at work, and has no rest or playtime, as this is taken up with drinking.
2. Occupational deprivation, which arises when external circumstances prevent the individual from using his capacities to the full, leading to an imbalance and failure to develop or maintain normal functioning. Social withdrawal, less time at work and with the family, breakdown of support systems and relationships are all part of the alcoholic's life.
3. Occupational alienation, which occurs when the person engages in activity which is not in accordance with the occupational nature of the culture or individual. The results are frustration, boredom, unhappiness and stress. Active, open, excessive drinking and solitary drinking bring about these effects. (The theory is described by Creek, 2002, p. 42.)

Without a doubt addressing these three issues can provide a sound basis for intervention by the occupational therapist. The responsibility for leading a sober life rests solely with the client, but the occupational therapist can help support attempts to address these three issues so that major change can take place. There must be a commitment to change and a lot of effort needs to 'go into changing the activity profile and developing a healthy, balanced lifestyle that fills the void left by not drinking. Skills and knowledge learnt in treatment must be put into use' (Wilcocks, 1992, p. 51).

Creek (2002) builds on the theories of White (1971), which are also applicable to the recovering alcoholic. Whilst the alcoholic was formerly intent on living a lifestyle based on activities which revolved around the use of alcohol, he now finds that he has an intrinsic drive to realize potential 'and exert an influence on the environment. It is drive which leads to the development of competence, as the individual tests his capacities on the outside world and gains confidence in his ability' (Creek, 2002, p. 41).

Models of intervention and occupational therapy

It is important to look at the models of treatment of alcoholism that are commonly used throughout the world in order to understand where occupational therapy is most effective.

The most commonly used and fashionable model for intervention is the Minnesota model, which is used by Alcoholics Anonymous (AA) worldwide, even in the remotest areas. This is a programme of 12 steps, the details of which can be found in the chapter by Chacksfield and Lancaster in Creek (2002, p. 521) or in literature obtained directly from the AA.

In whatever setting the occupational therapist works, these steps have proved to be very successful and must be thoroughly acknowledged by the occupational therapist, whose programme of skills training in all aspect of life fits in very well with the model. The alcoholic must always be encouraged to attend AA meetings as a vital means of support in addition to any other treatment.

Gorski (1989) has been a prolific writer in the field of alcoholism and describes six phases of treatment:

1. *Pretreatment/transition:* Recognition that there is a problem and the decision to seek help. Breakdown of denial which is often facilitated by family, employers and good friends.
2. *Stabilization:* Withdrawal crisis with possible delirium tremens (DTs) and epileptic-type fits. This can last from one to two weeks.
3. *Early recovery:* Learning to function without alcohol. First six months.
4. *Middle recovery:* Returning to a normal balanced lifestyle. Correction of neuro-transmitters. 1–2 years.
5. *Late recovery:* Personality change. Several years.
6. *Maintenance:* Sobriety/abstinence.

The occupational therapist can be involved in any of these stages of treatment in the following way:

- *Pretreatment/transition:* In the organization of and participation in the process of confrontation. This is a skill not usually taught at the undergraduate level of occupational therapy training but is important to learn if working with alcoholics in any setting. Confrontation is the start of intervention and can be used after relapse occurs. It is the firm but caring process of challenging a person about the drinking problem and presenting irrefutable facts about it. The purpose is to break through the denial and secure a promise of treatment. Details of this process can be found in Wilcocks (1992, p. 33).

- *Stabilization:* In this phase the occupational therapist makes contact with the client and gently begins to introduce the concept of treatment.
- *Early recovery:* This is the most dynamic stage for occupational therapy intervention as part of a team effort.
- *Middle recovery:* Aftercare in the form of support groups dealing with subjects such as life skills (stress management, social skills and assertiveness training, activity skills groups), relapse prevention and vocational rehabilitation.
- *Late recovery and maintenance:* Ongoing aftercare.

Occupational therapy intervention in early recovery

People with alcohol dependency or abuse are treated by occupational therapists in various settings, including:

- rural and urban community clinics
- outpatient clinics in rural and urban areas
- short-term treatment centres
- minimally in long-term treatment facilities
- in aftercare facilities such as recreation centres and private practices.

The general principles for therapy are the same for all areas.

The occupational therapist needs a firm but empathetic, supportive and understanding approach to the alcoholic patient. Her attitude should be positive and motivated towards complete sobriety and integration of the client back into normal society again. There is no room in the team for any member who has a hardened and unempathetic attitude towards alcoholism.

The occupational therapist working in a team, usually with a social worker, nurse and doctor, must fully understand that the person with the illness of alcoholism must never drink again. All studies on controlled drinking have been a failure. There has to be complete abstinence on the part of the client.

Assessment

The following assessment is useful in determining the extent of the problem and was devised at Riverfield Lodge Rehabilitation Centre in Gauteng, South Africa, in 1991:

Table 23.1 Psychological behavioural signs of alcoholism (Wilcocks et al., 1992)

	YES	NO
Using alcohol to enhance moods or as a 'pick-up' when down		
Using alcohol to boost confidence		
Drinking faster than, or more than, others		
Consistently drinking more than was originally intended		
Finding that alcohol is having a negative impact on social, emotional, physical or occupational functioning and, in spite of this, not being able to stop or control it		
Missing deadlines or important meetings		
Drop in work performance		
Forgetting things and not being able to concentrate		
Being supersensitive to constructive criticism		
Drinking alone		
Deterioration in relationships with colleagues, spouse and friends		
Feelings of remorse or guilt over drinking		
Using drinking as a central activity in life		

If working in the community or in short-term units, the assessment of clients should be quick and efficient and can take place during both group and individual sessions. Assessment also continues when treatment begins.

The following assessment tools can be used:

- The COPM (Canadian Occupational Performance Measure, 1998)
- Stress assessment (Crouch, 2003) and stress assessment (Piek et al., 1993)
- Leisure assessment (Chacksfield and Lindsay, 1999)
- Work assessment, Assessment of Motor and Process Skills (AMPS, Fischer 2001)
- Cognitive processes (Allen and Allen, 1987)
- Interests. The Interest Checklist (Matsutsuyu, 1969)
- Self-esteem and self-concept. Rosenberg Self-Esteem Inventory (Rosenberg, 1965).

Important aspects of the client, which should be assessed by the occupational therapist, include:

- the client's strengths

- physical problems which affect functioning such as gross and fine motor coordination, tremor, poor balance and gait, muscular weakness, emaciation and obesity, and peripheral neuritis
- all aspects of cognition, affect, self-concept, volition, body concept, insight, judgement and interpretation, decision making and problem solving. Problems that are frequently found in the alcoholic patient are:
  - Lack of emotional insight. Intellectual insight may be present and the client may be proficient at describing the effects of alcohol (the defence mechanism of intellectualization). The occupational therapist should recognize this defence, but realize that the client has no real understanding of his illness.
  - Preoccupation with alcohol and related problems.
  - Temporary short-term memory and concentration loss.
  - Inability to make decisions and to solve problems (toxic effect of alcohol as well as alcohol being used previously to assist in these functions).
  - Poor self-concept and self-esteem which is a major precipitating factor in alcoholism and also a result of the illness.
  - Free-floating anxiety or situation-based anxiety, and an inability to cope with stress.
  - Major depression (episode and disorder), dysthymia and bipolar disorder are frequently found in alcoholics. It is a vicious circle since the alcoholic drinks to 'drown his sorrows' and the alcohol, a central nervous system depressant drug, has a sedative effect, which increases the misery and depression. People in a hypomanic state also abuse alcohol.
  - Passive or active underlying aggression is frequently found in the alcoholic.
  - Poor frustration tolerance and an inability to delay gratification.
  - A tendency to lie and deceive which has been learnt whilst involved in the procuring of alcohol and during the denial process.
  - Poor social skills and in particular problems with being appropriately assertive.

All areas of functioning should be covered as follows:

- The client's ability to cope with personal hygiene, self-care and care of the environment. In some severe cases there is a general lack of self-care in the form of bodily hygiene and care of the environment. Conversely female clients tend to overdress and to use too much make-up to disguise the fact that they have been drinking. Their homes are often spotless and well kept and all the physical needs of the family are attended to. However the emotional needs of the family are sadly lacking. Male clients may have an inability to handle financial affairs and to budget adequately.

- The client's ability to cope in the social sphere, i.e. social awareness, communication with others and the formation of interpersonal relationships. Often the alcoholic is a socially minded, gregarious person. Friends, however, are often drinking friends or business drinking associates. This problem is one of the stumbling blocks to the patient's reintegration into the community after treatment. Secret drinkers, usually female, are less sociable.
- The client's ability to use free time constructively, if he uses it at all at present. Most alcoholics have no hobbies or pleasurable pastime activities other than drinking-associated activities such as parties, snooker or darts evenings, pub activities and spectator participation in sport. It is difficult to determine whether the alcoholic drinks because he has nothing better to do, or because his drinking pattern has eliminated any other type of free-time activity!
- The client's performance at work and the effect that the alcohol has had on his work performance, such as absenteeism, accidents, excessive medical care, decreased productivity and faulty decision making. If needed, a full work assessment can be undertaken, but this is not possible when the occupational therapist is working with large numbers in the community. Traditionally the alcoholic, when not under the influence of alcohol, is a very hard worker. The greatest problem is holding the job down when they are drinking, or being treated for the problem, and the lack of understanding of most employers.

Aims of treatment:
- To gain emotional insight into the illness of alcoholism.
- To encourage meaningful free time and leisure activities which could provide a replacement for periods of drinking alcohol.
- To improve the patient's self-concept by encouraging a feeling of self-worth.
- To assist in the handling of stress in an effective manner and to reduce anxiety.
- To provide a group setting where emotions can be expressed freely and where new behaviours and situations can be tried out, e.g. art groups and psychodrama.
- To treat specific difficulties such as depression, poor memory and concentration.
- To encourage long-lasting, mature interpersonal relationships.
- To carry out vocational rehabilitation where appropriate, and prepare the client for work.
- With the help of the social worker, help the client with financial affairs if this is a problem and, if necessary, help him look for employment.
- Where necessary attend to activities of daily living (ADL) such as self-care, home management, childcare.
- To build up physical fitness.
- To plan future goals related to a sober lifestyle.
- To plan for ongoing support and aftercare.

Treatment

Principles of handling

People with the illness of alcoholism are known to be manipulative and difficult to handle. Therefore it is important that the occupational therapist is one step ahead of the client the whole time, is assertive and open, and anticipates manipulation. It is important to confront the client in a non-aggressive manner when unacceptable behaviour, such as lying, occurs.

Firm limits have to be set on behaviour, yet the occupational therapist must be empathetic. Alcoholism is one of the most difficult of all conditions to overcome. Be understanding and consistent in approach and give the client time to talk.

The alcoholic tends to be a dependent person in all respects. It is part of the personality. Other dependencies often go hand in hand, such as smoking cigarettes, drugs and medication, eating certain foods and dependency on people. The occupational therapist must be aware of a dependent relationship developing between herself and the patient as this leads to manipulation with regard to such issues as favours, demands on time and avoiding responsibilities.

Structuring the treatment situation

This will depend very much on the treatment setting, but the same rules apply whether it is in a rural clinic or a private hospital:

- Clients may have to be treated individually at first, but group treatment is preferred because of the social context, and should be introduced as soon as possible.
- Strict control must be kept on tools and equipment. Make sure all tools are replaced before the client leaves the activity group.
- Most alcoholic clients work at a fairly high level of competency and are in a position to help prepare activities.
- As a precautionary measure, all noxious substances and alcohol-based substances such as methylated spirits, thinners, shoe polish and leather dyes should be kept locked away at all times. Activities such as glass painting should be avoided. Experience has shown that clients tend to sniff the volatile liquid excessively hoping to become 'high'.

Requirements of activities

This will depend on the client's level of activity participation (see chapter 1). Initially, when using creative activities for leisure time pursuits, use short-term, successful activities with a good end product. This raises the client's self-esteem and caters for poor frustration tolerance and lack of concentration. The cost of creative activities must be taken into consideration. It will depend on the socio-economic level and debt situation of the client.

There should be a good balance of activities incorporating both work and recreational activities. Recreational activities that are appropriate, meaningful and of a long-lasting quality should be introduced, which will assist in the replacement of drinking, e.g. sport.

Both individual and group activities should be planned.

Grading of activities

The grading of activity participation by the client in the occupational therapy programme will proceed as he recovers. Elements of responsibility, frustration, duration and complexity can be introduced gradually until the client is independent and ready to face the world.

The total treatment plan and OT

The occupational therapy treatment from the recovery stage onwards is rehabilitative in approach and is part of the wider intervention by a multidisciplinary team. This approach consists of educational programmes, socio-emotional group work, stress management and relaxation, life skills training, recreational activities including sport and creative/hobby activities, individual counselling by professional members of staff (including the occupational therapist) and religious counsellors, psychotherapy by the clinical psychologists and medical care.

Alcoholics Anonymous (AA) meetings are also usually part of the total programme.

Specific contributions by the occupational therapist

Group work

Stress management

Stress management is an integral part of the total approach to the treatment of the alcoholic. Many good programmes are available on this subject such as Ritchie (1985) and Fontana (1989) for more privileged clients, and new programmes which have been researched by Crouch (2003) for rural communities. The content of the course should cover the following subjects:

- stress and how it affects the body and mind as well as a person's functioning
- learning to balance the lifestyle and control stress
- stress and alcohol
- relaxation.

Social skills training

These groups should include training in both verbal and non-verbal communication. Special emphasis should be placed on assertiveness training so that the alcoholic can learn to be assertive without the use of alcohol. Controlling anger and aggression should be part of this training.

'Powerless' and 'damage' groups

This is a technique of group work specifically used for people with addictions and is often shared by the professionals in the team, e.g. the social worker and occupational therapist. The inference is that alcohol makes one powerless in the face of society and also damages body, spirit, relationships, families, etc.

Educational groups

These are groups that are also shared by the professionals in the team. Didactic sessions are known to have very little lasting value and contribute only to intellectual insight. Videos with an in-depth discussion are far more effective.

Psychodrama

According to Blatner (1992), psychodrama is an outstanding technique for helping the client gain insight into his problem. With a skilled occupational therapist, this is one of the most dynamic and powerful techniques. The client gains insight into himself, his behaviour, relationships and the problem of alcoholism. He is also able to test new behaviours and plan for the future. Occupational therapists in South Africa have postgraduate training in this technique available to them through the Occupational Therapy Association of South Africa (OTASA).

Free-time and recreational/leisure activities

The alcoholic client needs to adapt to a new lifestyle. As interest in free-time activities can provide a meaningful replacement for drinking, a certain amount of time every day should be devoted to active involvement in an activity other than work. (Alcoholics tend to become completely obsessed with work during the recovery process.) Clients with families should be encouraged to undertake activities that would be suitable to share with the family. Not only would this support the client in theri endeavour, but will improve family relationships. Examples of activities are:

* Creative activities such as woodwork, wood carving or wood burning, leatherwork, decoupage, printmaking of all kinds, fabric painting, pottery, sewing and painting. (These activities are often culturally bound and will differ from culture to culture.)

- Gardening and horticulture, e.g. vegetable gardening or exotic gardening such as growing orchids or roses.
- Sport with both active and passive participation. Sport is often associated with drinking and the client must be cautioned. Exercise in the form of walking or exercise groups.
- Involvement in social clubs, religious groups, AA groups and voluntary work.

Physical fitness

Physical training should be an integral part of the programme and should take place at the start of every day. Correct breathing and posture should be encouraged, as should attention to weight loss where applicable. General fitness and improved circulation will be achieved.

Regular exercise has been shown to improve mood and motivation, so it is extremely important to encourage appropriate exercise to balance the lifestyle of the alcoholic. Encouraging them to exercise after work takes them away from the most dangerous drinking time.

Vocational rehabilitation

Over the past few years occupational therapists have become highly trained and expert in vocational rehabilitation. It is a field of practice that is very important for the alcoholic. Returning the alcoholic to work, whether in the home or the open labour market, is an important achievement in the whole rehabilitation process.

The attitude of the employer towards the alcoholic has improved marginally and it is important, where possible, for the occupational therapist to work with the employer. Employers are encouraged to keep a client's job open whilst they are in rehabilitation. The occupational therapist must take care that the employer is understanding and that the contact does not place the client's job in jeopardy.

The housewife may require assistance with such issues as economical cooking, time planning, sewing and other home management skills. Important subjects such as child handling may have to be introduced into the occupational therapy programme.

Treatment of specific problems

Problems identified in the assessment such as poor memory, poor concentration, aggression and depression should be treated on an individual basis or in groups. Activities should be analysed for their potential to be therapeutic.

Financial management and budgeting

Occupational therapists working in the field of alcoholism such as Pienaar

(Crouch and Pienaar, 1984) have found that many clients have financial difficulties due to the excessive use of alcohol. Group sessions which deal with budgeting and financial control are extremely helpful. It may be useful to bring in an expert on the subject, so that clients can work out their own budgets and pinpoint difficulties.

Entertainments

Non-alcoholic barbecues and other social entertainment such as dances, where alcohol is usually served in the community, should form an integral part of the programme. Clients need to learn to enjoy themselves without the use of alcohol. This is a very difficult concept for them.

Goal-setting and forward planning

Rehabilitation is a long process for the alcoholic and it is essential for the occupational therapist to help plan the future. Goal-setting for both short-term and long-term goals is important, as well as implementing a commitment from the client to take part in supportive aftercare. It is also very important for the occupational therapist to discuss with the client his achievements thus far.

Aftercare

Treatment in a clinic or hospital is worthless unless a supportive aftercare system is firmly in place for the client.

Support groups should be provided by any treatment centre worth its salt. Clients should be able to attend both daytime and after-hours groups. They benefit greatly from returning to the treatment centre for support and updating. It also benefits and encourages clients who are still in the programme to meet those who have returned to a normal life again and who are coping with the addiction process.

Alternative venues are provided by the AA and religious groups, as well as private practitioners in the health professions.

Prevention and treatment programmes in poor communities: the occupational therapist's role

Alcoholism is a very serious problem in impoverished rural and urban communities in South Africa as well as in many developing countries. Occupational therapists working in these areas can follow the intervention guidelines already given in this chapter and where community rehabilitation workers and occupational therapy auxiliaries are available, work out an effective treatment plan. Although this situation relates to South Africa, many other countries have similar problems and it is anticipated that this information will be useful.

Target groups
Prevention is better than cure and the following groups in the community can be successfully targeted for education on alcoholism:

- community meetings for adults and youths
- literacy education groups
- women's leagues and self-help groups
- burial society groups
- care groups
- antenatal and well-baby clinics
- disabled persons
- school committees, for example a parent–teachers association (PTA)
- meetings of religious and political leaders
- alcoholics Anonymous (AA), available in many impoverished areas.

Teaching methods
Teaching about alcoholism can be carried in the following way:

- the use of role-play and by using puppets, talks and lectures. Small group work is most effective
- the use of posters, pamphlets, magazine articles and other media such as radio and TV
- the use of songs and music
- the use of drama and informal acting.

Providing alternatives to alcohol abuse
Alcoholism can be prevented in a large section of the community by providing adequate recreation and sports facilities as well as opportunities for workshops and skills training groups. Trying to counteract unemployment is a vast undertaking for the country but will greatly improve the incidence of alcoholism.

Case study: Mr M

Background

Mr M is 45 years old, the respected headmaster of a secondary school in Alexandra, a crowded, impoverished area close to Johannesburg in South Africa. He and his wife live in a better area, 5 km away from the school. They have two sons and a daughter who go to school in Johannesburg.

Mrs M has a morning job doing administrative work at their local Methodist church.

Being a headmaster in this school is extremely stressful. There are major problems with children playing truant, violence and stressed teachers.

One of the teachers brought a small bottle of brandy to him one day, which she had found in a classroom. With his strict Methodist upbringing, Mr M has never touched alcohol until recently. However, he found that a small tot of brandy after work, whilst still in his office, helped him relax after a very stressful day.

The tolerance factor of alcohol took hold and Mr M started using more and more of the brandy to get the same effect and he then found that a small tot in the morning helped him through the day. His wife became suspicious of something wrong when he was arriving home later and later in the evening. She noticed that he had become sullen and aggressive and was not his usual quiet and controlled self.

He began to withdraw from the staff at the school and his secretary often told the staff that Mr M was at a meeting and not available.

Late one afternoon after Mr M's secretary had left, the deputy head of the school came back to fetch something he had left behind. He saw that Mr M's office light was on and went in to investigate. He found Mr M in a highly inebriated state, incoherent and falling all over the room. He took Mr M home to his house and phoned Mrs M to tell her that they had a late meeting. Later that evening he took Mr M home. Mr M went straight to bed. In the morning, at school, the deputy head approached Mr M about the problem. Mr M totally denied any problem and told the deputy head to go away.

Intervention

The deputy head approached Mr M's wife, who gave him permission to phone a local alcohol rehabilitation clinic, where he spoke to the social worker. A plan was devised to confront Mr M in his office the next day. Members of the confrontation group consisted of the deputy head, Mrs M, the Methodist minister and the social worker. The social worker met with the group first to assist them in the confrontation.

Mr M was shocked to see the group walk into his office in the morning (before he had had his first drink). Behind a locked door, firm evidence was presented to Mr M about his problem. He agreed to be admitted to the clinic for rehabilitation on condition that the matter would be highly confidential and that his job would be held for him. The deputy head agreed to run the school in his absence and to say that Mr M was in hospital for an illness. His contribution to a medical insurance would help with the payment of treatment.

Occupational therapy

As part of the multidisciplinary team approach to treatment, Mr M met the occupational therapist whilst in the withdrawal/detoxification unit. She explained the purpose of the occupational therapy programme and what would be expected of him. He was also introduced to his psychotherapist and intensive counselling was started.

In two days Mr M was involved in gentle exercise, educational groups and stress management after a thorough assessment had been undertaken.

The aims of occupational therapy for Mr M were:

- To develop emotional insight into his problem.
- To learn to handle stress by changing to a balanced lifestyle of work, exercise and leisure/recreation (to be shared with his wife and family).
- To introduce leisure time activity.
- To discuss the work situation with special emphasis on assertive behaviour and anger management.
- To plan for involvement in aftercare including the clinic's aftercare programme and the local AA group.

The occupational therapy programme
In addition to the exercise, educational groups and stress management, Mr M was gently introduced to psychodrama and also to assertiveness training. He also joined the creative activity group and renewed his old interest in woodwork.

Before he was discharged after 14 days' treatment, the social worker asked Mrs M to come to a consultation between herself, Mr M and the occupational therapist. Guidelines for working with Mr M in his journey of sobriety were given, such as emotional support, enforcing the principles of stress management in terms of a balanced lifestyle and the extreme importance of supportive aftercare. Pointers to recognize relapse were discussed.

Mr M is back at work as headmaster, and at present is firmly entrenched in his aftercare. His wife and the deputy head are open with him about the problem and they talk about it frequently and encourage him in his ongoing rehabilitation. The minister gives him a handshake and wink, every Sunday morning at church!

Conclusion

Every recovering alcoholic is a mini miracle and sobriety is his most precious gift. He works with great courage and dedication to preserve and enhance his sobriety and no one, not the alcoholic nor his family should ever become complacent about it or take it for granted (Wilcocks, 1992, p. 59).

Alcoholism is an illness that can be successfully treated by a multidisciplinary approach. The occupational therapist's role in the total rehabilitation programme of the alcoholic is very specific and definable from a theoretical 'occupation' premise and is stimulating and rewarding. It is an area of practice that also has its disappointments and frustrations and these are related to relapse and manipulative behaviour on the part of the alcoholic. Once the occupational therapist has learnt to handle these difficulties, she becomes an important agent in helping the client start a new life.

In terms of the magnitude of this problem in many countries in the world, there is no doubt at all that occupational therapists must start to address the problem of alcoholism from a broad perspective. They must become involved in the legislative and decision bodies on the subject, as well as being part of the preventative and rehabilitation programmes at a primary healthcare level.

Questions

1. What is meant by substance dependence and how does this illness affect a person in all aspects of their occupational functioning?
2. What is relapse in the alcoholic? How can this be prevented?
3. Discuss three important aspects of occupational therapy intervention with the alcoholic.
4. Describe, giving aims of treatment, three types of group work that are successful in the treatment of the alcoholic.
5. Discuss the importance of aftercare for the alcoholic.
6. How can an occupational therapist be involved in preventative programmes for alcoholism at grassroots level?

Chapter 24
Occupational therapy intervention for drug-related disorders

LISA WEGNER

Global context

Drug use has become a major public and professional concern in almost every country in the world. The United Nations Drug Control Programme estimated 3.4 per cent of the world's population to be illicit (or non-medical) drug users (United Nations Office on Drugs and Crime, 2003). Cannabis is the most widely used drug worldwide, followed by heroin and cocaine. The main problem drugs in the late 1990s (as reflected by treatment demands) were cocaine in North and South America, opiates in Europe, Asia and Australia, and cannabis in Africa. Most countries are experiencing an increase in drug consumption, particularly amongst young people. 'Monitoring the Future' surveys conducted annually with 50,000 young people in the United States reported a doubling in the rates of illicit drug use during the early 1990s. However, in more recent years the surveys have shown that generally drug use has tended to stabilize, and in some instances even decrease (National Institute on Drug Abuse, 2003). The use of drugs can be associated with attitudinal factors such as perceived risk of harm, disapproval of drug use and perceptions of the availability of drugs.

South African context

The developing countries are particularly vulnerable to the increase in drug use because of the demands placed on the health system, as well as on society and the economy. A study of the prevalence of substance use amongst South African adolescents reported that cannabis use had almost doubled since 1990 (Flisher et al., 2003). The average age of people treated for cannabis use is 19–24 years, and the majority of users are male (Myers and Parry, 2003). A report by the Director of the Medical Research Council's Alcohol and Drug Abuse Research Group revealed that between 1996 and 2003, treatment demands for cannabis and heroin use increased by 11 per cent and 6 per cent respectively (Parry, 2003). Furthermore, the age of patients admitted to treatment centres decreased, reflecting an increase in drug use by adolescents and even children (Parry, 2003). These are worrying statistics given the lack of access to intervention by much of the population.

Many factors can be associated with an increased risk of drug use including individual, family, social, genetic and contextual factors (Gilvarry, 2000). In South Africa much of the population lives in disadvantaged areas lacking in resources. Social problems such as poverty, violence, crime and gangsterism further compound the situation. Adolescents living in these areas tend to experience relatively high levels of boredom in their leisure time (Wegner, 1998) as opportunities to become involved in healthy leisure activities are restricted by the lack of resources within the environment (Wegner and Magner, 2002). This situation increases the potential for substance use and other risk behaviours.

Drug use and abuse

Drug use refers to the general use of drugs and usually starts on an experimental basis. Experimentation can lead to *drug abuse*, where individuals use drugs despite knowing that the effects are harmful and dangerous. With repeated use over time *drug dependence* or addiction can occur. According to the DSM-IV-TR™, this is when individuals need to use increasing amounts of the drug to achieve the same effect (otherwise known as tolerance), and feel unable to perform daily tasks without using the drug (American Psychiatric Association, 2000). Withdrawal symptoms may be experienced if the drug is not used for some time. From an occupational perspective, people use drugs to enable, avoid or enhance occupation, as a coping mechanism, and to alter perception (Chacksfield and Lancaster in Creek, 2002). Drugs can be broadly classified according to the different effects they produce in the human body (see Table 24.1). Drugs are commonly consumed by smoking, inhalation, oral ingestion or injection.

Table 24.1 Classification of commonly abused drugs

Drug category	Examples	Primary effects	Common side-effects
Opiates/Opioids Narcotics	Morphine, Codeine, Heroin	Analgesic, decrease anxiety, sedation	Addiction, sharing needles may lead to HIV infection and hepatitis, death
Stimulants	Amphetamines (Appetite suppressants Stay-awake tablets) Cocaine, Crack (Cocaine plus heroin = 'speedball') Tik-Tik	Stimulant, pleasurable high, increased activity, loss of appetite	Highly addictive, irritability, weight loss, restlessness, sleep disturbances, mood swings, depression, social withdrawal, violence, heart and respiratory failure

Table 24.1 contd.

Drug category	Examples	Primary effects	Common side-effects
Hallucinogens	MDMA (Ecstasy) Lysergic acid diethylamide (LSD)	Stimulant, sense of pleasure and confidence, psychedelic	Panic attacks, insomnia, increased heart rate and blood pressure, sudden death
Depressants	Barbiturates Benzodiazepines	Sedation, relaxation	Addiction
Inhalants	Model glue, Spray paint, Petrol, Cleaning fluids	Relaxation; Creates 'a buzz'	Liver or kidney damage, convulsions, brain damage, peripheral neuropathy, sudden death
Other	Cannabis (also known as marijuana, dagga, pot, grass, weed, joint, hashish)	Euphoria, sense of relaxation, distorted perceptual and sensory processes, increased appetite (or 'munchies')	Psychological dependence, depersonalization, disorientation, acute panic attacks, paranoia
	Mandrax (Methaqualone and antihistamine) Known as a 'whitepipe' when smoked with cannabis	Same as above	Addiction, seizures coma, death

Intervention with drug-related disorders is a complex and lengthy process. Individuals can receive inpatient or outpatient treatment at state or private medical facilities, where the length of treatment may range from two weeks to six months, or even longer in some cases. This type of treatment is 'therapeutic' or 'rehabilitative' in nature. Intervention can also be 'preventative', where the focus is on increasing awareness about drugs and their harmful effects, and enabling people to stay drug-free. Prevention programmes usually occur in community settings such as clinics, libraries and schools. Support and advice is available from Narcotics Anonymous (NA) (website www.ukna.org; tel. 0881 300327). NA is a non-profit fellowship of recovering addicts who meet regularly to help each other stay clean. Related organizations provide support for family and friends affected by drug abuse. Many local religious organizations also offer assistance regarding drug addiction.

The occupational performance approach

The occupational performance approach is concerned with the dynamic interaction between the *person*, the *context* and his/her *occupations*

(Watson, 1997). Occupational performance refers to the hierarchy of roles, tasks and activities that allow the individual to organize his/her daily occupations (Christiansen and Baum in Watson, 1997). The occupational performance approach is a useful way of planning intervention for clients with drug-related disorders and will form the basis for discussion in this chapter. The case study illustrates how theory is applied in practice.

Referral

Individuals who are using drugs often tend to have limited insight into the damaging effects of drugs on their occupational performance. This may be combined with a desire to conceal the drug use from families and employers. Often an individual is referred for treatment after an incident such as an accidental overdose, or a warning from the school or employer triggers the individual or a family member to seek help. Clients can be referred for treatment by the usual referral sources, including doctors, social workers, psychologists, nurses, teachers, employers and family members. The courts may also refer people who have been involved in criminal activities associated with their use of drugs.

Case study – referral

Jack (24 years) was referred to a therapeutic drug rehabilitation unit by his doctor. He has been admitted as an inpatient for a period of six weeks. He will be able to go home for weekends from the third week. Jack used to live with his girlfriend and their three-year-old daughter, until the girlfriend broke up with him because of his drug use. He moved in with his parents, but conflict soon arose as his drugging habit escalated. His mother insisted that he see the family doctor.

Assessment

Clients may initially undergo a period of detoxification depending on the drugs used. Assessment by the multidisciplinary team starts during this time. The occupational therapist's role is to assess the impact of drug use on the client's occupational performance, and the extent of the dysfunction in his/her life. This can be done by drawing up the client's occupational performance profile (Watson, 1997). The American Occupational Therapy Association's Uniform Terminology for Occupational Therapy (in Neistadt and Crepeau, 1998) can be used to guide the assessment process. Assessment should be client-centred, where the occupational therapist helps the client identify the level of dysfunction within his/her performance areas and role fulfilment. It is important to consider the client's past, present and intended future performance.

The occupational therapist assesses the relevant performance compo-nents related to the client's deficits in the performance areas. With drug-related disorders the components that are commonly affected are cognitive integration, psychosocial skills and psychological components, but the client's physical status should also be assessed. Assessment of con-text includes temporal factors such as age and stage of development, as well as social, cultural, environmental and physical factors. The occupa-tional therapist should consider how the client's particular context affords him/her opportunities for performance, as well as how it demands particular behaviours from the client (Kielhofner, 1995).

The occupational performance profile can be compiled by means of the following methods of assessment. It may be necessary to adapt some of the methods according to the time available for assessment and the inter-vention context.

1. Interviewing the client: The Occupational Performance History Interview (OPHI) (Kielhofner, 1995) enables the occupational therapist to obtain information about the client's past and present occupational functioning. It covers five content areas:

   - organization of daily living routines
   - life roles
   - interests, values and goals
   - perceptions of ability and responsibility
   - environmental influences.

   By using the Canadian Occupational Performance Measure (COPM) the occupational therapist can assess which aspects of the performance areas the client considers important, as well as the client's satisfaction with his/her task performance (Law et al., 1994). This facilitates the establishment of meaningful goals for intervention.
2. Observation of occupational performance: Insight into performance can be obtained by observing the client's participation in structured settings such as groups, as well as in unstructured settings such as dur-ing mealtimes. The client's self-presentation, social interaction and ability to carry out tasks are all factors that can be observed.
3. Self-assessments and checklists: The client completes these independ-ently; therefore they are a useful tool for promoting insight and self awareness, and eliciting discussion. Examples are the Role Checklist and the Modified Interest Checklist (Kielhofner, 1995).

Case study – assessment

During her assessment interview, the occupational therapist starts build-ing a therapeutic relationship with Jack by engaging him in a conversation about his life. Jack tells her, 'Looking back on things now, the reason I didn't study further after finishing school was probably because of my drugging'. He says that his girlfriend supported him financially which made him feel 'less of a man'. The occupational therapist notices Jack's feelings of guilt. She asks him if he has any talents. He replies, 'I think I am quite creative, and I use this talent to make jewellery. I like using wire, beads and natural materials like shells and feathers. I've even made a bit of money selling some of my jewellery – but then I just use the money to buy drugs.'

Jack begins to talk about his history of drug-taking. He started drinking and smoking cigarettes when he was 14 years old, then progressed to smoking cannabis or 'dagga' as it is known in South Africa. He says, 'When I was about 17 years old, a friend showed me how to smoke a "white pipe". Do you know what that is? It's dagga mixed with crushed mandrax tablets which you put in a bottle neck and smoke. But the biggest mistake I made was to start sniffing cocaine two years ago – that caused a lot of problems in my life.'

Observations by the multidisciplinary team reveal Jack to be a quiet, passive person who does not interact much with the other patients in the unit, preferring to keep to himself. However, Jack tends to get frustrated and loses his temper easily, becoming verbally abusive.

Table 24.2 Case study – Occupational performance profile for Jack

Occupations	Person	Context
Roles Jack's significant life roles are father, boyfriend, son and worker. He has neglected these roles and has had difficulty performing according to role expectations. Therefore his role experience has been limited.	*Self-efficacy* Jack shows poor self-esteem and awareness, and lacks a consolidated self-concept/personal identity. Therefore his belief in his own capabilities (self-efficacy) is poor. He regards himself as a failure and feels that his problems are insurmountable.	*Temporal* Jack is in his mid-20s stage of intimacy versus isolation (Erikson, 1980). As such, he should be establishing his roles as partner, father and worker. He has recognized the need to stop using drugs.
Habits Jack's use of time has not been constructive. His days have lacked structure and planning, and are characterized by disorganization. Most of his time has been spent getting and using drugs, or recovering from the effects of drugs.	*Values* Jack has not been able to adhere to his value system as his need to obtain and use drugs has dominated his life. He feels very guilty about stealing money from his family, and verbally abusing his girlfriend.	*Social* Jack has strained relationships with his girlfriend and his parents. He has no friends apart from drug acquaintances. *Cultural* Jack identifies with the drug subculture. He has no strong spiritual beliefs.
Tasks and performance Jack has neglected the performance of routine tasks as expected by his roles.	*Interests* Jack has limited interests as drugs have been his only interest for many years.	*Physical* He lives at home with his parents although he would

Table 24.2 contd.

Occupations	Person	Context
Activities of daily living Neglected personal hygiene. Avoids social interaction with other people and has poor social skills. *Work and productive activities* Little or no experience in most aspects of home management tasks (cleaning, meal preparation, shopping, money management). Limited parenting skills. Is creative and shows talent as a jewellery-maker. Work habits are poor. *Leisure* Limited leisure interests apart from watching sport on television. Occasionally spends time designing jewellery.	*Goals* Jack wants to give up drugs and recognizes that he needs help to do this. He feels uncertain about the future, but thinks he might be able to develop his skill as a jewellery-maker. *Performance components* *Sensorimotor* Jack has poor endurance and is unfit. *Cognitive integration* Jack has some intellectual insight but no emotional insight. He has poor memory, a limited attention span and difficulties with problem solving and decision making. *Psychosocial skills* Poor interpersonal skills affect his ability to conduct himself appropriately in social situations. Has difficulty expressing his thoughts, feelings and needs. Resulting conflict in relationship with girlfriend and parents. Poor coping skills, e.g. handling stress and anxiety. Poor time management. Difficulty with self-control and anger management	prefer to be living with his girlfriend and child.

Intervention

The focus of intervention with drug-related disorders is on changing behaviour and lifestyle. This is achieved by enabling the client to:

- recognize the problem and its consequences
- admit the need for help and concentrate on learning to live with the problem in a constructive manner

- identify the changes that need to be made in lifestyle and behaviour
- translate this into action by making the necessary changes in order to develop a new way of life (Bekker, 2003).

Effective practice is always based on sound theoretical models. Models of intervention which have proven to be successful include the well-known Twelve Step Method of Alcoholics Anonymous, and the Stages of Change model developed by Prochaska and DiClemente (1986). The Stages of Change model assists the multidisciplinary team to understand the client's behaviour according to which stage he/she is in, and select appropriate treatment goals and activities for the stage. The client can be an active participant in the process of identifying the stage and setting realistic goals. The Stages of Change model recognizes that addicts move through six stages in their efforts to change their behaviour (Connors et al., 2001):

- *Pre-contemplation* – the person does not regard him/herself as having a problem and, therefore, is not usually in treatment. *'The only reason I'm here is because my wife says I have a drug problem.'*
- *Contemplation* – the person realises that his behaviour is a problem and thinks about changing; however he experiences ambivalence. *'Perhaps there have been times when my drugging has caused problems in my life.'*
- *Preparation* – the person resolves his ambivalence and makes the decision to change. *'I guess I am addicted to drugs and it's time to do something about it.'*
- *Action* – the person actively tries to change his behaviour. *'I have been trying to stop drugging and I'm here to find ways to help me do this.'*
- *Maintenance* – the person has successfully changed his behaviour and actively maintains the change. *'Now that I've managed to stop drugging I need to work hard at staying drug-free.'*
- *Relapse* – the person returns to the previous pattern of drug misuse. The Stages of Change model makes provision for relapse, acknowledging that people will most likely move through the stages several times before being able to maintain behaviour change on a long-term basis.

Occupational therapy intervention is 'directed at establishing a fit between the client's occupational roles, tasks, skills, abilities, and contextual demands' (American Occupational Therapy Association, 1994, in Watson, 1997, p. 20). Therefore intervention strategies used within an occupational performance approach are directed at the person, his occupations and context. Strategies may include (Watson, 1997):

- promoting a new lifestyle, way of living, and patterns of occupation
- engagement in purposeful therapeutic activities and occupations which are graded to promote competency, mastery and self-esteem

- improving skills and abilities in performance areas and components
- teaching new methods and skills, and providing opportunities to practise these
- counselling or educating relevant people within the community, work, school or home setting.

Outcome and goals of intervention

The intended outcome of occupational therapy intervention is that clients will achieve and maintain a lifestyle without the use of drugs. They will gain insight into their behaviour, and be equipped with relevant coping strategies and skills to improve their occupational performance in accordance with significant life roles. Drug-using activities will be replaced with constructive and satisfying activities. This will enhance their self-concept, enabling them to create meaning in their lives and preventing relapse.

Group intervention

Occupational therapy intervention with drug-related disorders occurs predominantly by means of group work. The occupational therapist should make use of the therapeutic factors inherent in groups, such as instillation of hope, universality, identification, altruism and interpersonal learning (Yalom, 1995) to shape desired behaviour. Members of the multidisciplinary team can be invited to co-facilitate the occupational therapy groups.

Orientation groups

During the orientation phase, new patients are first introduced to the environment of the facility and then to other patients and staff members. Orientation groups enable new patients to become familiar with the nature and goals of the programme, the rules of the facility, client rights and expectations. These groups are an opportunity for patients to commit themselves to the treatment process. It is useful to get the group members to establish their own set of norms, and sign a group contract. Patients who have been in the facility for longer can take responsibility for certain aspects of these groups.

Occupational groups

These are groups which focus on the therapeutic use of work, leisure and activities of daily living (ADL). A variety of treatment goals can be achieved by facilitating clients' participation in occupational groups, and altering the handling, structuring and grading principles for each client. It is not so much the type of activity, but more the expectations inherent within the objectives of the activity that are important in therapy. An important consideration is to make sure that all activities are culturally appropriate and relevant.

Table 24.3 Occupational groups, activities and objectives

Occupational group	Examples of activities	Objectives
Work	Craft activities such as woodwork, jewellery-making, paper crafts, fabric painting, wirework. Ward chores such as gardening, meal preparation, cleaning.	Develop worker role. Develop work habits. Develop work skills. Improve cognitive components (frustration tolerance, delay of gratification, memory, concentration). Develop responsibility. Improve self-esteem.
Leisure	Sports such as volleyball, aerobics, soccer, walking, jogging. Recreation, hobbies and games.	Identify and explore personal leisure interests, skills, activities and opportunities. Opportunity for relaxation. Improve self-esteem and self-concept. Improve physical health.
ADL	Meal preparation, shopping, budgeting, parenting, grooming, hygiene.	Develop and practise skills in relevant areas. Improve self-confidence and self-concept.

Intrapersonal skills groups

These groups focus on self-awareness, insight, values, goals, self-esteem and self-concept. People who have been abusing drugs for a long time often experience a delay in personal development. By considering the client's chronological and developmental stages, the occupational therapist can select appropriate activities to facilitate the client's ability to deal with developmental issues. This means that clients need to become aware of their intrapersonal strengths and weaknesses. They need to understand why they became addicted to drugs, and become aware of the damaging effects of their drug-taking behaviour on relatives, friends and their lives in general. They need to identify their values and set realistic short-term and long-term goals. Achievement of these goals will boost their self-esteem. These groups need to enable clients to create a new personal identity as non-drug users, and develop their self-concept. Evocative techniques such as art, poetry, music, creative writing and psychodrama may be used to achieve these goals. The occupational therapist should be prepared to handle cathartic expressions of feelings and emotions, which are an inevitable part of these groups.

Interpersonal skills groups

These groups aim to develop more effective communication, assertiveness and conflict resolution skills, thereby improving interpersonal relationships. The groups should be carefully graded, taking clients through a process of identifying their difficulties, learning effective skills and methods, practising these in the relatively safe environment of the group as well as in real life, and receiving feedback. Role play is a very useful technique to develop these skills. Clients should be encouraged to practise their new skills whilst participating in other aspects of the programme.

Coping skills groups

According to the needs of the client population, the occupational therapist may implement relevant coping skills groups including anger, stress and anxiety management. Relaxation groups can be held daily to expose clients to different methods of relaxation, and enable them to practise their relaxation skills.

Case study – intervention

On admission to the Unit, Jack is identified as being in the *Contemplation stage* according to the Stages of Change model. The priority goal of intervention at this stage is to resolve Jack's ambivalence about giving up drugs, and motivate him to stay in the drug rehabilitation unit. The multidisciplinary team uses the handling principles of support and encouragement at this stage.

Jack will participate in the following programmes:

- Orientation groups.
- Self-awareness – admitting to himself and others that he has a drug problem.
- Building insight – becoming aware of the problems caused by his addiction and resulting behaviour for himself and other people.

A few days after his admission, Jack verbalizes his decision to commit himself to the process of stopping his drug use, and seeking an alternative lifestyle. The team regards this as a sign that Jack is in the *Preparation stage*. Now the goal of intervention is to facilitate the *Action stage* by empowering Jack with the skills needed to overcome his drug addiction, thus boosting his self-esteem. At the same time, Jack will need to gain insight into the reasons for his addiction and the consequences of his drugging behaviour. As he does this, his self-concept will develop. Jack will be involved in the following groups:

- values clarification
- goal-setting
- insight building
- occupation (work, leisure and ADL)
- interpersonal skills groups
- coping skills (anger and stress management)

Team members remain supportive in their handling of Jack, but increase their expectations of performance and goal achievement. They also encourage Jack to take more responsibility in the unit. He returns home over weekends, where he has the opportunity to try out new skills and behaviours. He is also faced with challenges which he needs to negotiate. On Monday mornings, he reflects on his progress in a group.

Family groups

The family can become a vital support mechanism for the client as he reintegrates back into the community. Family relationships have often been damaged, and attention should be given to working with the client and the family members. This is usually the role of the psychologist or the social worker. The occupational therapist may counsel the family about issues such as structuring the daily routine, encouraging the client to find and maintain work, and the value of engaging in leisure pursuits.

Follow-up and support

The chances of relapse are far greater without careful planning for the period after discharge. The multidisciplinary team, including the client, needs to discuss follow-up and support options for the period following discharge. In preparation, the occupational therapist should run problem-solving and goal-setting groups where clients consider their future plans regarding issues such as accommodation, work and role fulfilment. Most importantly, clients should make realistic plans to structure their time with constructive, meaningful activities and occupations to replace drug-related activities.

Case study – follow-up and support

In preparation for the *Maintenance stage*, the goal of intervention during the week prior to discharge is to enable Jack to sustain his behaviour change and prevent relapse by equipping him with the necessary skills to cope after his discharge, and through realistic planning. During a group Jack says, 'I've realized what gives meaning to my life. I want my girlfriend and my daughter to give me another chance.' The psychologist runs a couple counselling session and Jack's girlfriend agrees to take him back. Jack feels he can be successful making and selling his jewellery. He commits himself to working for four hours every morning. He makes arrangements to run a stall at a local fleamarket on Saturday mornings. Jack asks his girlfriend if he can collect his daughter from childcare and take care of her in the afternoons. The occupational therapist and Jack discuss the expectations and responsibilities of being a father, and talk about ways of playing with young children. The occupational therapist encourages Jack to return to the unit to attend monthly support groups.

Community intervention programmes

As part of an emerging role in health promotion, occupational therapists are becoming involved in establishing intervention programmes aimed at decreasing drug abuse in communities by improving people's awareness about drugs and their harmful effects, and enabling them to stay drug-free. These programmes are often directed at children, adolescents and youth, and might involve parents, teachers and other relevant community members. Community intervention programmes should be based on the framework and principles provided by the World Health Organisation's Ottawa Charter for Health Promotion (1986). The Community Project Process Model (University of the Western Cape, 2002) is a guideline that can be used to develop community intervention programmes. The steps in the Process Model are explained in the case study.

Case study – A drug prevention life skills programme for adolescents

This programme aimed to address the problem of escalating drug use amongst adolescents

Community entry: Key stakeholders were identified. Parents, school principals and educators were invited to attend meetings to discuss the extent of the problem. People were invited to express their opinions and suggest strategies for addressing the problem.

Needs assessment: A community profile was drawn up by looking at the infrastructure and dynamics of the community. A needs assessment was done by looking at community composition, organization, structure, capacity, environment, services and policies. A needs analysis showed that the most prevalent need was for a life skills programme to be implemented as part of the high school curriculum. The programme is comprehensive: meaning that it would not just focus on drug use, but would teach relevant skills and foster positive development amongst learners. Stakeholders felt that schools were the best place to run such programmes because they offered relatively easy access to the adolescent population, and the infrastructure and availability of educators meant that the programme could be delivered more cost-effectively. However educators would require training to implement the programme.

Planning intervention

Outcome – in eight months a life skills programme will have been planned, implemented and evaluated at five schools in the community.

Objectives – occupational therapy students will plan a life skills programme which aims to reduce drug use by increasing awareness, teaching relevant skills, and promoting health and wellness in adolescents. Teachers will be invited to participate in programme planning. Parents at the schools will be invited to parent meetings to raise their awareness about the programme and about drug use in general. The programme will be implemented at five schools. Evaluation of the programme will occur by means of focus groups with educators and learners, and a parents' meeting.

Indicators: It is useful to have a list of indicators which act as a grade or measure of the success of the project over time. Indicators should be explicitly stated, for example: 'The life skills programme consisting of ten life skills lessons will be implemented at each school during the first school term.'

Intervention

Direct intervention – carry out all the activities and actions to do with the intervention. These must link with the objectives.

Indirect intervention – carry out all the activities and actions that are not a direct part of the intervention, for example phone calls, reading and travelling. These must also be planned for as they can be time-consuming.

Evaluation of intervention: Analyse the direct and indirect intervention as well as the indicators to evaluate what worked and what did not work. Involve community members and stakeholders where possible and give feedback to everyone involved.

Future planning: This should be realistic and feasible. It can be done using the What? When? Why? How? Where? Who? method.

Conclusion

The occupational performance approach is a useful method for planning and implementing occupational therapy with drug-related disorders. The occupational therapist considers the dynamic interaction between the person, his occupations and context. By drawing up an occupational profile, the occupational therapist assesses the impact of drug use on the client's occupational performance, and the extent of the dysfunction in his/her life. The profile takes into account the individual's roles, tasks, values, interests, goals, performance areas and components, within a temporal, social, cultural and physical context. The focus of intervention with drug-related disorders is on changing behaviour and lifestyle, and this occurs mainly through group work. The multidisciplinary team, including the client, needs to discuss follow-up and support options for the period following discharge. It is important that patients plan to structure their time with constructive, meaningful activities and occupations to replace drug-related activities. Community intervention programmes for drug-related disorders are directed at raising community awareness around the harmful effects of drugs, developing skills and preventing drug abuse. These programmes can be designed using the Community Project Process Model.

Questions

1. Discuss the diagnosis of *Substance Abuse* versus *Substance Dependence* (DSM-IV-TR™ (American Psychiatric Association, 2000)) by comparing how occupational performance may be affected. Use the American Occupational Therapy Association's Uniform Terminology document to assist you.
2. Work with a partner. Refer to the Occupational Performance History Interview or brainstorm relevant questions for an initial interview with a patient. Role-play your interview. Afterwards discuss how it felt to be in the roles of the interviewer and the patient.
3. Describe a treatment session for a group of patients who are in the Action stage, where the aim is to improve their insight about how drugging has affected significant people in their lives.
4. Outline a series of three groups for Jack, where the aim is to develop his skills in home management tasks. Explain how you would grade these sessions.
5. Discuss the importance of follow-up groups for patients. Brainstorm why people might NOT attend these groups. Suggest ideas to overcome these problems. Outline a structure for the monthly follow-up groups and suggest possible topics.
6. Plan a community intervention programme addressing drug abuse amongst adolescents in your own community, according to the steps outlined in the Community Project Process Model.

Chapter 25
Gerontology, psychiatry and occupational therapy

RAE LABUSCHAGNE

> Every man is in certain respects like all other men,
> like some other men
> like no other man. (Kluckhorn and Murray, 1953)

Relatively few occupational therapists choose to work with the elderly. Is it perhaps because the training of aspirant occupational therapists in the field of gerontology is generally inadequate? Whatever the reason, the results are that our elderly patients are not offered the best of the profession, while occupational therapists themselves are not aware of the rewards of working with geriatric clients. Unfortunately, ageism exists and the aged are persistently labelled negatively. A manifestation of this is the feeling that the elderly patient is likely to die within a short period of time, while a youthful patient has many more years ahead of them. Yet this is a misconception – with increased life expectancy in the Western world and in parts of Asia, an individual of 65 may well have another 15 or more years to live.

The occupational therapist who chooses to work in the field of geriatrics or gerontology needs to combine a love of the aged with enthusiasm and sound knowledge of the ageing process. Zarit (1980) says that in order to provide effective clinical services to older people, it is important to have knowledge in three broad areas: first, information on the ageing process and its impact on behaviour; second, a basic understanding of current mental health concepts and procedures, including diagnosis and treatment; and finally, knowledge of the specific clinical issues involved in working with older persons. Given the training of occupational therapists, the professional group ought to be well placed to fill the criteria as described by Zarit. Human individuality is stressed in the training, and nowhere in the practice of the profession is this clearer and more marked than in geriatric care. A more disparate group of people one could not wish to find! Apart from individual differences, remember that the cohort or generation to which an individual belongs has a profound influence on their life view, values and morals. In addition, changes occur in 'normal ageing', and superimposed on these are the various pathologies that occur in old age. This is what makes working with geriatric clients fulfilling and challenging.

Following Zarit's model, let us begin by investigating the ageing process itself.

Theories of ageing

Emotional theory of ageing

The ageing process has not only a physical impact, but many emotional and psychological implications for the older person. Some researchers feel that the last few years of an older person's life are characterized by losses (Buhler, 1961; Butler and Lewis, 1977). Occupational therapists need to be aware of those losses and of the fact that the extent and experiencing of the losses may be exacerbated by the individual being devalued and marginalized by society.

One impact of the losses is the reduction of elderly person's social participation. This loss continuum includes the children leaving home, loss of social roles, loss or reduction of income, death of siblings, friends, family and spouse, loss of sensory acuity and loss of mobility. The loss of control over one's life when one becomes frail and incapacitated, which frequently occurs, particularly with the institutionalized aged, may have far-reaching effects in negative feelings of self-worth and esteem. The world of the older person shrinks as he/she disengages, for whatever reason, from society, and the home and immediate environment become increasingly important. Routines and habits assume substantial roles as they add a sense of security and structure to the life of the older person. Occupational therapists should therefore be sensitive when suggesting changes to the environment and habits of clients, and should always consider the social and cultural heritage of the patient while creating opportunities for self-esteem and a sense of control.

Psychosocial theories of ageing

Maslow's theory (1987)

Maslow identified five groups of needs: physiological; security; love; self-esteem and lastly the need for self-actualization. Although these needs are hierarchically based, it does not imply that a higher need will be experienced only when the lower ranking needs are completely satisfied. Higher ranking needs may be experienced when a lower ranking need has been partially satisfied.

This theory is particularly apposite when working with all institutionalized clients, and in particular those suffering from Alzheimer's disease and related dementias, because it is far easier for caregivers to provide and cater for the two lower categories of needs than the need for love, esteem and self-actualization.

Rogers' phenomenological theory (1951)

Carl Rogers' phenomenological approach developed out of his experience with clients and is essentially person-centred. This approach is centred on the individual's experience of his world and himself and sees the striving for, and realization of, one's inherent potential as the goal of development. Self-concept – the congruence of the concept an individual has of himself and his potential – is central to Rogers' theory, i.e. how close the match is between the idea the individual has of himself and the reality of his abilities and potential.

Rogers states that self-worth results from being unconditionally accepted by others and by being allowed the freedom to be one's true self. The unconditional acceptance of the child is very important for developing as a secure, well-functioning adult, but this is equally applicable to the aged. Occupational therapists should remember that the value judgements and the evaluations they make of patients have a considerable effect on the patient's perceptions of self-concept and feelings of self-worth. They also need to consider how many facilities for the aged provide few or no opportunities for development and for striving for control over one's destiny. Control over the environment or one's own destiny is particularly difficult for frail, bedridden elderly who reside in a nursing home where the routine of the facility tends to accommodate the needs of the staff at the expense of the needs of the residents.

Erikson's theory of psychosocial development (1980)

This is a psychosocial theory in that it stresses the interaction between the inner qualities of the individual and the demands of their culture. Erikson's theory is considered to be of particular importance as it relates to the entire lifespan, dividing the human life into stages where each individual is faced with crises that they must overcome in order to develop further. Erikson's theory is basically an optimistic one, as the individual is able to recover from impaired development during the earlier stages of development.

The following is a summary of the stages, associated crises and the positive resolution:

1. Basic trust versus mistrust: synthesis leads to hope
2. Autonomy versus shame and doubt: synthesis leads to willpower
3. Initiative versus guilt: synthesis leads to purpose
4. Industry versus inferiority: synthesis leads to competence

5. Ego identity versus confusion: synthesis leads to fidelity
6. Intimacy versus isolation: synthesis leads to love
7. Generativity versus stagnation: synthesis leads to caring
8. Ego integrity versus despair: synthesis leads to wisdom.

The first six stages will be reviewed briefly. The last two stages are of primary concern.

Basic trust versus mistrust: resolution = hope
This coincides with the child's first year of life in which the child develops a sense of trust and hope if they are cared for, nurtured, given love, security and acceptance. Should this not happen, the child develops a sense of distrust.

Autonomy versus shame: resolution = willpower
This stage covers the second year of life. Autonomy develops as a child becomes capable of exercising willpower. This in turn leads to a child failing sometimes to master situations, and if not dealt with sympathetically and supportively, this can lead to a sense of failure and self-doubt.

Initiative versus guilt: resolution = purpose
This stage lasts approximately from ages three to six years. The young child is exposed to a variety of new situations and people, through which he has to learn about the rules of his society and culture. Should the child be supported during this phase and guided with compassion and tact, he will develop a sense of purpose.

Industry versus inferiority: resolution = competence
This phase coincides roughly with the primary school stage, and ends with puberty. The skills the child has learned in the previous stage are developed and polished in preparation for adulthood and if well learned, will help the child to achieve competence, mastery and success. If the child consistently fails, he will develop feelings of inferiority.

Ego identity versus role confusion: resolution = fidelity
This stage coincides with adolescence and the identity crisis experienced by teenagers. Teenagers explore various roles and options during this period. If a clear definition of identity is not achieved, commitment to adult roles and long-term objectives will be problematic.

Intimacy versus isolation: resolution = love
Erikson (1963, p. 263) defines intimacy as 'the capacity to commit ... to concrete affiliations and partnerships and to develop ethical strength to abide by such commitments, even though they may call for significant sacrifices and compromises'. The opposite of intimacy is isolation. Those

elderly people who have not had a life full of love and intimacy may feel isolated and left out of life if they have no loving memories to recall and savour.

Generativity versus stagnation: resolution = caring

This phase is thought to last from the age of approximately 25 years to 65 years and thus spans the major part of life. It is during this period that one establishes a work commitment and starts a family. The period is one of responsibilities, not just in a work situation, but in family relationships as well. A widening range of interests characterizes the stage. When the demands, responsibilities and relationships are integrated and balanced, it is exciting and demanding. Erikson (1997) says that at the end of this period the individual may feel an urge to withdraw somewhat, but that this may result in a feeling of not belonging and not being needed. Generativity, which comprises the major life involvement of active individuals, is not necessarily expected in old age.

Integrity versus despair: resolution = wisdom

Erikson (1963, p. 113) says of this final stage, 'Despair expresses the feeling that time is now too short for the attempt to start another life and to try out alternate roads'. When people have successfully passed through the previous stages, they are able to look back on their lives with satisfaction, to make sense of what has gone before. It is a time of introspection and a time of reviewing one's life, a time of making peace with the things we have done and the things we have left undone.

This phase of life demands compassion and understanding from the occupational therapist, as patients may be going through an intensely emotional experience as they review their lives. It is a task of the last period of life. Listen to the stories the patient relates. Often it is through the telling and retelling of personal encounters that someone is able to make sense of what has gone before. Often family members or friends say, 'Give my mother something to do. She just sits all day.' Respect the need to be introspective. The old person who has not made peace with herself and her life is very often the one who dies with unfinished business.

Disengagement theory of ageing

(Cumming and Henry, 1961)

This is a controversial theory, which was developed to explain why ageing persons separate from the mainstream of society. It is considered a mutual process of disengagement between the individual and society. Such a withdrawal keeps the elderly from becoming frustrated by maintaining roles they are no longer able to fulfil, while making place for younger people to fill these roles. It is thought that if the aged are forced to disengage from society, this results in dissatisfaction on the part of the aged. Should, however, the person himself/herself decide to give up certain roles, the disengagement need not necessarily be traumatic. Compare, for example, an older person who is forced to retire and one who does so voluntarily.

There is a fair amount of criticism for this theory as disengagement is not a universal phenomenon, i.e. it is not seen in all cultural groups and it does not account for the highly adjusted elderly people who are still actively engaged.

Activity theory of ageing

According to the activity theory, older people who are more socially active are more likely to adjust well to ageing (Lemon et al., 1972, pp. 511–523). The theory is based on the following propositions:

- Social activity is necessary for continued role enactment.
- Role enactment is essential for a positive self-image.
- People who have a wide range of activities have more opportunity to reaffirm their positive self-image.
- People who have a wide range of roles have more opportunities for role enactment, which is the substance of self-image and self-concept.

Critics argue that the ageing process is too complex to be characterized by such a simplistic formulation. Still, as an occupational therapist it is important to take the past life of the patient into consideration – if the person was a loner all his life and pursued solitary interests, it is highly unlikely that his life satisfaction and self-concept will be reinforced by becoming actively involved in a number of roles, particularly if it is against his wishes.

Psychogeriatrics

Occupational therapists will encounter two main areas of interest in psychogeriatrics, or the psychiatry of the elderly: dementias and affective disorders, e.g. depression. Both areas offer unique challenges to the occupational therapist. In addition occupational therapists need to be aware of the fact that conditions such as Alzheimer's disease and depression do not exist as isolated conditions and there may well be concomitant illnesses in ageing patients.

Depression

Unfortunately, depression is a common disorder in the elderly. Whether older people become more susceptible to depression as they age is questionable, but the losses which occur during the ageing process, which may range from changes in health status to loss of family home, spouse, income and so on, often precede a depressive episode. (It is likely that similar losses would adversely affect younger individuals in the same way, but for many older people these losses may be experienced in a condensed period of time and the individual may feel highly vulnerable.) It is sad that depression in the elderly often goes untreated by doctors, and unrecognized by friends, families and carers who assume that old age is itself a miserable state. The elderly themselves may resist seeking help from psychologists, psychiatrists or counsellors because of their own biases against mental health services and professionals. Importantly, acute as well as mild depressions in the aged generally react well to therapy and medication.

Dementia

Dementia is a syndrome or collection of symptoms which the Geriatrics Committee of the Royal College of Physicians of London defines as follows (Editorial in Lancet, 1981):

> Dementia is the global impairment of the higher cortical functions including memory, the capacity to solve the problems of day-to-day living, the correct use of perceptuo-motor skills and the control of emotional reactions, in the absence of gross clouding of consciousness. The condition is often irreversible and progressive.

Dementias present a different kind of challenge to depression, particularly when gross deterioration has taken place. Of all the dementias, Alzheimer's Disease and Related Disorders (ADRD) is the most prevalent among the aged.

With the deficits that occur with ADRD, caregivers, particularly in facilities where 24-hour care is provided, tend to concentrate on the basic physiological needs of the individual. These needs – as well as those of security as described by Maslow (1970) – are generally adequately covered.

However, the more esoteric needs of the individual, such as a sense of belonging and acceptance, opportunities that foster feelings of self-esteem and self-actualization and achieving a sense of integrity, are ignored; considered too much of a challenge, or simply impossible to fill, given the pathology present and the demands an effective programme would place on the staff. In many facilities for the aged, and particularly for psychogeriatric patients, there is a feeling of hopelessness and futility on the part of the staff.

It is these higher needs that embody the uniqueness of the individual and acknowledge the fact that, despite gross deterioration in many areas, both cognitive and functional, the needs are real and present. Satisfying these needs, in the face of an inexorable passage of the illness and of the life course itself, becomes the challenge to occupational therapists. The need to live until we die holds true for all of us, no matter how ill or how old.

Treatment of Alzheimer's Disease and Related Disorders (ADRD)

Erikson says of the last phase of life that the individual strives to achieve a sense of integrity versus despair. Imagine, then, patients with ADRD who have even less control over their lives than the physically frail elderly who can express their preferences and needs and may be given the opportunity to realize them and achieve a sense of integrity and self-actualization. Choices, however limited, should still be offered to the ADRD client.

Providing ongoing care and treatment

Occupational therapists cannot give up on their ageing patients. One has to stop and ask oneself to what extent the decline in mental capacity is a result of lack of stimulation, of passivity, exclusion and loss of familiar people and environment. Coupled with the sensory deterioration that accompanies 'normal' ageing is an overwhelming sense, in many professionals, that nothing can be done for the elderly patient suffering from dementia. By not individualizing treatment of and approaches to the ADRD client the professional merely assumes that the clients are all the same. Occupational therapists often fail to do regular assessments of aged patients to determine their weaknesses as well as their strengths. They also fail to recognize, celebrate, nurture and encourage the islands of health that Brodaty (1999, pp. 18–32) so poignantly describes when he speaks of the process of dementias:

> The loss of brain tissue caused by a dementia can be likened to the erosion of a landscape caused by advancing water. In most the continent of memory is washed away. In some language disappears first. In others ... loss of executive type functions, such as planning and organisation, may dominate the early picture. Often there are islands of lands unaffected by the advancing tide of Alzheimer's disease until the late stages. ... The sequence of the erosion of these land masses does not always follow the classical pattern...

After a thorough assessment and a review of premorbid strengths, the primary goal of intervention should be to help patients function on as high a level as is possible, to exercise as much control over their lives as possible and to maintain and preserve 'the islands of health' and to encourage the development of others.

Essential factors in the treatment of ADRD

Assessing cognitive, memory and physical levels

Thorough assessments of the cognitive, memory and physical levels must also be done on an ongoing basis and should be complemented by ongoing observation and reporting. These assessments form the basis of any planned activities.

An awareness of the symptoms of the illness and their manifestation is extremely important for any assessment to be done. The guidelines below outline the problematic abilities of the ADRD patient, as well as the influence these have on possible activities.

Abstract thought

The ADRD patient has problems with logic, insight and abstract concepts and ideas. Activities are more likely to be successful when the occupational therapist breaks them down into their simplest and most concrete steps and demonstrates one step at a time.

Concentration and attention

Sustained concentration and attention become problematic and the ability to initiate and sustain an activity and to bring it to its logic conclusion is impaired. Activities should be tailored to the attention and concentration span of individual clients. If even just one step of an activity is completed and enjoyed by the client, then one may say that it has been successful. (The fact that activities are short and may not occupy the major part of the day is very often problematic for families who are concerned about their family member not being busy all day. Education of families about the illness and about the ageing process is important.)

Executive functioning

This is divided primarily into four components:

1. *Volition* refers to 'the complex process of determining what one needs or wants and conceptualising some kind of future realisation of that need or want' (Lezak, 1995, p. 651).
2. *Planning* refers to 'the identification and organisation of the steps and elements (e.g. skills, materials, other persons) needed to carry out an intention or achieve a goal' (Lezak, 1995, p. 655).
3. *Purposive action* is 'the translation of an intention or plan into productive, self-serving activity requires the actor to initiate, maintain, switch, and stop sequences of complex behaviour in an orderly and integrated manner' (Lezak, 1995, p. 658).
4. *Effective performance:* 'a performance is as effective as the performer's ability to monitor, self correct, and regulate the intensity, tempo, and other qualitative aspects of delivery' (Lezak, 1995, p. 674).

Given the complex components of executive functioning, the occupational therapist needs to take care not to set the client up for failure, but rather set the client up to achieve. This is only possible if assessments are accurate and sensitive and if activities are broken into their simplest steps, with the occupational therapist very often demonstrating and acting as the initiator for those people who have no volition or are not able to initiate an idea, movement or action themselves. For example, if the patient/client demonstrates apraxia, the occupational therapist may hold the client's hand and demonstrate the movement or action needed. Often the client may not be able to complete all the steps of the activity, but whatever he can do should be encouraged and the occupational therapist should help and support throughout the activity.

Activities with the aged are more likely to succeed if they fall within the field of reference and experience of the individual. The occupational therapist once again needs to have an accurate history of the individual as a tool to planning meaningful activities.

Interacting with people who have cognitive impairments

Nissenboim and Vroman (2000, pp. 34, 35) recommend the following four steps when planning interactions with people who have cognitive impairments:

1. *Familiarizing:* The occupational therapist describes the object while the patient familiarizes himself/herself with it and is encouraged to use all appropriate senses in the familiarization process such as hearing, feeling and touching.
2. *Naming:* In this step the occupational therapist names the object(s) being handled, and encourages the person to do so. Nissenboim and Vroman (2000) stress that no pressure should be placed on the person and that he/she needs to receive approbation and recognition for an attempt to respond.
3. *Demonstrating:* Visual, tactile and auditory focus are provided here by the occupational therapist. Occupational therapists need to remember that executive functioning is a problem with cognitively impaired people, so that any activity should be broken down into its simplest steps and be performed as discrete activities.
4. *Encouraging and rewarding:* We all need to be encouraged and rewarded for efforts made. Recognition of a person's attempt to participate is essential for self-esteem. The occupational therapist should include her feelings as well as this forms a bond and creates a feeling that the interaction has been a participatory one and satisfying to both the client and the therapist.

Creating an appropriate therapeutic environment

By providing a calm, relaxed atmosphere with a consistent routine that is geared to the habits and strengths of the individuals in the unit, the occupational therapist is able to encourage the individual to function optimally with self-respect in an atmosphere of trust and security. If the routine is staff- and not patient-orientated, it may well defeat the purpose.

It is important to take into account the normal sensory deficits of ageing; for example, more lighting is needed for the older eye, older eyes are sensitive to glare, etc.

However, the physical environment should compensate not only for sensory deficits and losses, but for cognitive ones as well. An appropriate environment should be:

- consistent and predictable
- unambiguous, with discrete areas clearly defined for various activities and functions (e.g. furniture may give clues as to the use of the space)
- one that provides neither too much nor too little stimulation
- sensitive to the declining abilities of the individual, and make an attempt to compensate for these
- small rather than large
- one in which the individual is able to functional optimally
- one which preserves skills
- one which encourages optimal use of skills and abilities
- one which will compensate for cognitive and memory loss by providing cues (e.g. for spatial orientation)
- one in which the person feels safe
- one which allows for habits and customs of a lifetime
- one which encourages and preserves long-term memories and relationships
- appropriate for adults, as your patients should continue to function as such
- reflective of the experience of particular cohorts and cultures
- one that encourages the residents to want to participate in familiar activities such as bed making (use duvets which are simple to pull up), setting tables, removing dishes, dusting, sweeping, etc.

Promotion of awareness and orientation

It is also important for the therapeutic environment to promote orientation and maximize awareness. Possible techniques are to:

- use simple unambiguous signs, as residents may not be able to comprehend complex language
- place signs at eye level
- use bright, contrasting colours
- create personalized doors to make each patient's room more relevant and understandable to the residents (e.g. hang favourite photographs or personal mementoes on the bedroom door and make sure that they are securely attached to the door or wall)
- follow a regular schedule by doing the same activities in the same location (routine and familiarity are important)
- create purpose-specific rooms if possible so that residents always know what to expect when they enter (e.g. do not have the dinning room doubling as an activity room)

- make areas such as the bathrooms and lounges easily visible and accessible
- disguise exits and underplay the visibility of rooms that the residents should not use (one may do this by attaching mirrors, hanging curtains or posters in front of the doors, etc.)
- All furniture and bathroom equipment such as beds, easy chairs, toilets and showers, etc., should be so designed to promote the physical independence of the clients.

Sensory stimulation

Another area to note is that of sensory stimulation, which should be sensitive to over- and under-load. By in-depth assessments of the clients, occupational therapists can determine each person's particular level. It is a challenge to provide a balance so that the individual is not subjected to overload or, conversely, sensory deprivation. Loud noises, whether music, talk or housekeeping sounds, untidy and disorderly rooms and materials and equipment that are not stored neatly, or not stored at all, can distract the resident who may already have a short attention span. When carrying out an activity, make sure that only the materials and equipment for that specific activity are visible. Limit the extraneous distractions as far as possible.

Building up an individual life history

In order to achieve these goals, the occupational therapist needs to gain as complete a picture as possible of the client prior to their illness and admission. Consultation with the former primary caregiver is essential in building up a picture and history of the individual. The client's likes, dislikes, personal habits and interests, strengths and weaknesses need to be part of the profile of the individual. Included in the initial interview with the primary caregiver should be the following:

- How does the client prefer to be addressed? Does he/she have a nickname?
- Sleeping patterns.
- Bathtime routine (e.g. Does he/she prefer to shower? Is this a morning or evening routine? Does he shave before or after bathing/showering? Does he/she use a mug of water when brushing his/her teeth, or cup the water for rinsing in his/her hands?)
- Eating patterns (e.g. Is the main meal at midday or in the evening? Does the client have a snack before going to bed in the evening? What are his/her favourite foods? What food does he/she dislike most?)
- Method of dressing (e.g. Does the client first put on his shirt and then his socks?)
- What are the client's bladder and bowel habits?
- What hobbies and interests did/does the client have? (e.g. music, reading, woodcarving, knitting, singing, ballroom dancing, etc.)

- What was the client's profession?
- Family details (e.g. How long has the client been married? What does he/she call his/her spouse? How many children, grandchildren does he/she have? How many siblings does the client have and what are their names?)
- Personal history (e.g. What is the client's home address? Where did he grow up? What did his father do? Where did he go to school? What was his first or home language?)
- What was the client's premorbid personality? Was he/she introverted or extroverted?

Possible activities and treatments

Activities should be based on previous skills and interests, as well as an awareness of the socio-economic and cultural background of the client. The current functional and intellectual levels of the clients should be kept in mind at all times, thus re-emphasizing the need for ongoing assessments and monitoring. Generally, occupational therapists need to develop a well-rounded programme that includes the following: physical activity, cognitive and memory stimulation, and social activities. The wholeness of the individual should be remembered and celebrated at all times.

Activities of daily living (ADL)

Activities and actions which are based on habit and have well-established patterns must continue as far as possible. Encourage clients to follow and use habits which are intact. (The occupational therapist should use the information from the personal history to develop these activities, e.g. dressing, eating, and bathing habits.) It is important to be aware of the client's personal habits and to set up his/her programme so that the demands and rituals of life prior to the onset of the illness are familiar and comfortable. This of course demands from the staff an awareness of each patient/client and a willingness to let convenience and facility routines be secondary to the individual needs of the clients.

Rote learning

Activities based on rote learning such as old songs, poems, dances, etc., should be encouraged. Participating in such activities engenders a sense of achievement and wellbeing.

Reality orientation (RO)

Orientation to time, place and person is stressed in most of the literature on treating dementias. Zarit (1980, p. 375) points out: 'Not knowing where one is, or the date, is a symptom of significant degrees of brain dysfunction.' On the other hand, he goes on to say that knowing the date does not lead to long-term improvements in behaviour. Bowlby (1993, pp. 92–93) mentions that: 'In the light of the current research findings and knowledge about ADRD, reality *orientation* should now be more properly known and implemented as reality *reassurance*' and the orientating information should be provided to reassure the client and 'not for repetition and recall'. It is far more effective to address the feelings experienced by the client than to address the accuracy of their perceptions. This is particularly pertinent in handling a client who experiences paranoid symptoms. Still, reality orientation forms an important part of any treatment programme for dementias. There are three aspects to reality orientation:

1. *24-hour reality orientation*

   Emphasizing orientation to time, place and person with every interaction was regarded by Dr James Folsom (1968) as crucial to this approach. Each time the client offers an appropriate response, he is rewarded with praise and support. To constantly correct cognitively impaired and in particular ADRD sufferers and orientate them to reality can be extremely distressing for the clients. However, one can incorporate reality and factual information in one's conversation with the client, but as with all interaction and verbal conversation with ADRD sufferers try to pare down conversation and avoid being verbose. It is not ethical to patronize or 'play along'. Instead, it is possible to distract the client or build on the situation. The knowledge that one has of the client is extremely important, so that if, for example, the client asks for his/her mother, long dead, one is able to say, 'Your mother's name was Marie. Let's go and look at the photo you have of her.'

2. *Classroom reality orientation*

   This activity is based on small groups and takes place in a classroom situation. These classroom situations tend give the staff structure and may well be more beneficial to staff than to clients, as the staff feel that they are 'doing something'. It may well be better to incorporate reality into all dealings with clients rather than setting up an artificial situation which has little bearing on reality.

3. *Attitude therapy*

   This is the third component of reality orientation. Depending on the client, a specific approach and response to each individual client is recommended. This consistency is thought to provide security for clients in that they are handled and approached in an unambiguous and consistent manner. This approach demands discipline and training on the part of the staff and is particularly difficult to maintain where there is rapid staff turnover.

   Rather than adhere strictly to these approaches, the occupational therapist should use cues to orientate clients in a natural and unstructured way. One should naturally introduce reality into everyday interactions with clients, and a therapeutic environment as described above is very important.

Reminiscence therapy

Reminiscence work focuses on long-term memory. Of all the approaches to working with cognitively impaired geriatric patients, and particularly those who have ADRD, reminiscence is one that certainly encourages participation and fosters opportunities for self-esteem and recognition and identity. If we consider Maslow's hierarchy of needs, then reminiscence is one approach that attempts to fulfil these needs. It demands from the staff that they become acquainted with a detailed life history of their clients they care for. This knowledge often changes the way in which the elderly are regarded by the staff. In a way, the staff becomes the memory bank of the client and a knowledge of the past gives us indications of activities that are likely to be meaningful to our clients.

Because people suffering from dementia have difficulty in initiating activities, occupational therapists need to expose them to activities that have relevance to them and their experience. There are, of course, experiences and life passages relevant to all people and working from that basis, occupational therapists can draw up reminiscence groups and activities that can allow for individual experiences and differences. For

Table 25.1 Sensory stimulation relating to themes

Themes	Sensory stimulation
Babies and childhood	Look at photos as babies; family photos, photos of home town, etc. Baby powder, old-fashioned feeding bottles, baby shawls, etc. can be passed around and handled. Pass around and shake baby rattles, smell baby powder. Have a young mother and her baby attend the group. Sing familiar lullabies. Recite nursery rhymes.
School days	Look at school photographs. Bring school uniforms. Pass around slates and stylus, inkwells, pens with nibs, chalk, etc. Look at sporting equipment, toys: tops, marbles, etc. Sing songs of childhood, recite poems, etc. Discuss forms of transport – show pictures of cars, buses and trains.
Young adulthood	Look at photographs, especially of fashions, including shoes, clothes, handbags and hats of the appropriate era. Also handle hair curlers and crimping irons. Let participants try on items of clothing, etc. This usually leads to discussions about courting and marriage. Sing popular songs of the era and listen to music. Discuss trends and popular fads of the time. Discuss forms of transport – show pictures of cars, buses, etc.

Table 24.1 contd.

Themes	Sensory stimulation
Adult life	Discuss work, family and rearing children.
	Look at photographs and handle common objects used in homes and found in homes, such as a rolling pin, washboard, flat iron, tools and old household appliances.
	Discuss first homes and housing – show pictures and ask for photos of family homes.
	Bake favourite biscuits, etc.
	Look at examples of various hand crafts: tatting, embroidery, knitting, etc. Discuss hobbies.
	Sing popular songs and listen to music of that era.

example, the occupational therapist could deal with the following themes with concomitant activities:
From all of the above, the occupational therapist can create opportunities for various activities that have relevance and are familiar to those participating in the reminiscence groups. Be aware of the danger of over-stimulation when introducing activities based on sensory stimulation.

Conclusion

Working with the aged is one of the most exciting fields of occupational therapy. It is here that the occupational therapist plays a vital role in making the last period of life meaningful and purposeful despite pathology.

Questions

1. Briefly discuss creating a therapeutic environment for people experiencing disorientation.
2. Discuss the approach to interaction with people who have cognitive impairments as set out by Nissenboim and Vroman.
3. Discuss the four elements of executive functioning and how it would influence your approach to activities.
4. Explain how you could develop an activity programme to stimulate long-term memories.
5. Which elements would you include in a well-rounded programme for clients with Alzheimer's disease?
6. Draw up a form with questions you would consider helpful in establishing the facts of the client's life history.

References

Ackerman TF (1996) Why doctors should intervene. In TA Mappes and D de Grazzia, Biomedical Ethics. 4th edn. pp.73–77. New York: McGraw-Hill.

Agnew Pl, Poulsen A and Maas F (1985) Attitudes and knowledge of occupational therapy clinicians and students regarding the sexuality of disabled people. Australian Occupational Therapy Journal 32(2): 54–61.

Ahrens CS, Lane Frey J, Senn Burke SC (1999) An individualised job engagement approach for persons with severe mental illness. Journal of Rehabilitation Oct./Nov./Dec. 1999: 17–24.

Alers VM, de Freitas J (unpublished) Self respect and sexuality interactions (Johannesburg), adapted from LW Pedretti and MB Early (2001) Occupational Therapy: Practice Skills for Physical Dysfunction. 5th edn. St Louis: Mosby.

Alers V, Smuts B (2002) The development and evaluation of an experiential approach to teaching occupational therapy groupwork. South African Journal of Occupational Therapy 32(3).

Allen CK, Allen RC (1987) Cognitive disabilities: measuring the consequences of mental disorders. Clinical Psychiatry 48(5): 185–190.

American Psychiatric Association (APA) (1996) Policy Guidelines: HIV and Inpatient Psychiatric Units. Reference No. 960012. Washington, DC: APA.

American Journal of Occupational Therapy (2002) Guide for supervision of occupational therapy personnel, American Journal of Occupational Therapy 48(11): 1045–1046.

American Journal of Occupational Therapy (2000) Code of Ethics Volume 54(6) Nov./Dec.: 614–621.

American Journal of Occupational Therapy (2000) Supplement: Practice Guideline for the Treatment of Patients with HIV/AIDS. 157(11): 1–55.

American Occupational Therapy Association (1989) Entry level role delineation for OTRs and COTAs. American Journal of Occupational Therapy 44(12): 1091–1102.

American Occupational Therapy Association (1994) Uniform terminology for occupational therapy. 3rd edn. American Journal of Occupational Therapy 48(11): 1047–1054.

American Occupational Therapy Association (1999) Guide for Supervision of Occupational Therapy Personnel in the Delivery of Occupational Therapy Services. Official Position Paper, American Journal of Occupational Therapy 53: 592–594.

American Occupational Therapy Association (2002) Practice Framework Glossary. American Journal of Occupational Therapy 56(6): 667–668.

American Psychiatric Association (1994) Diagnostic and Statistical Manual of Mental Disorders. 4th edn. (DSM-IV) Washington: American Psychiatric Association.

American Psychiatric Association (2000) Diagnostic and Statistical Manual of Mental Disorders. 4th edn. (DSM-IV-TR™) Washington: American Psychiatric Association.

Andrews J (2000) The value of reflective practice: A student case study. British Journal of Occupational Therapy 63(8).

Angold A (2002) Diagnostic interviews with parents and children, in M Rutter and E Taylor (eds) Child and Adolescent Psychiatry. 4th ed. Oxford: Blackwell Science Ltd.

Anthony WA (1994) Characteristics of people with psychiatric disabilities that are predictive of entry into the rehabilitation process and successful employment. Psychosocial Rehabilitation Journal 17(3): 3–13.

Arns PG, Linney JA (1993) Work, self and life satisfaction for persons with severe and persistent mental disorders. Psychosocial Rehabilitation Journal 17(2): 62–79.

Astin JA (1997) Stress reduction through mindfulness meditation: Effects of psychosocial symptomatology, sense of control and spiritual experiences. Psychother Psychosom 66: 97–106.

Atkinson RL, Atkinson RC, Smith EE, Bem DJ, Hilgard ER (1990) Introduction to Psychology. 10th edn. New York: Harcourt Brace Jovanovich.

Axline V (1989) Play Therapy. New York: Churchill Livingstone.

Ayres AJ (1972) Southern California Sensory Integration Tests Manual. Los Angeles: Western Psychological Services.

Ayres AJ (1975) Southern California Postrotary Nystagmus Test (SCPRNT). Los Angeles: Western Psychological Services.

Ayres AJ (1979) Sensory Integration and the Child. Los Angeles. Western Psychological Services.

Ayres AJ (1979/1981) Sensory Integration and the Child. Los Angeles: Western Psychological Services.

Ayres AJ (1983) Sensory Integration and Learning Disorders. 8th edn. Los Angeles: Western Psychological Services.

Ayres (1986) SAISI Research Committee, Clinical Observation. Adapted from Ayres J (1986).

Ayres AJ (1989) Sensory Integration and Praxis Tests. Los Angeles: Western Psychological Services.

Ayres AJ and Tickle LS (1980) Hyperresponsivity to touch and vestibular stimuli as a predictor of positive response to sensory integration procedures by autistic children. American Journal of Occupational Therapy 34: 375–381.

Banks B, Charleston S, Grossi T, Mank D (2001) Workplace supports, job performance, and integration outcomes for people with psychiatric disabilities. Psychiatric Rehabilitation Journal 24(4): 389–396.

Bannister A, Huntington BA (2002) Communicating with Children and Adolescents. Action for Change. London: Jessica Kingsley Publishers.

Barbour RS (1994) The impact of working with people with HIV/AIDS: A review of literature. Journal of Social Science Medicine 39(2): 221–232.

Barker RL, Branson DM (2000) Forensic Social Work. 2nd edn. New York: The Haworth Press.

Barlow DH, Durand VM (1998) Abnormal Psychology: An Integrative Approach. 2nd edn. Washington: Brooks/Cole Publishing Company.

Barnard P (2003) Vona du Toit's Model of Creative Ability applied to Paediatrics. Unpublished Undergraduate course notes, University of Witwatersrand, Johannesburg.

Barnes MA (1996) The Healing Path with Children: An Exploration for Parents and Professionals. Ireland: Viktoria Fermoyle and Berrigan Publishing House.

Barnitt RE (1993) Deeply troubling questions: The teaching of ethics in under-graduate courses. British Journal of Occupational Therapy 56(11): 401–406.

Barnitt RE (1993) What gives you sleepless nights? Ethical practice in occupation-al therapy. British Journal of Occupational Therapy 56(6): 207–212.

Baron K, Kielhofner G, Goldhammer V, Wolenski J (2002) User's Manual of the Occupational Self Assessment. Chicago: Model of Human Occupation Clearinghouse.

Baron KB (1987) The model of human occupation: A newspaper treatment group for adolescents with conduct disorder. Occupational Therapy in Mental Health 7(2): 89–104.

Barrett M (1999) Sexuality and Multiple Sclerosis. 3rd edn. Ontario: Multiple Sclerosis Society of Canada.

Barrow OJ (1999) The Criminal Procedure Act 51 of 1977. 11th edn. Cape Town: Juta and Co. Ltd.

Barton R (1976) Institutional Neurosis. Bristol: John Wright and Son Ltd.

Baum CM, Edwards DF (2001) The Washington University Activity Card Sort, Washington University Press.

Bayley N (1995) Bayley Scale for Infant Development. 2nd edn. The Psychological Corporation.

Beardslay Tim (1998) Coping with HIV's ethical dilemmas. Scientific American 7(98): 86–88. Online available from www.genethik.de/aids.aids09.htm. (accessed 8/6/2003).

Beauchamp IL, Childress JF (1994) Principles of Biomedical Ethics. 4th edn. Chapters 3–6. New York: Oxford University Press.

Beck AT, Emery G (eds) (1985) Anxiety Disorders and Phobias: A Cognitive Perspective. New York: Basic Books.

Beery EB (1997) The Beery-Buktenica Developmental Test of Visual-Motor Integration. New Jersey: Modern Curriculum Press.

Beery KE (1997) The Developmental Test of Visual-Motor Integration 4th Edition. San Antonio. Psychological Corporation

Bekker C (2003) What to expect. www.steppingstones.co.za/article-treatment_programmes.asp (accessed 9/10/2003).

Berk RA, DeGangi GA (1983) DeGangi-Berk Test of Sensory Integration. Los Angeles: Western Psychological Services.

Beyers D, Vorster C (1991) Groepterapie en praktyk. Unpublished study guide.

Blanche EI, Botticelli TM, Hallway MK (1998) Combining Neuro-Developmental Treatment and Sensory Integration Principles: An Approach to Pediatric Therapy. USA: Therapy Skill Builders.

Blatner A (1992) Foundations of Psychodrama. Theory and Practice. 3rd edn. New York: Springer Publishing Co.

Bloomer SL, Williams JP (1986) The Bay Area Functional Performance Evaluation (BaFPE). San Francisco: USCF.

Bodenheimer C, Kerrigan AJ, Garber SI, Monga TN (2000) Sexuality in persons with lower extremity amputations. Disability and Rehabilitation 22(9): 409–415.

Bond GR (1992) Vocational rehabilitation. In RP Liberman (ed) Handbook of Psychiatric Rehabilitation, pp.244–263. New York: Macmillan Press.

Bond GR, Drake RE, Mueser KT, Becker DR (1997) An update on supported employment for people with severe mental illnesses. Psychiatric Services 48(3): 335–346.

Bothwell R (1998) The anxious patient. In SE Baumann (ed) Psychiatry in Primary Health Care. Cape Town: Juta and Co.

Botterbusch KF (1982) A Comparison of Commercial Vocational Evaluation Systems. 2nd edn. Menomonie, WI: Materials Development Center, Stout Vocational Rehabilitation Institute, University of Wisconsin-Stout.

Bowlby C (1993) Therapeutic Activities with Persons Disabled by Alzheimer's Disease and Related Disorders. Githersburg, MD: Aspen Publishers.

Bowlby J (1988) A Secure Base. New York: Basic Books.

Branch J (2003) Tara H Moross Centre – Notes on Elements of Psychotherapy Unit (unpublished). Johannesburg.

British Journal of Occupational Therapy (2001) Code of Ethics. College of Occupational Therapists 64(2): 612–617.

Brodaty H (1999) The role of the GP in the management of Alzheimer's disease. Modern Medicine of South Africa 21(9): 18–32.

Brollier C, Hamrick N, Jacobson B (1994) Aerobic exercises: A potential occupational therapy modality for adolescent with depression. Occupational Therapy in Mental Health 12(4): 19–28.

Brown DG, Zinkin LM (1994) The Psyche and the Social World. London: Routledge.

Bruce MA, Borg B (1993) Psychosocial Occupational Therapy. Frames of Reference for Intervention. 2nd edn, p.130. New Jersey: Slack Inc.

Bruininks RH (1978) The Bruininks-Oseretsky Test of Motor Proficiency. Circle Pines MN: American Guidance Service Publishing.

Buhler C (1961) Meaningful life in the mature years. In RW Kleemeier (ed) Ageing and Leisure. New York: Oxford University Press.

Bundy AC, Lane SJ, Murray EA (2002) Sensory Integration Theory and Practice. 2nd edn. Philadelphia: FA Davis Company.

Burns RB (1987) The Secrets of Getting a Job. Cape Town: College Tutorial Press.

Butler RN, Lewis MI (1977) Ageing and Mental Health. St Louis: Mosby.

Buys TM (1993) Vocational evaluation. Unpublished paper presented at Refresher Course in Vocational Rehabilitation, 18 March 1993, Pretoria University, South Africa.

Canadian Association of Occupational Therapy (1991) Occupational Therapy for Client-centred practice. Toronto ON: CAOT Publications ACE.

Canadian Association of Occupational Therapists (2003) Guidelines for Supervision of Assigned Occupational Therapy Service Components. Available from: www.caot.ca/index.cfm?ChangeID=1andpageID=579.

Carey P, Farrell J, Hui M, Sullivan B (2001) Heyde's Modapts. A Language of Work. Brisbane, Australia: Heyde Dynamics Pty Ltd.

Carrier, C., Dutton, H and Lee, R. (2002) In Department of Health and Rehabilitation Sciences. University of Cape Town, Cape Town.

Carver CS, Scheier MF, Weintraub JK (1989) Assessing coping strategies: a theoretically-based approach. Journal of Personality and Social Psychology 56(2): 267–83.

CASE (Community Agency for Social Enquiry) (1995) National Household Survey. South Africa.

CASE (Community Agency for Social Enquiry) (1999) We also Count. The extent of moderate to severe reported disability and the nature of the disability experience in South Africa. Johannesburg, South Africa.

Case Smith J (ed) (2001) Occupational Therapy for Children. 4th edn. St Louis: Mosby.

Cassidy J, Shaver PR (1999) The Handbook of Attachment: Theory, Research and Clinical Applications, New York and London: Guildford Press.

Casteleijn JM (2001) The Measurement of Properties of an Instrument to assess the level of Creative Participation – Masters thesis. Pretoria: University of Pretoria.

Center for Psychiatric Rehabilitation, Boston University (1998) Handling your psychiatric disability in work and school: potential accommodations on the job.

Chacksfield J, Lancaster J (2002) Substance misuse. In J Creek (ed) Occupational Therapy and Mental Health. 3rd edn. London: Churchill Livingstone.

Chacksfield JD, Lindsay SJE (1999) The reduction of leisure in alcohol addiction. Paper presented at the College of Occupational Therapists Conference.

Checkly S (1998) The Management of Depression. Oxford: Blackwell Science Ltd.

Chiland C, Young JG (1992) New Approaches to Mental Health from Birth to Adolescence. New Haven, CT: Yale University Press.

Chimera C (2002) The Yellow Brick Road: Helping children and adolescents to recover a coherent story following abusive family experiences. Facilitated contact with birth parents using the Therapeutic Spiral Model™. In A Bannister and A Huntington Communicating with Children and Adolescents. Action for Change. London: Jessica Kingsley.

Chimera C (2003) (Unpublished) The Yellow Brick Road. A Workshop on Intensive Attachment Therapy: Addressing the narrative process in action with traumatised children and their families. Midrand, Gauteng, South Africa.

Christiansen C, Baum C (1997) Occupational Therapy: Enabling Function and Well-being. 2nd edn. New Jersey: Slack Inc.

Christiansen C, Townsend E (2004) Introduction to Occupation: The Art and Science of Living. New Jersey: Prentice Hall.

Clancy H, Clark M (1990) Occupational Therapy with Children. Melbourne: Churchill Livingstone.

Clark F, Ennevor BL, Richardson PL (1996) A grounded theory of techniques for occupational storytelling and story making. In R Zemke and F Clark (eds) Occupational Science: The Evolving Discipline. Philadelphia: FA Davis.

Clark F, Zemke R, Frank G, Parham D, Neville-Jan A, Hedricks C, Carson M, Fazio L, Abreu B (1993) Dangers inherent in the partition of occupational therapy and occupational science. American Journal of Occupational Therapy 47: 184–186.

Clarke E and Peters S (1994) The Scorable Self-care Evaluation (SCORE). New Jersey: Slack Inc.

Clarke L (2003). Help for young lives on the line. Sunday Tribune (S.A.) 12 October, p.5.

Code of Good Practice on Key Aspects of the Employment of People with Disabilities (this code is attached to the Employment Equity Act (Act No. 55 of 1998) of South Africa). www.labour.gov.za/docs/legislation/eea/codegoodpractise.htm.

Cohen S, Kamarck T, Mermelstein R (1983) A global measure of perceived stress. Journal of Health and Social Behaviour 24: 385–96.

Colarusso R, Hammill D (1972) Motor-Free Visual Perception Test (MVPT). Novato, CA: Academic Therapy Publications.

Coleman JC (1969) Psychology and effective behaviour. Glenview, IL: Foresman and Co.

Collins English Dictionary (1979) London and Glasgow: Collins.

Commission on Accreditation of Rehabilitation Facilities (1991) Work hardening programs. In Standards Manual for Organizations Serving People with Disabilities. Tucson, AZ: CARF.

Concha M and Lorenzo T (1993) The prevalence of disability in a rural area of South Africa, with special reference to moving disabilities. South African Journal of Occupational Therapy 23(2): 6–15.

The Concise Oxford Dictionary: New Edition (1975) (6th edn). Oxford: Clarendon Press.

Connors GJ, Donovan DM, DiClemente CC (2001) Substance Abuse Treatment and the Stages of Change: Selecting and Planning Interventions. New York: Guilford Publications, Inc.

Cooper CL (1981) The Stress Check. New Jersey: Prentice Hall.

Coopersmith S (1981) The Antecedents of Self-esteem. Revised edn. Novato, CA: Consulting Psychologists Press.

Copperman LE, Forwell SJ, Hugos L. (2003) In CA Trombley and M Vining Radomsky (eds) Occupational Therapy for Physical Dysfunction. 5th edn, p.905. Philadelphia: Lippincott H. Williams & Williams.

Corey MS, Corey G (1997) Groups. Process and Practice. 5th edn. New York: Brooks/Cole Publishing Company.

Cornish PM (1975) Activities for the Frail Aged. New York: Potentials Development for Health and Aging Services Inc.

Cossa M (2003) Therapeutic spiral Model and Adolescents: A Developmental Perspective. www.therapeuticspiral.org/articles (accessed 5/2/2004).

Couldrik L (1998a) Sexual issues: an area of concern for occupational therapists? British Journal of Occupational Therapy 61(11): 493–496.

Couldrik L (1998b) Sexual issues within occupational therapy, Part 1: Attitudes and practice. British Journal of Occupational Therapy 61(12): 538–543.

Couldrik L (1999) Sexual issues within occupational therapy, Part 2: Implications for education and practice. British Journal of Occupational Therapy 62(1): 26–30.

Cox M (2002) The Six TSM Structures for Safety. www.therapeuticspiral.org/articles/6tsm-structures.htm.

Creek J (ed) (1988) Occupational Therapy: New Perspectives. London: Whurr Publishers.

Creek J (1990) Occupational Therapy and Mental Health. Edinburgh: Churchill Livingstone.

Creek J (2002) How Therapists Think in Practice. Course notes.

Creek J (ed) (2002) Occupational Therapy and Mental Health. 3rd edn. London: Churchill Livingstone.

Crepeau EB, Cohn ES, Boyt Schell BA (eds) (2003) Willard and Spackman's Occupational Therapy 10th Edition. Philadelphia: Lippincott, Williams and Wilkins.

Crossley ML (1997) 'Survivors' and 'Victims': Long-term HIV positive individuals and the ethos of self empowerment. Journal of Social Science and Medicine 45(12): 1863–1873.

Crouch RB (2003) Stress assessment. PhD Thesis, Medical University of South Africa (MEDUNSA).

Crouch RB, Alers VM (1997) Occupational Therapy in Psychiatry and Mental Health. 3rd edn. Cape Town: Maskew Miller Longman (Pty) Ltd.

Crouch RB, Pienaar R (1984) An Occupational Therapy Group Programme with Alcoholic Patients. Proceedings of National Congress of SAAOT 26–29 June 1984.

Cumming E, Henry W (1961) Growing Old: The Process of Disengagement. New York: Basic Books.

Cynkin S, Robinson AM (1990) Occupational Therapy and Activities Health: Towards Health through Activities. Boston: Little, Brown & Co.

Dada MA, McQuoid-Mason DJ (2001) Introduction to Medico Legal Practice. Durban: Butterworths.

Davies S, Stewart A (1987) Nutritional Medicine. The Drug-Free Guide to Better Family Health. London: Pan Books.

De Witt MW, Booysen MI (eds) (1995) Socialisation of the Young Child. Selected Themes. Pretoria: JL van Schaik. South Africa.

De Witt PA (1994) Assessment of the Levels of Creative Ability. Pretoria: Marie and Vona du Toit Foundation.

De Witt PA (2002) The occupation in occupational therapy. South African Journal of Occupational Therapy 32(3): 2–7.

De Witt PA (2003) Investigation into the criteria and behaviour used to assess task concept. South Africa Journal of Occupation Therapy 33(1): 4–7.

Deane N (2003) Disability claims rise and productivity falls as HIV/AIDS takes its toll in the workplace. Mail and Guardian 19(39) (26 Sept.–2 Oct.).

Decosas J (2002) Correspondent: HIV/AIDS in Africa. The Lancet 360(30): 1786–1787.

DeGangi G (2000) Pediatric Disorders of Regulation in Affect and Behavior: A Therapist's Guide to Assessment and Treatment. USA: Academic Press.

De Gangi GA, Belzar-Martin LA (in press) The sensorimotor history questionnaire for preschoolers. Journal of Developmental and Hearing Disorders 2.

DeGangi GA, Poisson S, Sickel RZ, Wiener AS (1995) Infant/Toddler Symptom Checklist 7–30 months. San Antonio, TX: The Psychological Corps/Therapy Skill Builders.

DeGangi GA, Greenspan, SI (1989) Test of sensory function in infancy. Los Angeles: Western Psychological Services.

Dennison ST (1998) Activities for Adolescents in Therapy. Springfield, IL: Charles C Thomas Publisher.

Department of Health (1997a) Year 2000 Health Goals, Objectives and Indicators for South Africa. In: The White Paper for the Transformation of the Health System of South Africa, Pretoria: Department of Health.

Department of Health (1997b) White Paper on an Integrated National Disability Strategy. Government Press, Pretoria, South Africa.

Department of Health (2000) 'Rehabilitation Services – Basic considerations' and 'Community Based Rehabilitation – service description'. Pretoria: Department of Health.

Department of Health (2000) National Rehabilitation Policy. Pretoria: Government Printer.

Department of Health (2003) National Psychosocial Rehabilitation Policy. Pretoria: Government Printer.

Desisto MJ, Harding CM, McCormick RJ, Ashikaga T, Gautam S (1995a) The Maine-Vermont three decade studies of serious mental illness: matched comparison of cross-sectional outcome. British Journal of Psychiatry 167: 331–338.

Desisto MJ, Harding CM, McCormick RJ, Ashikaga T, Brooks GW (1995b) The Maine-Vermont three decade studies of serious mental illness: longitudinal course comparisons. British Journal of Psychiatry 167: 338–342.

Diller L (1994) Finding the right treatment combinations: Changes in rehabilitation over the past five years. In A Christensen, BP Uzzell (eds) Brain Injury and Neuropsychological Rehabilitation – International perspectives, pp. 1–15. New Jersey: Lawrence Erlbaum.

Dolan C, Concha ME, Nyathi E (1995) Community rehabilitation workers: do they offer hope to disabled people in South Africa's rural areas? International Journal of Research 18(3): 187–200.

DPSA (Disabled People South Africa) (2001). Pocket Guide on Disability Equity. An Empowerment Tool. Cape Town: DPSA Parliamentary Office.

du Toit HJV (1968) A technique for the early introduction of a work-related occupational therapy program for the patient who will retain significant residual disability. Pretoria: Pretoria College of Occupational Therapy.

du Toit HJV (1972) The restoration of activity participation leading to work participation. South African Journal of Occupational Therapy 2.

du Toit HJV (1974) An investigation into the correlation between volition and its expression. South African Journal of Occupational Therapy 6–10.

du Toit HJV (1974) The Background to the Evaluation and Improvement of Creative Participation. Johannesburg: National Council for the Care of Cripples.

du Toit HJV (1980) Patient Volition and Action in Occupational Therapy. Pretoria: Vona and Marie du Toit Foundation.

du Toit HJV (1980) The implementation of a program aimed at evaluating the current level of creative ability in an individual and stimulating the growth of his creative ability which leads to work capacity. Johannesburg: National Council for the Care for Cripples.

du Toit V (1991) Patient Volition and Action in Occupational Therapy. 2nd edn. Pretoria: Vona and Marie du Toit Foundation.

Duncan M (2004) Promoting mental health through occupation. In R Watson and L Swartz (eds) Transformation through Occupation. London: Whurr Publishers.

Duncan M, Watson R (2004) Transformation through occupation: a prototype. In R Watson and L Swartz (eds) Transformation through Occupation. London: Whurr Publishers.

Dunn W (1999) Sensory Profile: User's Manual. London: Psychological Corporation.

Dunn W, Brown C, McGuigan A (1994) The ecology of human performance: A framework for considering the effects of context. American Journal of Occupational Therapy 48: 595–607.

Durlak JA (1997) Successful Prevention Programs for Children and Adolescents. New York: Plenum Press.

Dusek JB (1987) Adolescent Development and Behaviour. New Jersey: Prentice-Hall International.

Dwivedi KN (1993) Group Work with Children and Adolescents: A Handbook. London: Jessica Kingsley Publishers, Ltd.

Earls F, Mezzacappa E (2002) Conduct and Oppositional Disorders. In M Rutter and E Taylor (eds) Child and Adolescent Psychiatry. 4th edn. Oxford: Blackwell Science Ltd.

Early J (2002) Healing through relationship in an interactive Gestalt group. www.early.org/group%20therapy/healingthrough-relationship.htm (29 June 2002).

Edmans J (1998) An investigation into stroke patients resuming sexual activity. British Journal of Occupational Therapy. January. Vol 61(1): 36–38.

Elpers R, in HI Kaplan, BJ Sadock (2000) Comprehensive Textbook of Psychiatry. 7th edn. New York: Lippincott Williams and Wilkins

Emery RE, Lauma-Billings (2002) Child abuse. In M Rutter and E Taylor (eds) Child and Adolescent Psychiatry. 4th edn. Oxford: Blackwell Science Ltd.

Engelbrecht E, Kreigler SM, Booysen MI (1996) Perspectives on Learning Difficulties. JL van Schaik. Pretoria.

Erikson EH (1963) Childhood and Society. New York: Norton.

Erikson EH (1980) Identity and the Life Cycle. New York: Norton.

Erikson EH (1997) The Life Cycle Completed. New York: Norton.

Evans J (1985) Performance and attitudes of occupational therapists regarding sexual habilitation of pediatric patients. The American Journal of Occupational Therapy. Vol 39(10): 664–671.

Evans J (1987) Sexual consequences of disability: Activity analysis and performance adaptation. Occupational Therapy in Health Care. Spring. Vol 4(1): 149–154.

Falconer JA (1998) Stress management following brain injury: Strategies for families and caregivers. Cognitive-behavioural brain injury rehabilitation. Behaviour management in residential brain injury settings. Living with brain injury: Post-rehabilitation recovery. Developing a low-cost brain injury rehabilitation program: Guidelines for family members. Recovering from brain injury: A continual process. www.brain-train.com/articles/npvsvoc.htm.

Farmer P, Leandre F, Mukherjee JS, Claude MS, Nevil P, Smith-Fawzi MC, Koenig SP, Castro A, Becerra M, Sachs J, Attaran A and Kim JY (2001) Community-based approaches to HIV treatment in resource poor settings. Lancet 358(9279): 404–409.

Faure M and Richardson A (2002) Baby Sense: Understanding Your Baby's Sensory World – The Key to a Contented Child. Singapore: Metz Press.

Figley CR (ed) (1995) Compassion Fatigue. Coping with Secondary Traumatic Stress Disorder in Those who Treat the Traumatized. New York: Brunner Mazel.

Finlay L (1997) The Practice of Psychosocial Occupational Therapy. 2nd edn. United Kingdom: Stanley Thornes Ltd.

Fischer AC (2001) Vol. 1, Development, Standardisation and Administration Manual, Vol. 2, User Manual. 4th edn. Fort Collins, CO: 3 Star Press.

Fisher AG, Murray EA, Bundy AC (1991). Sensory Integration: Theory and Practice. Philadelphia: FA Davis.

Flisher AJ, Parry C, Evans J, Muller M and Lombard C (2003) Substance use by adolescents in Cape Town: prevalence and correlates. Journal of Adolescent Health 32: 58–65.

Folsom JC (1968) Reality orientation for the elderly patient. Journal of Geriatric Psychiatry 1: 291–307.

Folstein MF, Folstein SE and Mchugh PR (1975) Mini-mental state examination, a practical method of grading the cognitive state of patients for the clinician. Journal of Psychiatric Research 12: 189–198.

Fontaine KI (1991) Unlocking sexual issues. Nursing Clinics of North America 26(3): 737–743.

Fontana D (1989) Managing Stress. London: Routledge Ltd.

Fouché LO (2001) Unpublished Master's dissertation. Pretoria: University of Pretoria.

Foulder-Hughes I (1998) The educational needs of occupational therapists who work with adult survivors of childhood sexual abuse. British Journal of Occupational Therapy 61(2): 68–74.

Fourie M (2002) Occupational of Women Living in Poverty. Master's Dissertation. School of Health and Rehabilitation Sciences; Division Occupational Therapy. Cape Town: University of Cape Town.

Frances A, Pincus HA, First MB (1995) Diagnostic and Statistical Manual of Mental Disorders. 4th edn. Washington: American Psychiatric Association

Freeman M (1992) Negotiating the future of traditional healers in SA – differences and difficulties. Critical Health 40.

Freire P (1974) Education: The Practice of Freedom. London: Writers and Readers Co-operative.

Freud S (1936) The Problem of Anxiety. New York: Norton.

Frieg A and Hendry JA (2002) Disability grant and recipients and caregiver utilisation. South African Journal of Occupational Therapy 32(2): 15–18.

Galder Gath D and Mayou R (1996) Oxford Textbook of Psychiatry. Oxford: Oxford University Press.

Galvaan R (2000) The Live-in Domestic Worker's Experience of Occupational Engagement. Master's Dissertation. School of Health and Rehabilitation Sciences; Division Occupational Therapy. Cape Town: University of Cape Town.

Gardner MF (1996) Test of Visual-Perceptual Skills (non-motor) (Revised) Burlingame, CA: Psychological and Educational Publications.

Gardner M (2002) Cognitive approaches. In J Creek (ed) Occupational Therapy and Mental Health. London: Churchill Livingstone.

Garske GG, Stewart JR (1999) Stigmatic and mythical thinking: Barriers to vocational rehabilitation services for persons with severe mental illness. Journal of Rehabilitation Oct./Nov./Dec: 4–8.

Gil I (1996) Treating Abused Adolescents. New York: The Guilford Press.

Gillis LS (1986) Guidelines in Psychiatry. 3rd edn. Cape Town: Juta and Co.

Gilman S and Newman SW (1992) Essentials of Clinical Neuroanatomy and Neurophysiology. 9th edn. Philadelphia: FA Davis.

Gilvarry E (2000) Substance abuse in young people. Journal of Child Psychology and Psychiatry 41: 55–80.

Goldberg D, Williams P (1988) A User's Guide to the General Health Questionnaire. Windsor: NFER-Nelson.

Gorski T (1989) Passages Through Recovery, An Action Plan for Preventing Relapse (Hazelden Recovery Series). Iowa: Hazelden Information Education.

Greenspan, SI (1992) Infancy and Early Childhood: The Practice of Clinical Assessment and Intervention with Emotional and Developmental Challenges. Madison, CT: International Universities Press.

Grinfeld MJ (1997) EEOC issues ADA guidelines for mentally disabled. Psychiatric Times XIV(6).

Gronwall D, Wrightson P and Waddell P (1999) Head Injury – The Facts. 2nd edn. Auckland, New Zealand: Oxford University Press.

Group for the Advancement of Psychiatry, Formulated by the Committee on Psychiatry and the Law (1991) The Mental Health Professional and the Legal System. New York: Brunner Mazel.

Gutman S (2001) Traumatic brain injury. In Pedretti LW, Early MB (Eds) Occupational Therapy – Practice Skills for Physical Dysfunction, 5th edn. St. Louis, Missouri: Mosby, Inc., pp.671–701.

Gutterman L (1990) A day treatment programme for persons with AIDS. American Journal of Occupational Therapy 44(3): 234–237.

Gutterman L (2001) HIV infection and AIDS. In LW Pedretti and MB Early (eds) Occupational Therapy Practice Skills for Physical Dysfunction. 5th edn. St Louis, London: Mosby, p.1018.

Hagedorn R (1992) Occupational Therapy: Foundations For Practice: Models, Frames of Reference and Core Skills. Edinburgh: Churchill Livingstone.

Hagedorn R (1997) Foundations for Practice in Occupational Therapy. 2nd edn. Edinburgh: Churchill Livingstone.

Ham JR, Fenech AM (2002) Continuing professional development for occupational therapy support workers. British Journal of Occupational Therapy 65(5): 227–228.

Hammell KW (2001) Intrinsicality: Reconsidering spirituality, meaning(s) and mandates. Canadian Journal of Occupational Therapy June: 186–194.

Hammill DD, Bryant BR (1986) Detroit Test of Learning Aptitude – Primary. Austin, TX: PRO-ED.

Hammill DD, Pearson NA, Voress JK (1993) Developmental Test of Visual perception. 2nd Edn. Austin, TX: PRO-ED.

Harding C (1997) Some things we've learned about vocational rehabilitation of the seriously and persistently mentally ill. www.akmhcweb.org/ncarticles/Vocational%2520Rehab.htm.

Harding CM, Strauss JS, Hafez H, Lieberman PB (1987) Work and mental illness: I. Towards an integration of rehabilitation process. Journal of Nervous and Mental Disease 175(6): 317–327.

Harris DB (1963) Goodenough-Harris Drawing Test. Harcourt Brace Jovanovich Inc., USA.

Harrison P, Oakland T (2003) Adaptive Behavior Assessment System. San Antonio, TX: Psychological Corporation.

Harter S (1983) Developmental perspectives on the self. In PH Mussen (ed) Handbook of Child Psychology. New York: Wiley, pp.275–385.

Harter S (1985) The Self-perception Profile for Children. Denver, CO: University of Denver.

Haslett C, Chilvers ER, Hunter JA, Boon N (1999) Davidson's Principles and Practice of Medicine. Edinburgh: Churchill Livingstone, pp.87–107.

Hasselkus BR (2002) The Meaning of Everyday Occupation. New Jersey: Slack Inc.

Haug H, Rossler W (1999) Deinstitutionalisation in central Europe. Eur Arch Psychiatry Clinical Neuroscience 249(3): 115–122.

Hay J, Byrne C, Cohen G, Schmuck ML (1996) An 18 month follow-up of an inter-disciplinary human sexuality workshop. Canadian Journal of Occupational Therapy 63(2): 129–132.

Health Professions Council of South Africa (1984) Rules for Registration of Occupational Therapy Technicians: Professional Board Notice: 533 of 1984. Pretoria: Health Professions Council of South Africa.

Health Professions Council of South Africa (1992a) Regulations Defining the Scope of the Profession of Occupational Therapy: Regulation 2145 of 31 July 1992. Pretoria: Health Professions Council of South Africa.

Health Professions Council of South Africa (1992b) Rules Specifying Acts or Omissions in Respect of which Disciplinary Steps may be taken. Regulation 1379 of 12 August 1994 (includes ethical rules, currently on review). Pretoria: Health Professions Council of South Africa.

Health Professions Council of South Africa (1994) Rules for Registration of Occupational Therapy Auxiliaries. Professional Board Notice: 44 of 1994. Pretoria: Health Professions Council of South Africa.

Health Professions Council of South Africa (2003) Professional Board for Occupational Therapy and Medical Orthotics/Prosthetics. Policy Statement: Occupational Therapy Auxiliary and Technician categories of practitioners – Training and Practice, November 2003. Professional Board for Occupational Therapy and Medical Orthotics/Prosthetics. Pretoria: Health Professions Council of South Africa.

Heggenhougen HK, Shore L (1986) Cultural components of behavioural epidemiology: Implications for primary health care. Social Science Medicine 22(11): 1235–1245.

Hemphill BJ (ed) (1982) The Evaluative Process in Psychiatric Occupational Therapy. New Jersey: Slack Inc.

Hemphill BJ (ed) (1998) Mental Health Assessment in Occupational Therapy. New Jersey: Slack Inc.

Henderson S (1998) Frames of references utilised in the rehabilitation of individuals with eating disorders. Canadian Journal of Occupational Therapy 66(1): 43–51.

Henderson SE, Sugden DA (1992) The Movement Assessment Battery for Children. London: The Psychological Corporation.

Henley E, Twible R (2001) The value of physiotherapy and occupational therapy in community based rehabilitation. Asia and Pacific Journal on Disability. www.dinf.ne.jp/doc/prdl/othr/apdrj/z13fm0100/z13fm0105.htm (accessed 2/05/2002).

Hill SW (1995) The prediction of vocational outcomes in schizophrenia: Do diagnosis and symptomatology really matter? A review of the literature. www.angelfire.com/oh/avalanchDiode/SCHZWRK.html (accessed 10/6/2003).

Hocking C (2000) Occupational science: a stock take of accumulated insight. Journal of Occupational Science 7: 58–67.

Hoge RD (1999) Assessing Adolescents in Educational, Counselling and other Settings. New Jersey: Lawrence Erlbaum.

Holland K (1993) Occupational Therapy Support Staff, A Challenge Facing Occupational Therapy? Paper presentation. South African Association of Occupational Therapists Congress, University of Pretoria, July 1993.

Holland K (2001) A study to identify stressors perceived by Health Science lecturing staff in a school at a South African University. MEd Dissertation (Tertiary Education), pp. 82–83. Natal, South Africa: Natal University.

Holmes, P (2002) The Use of Action Methods in the Treatment of the Attachment Difficulties of Long-term Fostered and Adopted Children. In A Bannister, A Huntington, Communicating with Children and Adolescents: Action for Change. London and Philadelphia: Jessica Kingsley.

Holmes TH, Rahe RH (1967) The Social Adjustment Rating Scale. Journal of Psychosomatic Research 11: 213–218.

Holsten E (1985) Comparison of Vona du Toit's Theory with Other Theories on Motivation and Action. Pretoria: Vona and Marie du Toit Foundation.

Homer SL, Sehayek G (1995) The challenge of rural mental health. South African Congress for Occupational Therapy, Cape Town, July.

Hopkins HL, Smith HD (1988) Willard and Spackman's Occupational Therapy. 7th edn. Philadelphia: JB Lippincott Co.

Hopkins HL, Smith HD (1993) Willard and Spackman's Occupational Therapy. 8th edn. Philadelphia: JB Lippincott Co.

Howard M, Bleiberg J (1997) Manual of behaviour management strategies for traumatically brain injured adults in Diagnostics and treatment protocols: General management approaches and philosophy website www.nbia.nf.ca/general_management_approaches_&_philosophy.htm

Howe D (1995) Attachment Theory for Social Work Practice. London and Basingstoke: Macmillan.

Hudgins KM (1998) The Therapeutic Spiral Model. Developmental Repair. http://www.therapeuticspiral.org/articles (5/02/04).

Hudgins KM (2002) Experiential Treatment for P.T.S.D. The Therapeutic Spiral Model. New York: Springer Publishing Company.

Hudgins KM, Drucker K, Metcalf K (2000) The 'Containing double': A clinically effective psychodrama intervention for PTSD. British Journal of Psychodrama and Sociodrama 15(1): 58–77.

Hudnall Stamm BH (Ed.) (1999) Secondary Traumatic Stress – Self Care Issues for Clinicians, Researchers and Educators 2nd edn. Maryland USA: Sidran Press.

Hughes DA (1997) Facilitating Developmental Attachment, New Jersey and London: Jason Aronson Inc.

Hursh NC (1997) Essential competencies in industrial rehabilitation and disability management practice: A skills-based training model. In DE Shrey and M Lacerte (eds) Principles and Practices of Disability Management in Industry. Winter Park, FL: GR Press Inc, pp.303–352.

ICD-10 (1992) The ICD-10 Classification of Mental and Behavioural Disorders Geneva: World Health Organization.

International Labour Organization (ILO) (1981). Vocational Rehabilitation and the Employment of the Disabled: A Glossary. Geneva: ILO.

International Labour Organization (ILO) (1985) Basic Principles of Vocational Rehabilitation of the Disabled. 3rd edn. Geneva: ILO.

Jacobs H, Wissusik D, Collier R, Stackman D, Burdeman (1992) Correlations between psychiatric disabilities and vocational outcome. Hospital and Community Psychiatry 43: 365–369.

Jacobs K (1985) Occupational Therapy: Work-related Programs and Assessments. 2nd edn. Boston: Little, Brown and Co.

Jacobs K (1993) Work assessments and programming. In HL Hopkins and HD Smith (eds) Willard and Spackman's Occupational Therapy. Philadelphia: JB Lippincott Company, pp.226–248.

Jacobson K (1985) Occupational Therapy: Work-related Programs and Assessments. New York: Little, Brown and Co.

Jamison KR (1997) An Unquiet Mind. London: Picador.

Johnston M, Wright S, Weinman J (1995) A Guide to Measurement in Health Psychology. London: NFER-Nelson.

Jooste E (1980) Skeppende vermoe. South African Journal of Occupational Therapy 10(1).

Joubert R (1982) The correlation between sensory deprivation and creative ability. South African Journal of Occupational Therapy 1(1).

Joubert RWE, Van Der Reyden D (2003) A survey to explore moral and ethical dilemmas facing occupational therapists treating HIV/AIDS patients in rural and urban hospitals in KwaZulu Natal. Unpublished (June). Department of Occupational Therapy, University of Durban-Westville, Durban.

Jung CG (1933) Modern Man in Search of Soul. New York: Harcourt.

Kaplan HI, Sadock BJ (2000) Comprehensive Textbook of Psychiatry. 7th edn. Philadelphia: Lippincott Williams & Wilkins.

Kaplan HI, Sadock BJ (1998) Kaplan and Sadock's Synopsis of Psychiatry: behavioural sciences/clinical psychiatry, 8th edn. Baltimore: Lippincott Williams & Wilkins.

Kaplan HI, Sadock BJ, Grebb JA (1998) Synopsis of Psychiatry. 8th edn. New York: Williams & Wilkins.

Kaplan HS (1974) The New Sex Therapy. 6th edn. New York: Brunner Mazel.

Karp CL, Butler TL, Bergstrom SC (1998) Activity Manual for Adolescents. London: Sage Publications.

Keable D (1989) The Management of Anxiety: A Manual for Therapists. Edinburgh, New York: Churchill Livingstone.

Keeney BP (1983) Aesthetics of Change. New York: The Guilford Press.

Kellerman PF, Hudgins MK (eds) (2000) Psyxchodrama with Trauma Survivors: Acting Out Your Pain. London: Jessica Kingsley.

Kennedy L (1997a) The role of the occupational therapist in personal injury litigation – Part I. Economica Ltd, The Expert Witness Newsletter 2(3). Downloaded from www.economica.ca/ew23p3.htm (accessed 5/6/2003).

Kennedy L (1997b) The role of the occupational therapist in personal injury litigation – Part II. Economica Ltd, The Expert Witness Newsletter 2(4). Downloaded from www.economica.ca/ew23p3.htm (accessed 5/6/2003).

Kennedy M (1987) Occupational therapists as sexual rehabilitation professionals using the rehabilitative framework of reference. Canadian Journal of Occupational Therapy. 54(4): 189–193.

Kennerly H (1995) Managing Anxiety. A Training Manual. Oxford: Oxford University Press.

Kielhofner G (1985) The Model of Human Occupation. 1st edn. Baltimore: Williams & Wilkins.

Kielhofner G (1992) Conceptual Foundations of Occupational Therapy. Philadelphia: FA Davis.

Kielhofner G (1995) A Model of Human Occupation: Theory and Application. 2nd edn. Baltimore: Williams & Wilkins.

Kielhofner G (1997). Conceptual Foundations of Occupational Therapy. Philadelphia: FA Davis.

Kielhofner G (2002) A Model of Human Occupation: Theory and Application. 3rd edn. Baltimore: Lippincott & Wilkins.

Kielhofner G, Mallinson T, Crawford D, Nowak M, Rigby M, Henry A et al. (1998) User's Manual for the Occupational Performance History Interview OPHI-II. Chicago: Model of Occupational Performance Clearinghouse.

Kilsby M, Beyers S (1996) Engagement and interaction: a comparison between supported employment and day service provision. Journal of Intellectual Disability Research 40(4): 345–357.

King LJ (1974) A sensory integration approach to schizophrenia. American Journal of Occupational Therapy 28: 529–536.

Kingsley P, Molineux M (2000) True to our philosophy? Sexual orientation and occupation. British Journal of Occupational Therapy. 63(5): 205–210.

Kissling W and Baum LJ (1994) Prelapse Programme. Johannesburg: Lundbeck South Africa.

Klein RM, Bell B (1979) Klein-Bell Activity of Daily Living Scale. Seattle University of Washington: Division of Occupational Therapy.

Kleyn D, Viljoen F (1998). Beginner's Guide for Law Students. 2nd edn. Cape Town: Juta.

Kluckhorn C, Murray HA (1953) A conception of personality. In C Kluckhorn, HA Murray and DM Schneider (eds) Personality in Nature, Society and Culture. New York: Knopf.

Kniepmann K (1997) Prevention of disability and maintenance of health. In C Christiansen and C Baum (eds) Occupational Therapy: Enabling Function and Well-being. 2nd edn. New Jersey: Slack Inc.

Kramer P, Hinojosa J (1999) Frames of Reference for Pediatric Occupational Therapy. 2nd edn. Philadelphia: Lippincott Williams & Wilkins.

Kriel E (2003) Helping the sexually abused child: Seminar, Pretoria.

Kromberg JGR, Christianson AL, Manga P, Zwane ME, Rosen E, Venter A, Homer S (1997) Intellectual disability in rural black children in the Bushbuckridge district of South Africa. Southern African Journal of Child and Adolescent Mental Health 9(1).

Kruger H (2001, August) The pre-trial meeting. Presentation to Medicolegal Workshop, Institute of Occupational Therapists in Private Practice (INSTOPP), Centurion, South Africa.

Kübler-Ross E (1973) On Death and Dying. London: Routledge.

Kuldau JM, Dirks SJ (1977) Controlled evaluation of a hospital originated community transitional system. Archives of General Psychiatry 34: 1331–1340.

Landreth G (1991) Play Therapy, The Art of the Relationship. Muncie, IN: Accelerated Development.

Laurence O and Gostin JD (1995) Confidentiality vs Duty to Warn: Ethical and Legal Dilemmas in the HIV Epidemic. September. JIAPAC.

Lavery JV, Boyle J, Dickens BM, Macleod H, Singer PA (2001) Origins of desire for euthanasia and assisted suicide in people with HIV-1 or AIDS: A qualitative study. The Lancet 58(4): 362–367.

Law MC, Baptiste S, Carswell A, McColl MA, Polatajko H and Pollock N (1991) The Canadian Occupational Performance Measure. Toronto: Canadian Association of Occupational Therapy.

Law M, Baptiste S, Carswell A, McColl MA, Polatajko H, Pollock N (1994) Canadian Occupational Performance Measure. 2nd edn. Toronto: CAOT Publications ACE.

Law M, Baptiste S, Carswell A et al. (1998) Canadian Occupational Performance Measure (COPM) 3rd edn. Ottawa: CAOT Publications ACE

Law M, Baum C, Dunn W (2001) Measuring Occupational Performance: Supporting Best Practice in Occupational Therapy. New Jersey: Slack Inc.

Law M, Cooper B, Strong S, Stewart D, Rigby P, Letts L (1996) The person-environment-occupation model: a transactive approach to occupational performance. Canadian Journal of Occupational Therapy 63: 9–23.

Lehman AF (1995) Vocational rehabilitation in schizophrenia. Schizophrenia Bulletin 21(4): 645–656.

Lemon BW, Bengston VL, Peterson JA (1972) An exploration of the activity theory of ageing: activity types and life satisfaction among in-movers to a retirement community. Journal of Gerontology 27: 511–523.

Leonardelli C (1998) Milwaukee Evaluation of Daily Living Skills (MEDLS). In B Hemphill (ed) Mental Health Assessment in Occupational Therapy. New Jersey: Slack Inc.

Lewis S (1999) An Adult's Guide to Childhood Trauma. Understanding Childhood Trauma in South Africa. Cape Town: David Philip Publishers.

Lezak MD (1995) Neurological Assessment. New York: Oxford University Press.

Libermann D, Koperlowitz L, Smith JM (2000) In HI Kaplan and BJ Sadock Comprehensive Textbook of Psychiatry. 7th edn. New York: Lippincott Williams & Wilkins.

Linehan M (1993) Skills Training for Treating Borderline Personality Disorders. New York: Guildford Press.

Loftus EF (1980) Memory. Reading, MA: Addison-Wesley.

Lougher L (2002) Child and Adolescent Mental Health Services. In J Creek (ed) (2002) Occupational Therapy in Mental Health. 3rd edn. London: Churchill Livingstone, p. 393.

Louw DA (1990) Menslike Ontwikkeling. 2nd edn. Pretoria: Haum.

Louw DA (1998) Human Development. 2nd edn. Pretoria: Haum Tertiary.

Luger R, Sherry K, Vilikazi B, Wonnacott H, Galvaan R (2003) A struggle for identity: domestic workers, ubuntu and 'time-off' occupations. South African Journal of Occupational Therapy 33: 11–14.

Lysack C, Kaufert J (1994) Comparing the origins and ideologies of the independent living movement and community based rehabilitation. International Journal of Research 17: 231–240.

MacLennan BW, Dies KR (1992) Group Counselling and Psychotherapy with Adolescents. 2nd edn. New York: Columbia University Press.

Madden CA, Mitchell VA (1993) Professions' Standards and Competence: A Survey of Continuing Education for the Professions. Bristol: University of Bristol.

Mail and Guardian, 19(32) (8–14 Aug. 2003).

Mail and Guardian, 19(35) (29 Aug. to 4 Sept. 2003).

Malcome C (2003) Choosing a theoretical framework for data constitution and analysis. DEd. Seminar, University of Durban-Westville, 7 Sept. (Unpublished).

Mancuso LL (1990) Reasonable accommodations for workers with psychiatric disabilities. Psychosocial Rehabilitation Journal 14(2): 3–19.

Mann JM, Tarantola DJM (1998) HIV 1998: The Global Picture. Scientific American 7(98): 62–63. www.genethik.dw/aids/aid01.htm (accessed 8/6/2003).

Mannion E (1996) Resilience and burden in spouses of people with mental illness. Psychiatric Rehabilitation Journal 20(2): 13–61.

Mapham K, Lawless N, Abbas M, Ross-Thompson N, Duncan M (2004) The play and leisure profiles of children in Lavender Hill. South African Journal of Occupational Therapy 34(2): 7–12.

Mappes TA, De Grazzia D (1996) Biomedical Ethics. 4th edn. New York: McGraw-Hill Inc.

Marshak L, Bostick D, Turton L (1990) Closure outcomes for clients with psychiatric disabilities served by the vocational rehabilitation system. Rehabilitation Counselling Bulletin 33: 247–250.

Marshal F Folstein et al. (2001) The Mini Mental State Examination (MMSE). New York: Psychological Corporation.

Masilela TC, Macleod C (1998) Social support. Its implications in the development of a community based mental health programme. South African Journal of Occupational Therapy 27(2): 11–16.

Masilela TC, Macleod C, Sehayek G, Tollman S, Malomane E, Homer S (1996) Monograph: an assessment of the mental health needs of communities in the Agincourt subdistrict of Bushbuckridge, Mpumalanga Province. Unpublished monograph. Health Systems Development Unit. Johannesburg: University of the Witwatersrand.

Maslow AH (1987) Motivation and Personality. 3rd edn. London: Harper.

Matsutsuyu JS (1969) The interest checklist. American Journal of Occupational Therapy 23(4): 323–328.

Mattingly C (1991) What is clinical reasoning? American Journal of Occupational Therapy 45(11): 979–986.

Mattingly C (1998) Healing Dramas and Clinical Plots: The Narrative Structure of Experience. Cambridge: Cambridge University Press.

Mattingly C, Fleming MH (1994) Clinical Reasoning: Forms of Enquiry in a Therapeutic Practice. Philadelphia: FA Davis.

Max-Neef MA (1991) Human Scale Development. London: The Apex Press.

McAlonan S (1996) Improving sexual rehabilitation services: The patient's perspective. American Journal of Occupational Therapy 50(10): 826–834.

McColl MA (1997) Social support and occupational therapy. In C Christiansen and C Baum (eds) Occupational Therapy: Enabling Function and Well Being. New Jersey: Slack Inc.

McColl M (2000). Spirit, occupation and disability. Canadian Journal of Occupational Therapy Oct.: 217–228.

McGee JJ, Menolascino JF (1991) Beyond Gentle Teaching: A Nonaversive Approach to Helping Those in Need. London: Plenum.

McGuire D (2003) Neurologic Manifestations of HIV – HIV Insite Knowledge Base Chapter, June, pp. 2–25. www.hivinsite.ucsf.edu/InSite (accessed 8/6/2003).

McQuoid-Mason DJ, Dada MA (1999) A guide to forensic medicine and the law. Module 7, Medical Law and Ethics, Independent Medico-Legal Unit. Durban: University of Natal.

McQuoid-Mason DJ, Dada MA (eds) (2001) Legal Aspects of Medical Practice: An Introduction to Medico-legal Practice. Durban: Butterworths.

McWilliams S (1997) Head injury. In A Turner, M Foster and SE Johnson (eds) (1997) Occupational Therapy and Physical Dysfunction: Principles, Skills and Practice. 4th edn, pp. 463–479. New York: Churchill Livingstone.

Mendis P (1994) Disability prevention and rehabilitation. Chapter 55 in KS Lankinen, S Bergstrom, PH Makela, M Peltomaa. Health and Disease in Developing Countries. London: Macmillan.

Meninger W in HI Kaplan and BJ Sadock (2000) Comprehensive Textbook of Psychiatry. 7th edn. New York: Lippincott Williams & Wilkins.

Mental Health Act (Act No. 18 of 1973). Department of Health – Republic of South Africa. Pretoria: Government printers.

Mental Health Care Act (Act No. 17 of 2002). Pretoria: Government printers.

Meyer A (1922) The philosophy of occupational therapy. Archives of Occupational Therapy 1: 1–10.

Meyer, Moore and Viljoen (1988) Persoonlikheidsteorieë van Freud tot Frankl. Johannesburg: Lexicon Publishers.

Miller, LJ (1988) Miller Assessment for Preschoolers (MAP). San Diego: Harcourt Brace Jovanovich.

Miller LJ (1993) FIRSTSTEP Screening Test for evaluating preschoolers. San Antonio, TX: The Psychological Corporation.

Miller RJ, Walker KF (1993) Perspectives on Theory for the Practice of Occupational Therapy. MD: Aspen Publishers Inc.

Miller WT (1984) An occupational therapist as a sexual clinician in the management of spinal cord injuries. Canadian Journal of Occupational Therapy 51(4): 172–175.

Millon T (1984) On the renaissance of personality assessment and personality theory. Journal of Personality Assessment 48.

Milne D (1992) Assessment: A Mental Health Portfolio. London: NFER-Nelson.

Minuchin S (1974) Families and Family Therapy Library of Congress Catalogue. Card N0 8/ Cambridge, MA: Harvard University Press.

Missiuna C, Pollock N (2000) Perceived efficacy and goal setting in young children. Canadian Journal of Occupational Therapy 67(2): 100–108.

Modiba P, Porteus K, Schneider H, Gunnarsson V (2000) Community mental health service needs: a study of service users, their families and community leaders in the Moretele District, North West Province. Centre for Health Policy. Johannesburg: University of the Witwatersrand.

Monasterio EB (2002) Enhancing resilience in the adolescent. Nursing Clinic of North America 37: 373–379.

Monga TN, Tan G, Ostermann HJ, Monga U, Grabois M (1998) Sexuality and sexual adjustment of patients with chronic pain. Disability and Rehabilitation 20(9): 317–329.

Montemayor R, Adams GR, Gullotta TP (1990) From Childhood to Adolescence: A Transitional Period? pp. 269–287. London: Sage.

Morrison J, Anders TF (1999) Interviewing Children and Adolescents. New York: Guilford Press.

Mosey AC (1973) Activities Therapy. New York: Rana Press.

Mosey AC (1982) Three Frames of Reference for Mental Health. New Jersey: Charles B. Slack

Mpe NF (2001) Unpublished Masters dissertation. Pretoria: University of Pretoria.

Murray CJL, Lopez AD (1994) Quantifying disability: data, methods, and results. World Health Organization 72(3): 481–494.

Murray-Slutsky MS, Paris BA (2000) Exploring the Spectrum of Autism and Pervasive Developmental Disorders. San Antonio, TX: Therapy Skill Builders.

Myers B, Parry C (2003) Fact Sheet – Cannabis and Mandrax Use in South Africa www.sahealthinfo. org/admodule/cannabis.htm (accessed 12/6/2003).

NAEYC Position Statement (1997) Principles of child development and learning that inform developmentally appropriate practice: Developmentally Appropriate Practice in Early Childhood Programs Serving Children from Birth through Age 8 National Association for the Education of Young Children www.naeyc.org/about/position/dap3.htm.

National Council on Disability (2000) From Privileges to Rights: People Labelled with Psychiatric Disabilities Speak for Themselves. Available: www.ncd.gov/publications/publications.html (accessed 12/9/2003).

National Health Research and Development Programme, Health and Welfare (1993) Role and Use of Support Personnel in the Rehabilitation Disciplines. Project #6609-1830-RP. Edmonton: University of Alberta.

National Institute on Drug Abuse. High School and Youth Trends www.nida.nih.gov/Infofax/HSYouthtrends.html (accessed 7/10/2003).

Neistadt M (1986) Sexuality counselling for adults with disabilities: a module for an occupational therapy curriculum. American Journal of Occupational Therapy 40(8): 542–545.

Neistadt M (1998) Teaching clinical reasoning as a thinking frame. American Journal of Occupational Therapy 52(3): 221–228.

Neistadt ME, Crepeau EB (1998) Willard and Spackman's Occupational Therapy. 9th edn. Philadelphia: Lippincott-Raven.

Nelson RR, Condrin JL (1987) A vocational readiness and independent living skills program for psychiatrically impaired adolescents. Occupational Therapy in Mental Health 7(2): 23–38.

Nissenboim S, Vroman C (2000) The Positive Interactions Program of Activities for People with Alzheimer's Disease. Baltimore: Health Professions Press.

Noble JH, Honberg RS, Hall LL, Flynn LM (1997) A legacy of failure: The inability of the Federal-State Vocational Rehabilitation System to serve people with severe mental illnesses. National Alliance for the Mentally Ill (NAMI), www.nami.org/update/legacy.htm (accessed 6/4/2003).

Norman K, Ramnarain B, Thomson C (2003) An exploration into the daily life tasks of orphaned children living within an AIDS affected community. Undergraduate Occupational Therapy dissertation (unpublished). Durban: University of Durban-Westville.

Northcott R, Chard G (2000) Sexual aspects of rehabilitation: the client's perspective. British Journal of Occupational Therapy 63(9): 412–418.

Novak PP, Mitchell M (1988) Professional involvement in sexuality counselling for patients with spinal cord injuries. American Journal of Occupational Therapy 42(2): 105–112.

O'Brien et al. (2000) The impact of occupational therapy on a child's playfulness. Occupational Therapy in Healthcare 12(2/3): 39–51.

O'Bryan A, Simons K, Beyer S, Grove B (2000) A Framework for Supported Employment. York: Joseph Rowntree Foundation.

Oaklander V (1988) Windows to our Children: A Gestalt Therapy to Children and Adolescents. New York: The Gestalt Journal Press.

Oaklander V (1999) Group play therapy from a Gestalt perspective. In DS Sweeney and LE Hofmeyer (eds) The Handbook of Group Play Therapy: How to do it, how it works, whom it's best for. San Francisco: Jossey-Bass, pp.162–175.

Occupational Therapists in Life Assurance (OTLA) (undated) Guidelines for occupational therapy evaluations and reports. Booklet sponsored by Momentum Risk Management Consultancy, South Africa.

Occupational Therapy Association of South Africa (1999) Occupational Therapy Support Staff. Their Role and Function. Pretoria: Occupational Therapy Association of South Africa.

Occupational Therapy Practice Framework: Domain and Process (2002) The American Journal of Occupational Therapy 56(6): 609–639.

Oetter P, Richter EW, Frick SM (1995) Motor Oral Respiration and Eyes. Integrating the Mouth with Sensory and Postural Functions. 2nd edn. Hugo, MN: PDP Press.

Offord DR, Benett KJ (2002) Hospital and community psychiatry. In M Rutter and E Taylor (eds) Child and Adolescent Psychiatry. 4th edn. Oxford: Blackwell Science Ltd.

Oser A (1997) Star Power for Preschoolers: Learning Life Skills Through Physical Play. St Paul, MN: Redleaf Press.

Packer B (1995) Appropriate Paper Based Technology (APT) A Manual. London: Intermediate Technology Publications.

Pandya SK (1997) Patients testing positive for HIV – ethical dilemmas in India. Issues in Medical Ethics 5(2): 49–55 (Mumbai: SNDT Churchgate).

Parham D, Mailloux Z, Smith-Roley S (2000) Sensory processing and praxis in high functioning children with autism. Paper presented at Research 2000, 4–5 February, Redondo Beach, CA.

Parham DL, Fazio LS (1997) Play in Occupational Therapy for Children. St Louis: Mosby.

Parry C (2003) The Changing Face of Drug Abuse in Cape Town: 1996–2003. http://www.mrc.co.za/pressreleases/2003/28pres2003.htm (accessed 7/10/2003).

Partridge C, Johnston M (1989) Perceived control of recovery from physical disability: measurement and prediction. British Journal of Clinical Psychology 28: 53–9.

Patel V (2003) Where There is No Psychiatrist. A Mental Health Care Manual. The Royal College of Psychiatrists. Glasgow: Gaskell, Bell and Bain Ltd.

Patti L, Harrison, Thomas Oakland (2000) Adaptive Behaviour Assessment System (ABAS). USA: Psychological Corporation.

Paul R (1996) Using Intellectual Standards to Assess Student Reasoning. OH: Center for Critical Thinking.

Payne MJ, Greer DI, Corbin DE (1988) Sexual functioning as a topic in occupational therapy training: A survey of programs. The American Journal of Occupational Therapy. 42(4): 227–230.

Pedretti LW, Early MB (2001) Occupational Therapy: Practice Skills for Physical Dysfunction. 5th edn. St Louis: Mosby.

Perry B (1995) Maltreated Children: Experience: Brain Development and the Next Generation. New York: WW Norton.

Peterson JS (1995) Talk with Teens about Feelings, Family, Relationships and the Future. Minneapolis: Free Spirit Publishing.

Petrick M, Homer S, Evans R (1999) Workshop report: Are therapists aware of the needs of people with disabilities? South Africa Journal of Physiotherapy 55(1): 26–28.

Piek S, Crouch RB, Venter E (1993) Stress Assessment. Unpublished. RB Crouch, PO Box 95657 Grantpark 2051 South Africa.

Piers EV, Harris DB (1984) Revised Manual for the Piers–Harris Children's Self-Concept Scale Los Angeles: Western Psychological Services.

Pizzi Assessment of Productive Living (2003) In M Pizzi, A Burkhardt Occupational Therapy for Adults with Immunological Diseases: Aids and Cancer, p. 826.

Pizzi Holistic Wellness Assessment (2001) In B Velder, P Wittman (eds) Occupational Therapy in Health Care (Special issue on community-based practice) 13: 51–66, Binghampton, NY: Hawthorn Press.

Pizzi M (1990) The transformation of HIV infection and AIDS in occupational therapy: Beginning the conversation. American Journal of Occupational Therapy 44(4): 199–203.

Pizzi M (1992) Women, HIV infection and AIDS: Tapestries of life, death and empowerment. American Journal of Occupational Therapy 46(11): 1021–1026.

Pizzi M, Burkhardt A (2003) Occupational Therapy for Adults with Immunilogical Diseases: AIDS and Cancer. In EB Crepeau, ES Cohn, BA Boyt Schell (eds) Willard and Spackman's Occupational Therapy. 10th edn, pp. 821–826. Philadelphia: Lippincott, Williams & Wilkins.

Polkinghorne D (1991) Narrative and self concept. Journal of Narrative and Life History 1: 135–153.

Powell TJ, Enright SJ (1991) Anxiety and Stress Management. London: Routledge.

Power MJ, Champion LA, Aris SJ (1988). The development of measure of social support: the Significant Others Scale (SOS). British Journal of Clinical Psychology 27: 349–58.

Pratt J, McFadyen A, Hall G, Campbell M, McLay D (1997) A review of the initial outcomes of a return-to-work programme for police officers following injury or illness. British Journal of Occupational Therapy 60: 253–267.

Pretorius HW (1995) Mental disorders and disabilities across cultures: a view from South Africa. The Lancet 345: 534.

Pretorius L (1998) An overview of legislation impacting on CBR. Paper presentation. CBR Management Course. Institute of Urban Primary Health Care, Johannesburg, Gauteng, South Africa.

Prochaska JO, DiClemente CC (1986) Towards a comprehensive model of change. In RJ Miller and N Heather (eds) Treating Addictive Behaviours: Processes of Change. London: Plenum.

Profis M (1992) Personality Disorders – Unpublished notes.

Radebe M (2004) Tok tok or talk talk: A playful way of communicating about serious things. Abstract and presentation at the 2nd National Conference on Victim Empowerment: Ten Years of Democracy – From Victims' Needs to Victims' Rights. Durban.

Randall L (2002) Psychosocial aspects of functional capacity evaluations. Unpublished paper presented at Vocational Rehabilitation Workshop, 25 April, Pretoria University, South Africa.

Randall L (2003) 'Disability Equity', pages D03/001-D03/018. Labour Law Handbook for Managers. Johannesburg: Fleet Street Publications.

Randall L (1999) (unpublished) Lecture notes compiled for Clinical Reasoning lecture for undergraduate occupational therapy students, South Africa.

Reed KL (1984) Models of Practice in Occupational Therapy. Baltimore: Williams & Wilkins.

Reed KL (1991) Quick Reference to Occupational Therapy, pp. 366–370. MD: Aspen Publishers.

Reed KL, Sanderson SN (1992) Concepts of Occupational Therapy. 3rd edn. Baltimore: Williams & Wilkins.

Reed KL, Sanderson SN (1999) Concepts of Occupational Therapy. 4th edn. Baltimore: Lippincott Williams & Wilkins

Remocker AJ, Storch ET (1982) Action Speaks Louder – a Handbook of Non-verbal Group Techniques. 3rd edn. Edinburgh: Churchill Livingstone.

Reynolds WM, Kobak KA (1995) Hamilton Depression Inventory (HDI) Professional Manual. Odessa, FL: PAR (Psychological Assessment Resources).

Ribeiro KL (2001) Client-centred practice: Body, mind and spirit resurrected. Canadian Journal of Occupational Therapy, April: 65–69.

Riddell S (2002) Work Preparation and Vocational Rehabilitation: A Literature Review. Glasgow: Strathclyde Centre for Disability Research.

Ritchie J (1985) Helping People to Unwind. NSW, Australia: Lifestyles Promotions Unit Dept. of Health.

Robertson B, Allwood C, Giagino C (2001) Textbook of Psychiatry of Southern Africa. Oxford: Oxford University Press.

Rogers CR (1951) Client-centered Therapy: Its Current Practice, Implications and Theory. Boston: Houghton Mifflin.

Rogers, C (1977) Carl Rogers on Personal Power. New York: Delacorte.

Rogers ES, Anthony WA, Cohen M, Davies RR (1997) Prediction of vocational outcome based on clinical and demographic indicators among vocationally ready clients. Community Mental Health Journal 33(2): 99–112.

Roper M (1985) Value clarification. South African Journal of Occupational Therapy 15: 21–24.

Rosenberg J (1965) Society and Adolescent Self-Image. Princeton, NJ: Princeton University Press.

Rosenberg B (1973) The work sample approach to vocational evaluation. In RE Hardy, JG Cull (eds). Vocational evaluation for rehabilitation services. Springfield, IL: Charles C Thomas.

Rosenberg M (1989) Society and the Adolescent Self-image (reprint edition). Middletown, CT: Wesleyan University Press.

Rustad RA, De Groot TL, Jungkunz ML, Freeberg KS, Borowick LG, Wanttie AM (1993) Cognitive Assessment of Minnesota (CAM). New York: Therapy Skill Builders.

Rutter M, Taylor E (2002) Child and Adolescent Psychiatry. 4th edn. Oxford: Blackwell Publishing.

Ryan SE (ed) (1986) The Certified Occupational Therapy Assistant – Roles and Responsibilities. New Jersey: Slack Inc.

Sachs D, Labovitz DR (1994) The caring occupational therapists: scope of professional roles and boundaries. American Journal of Occupational Therapy 48: 997–1005.

Sadock BJ, Sadock VA (2003) Kaplan and Sadock's Synopsis of Psychiatry: Behavioural sciences/clinical psychiatry. 9th edn. Lippincott, Williams & Wilkins.

Sands M (2003) The occupational therapist and occupational therapy assistant partnership. In E Crepeau, ES Kohn, BA Boyt-Schell. Willard and Spackman's Occupational Therapy. 10th edn. Philadelphia: Lippincott, Williams & Wilkins, pp.147–152.

Sarason IG, Sarason BR, Shearin EN, Pierce GR (1987) A brief measure of social support: practical and theoretical implications. Journal of Social and Personal Relationships 4: 497–510.

Saury R (2003) Story and Healing in Action: New Methods for Fostering Heart-to-heart Dialogue about Race. Multicultural Education. Caddo Gap Press. Winter 2003: 11(2): 49–54.

Schaaf RC, Anzalone MA, Burke JP (2001) The Sensory Integration Observation Guide. In S Smith Roley, E Blanche, RC Schaaf, Understanding the Nature of Sensory Integration with Diverse Populations. San Antonio, TX: Psychological Corporation.

Schaefer CF (ed) (1976) The Therapeutic Use of Child's Play. New York: Jason Aronson Inc.

Scheier MF, Carver CS (1985) Optimism, coping and health: assessment and implications of generalized outcome expectancies. Health Psychology 4: 219–47.

Schkade JK, Schultz S (1992) Occupational adaptation: towards a holistic approach for contemporary practice, part 1. American Journal of Occupational Therapy 46: 829–837.

Schön D (1983) The Reflective Practitioner: How Professionals Think in Action. New York: Basic Books.

Scott AD, Dow PW (1995) Traumatic brain injury. In CA Trombly (ed) Occupational Therapy for Physical Dysfunction. 4th edn. Baltimore: Williams & Wilkins, pp.705–733.

Scott DW, Katz N (1988) Occupational Therapy in Mental Health: Principles in Practice. London: Taylor and Francis.

Scott J, Mark G, Williams J, Beck, Aaron T (1989) Cognitive Theory in Clinical practice – An Illustrative Case Book. London: Routledge.

Selye H (1974) Stress without Distress. Philadelphia: Lippincott.

Senior L, Hopkins K (1998) Growing Up with a Smile. Johannesburg: Smile Education Systems (Pty) Ltd.

Sholle-Martin S (1987) Application of the model of human occupation: Assessment in child and adolescent psychiatry. Occupational Therapy in Mental Health 7(2): 3–22.

Shrey DE, Lacerte M (eds) (1997) Principles and Practices of Disability Management in Industry, pp. 627/55–105. Winter Park, FL: GR Press Inc.

Siegel BS (1989) Peace, Love and Healing. New York: Harper and Row.

Sim J (1996) Client confidentiality: Ethical issues in occupational therapy. British Journal of Occupational Therapy 59(2): 56–61.

Sinani/KwaZulu-Natal Programme for Survivors of Violence (2003) Pamphlets. 1 How trauma affects us. 2 How people recover from trauma. 3 What can communities do to break the cycle of violence? 1204 Sangro House, 417 Smith Street, Durban: South Africa.

Sinclair K (2003) A Model for the Development of Clinical Reasoning in Occupational Therapy. PhD thesis, Hong Kong Polytechnic University.

Smith (2003) Managing the Somatoform disorders. CME Your South African Journal of Continuing Professional Development 21(3): 156–160.

Smith Roley SS, Blanche EI, Schaaf RC (2001) Understanding the Nature of Sensory Integration with Diverse Populations. San Antonio, TX: Therapy Skills Builders/Harcourt Health Sciences Co.

Snyman CR (1995) A Draft Criminal Code for South Africa. Cape Town: Juta and Co. Ltd.

Snyman CR (1999) Strafreg. 4th edn. Durban: Butterworths.

Solarsh B, Katz B, Goodman M. (1990) Strive Towards Achieving Results Together Integrated Programme – START. Johannesburg, South Africa: Sunshine Centre Association.

Solomon MF, Siegel DJ (eds) (2003) Healing Trauma: Attachment, Mind, Body and Brain. New York and London: WW Norton.

South African Association of Occupational Therapists (1989) Supervision of Qualified Support Staff. Policy document. Pretoria: South African Association of Occupational Therapists.

South African Federal Council on Disability (1999) Accommodation considerations for people with psychiatric disabilities. www.ability.org/za/accommodations/psychiatric/considerations.html (accessed 6/5/2003).

South African Medical Association (2001) Human Rights and Ethical Guidelines on HIV: A manual for medical practitioners. Policy approved by the Human Rights, Law and Ethics Committee and Board of Directors, November.

Sroufe LA, Cooper RG, De Hart GB (1992) Child Development: Its Nature and Course. 2nd edn. New York: Knopf.

Stagnitti K, Unsworth, CA, Rodger S (2000) Development of an assessment to identify play behaviours that discriminate between the play of typical preschoolers and preschoolers with pre-academic problems. Canadian Journal of Occupational Therapy 67(5): 291–303.

Stein F, Cutler SK (2002) Psychosocial Occupational Therapy – A Holistic Approach. New York: Thomson Learning.

Stern D (1985) The Interpersonal World of the Infant. New York: Basic Books.

Steward B (1997) Employment in the next millennium: the impact of changes in work on health and rehabilitation. British Journal of Occupational Therapy 60: 268–272.

Stock Kranowitz C (1998) The Out-of-Sync Child: Recognizing and Coping with Sensory Integration Dysfunction. New York: Skylight Press.

Stock Kranowitz C (2003) The Out-of-Sync Child Has Fun: Activities for Kids with Sensory Integration Dysfunction. New York: The Berkley Publishing Group.

Stone JH, Roberts M, O'Grady J, Taylor AV, O'Shea K (2000) Faulk's Basic Forensic Psychiatry. 3rd edn. London: Blackwell Science.

Storey K, Horner RH (1991) Social interaction in three supported employment options: a comparative analysis. Journal of Applied Behaviour Analysis 24: 349–360.

Strauss JS, Hafez H, Lieberman P, Harding CM (1985) The course of psychiatric disorder: III. Longitudinal principles. American Journal of Psychiatry 142(3): 289–296.

Strong S (1998) Meaningful work in supportive environments: experiences with the recovery process. American Journal of Occupational Therapy 52: 31–38.

Swartz L (1998) Culture and Mental Health: A Southern African View. Cape Town: Oxford University Press.

Sykes Wylie M (2004) The limits of talk: Bessel van der Kolk wants to transform the treatment of trauma. Psychotherapy Networker 28(1): 30–41.

Szabo CP (1995) Adolescent depression. Continuing Medical Education Journal 13(11): 1329–1333.

Szabo CP (1996) Adolescent psychiatry – inpatient diagnostic trends. South African Medical Journal 86(6; Suppl): 746.

Tarasoff vs. Regents of University of California, California Supreme Court, (1976) Cal. Sct. 17 CalRep, 3rd Series 425.

Thorburn MJ (2000) Training of CBR personnel: current issues–future trends. Asia and Pacific Journal on Disability 11(1).

Toscani MF, Hudgins MK (1996) Trauma survivors' intrapsychic role atom: including prescriptive roles (monograph) Charlottesville VA: The Centre for Experiential Learning.

Townsend E (1999) Enabling occupation in the 21st century: making good intentions a reality. Australian Occupational Therapy Journal 46: 147–159.

Townsend E (2000) Enabling occupation. Journal of Occupational Science 7(1): 42–43.

Townsend E, Wilcock A (2004) Occupational justice. In CH Christiansen and E Townsend (eds) Introduction to Occupation: The Art and Science of Living. New Jersey: Prentice Hall.

Trombly CA (1995) Occupation: purposefulness and meaningfulness as therapeutic mechanisms. American Journal of Occupational Therapy 49: 960–972.

Tryssenaar J (1995) Interactive journals: an educational strategy to promote reflection. American Journal of Occupational Therapy 49(7): 695–702.

Tsang H, Lam P, Ng B, Leung O (2000) Predictors of employment outcomes for people with psychiatric disabilities: A review of the literature since the mid '80's. Journal of Rehabilitation 66(2):19–31.

Tulloch S (ed) (1993) Reader's Digest Oxford Complete Word Finder. London: Readers Digest Association Limited.

Turner A, Foster M, Johnson SE (1999) Occupational Therapy and Physical Dysfunction: Principles, Skills and Practice. 4th edn. New York: Churchill Livingstone.

Tuttle J, Melnyk BM, Loveland-Cherry C (2002) Adolescent drug and alcohol use: Strategies for assessment, intervention and prevention. Nursing Clinic of North America 37: 443–460.

UNDP (1993) Guide on Evaluation of Rehabilitation Programmes for Disabled People. First Draft. Geneva: UNDP.

United Nations Department of Public Information (1994) The Standard rules on the Equalisation of Opportunities for Persons with Disabilities. Resolution 48/96 of the 48th Session of the United Nations General Assembly. United Nations. New York, NY.

United Nations Office on Drugs and Crime. Drug Abuse and Demand Reduction www.unodc.org/unodc/en/drug_demand_reduction.html   (accessed 7/10/2003).

University of the Western Cape, Department of Occupational Therapy (2002) Community Project Process Model. Unpublished document.

US Department of Health, Education and Welfare (1989) Mental Retarded Activities of the US Department of Health, Education and Welfare. Washington: US Government Printing Office.

Van der Kolk BA (1994) The body keeps the score: memory and the emerging psychobiology of post traumatic stress. Harvard Review of Psychiatry 1: 253–265.

Van der Kolk BA (2002) In terror's grip: healing the ravages of trauma. Cerebrum, 4: 34–50. NY: The Dana Foundation.

Van der Kolk BA, Fisler R (1995) Dissociation and the fragmentary nature of traumatic memories: overview and exploratory study. Journal of Traumatic Stress, 8: 505–525.

Van der Kolk BA, Hopper JW, Osterman JE (2001) Exploring the nature of traumatic memory: combining clinical knowledge with laboratory methods. Journal of Aggression, Maltreatment and Trauma 4: 9–31; and Freyd JF, DePrince AP (eds) Trauma and Cognitive Science (pp. 9–31). Binghamton, NY: Haworth Press.

Van der Kolk BA, Pelcovitz D, Roth S, Mandel FS, Msfarlane A, & Herman JL (1996) Dissociation, somatization, and affect dysregulation: the complexity of adaptation of trauma. American Journal of Psychiatry, 153(Suppl): 83–93.

Van der Reyden D (1992) Workshop – Supervision of Support Staff. Durban, South Africa: University of Durban-Westville.

Van der Reyden D (1993) Workshop – Legal and Ethical Issues. Workshop notes. Durban.

Van der Reyden D (1994) Creative Ability Proceedings of Creative Ability Workshop, Pretoria.

Van der Reyden D (1995) Supervision of Support Staff. Paper presentation National SAAOT Congress, Bloemfontein, South Africa.

Van der Reyden D (2000) Supervision. In M Conlan and A Nott (eds) Occupational Therapy Training Manual for Auxiliaries, pp. 443–49. Pretoria: Occupational Therapy Association of South Africa.

Van der Reyden D, Duncan M (1997) Workshop – The Occupational Therapist/ Occupational Therapy Auxiliary Supervisory Relationship Dilemma. Workshop notes, Occupational Therapy Association of South Africa Congress, Durban.

Van der Reyden D, Holland K (2000) Occupational therapy ethics. In M Conlan and A Nott (eds) Occupational Therapy Training Manual for Auxiliaries, pp. 19–32. Pretoria: Occupational Therapy Association of South Africa.

Van Niekerk L (1998) A perspective on role definition. South African Journal of Occupational Therapy 28: 2–5.

Vance HB, Pumariega A (2001) Clinical Assessment of Child and Adolescent Behaviour, p.5. New York: John Wiley and Sons.

Varney-Blackburn J (1985) Breakthrough! The reduction of self-injurious behaviour and other problems related to mental retardation and autistic behaviour in children. South African Journal of Occupational Therapy 15: 27–30.

Visier L (1998) Sheltered employment for persons with disabilities. International Labour Review 137(3): 347–365.

Wallston KA, Wallston BS, DeVellis R (1978) Development of the multidimensional health locus of control (MHLC) scales. Health Education Monographs 6: 161–70.

Watson D, Clark LA, Tellegen A (1988). Development and validation of brief measures of positive and negative affect: the PANAS Scales. Journal of Personality and Social Psychology 54: 1063–70.

Watson DE (1997) Task Analysis: An Occupational Performance Approach. Bethesda, MD: The American Occupational Therapy Association.

Watson M, Greer S (1983). Development of a questionnaire measure of emotional control. Journal of Psychosomatic Research 27: 299–305.

Webber G (1995) Gentle teaching, human occupation, and social role valorisation. The British Journal of Occupational Therapy 58: 261–263.

Wegner L (1998) The relationship between Leisure Boredom and Substance Use amongst High School Students in Cape Town. Unpublished thesis. Cape Town: University of Cape Town.

Wegner L, Magner I (2002) Is leisure an occupational concern? Understanding leisure in adolescents. Paper presented at the 13th WFOT World Congress of Occupational Therapists, June 2002, Sweden.

Weinstein B, Schossberger JA (1964) Therapeutic progress as reflected in work and creativity (unpublished).

Wenar C, Kerig P (2000) Developmental Psychopathology. From Infancy Through Adolescence. McGraw-Hill Companies Incorporated (International edition).

Western Cape Education Department (2000) Abuse No More – Dealing Effectively with Child Abuse. WCED Western Cape, South Africa.

White M (1991) Deconstruction and therapy. Adelaide: Dulwich Centre Newsletter 3: 21–40.

White M (1995) Re-authoring Lives: Interviews and Essays. Adelaide: Dulwich Centre Publications.

White RW (1971) The urge towards competence. American Journal of Occupational Therapy 25(6): 271–274.

Whiteford G, Townsend E, Hocking C (2000) Reflections on a Renaissance of Occupation. Canadian Journal of Occupational Therapy 67(1): 61–69.

Wiener J (1991) Textbook of Child and Adolescent Psychiatry. Washington: American Psychiatric Press.

Wilbarger P, Wilbarger JL (1991) Sensory Defensiveness in Children Aged 2–12. An Intervention Guide for Parents and Other Caretakers. Santa Barbara, CA: Avanti Education Programs.

Wilcock A (1993) A theory of human need for occupational. Journal of Science of Occupation 1: 17–24.

Wilcock AA (2001) Occupational science: the key to broadening horizons. British Journal of Occupational Therapy 64: 412–416.

Wilcock AA (1998a) An Occupational Perspective of Health. New Jersey: Slack Inc.

Wilcock AA (1998b) Reflections on doing, being and becoming. Canadian Journal of Occupational Therapy 65: 248–256.

Wilcock AA, Townsend E (2000) Occupational justice. Journal of Occupational Science 7: 84–86.

Wilcocks L (1992) Alcohol Abuse. How to Help Someone You Love. Johannesburg: Aspen-Oak Associates cc. PO Box 56278, Pinegowrie 2123 South Africa.

Wilcocks L, Edmunson L, Hannon A (1992) Psychological Behavioural Signs of Alcoholism. (Unpublished). Johannesburg: Riverfield Lodge.

Williams GH and Wood PHN (1982) Sex and disablement. What is the problem and whose problem is it? International Rehabilitation Medicine 4(2): 89–96.

Williams MS, Shellenberger S (1996) How Does Your Engine Run?: A Leader's Guide to The Alert Program for Self-Regulation. Albuquerque, NM: Therapy Works Inc.

Willoughby C, King G, Polatajko H (1996) A therapist's guide to children's self-esteem. The American Journal of Occupational Therapy 50(2):124–131.

Willson M (1983) Occupational Therapy in Long-term Psychiatry. Edinburgh: Churchill Livingstone.

Wilson A, Lightbody P, Riddell S (1999) A flexible gateway to employment? An evaluation of Enable Service's traditional and innovative forms of work preparation. Glasgow: Strathclyde Centre for Disability Research.

Wilson EB (1998) Occupational Therapy for Children with Special Needs. London: Whurr Publishers.

Wilson M (1984) Occupational Therapy in Short-term Psychiatry. Harlow: Longman Group Ltd.

Wilson M (1996) Occupational Therapy in Short-term Psychiatry. 3rd edn. New York: Churchill Livingstone.

Winston ME (1996) AIDS confidentiality and the right to know. In TA Mappes and D deGrazzia (eds) Biomedical Ethics. 4th edn, pp.169–177.

Wonnacott H (2003) Facing Up: A Community Occupational Enrichment Programme. Proceedings of the 3rd International Congress of Occupational Therapy Africa Regional Group (OTARG) Kenya.

Woods Nf. (1984) Human Sexuality in Health and Illness. 3rd edn. Toronto: Mosby.

World Health Organization (1978) Declaration of Alma-Ata: Primary Health Care. Geneva: WHO.

World Health Organization (1986) Ottawa Charter for Health Promotion. Geneva: WHO.

World Health Organization (1992) The ICD-10 Classification of Mental and Behavioural Disorders. Geneva: WHO.

World Health Organization (1992) International Statistical Classification of Diseases and Related Health Problems. 10th revision, Vol. 1. Geneva: WHO.

World Health Organization (1994) International Statistical Classification of Diseases and Related Health Problems. 10th revision. Vol. 3. Geneva: WHO.

World Health Organization (1996) Psychosocial rehabilitation: a consensus statement. Geneva: WHO.

World Health Organization (2001a) International Classification of Functioning, Disability and Health: ICF Short version. Geneva: WHO.

World Health Organization (2001b) Mental Health Policy Project. Policy and Service Guidance Package. Geneva: WHO.

Xie H, Dain BJ, Becker DR, Drake RE (1997) Job tenure amongst persons with severe mental illness. Rehabilitation Counselling Bulletin 40(4): 230–239.

Yallop S and Fitzgerald (1997) Exploration of occupational therapist' comfort with client sexuality issues. Australian Occupational Therapy Journal 44: 53–60.

Yalom ID (1985) The Theory and Practice of Group Psychotherapy. 4th edn. New York: Basic Books Inc.

Yerxa EJ (1993) Occupational science: a new source of power for participants in occupational therapy. Occupational Science: Australia 1: 3–9.

Yerxa EJ (1998) Health and the human spirit for occupation. American Journal of Occupational Therapy 52: 412–418.

Zarit SH (1980) Ageing and Mental Disorders. New York and London: Macmillan.

Zemke R, Clark F (eds) (1996) Preface. In Occupational Science: The Evolving Discipline. Philadelphia: FA Davis.

Zhao T, Kwok J (1997) A report on a research study to develop guidelines for CBR evaluation. Asia and Pacific Journal on Disability 1(1).

Zigmond AS, Snaith RP (1983). The Hospital Anxiety and Depression Scale. Acta Psychiatrica Scandinavica 67: 361–70.

Zola IK (1982) Denial of emotional needs to people with handicaps. Archives of Physical Medicine and Rehabilitation 63(2): 63–67.

Websites

Alcoholics Anonymous www.alcoholics-anonymous.org (accessed 10/10/2003).

Introduction to Mental Retardation, www.thearc.org, The Arc, USA (accessed 01/25/2004).

National Council on Disability www.psych.org/psych/htdocs/public_info/bill_rights.html

South African Department of Labour: www.labour.gov.za/docs/legislation

The Expert Witness Institute (United Kingdom): www.ewi.org.uk

The Society of Expert Witnesses (United Kingdom): www.sew.org.uk

The Academy of Experts (United Kingdom): www.academy-experts.org.uk

The Expert Witness Newsletter (Canada): www.economica.ca

The Expert Witness Network (USA): www.witness.net.html

Trauma Survivor Treatment www.therapeuticspiral.org (accessed 06/08/2003).

Traumatic Brain Injury www.nbia.nf.ca/general_management _approaches_and_ philsophy.htm

Vocational Rehabilitation www.ability.org.za/accommodations/psychiatric/considerations.html (accessed 6/5/2003).

Vocational Rehabilitation www.bu.edu/cpr/jobschool/potentialjob.html (accessed 6/5/2003).

www.CuttyhunkRose/inspirations (Starfish, accessed 2/5/2003).

www.dwp.gov.uk/jad/2002/wae136rep.pdf. (accessed 06/06/2003).

www.livingwithanxiety.com (accessed 12/9/03).

www.panicportal.com (accessed 12/9/03).

www.psychiatrictimes.com/p970601.html (accessed 6/5/2003).

Index

Page numbers in *italics* refer to tables or illustrations.
OT refers to occupational therapy.